Second Edition

SWINE in the
LABORATORY

Surgery, Anesthesia, Imaging, and Experimental Techniques

Second Edition

SWINE in the LABORATORY

Surgery, Anesthesia, Imaging, and Experimental Techniques

M. Michael Swindle, DVM, DACLAM, DECLAM
Medical University of South Carolina
Charleston, SC

Illustrator: Richard Hughes, AA, LATg
Medical University of South Carolina
Charleston, SC

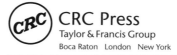
CRC Press
Taylor & Francis Group
Boca Raton   London   New York

CRC Press is an imprint of the
Taylor & Francis Group, an informa business

CRC Press
Taylor & Francis Group
6000 Broken Sound Parkway NW, Suite 300
Boca Raton, FL 33487-2742

International Standard Book Number-10: 0-8493-9278-0 (Hardcover)
International Standard Book Number-13: 978-0-8493-9278-8 (Hardcover)

Library of Congress Cataloging-in-Publication Data

Swindle, M. Michael.
   Swine in the laboratory : surgery, anesthesia, imaging, and experimental techniques / M. Michael Swindle. -- 2nd ed.
      p. ; cm.
   Rev. ed. of: Surgery, anesthesia, imaging, and experimental techniques in swine. 1998.
   Includes bibliographical references and index.
   ISBN-13: 978-0-8493-9278-8 (Hardcover : alk. paper)
   ISBN-10: 0-8493-9278-0 (Hardcover : alk. paper)
   1. Surgery, Experimental. 2. Swine--Surgery. 3. Swine as laboratory animals. 4. Veterinary anesthesia. I. Surgery, anesthesia, and experimental techniques in swine. II. Title.
   [DNLM: 1. Swine--surgery. 2. Anesthesia--veterinary. 3. Animals, Laboratory. 4. Surgery, Veterinary--methods. 5. Surgical Procedures, Operative. QY 60.S8 S9773sa 2007]

RD29.5.S94S944 2007
617.0072'4--dc22
                                         2006102924

Visit the Taylor & Francis Web site at
http://www.taylorandfrancis.com

and the CRC Press Web site at
http://www.crcpress.com

Dedication

To my wife, Paula, and my daughters, Katelyn and Ashley

Preface

This book is an expanded and updated version of *Surgery, Anesthesia and Experimental Techniques in Swine* which was published in 1998. Over the years I have kept a file of questions and communications concerning the use of swine as animal models that arose from readers of that publication. We also hold annual training classes for swine users which have involved discussion and demonstration of many models and surgical techniques that have not yet been published in another format. Answers to all of the questions I have been asked from these sources are included in this edition. The purpose of the book is to provide a practical technical guide for the use of swine in biomedical research. The primary target audience is investigators, veterinarians, and technicians using swine for experimental procedures. Some of the information may be useful for veterinarians in agricultural practice.

Predominantly this book provides information on models produced by surgical or other invasive procedures. There is a presumption that physicians and scientists will have at least a rudimentary knowledge of the fundamental principles of surgery. It is impossible to fully describe all the models that can be developed in this species; however, there should be enough detail to provide basic principles of performing experiments with an organ or system of interest.

There are new chapters on toxicology and radiobiology that were not included in the previous edition. The toxicology chapter was written by Ove Svendsen, DVM, PhD, from the Royal Veterinary and Agricultural University in Copenhagen, Denmark. Professor Svendsen is recognized as one of the leading authorities on the use of minipigs in toxicology. The number of tables of normal values has been greatly expanded both in the chapters and in the appendix. Dr. Guy Bouchard from Sinclair Research Center supplied much of the information for Yucatan, Hanford, and Sinclair minipigs. Dr. Nanna Grand, Dr. Niels Christian-Ganderup, and Lars Ellegaard of Ellegaard Göttingen Minipigs were very helpful in supplying me with the information on their minipig. Anatomic and physiologic details have also been expanded. Much of this information has never been published in any other format. The sections on anesthesia and perioperative care have been updated substantially. In particular, I have attempted to provide practical information concerning postoperative care for the more complex models. The issues concerning anesthesia and perioperative care have been the primary source of questions I have received over the years.

Of particular note is the addition of magnetic resonance imaging, computerized tomography, and positron emission tomography. The DVD attached to this book contains images collected by these techniques. I owe a great deal of gratitude to my colleagues from the PET Center and Aarhus University Hospitals in Aarhus, Denmark, for this contribution. This effort was led by Aage Kristian Olsen, DVM, PhD, and his colleagues. I owe a debt of gratitude to Jens C. Djurhuus, MD, who helped to coordinate this effort through his position as professor and director of the Institute of Experimental Clinical Research at Aarhus University Hospital (Skejby Sygehus). I would also like to express my appreciation to Frederik Dagnaes-Hansen, DVM, PhD, for continuing to invite me to participate in his training activities in Aarhus as well. This continued collaboration has been very helpful to me.

Michael Sturek, PhD, and colleagues from Indiana University have added a chapter with information on the unique Ossabaw pig along with scanning images that are included on the DVD. This is the first time this information has been published.

Most of this book was written by me as a sole author; however, I received input from my fellow faculty members at the Medical University of South Carolina. In particular, Robert Hawes, MD, from the Digestive Diseases Center added a great deal of detail in the section on endoscopy. Other faculty members in the Department of Comparative Medicine were also helpful to me in this endeavor with advice and editorial comments. Sarah Bingel VMD, PhD, contributed histologic images of normal tissues. Kathy Laber, DVM, MS, and Alison Smith, DVM, aided me with editorial comments. Other colleagues have supplied me with photos from their work and they are credited in the photo captions they supplied.

My primary interest in publishing this textbook is to decrease the learning curve associated with using swine as models. The default terminology and names of structures is based upon veterinary terminology rather than human, which may initially cause some confusion with some, but the meaning should be clear. It is hoped that my ideas and suggestions will contribute to the appropriate and humane use of swine in biomedical research.

About the Author

M. Michael Swindle, DVM, is the director of the Division of Laboratory Animal Resources and professor and chairman in the Department of Comparative Medicine at the Medical University of South Carolina. He also holds a Professorship in the Department of Surgery.

Dr. Swindle received his BS degree (1968) and his DVM degree (1969), both from Texas A&M University and is a diplomate of the American College of Laboratory Animal Medicine (1982) and a de facto specialist, European College of Laboratory Animal Medicine (2001). He was in the U.S. Army Veterinary Corps from 1969 to 1972; in private veterinary practice from 1972 to 1979; and at Johns Hopkins Medical School from 1979 to 1985.

He has served the following professional organizations either as a member of the board of directors, committee chairman, and/or officer: American Association for the Accreditation of Laboratory Animal Care; American Association for Laboratory Animal Science; American College of Laboratory Animal Medicine; American Heart Association; Academy of Surgical Research; S.C. Consortium for Comparative Medicine; American Society of Laboratory Animal Practitioners; DHHS Secretary's Advisory Committee on Xenotransplantation; European College of Laboratory Animal Medicine. He is the recipient of the Smithy Research Award from the American Heart Association-SC Affiliate, the Von Recum Award from the Academy of Surgical Research, the Markowitz Award for Contributions to Experimental Surgery, the Brewer Scientific Achievement Award from the Animal Association for Laboratory Animal Science, and the American Society of Laboratory Animal Practitioners Excellence in Research Award.

His many publications and presentations are mainly in the areas of experimental surgery, anesthesia, and swine as animal models. He currently serves on the editorial boards of the *Journal of the American Association for Laboratory Animal Science*, *Comparative Medicine*, and the *Journal of Investigative Surgery*. He continues to be active in research and teaching activities using porcine models.

Contributors

Mouhamad Alloosh, MS, MD
Department of Cellular & Integrative
    Physiology
Indiana University School of Medicine
Indianapolis, Indiana

I. Lehr Brisbin, Jr., PhD
University of Georgia
Savannah River Ecology Laboratory
Aiken, South Carolina

James P. Byrd, BS
Department of Cellular & Integrative
    Physiology
Indiana University School of Medicine
Indianapolis, Indiana

Jason M. Edwards, BS
Department of Cellular & Integrative
    Physiology
Indiana University School of Medicine
Indianapolis, Indiana

Robert H. Hawes, MD
Digestive Diseases Center
Medical University of South Carolina
Charleston, South Carolina

Richard Hughes, LATg
Division of Laboratory Animal Resources
Medical University of South Carolina
Charleston, South Carolina

Svend Borup Jensen, MPhil, PhD
PET Center
Aarhus University Hospitals
Aarhus, Denmark

Pamela G. Lloyd, PhD
Department of Cellular & Integrative
    Physiology
Indiana University School of Medicine
Indianapolis, Indiana

Keith L. March, MD, PhD
Departments of Cellular & Integrative
    Physiology and
Biomedical Engineering
Indiana Center for Vascular Biology and
    Medicine
Indiana University School of Medicine
Indianapolis, Indiana

Michael A. Miller, PhD
Department of Radiology and
Indiana Center of Excellence in Biomedical
    Imaging
Indiana University School of Medicine
Indianapolis, Indiana

Eric A. Mokelke, PhD
Guidant CRM
Emerging Technology
St. Paul, Minnesota

Ole Lajord Munk, MSc, PhD
PET Center
Aarhus University Hospitals
Aarhus, Denmark

Aage Kristian Olsen, DVM, PhD
PET Center
Aarhus University Hospitals
Aarhus, Denmark

Kasper Pedersen
PET Center
Aarhus University Hospitals
Aarhus, Denmark

Michael Sørensen, MD
PET Center
Aarhus University Hospitals
Aarhus, Denmark

Michael Sturek, PhD
Department of Cellular & Integrative
  Physiology
Indiana University School of Medicine
Indianapolis, Indiana
and
Purdue University
West Lafayette, Indiana

M. Michael Swindle, DVM
Department of Comparative Medicine
Medical University of South Carolina
Charleston, South Carolina

Ove Svendsen, DVM, PhD
Department of Veterinary Pathobiology
Royal Veterinary and Agricultural University
Copenhagen, Denmark

Johnathan D. Tune, PhD
Department of Cellular & Integrative
  Physiology
Indiana University School of Medicine
Indianapolis, Indiana

James Wenzel, BS, MEd
Department of Cellular & Integrative
  Physiology
Indiana University School of Medicine
Indianapolis, Indiana

Dora Zeidler
Aarhus University
Aarhus, Denmark

Contents

1 Biology, Handling, Husbandry, and Anatomy

INTRODUCTION

Swine are used extensively in biomedical research with a significant increase in recent decades. They are replacing other mammalian species such as the dog as animal models, while also being developed as a model on their own merit. Swine have become accepted as a general surgical model. This increased use of swine in the laboratory would not have occurred if technical procedures for handling, husbandry, and anesthetizing the species were not refined during the same time period.

Major symposia on the use of swine in biomedical research have been organized in the last few decades, and their proceedings have resulted in books providing a vast amount of baseline information on the species (Swindle, 1992; Tumbleson, 1986; Tumbleson and Schook, 1996). Much of the discussion in these books is based on particular laboratory models and may not provide enough detailed information overall for persons not familiar with the species.

Other reference books on swine provide information on specific experimental fields (Lindberg and Ogle, 2001; Pond and Mersmann, 2001; Stanton and Mersmann, 1986; Swindle, 1983) in addition to the general references on anatomy and biology given in this chapter. Technical guidelines and health-care programs for managing swine in research have also been published (Bollen et al., 2000; Swindle et al., 2003; Laber et al., 2002).

This textbook is an updated and expanded edition of *Surgery, Anesthesia, and Experimental Techniques in Swine* (Swindle, 1998). The purpose of the book and this chapter, in particular, is to provide concise technical data on the use of swine in the laboratory, with an emphasis on surgically produced models. Tables of normal values are included in the appendix as well as within the various system chapters.

BREED SELECTION

All domestic and miniature swine are *Sus scrofa domestica*, as are many of the feral strains of swine found throughout the world. However, they differ substantially from each other in appearance, behavior, and size. Within this textbook, all commercially available breeds of swine raised mainly for meat production are referred to as domestic farm breeds, unless the breed is of particular importance to the model being described, when the breed is mentioned. The most common breeds of domestic swine found in the literature are Yorkshire, Landrace, Duroc, and crossbred animals. Breeds of miniature swine are either naturally occurring or commercially raised for research or pet-keeping. Miniature swine are referred to by their particular breed if it is mentioned in the references. The most commonly used breeds of miniature swine that are commercially available, which appear in recent biomedical literature, are the Yucatan miniature (Figure 1.1) and micro varieties; the Hanford (Figure 1.2), the Göttingen (Figure 1.3), the NIH, and the Sinclair S-1 (Hormel) (Figure 1.4). Other breeds of miniature pigs are available in limited markets and are not widely cited in the literature currently. These include the Ossabaw (Figure 1.5), Banna, Ohmini, Pitman-Moore, Chinese Dwarf, Meishan, Vietnamese potbellied (Figure 1.6), and the Panepinto, to name a few. Some of these were the foundation stock for miniature breeds currently in use, such

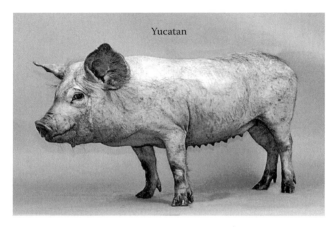

FIGURE 1.1 Yucatan miniature pig. (Courtesy of Sinclair Research Center.)

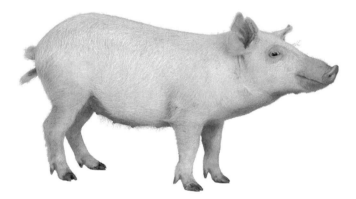

FIGURE 1.2 Hanford miniature pig. (Courtesy of Sinclair Research Center.)

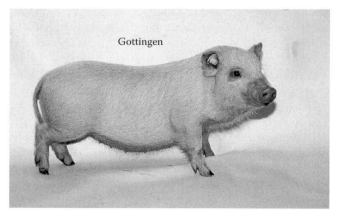

FIGURE 1.3 Göttingen miniature pig. (Courtesy of Ellegaard Minipigs Denmark.)

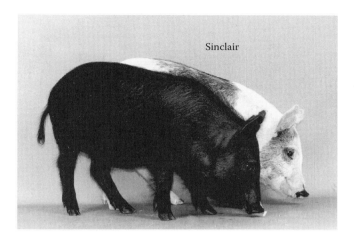

FIGURE 1.4 Sinclair S-1 miniature pig. (Courtesy of Sinclair Research Center.)

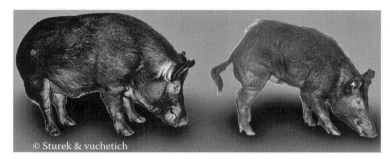

FIGURE 1.5 Ossabaw miniature pig. Obese (left) and thrifty (right) phenotypes. (Courtesy of Michael Sturek, PhD, University of Indiana.)

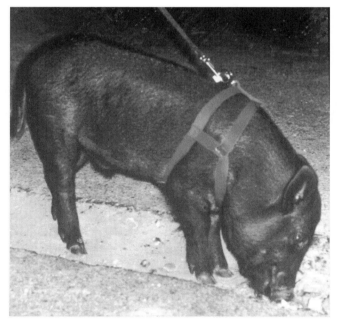

FIGURE 1.6 Vietnamese potbellied miniature pig.

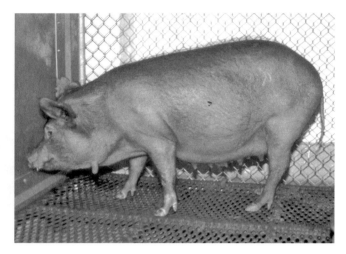

FIGURE 1.7 Sexually mature Yucatan pig on a plastic coated expanded metal floor.

as the Hanford, Sinclair, and Göttingen. Panepinto (1986) has written a summary of the derivation of various breeds of miniature swine. Of the breeds currently important to biomedical research, as listed previously, only the Yucatan and Ossabaw are naturally occurring miniature breeds.

The main difference between commercial breeds and miniature breeds is size at sexual maturity. Miniature breeds were purposely developed to provide a slower-growing porcine model that would be manageable at sexual maturity. Domestic swine exceed 100 kg body weight at sexual maturity and will continue to grow at an accelerated rate that is breed and diet related. It is not unusual to have a domestic pig at 12 months of age exceed 200 kg. In contrast, most breeds of miniature pigs weigh 12 to 45 kg at sexual maturity (Figure 1.7) (Fisher, 1993; Swindle et al., 1994).

It is neither cost effective nor user friendly to attempt to use domestic breeds as chronic models merely to save money on the purchase price. The higher cost of feed, husbandry considerations, and personnel safety issues quickly negate any perceived savings. Also, the rate of growth of domestic swine on long-term projects scientifically skews the results unless growth is part of the hypothesis. Rather, the breed of animal should be selected on the basis of biological characteristics necessary to conduct the experimental study. Table 1.1 represents a growth chart of estimated weights for various breeds of swine. Variations from this chart due to individual genetics, nutrition, gender, health status, and environmental conditions are possible. Species-specific growth charts are included in the appendix.

All investigators should describe accurately the swine used in their particular research in the materials and methods section of manuscripts. Essential information for meaningful comparison to other studies includes the anesthetic methods, breed, weight, age, and gender. Information that may be important in particular research protocols or for some journals includes the source of the animal, its health status, a description of the housing environment and diet, and pertinent genetic information. A recent attempt has been made to standardize the description of animal studies in cardiopulmonary resuscitation research because of the problems associated with making meaningful comparisons of results between laboratories (Idris et al., 1996). This document may be helpful as a blueprint for other areas of research that require comparisons between laboratories.

BIOLOGY

In the appendix, Table A.1–Table A.9 and Table A.31–Table 36 provide biological values for growth, development, and body weights of miniature swine used in research. If a particular breed of pig is not listed in the tables, then the comparison to the normals should be based on age. Within this

TABLE 1.1
Relative Body Weights and Growth of Domestic and Miniature Pigs

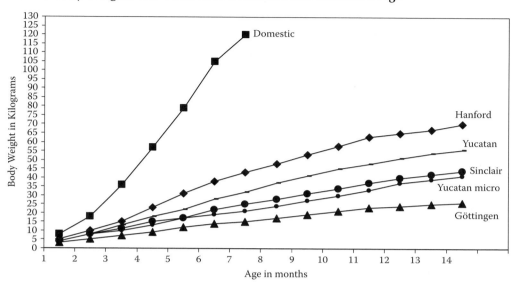

chapter, only the general biological characteristics of swine that should be of practical importance to biomedical researchers and laboratory animal personnel are discussed. A complete reference book on the biology of domestic swine has been published (Pond and Mersmann, 2001), and information on the biology and diseases of domestic swine with an emphasis on data important to commercial production of food animals is also available (Straw et al., 1999). Reference books have been written on the Vietnamese potbellied pig for pet owners and veterinary practitioners (Boldrick, 1993; Reeves, 1993). Additional information is provided in the system chapters and the appendix of this book.

TAXONOMY AND NOMENCLATURE

Swine are ungulate (hoofed) mammals. The taxonomic classification of the species used in research is as follows:

Phylum: Chordata
Class: Mammalia
Order: Artiodactyla
Family: Suidae
Genus: Sus
Species: scrofa
Subspecies: domestica.

Agricultural terminology is typically used in the literature and may cause some confusion to investigators not familiar with the terms. Some common definitions are listed as follows:

Swine	Refers to the whole species or multiple animals
Pig	Newborn animal; sometimes used interchangeably with swine, or to denote a single animal
Shoat	Weaned animal

Gilt	Immature female
Sow	Sexually mature female
Barrow	Castrated male
Boar	Sexually mature male
Farrowing	Parturition, giving birth to piglets
Porcine	Adjective used to describe anything pertaining to swine
Sounder	Herd of wild swine

REPRODUCTION

The sow has a bicornuate uterus and is polytocous. Their chromosome number is $2N = 38$. The gestation period is typically 114 d (range, 110–116 d) for the larger breeds, with that of miniature breeds usually shorter by a few days. Swine are weaned around 4–6 weeks of age (range, 3–8 weeks) and may start to eat solid food (creep feed) as early as 2–3 weeks of age.

The average estrous cycle is 21 d (range, 18–24 d), with estrus being typically 2 d (range, 1–5 d). In commercial operations, sows are usually mated twice when they are showing vulvar swelling and willingly accept the boar. Ovulation occurs 30–36 h after the onset of estrus.

Sexual maturity ranges from 3–7 months, most miniature breeds being sexually mature at 4–6 months of age. Sows will rebreed as soon as 3–9 d after parturition and may have approximately two litters per year for 5–6 years (Frandsson, 1981). The litter size varies greatly between breeds and may range from 4 to 20. However, attrition of the newborn may substantially reduce the number of animals weaned. In general, litter size is reduced with miniature swine.

In the appendix, Table A.37–Table A.43 provide reproductive values for miniature swine.

GROWTH AND DEVELOPMENT

The birth weight of pigs depends on the breed, nutritional status of the sow, and size of the litter, and ranges from 0.5 kg in smaller miniature pigs to 1–2 kg in domestic swine (Fisher, 1993; Swindle et al., 1994).

Newborn pigs require an external heat source such as a heat lamp to provide an ambient temperature that is close to normal body temperature to prevent cold stress. They do not have brown fat, nor do they metabolize glycogen and lipid stores for thermal control. This ability to regulate temperature gradually improves with physiological maturity over the first few days of life (Committees to Revise the Guide for the Care and Use of Animals in Agricultural Research and Teaching, 1999). Pigs are mobile shortly after birth. They nurse almost hourly in the first few days of life. In large litters, they may have to compete with littermates for adequate nutrition, depending upon the number of nipples on the sow.

The growth rate of domestic swine is significantly different from that of miniature breeds. Domestic swine are bred and managed so as to grow to 100–110 kg of body weight within 150–200 d of age. Their daily weight gain can be between 0.2 and 1.0 kg depending upon husbandry and nutritional circumstances within a particular age group. The weight range of 12–45 kg for miniature breeds at the same age provides a vivid contrast of the differences in growth rate (Fisher, 1993; Swindle et al., 1994).

The epiphyses of the long bones are not completely closed in domestic swine until approximately 3.5 years. Miniature swine vary depending upon the stature of the animal. For example, Yucatan microswine have epiphyseal closure at 1.5–2.0 years, whereas standard Yucatans have closure at 3.0–3.5 years.

Even though the commercial life span of domestic swine is less than 6 months for meat production and less than 5 years for breeding stock, their general life span may be 15–25 years depending upon the breed and environmental circumstances.

NUTRITION

Swine are true omnivores and will consume a wide variety of diets and test substances. Specific test diets, such as those for inducing atherosclerosis, are discussed with model descriptions in this book when appropriate.

Commercial pig food is designed to enhance the growth rate of domestic swine and may contain food additives such as antibiotics or growth stimulants. The feeding of various rations to swine within particular weight groups is a science based on optimum muscle growth. As a general guideline, commercially raised swine require metabolizable energy intake for the indicated weights as follows (in kcal/d): 3265 (10–20 kg), 6050 (20–50 kg), 8410 (50–80 kg) (National Research Council, 1998).

Ad libitum feeding of swine for long-term projects may produce obesity without any particular gain in nutritional value. Because this rapid weight gain is undesirable in miniature swine, commercial feed manufacturers have developed diets specifically for these breeds, which can also be fed to farm pigs used in research. The diets are designed to limit weight gain without causing nutritional deficiencies, which may occur if regular commercial diets are restricted only on a weight or volume feeding basis. Vitamin E or selenium content is of importance to swine and deficiencies can lead to cardiac and hepatic pathology. Experience has shown that the feeding of miniature swine diets to domestic swine does not cause nutritional disorders; however, chronically housed animals should have their body weight and general condition monitored (Fisher, 1993; Swindle et al., 1994; Bollen, 2001).

Generally, miniature pig diets are lower in protein and higher in fiber than commercial diets. Usually, the diets are made in three formulations: starter diet, grower diet, and breeder and lactation diet. Starter feeds (creep feed) are usually fed free choice within the first few weeks of life. The other diets, rations containing 3–3.2 kcal/g of metabolizable energy, are then usually fed at a rate of 2–3% of body weight per day. The formula used for calculating metabolizable energy (ME) for growth in body weight (BW) is ME = 2.52 × BW 0.63 for swine (Bollen et al., 2000). For most feeds, this calculates to approximately 0.2 to 2.5 kg of feed per day for swine in a weight range of 5–55 kg. Table 1.2 and Table 1.3 give two examples of how to chart the amount of ration to be fed for the guidance of animal caretakers. The chart values will differ between manufacturers of rations. The manufacturer's recommendations should be followed. Swine can be fed either the entire day's ration in a single feeding, or the calculated ration can be split into two feedings a day (National Research Council, 1998).

Gender differences in minipigs have been described in a study in which females were found to have a higher percentage of nitrogen retention and a higher percentage of body fat than males in the Göttingen breed (Bollen, 2001).

TABLE 1.2
Sample Feeding Chart for Minipigs

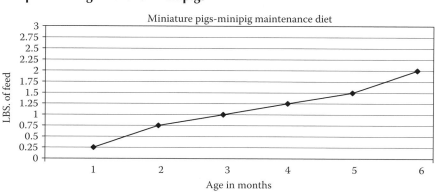

TABLE 1.3
Sample Feeding Chart for Farm Pigs

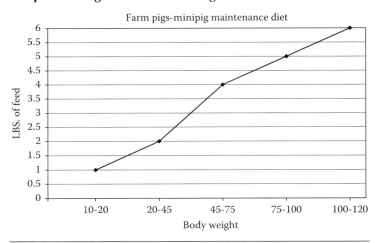

Swine require water of approximately 2.5 l/1.0 kg of feed consumed. This is best supplied with an automated watering system. If bowls are utilized, they should be attached to the side of the cage to prevent spillage and soiling. In this situation, water should also be mixed with the food to ensure adequate hydration. Automatic watering devices need to be checked daily for function. Water restriction can lead to sodium toxicosis ("salt poisoning"), which is characterized by encephalitic symptoms due to development of eosinophilic encephalomyelitis (Laber et al., 2002; Swindle et al., 2003).

Newborn swine are also susceptible to development of microcytic and hypochromic anemia when raised indoors without access to soil. This is prevented by routinely administering 100–200 mg of Fe dextran intramuscularly within 48 h of birth.

Presurgical fasting of 8–12 h will empty the stomach and small intestine; the colon usually requires 48–72 h. If a prolonged fast is required for some procedures, nutrition may be maintained by providing flavored oral electrolyte and glucose solutions commercially available from grocery stores (i.e., Gatorade®, Gatorade, Chicago, IL). These liquids do not interfere with endoscopic or laparoscopic procedures because they do not leave residue. Bedding and chewable objects should be removed from the cage of an animal being fasted for surgery (Swindle, 1983; Swindle et al., 1994).

In the appendix, Table A.3 provides guidelines for feeding and nutrition of miniature swine.

HEMATOLOGY

Hematologic and plasma biochemical values for swine vary to some degree with environmental conditions, health status, breed, age, and gender. However, normal values are generally comparable, and tables of values from various breeds of swine are included in the appendix.

Several general statements may be made concerning these values in swine. The hematocrit is physiologically low in neonatal swine, which requires the administration of iron dextran injections (100 mg i.m.) during the nursing period. Swine generally have a higher percentage of neutrophils than lymphocytes, but this can be variable (Pond and Mersmann, 2001). The blood volume of adult swine is 61–68 ml/kg. Their blood clotting pathway is similar to that of humans. They are considered to have 16 blood group antigens, A–P (EAA–EAP), but the antigens are generally weak (Feldman et al., 2000). They have approximately 80% homology with human erythropoietin amino acids but have low levels at birth (David et al., 2002).

In the appendix, Table A.10–Table A.30 provide hematology and serum chemistry values for miniature swine.

BEHAVIOR

Swine are social animals and prefer to be in contact with other members of their own species. To avoid stress and potential disease transmission in the laboratory setting, they should not be mixed with other species. They can be housed in socialized groups; however, dominance fighting will occur when new animals are introduced into the group. Single-housed animals should be able to see animals in other pens; this can be accommodated by using vertically slatted cage sides to allow them to see and touch each other. Dominant animals will bite the tails and ears of submissive animals, especially at feeding time. This can be minimized by housing problem animals separately and by providing longer or separate feeding troughs (Committees to Revise the Guide for the Care and Use of Animals in Agricultural Research and Teaching, 1999; Fisher, 1993; Panepinto, 1986; Swindle et al., 1994).

Swine cannot bend to groom themselves and will scratch against the side of the cage. They tend to be cannibalistic if a sick or injured animal is housed with them. For this reason, it is best for animals that have had surgery to be housed singly.

Swine develop a dunging pattern and will defecate at the opposite end of the cage from where they are fed. The cage should therefore be designed to have their food and water separate from the area where they are supposed to defecate.

Swine primarily are sedentary animals and will seldom exercise on their own. Generally, they will only move when aroused by activity such as feeding or the introduction of personnel or new swine. They tend to move around the perimeter of their area of confinement rather than in the center.

Swine have a rooting behavior and like to use their snouts to dig through bedding or pastures. In artificial environments, such as those likely to be found in research institutions, it is best to provide them with toys. Large Teflon balls can be used to provide objects that can be rooted and thrown, and they are easily sanitized. Swine also like to pull on objects such as chains hung from the ceiling or roof of the cage. However, these objects for psychological well-being (Figure 1.8 and Figure 1.9) must be carefully selected to minimize damage to the cage or animal (Panepinto, 1986; Swindle et al., 1994).

HUSBANDRY

In the U.S., two sets of regulatory guidelines exist for laboratory swine: one for biomedical research (Public Health Service, 1996) and another for agricultural research (Committees to Revise the Guide for the Care and Use of Animals in Agricultural Research and Teaching, 1999). These guidelines are contradictory for specified cage size. The cage sizes recommended are listed in Table 1.4 and Table 1.5. Guidelines from other countries are generally close to these two standards, and the Council of Europe (2006) has recently revised their standards (Table 1.6).

No consensus exists on the best type of caging to use for swine in a laboratory setting. Most research facilities are not dedicated to swine housing and require flexibility in housing other types of large animals in the same facility. Some general standards related to research housing are discussed later in this chapter.

Swine require flooring that provides for secure footing and a surface for wearing down their hooves. The flooring also needs to be easily sanitized. Swine can become stressed with slippery flooring and develop such symptoms as stress ulcers. Several types of flooring have been used with different degrees of success. Concrete or seamless epoxy floors should have grit added to provide for secure footing. These types of floors are best utilized with deep bedding of wood shavings or straw. These floors plus the bedding provide an outlet for the rooting behavior of the species.

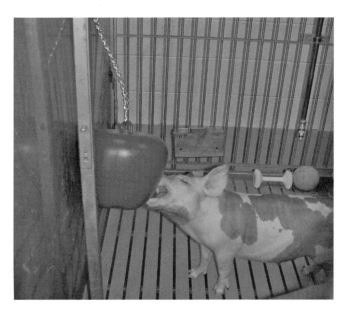

FIGURE 1.8 Yucatan pig in a cage with automatic water, attached feeder, and enrichment toys.

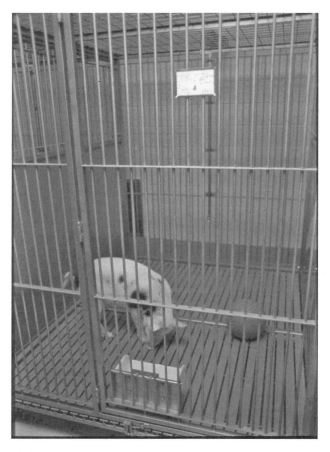

FIGURE 1.9 Yucatan pig in a typical pen.

TABLE 1.4
Space Requirements — ILAR Guide

Animals in Enclosure	Weight (kg)	Floor Area per Animal	
		ft^2	m^2
1	<15	8.0	0.72
	Up to 25	12.0	1.08
	Up to 50	15.0	1.35
	Up to 100	24.0	2.16
	Up to 200	48.0	4.32
	>200	≥60.0	5.4
2–5	<25	6.0	0.54
	Up to 50	10	0.9
	Up to 100	20	1.8
	Up to 200	40	3.6
	>200	≥52	4.68
>5	<25	6.0	0.54
	Up to 50	9.0	0.81
	Up to 100	18.0	1.62
	Up to 200	36.0	3.24
	>200	≥48.0	4.32

Source: Adapted from the *Guide for Care and Use of Laboratory Animals.* Copyright (1996) by the National Academy of Sciences. Courtesy of the National Academy Press, Washington, D.C. With permission.

TABLE 1.5
Minimum Floor Area Recommendations for the Animal Zone for Swine Used for Agricultural Research and Teaching

Stage of Production	Individual Pigs (per pig)		Groups of Pigs (per pig)	
	m^2	ft^2	m^2	ft^2
Litter and lactating sow, pen	3.15	35	—	—
Litter and lactating sow, sow portion of crate	1.26	14	—	—
Nursery, 3 to 27 kg (7 to 60 lb) of body weight	0.54	6	1.6–37	1.7–4.0
Growing, 27 to 57 kg (60 to 125 lb) of body weight	0.90	10	0.37–0.56	4.0–6.0
Finishing, 57 to 104 kg (125 to 230 lb) of body weight	1.26	14	0.56–0.74	6.0–8.0
Late finishing, 105 to 125 kg (231 to 275 lb) of body weight	1.26	14	0.74–0.84	8.0–9.0
Mature adults	1.26	14	1.49	16.0

Source: Adapted from the *Guide for the Care and Use of Agricultural Animals in Agricultural Research and Teaching.* Copyright (1999) by the Committees to Revise the *Guide for the Care and Use of Agricultural Animals in Agricultural Research and Teaching,* Savoy, IL. With permission.

TABLE 1.6
Pigs and Minipigs: Minimum Enclosure Dimensions and Space Allowances

Weight (kg)	Minimum Enclosure Size[a]		Minimum Floor Area per Animal		Minimum Lying Space per Animal (in thermoneutral conditions)	
	m²	ft²	m²	ft²	m²	ft²
Up to 5	2.0	22.2	0.20	2.2	0.10	1
Over 5 to 10	2.0	22.2	0.25	2.7	0.11	1.2
Over 10 to 20	2.0	22.2	0.35	3.8	0.18	1.9
Over 20 to 30	2.0	22.2	0.50	5.4	0.24	2.6
Over 30 to 50	2.0	22.2	0.70	7.5	0.33	3.6
Over 50 to 70	3.0	32.3	0.80	8.6	0.41	4.4
Over 70 to 100	3.0	32.3	1.00	10.8	0.53	5.7
Over 100 to 150	4.0	43.0	1.35	14.5	0.70	7.5
Over 150	5.0	53.8	2.50	26.9	0.95	10.2
Adult (conventional) boars	7.5	80.7			1.30	14.0

[a] Pigs may be confined in smaller enclosures for short periods of time, for example, by partitioning the main enclosure using dividers, when justified on veterinary or experimental grounds, i.e., for monitoring individual food consumption.

Source: Adapted from European Convention for the Protection of Vertebrate Animals Used for Experimental and Other Scientific Purposes, Council of Europe — ETS No. 123: Appendix A (http://conventions.coe.int/Treaty/EN/Treaties/Html/123-T11.htm).

Plastic-coated metal grid floors provide good sanitation, especially if they are raised above the floor level (Figure 1.7). However, swine will pull the plastic off the metal with the first sign of a tear. In the author's experience, diamond-shaped grids of approximately 5/8 in. openings provide best all-around conditions for housing swine of multiple sizes. Newer fiberglass slatted-rail types of flooring can be used in the same manner as expanded metal floors (Figure 1.8). They provide good sanitization and are not easily damaged. They are also lighter and can be removed easily for sanitization. In the author's experience, the slats should have a width of 1.75 in. (4.4 cm) with a space of 0.25 in. (0.64 cm) between slats. These grids can also be manufactured to provide a light-medium gritty surface to provide for hoof wear. Rails and grids can be manufactured from aluminum and wood; however, care must be taken to make sure that the floors will support the weight of large animals and that they can be easily sanitized. Wood is inappropriate except for some agricultural settings. If the flooring does not cause wear on the hooves of chronically housed animals, then they will have to be trimmed with hoof nippers approximately every 3 to 6 months. A typical caging system for swine and other large animal species is depicted in Figure 1.8–Figure 1.10.

Swine do not climb, but they may stand on their rear legs and lean against the cage to see other animals in some circumstances. They also use the sides of the cage to scratch themselves. If they cannot see other animals, they will use their snouts to try to open the cage. Also, if there is any loose-fitting area of the cage, swine will manipulate it with their snouts; consequently, the cage should be sturdy and free of any surface that can be manipulated or torn by the animals. Chain-link fencing can be used for small swine, but care should be taken to ensure that the sides of the cage meet the flooring securely to prevent animals from catching their hooves. If aluminum or stainless steel sides are used, the edges should be rounded and the bars sturdy. Vertical bars are preferred for swine and ruminants; however, these will not be as satisfactory for dogs. Cages can be manufactured to provide solid side panels that can be used to replace slotted panels when required.

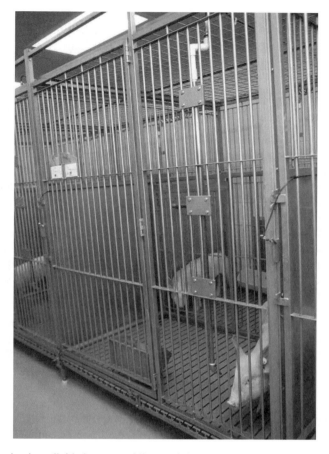

FIGURE 1.10 Farm pigs in a divided pen providing social contact.

Food bowls should be secured to either the side of the cage or to the floor. Easily sanitized stainless steel or Teflon feeders are preferable to the rubber feeders frequently used in agricultural settings. When the feeders are attached to the sides of the cage, guillotine-type closures should be avoided. In its anxiety to eat, the pig may slam it shut and injure the caretaker when food is being delivered.

Swine readily utilize automated watering systems, which are preferred to the use of water bowls because they provide a constant source of water without contamination and cannot be spilled like bowls. If bowls are utilized, they should be secured to the side of the cage. Water deprivation can result in dehydration and a clinical presentation of sodium toxicosis, which may be fatal (Straw et al., 1999). For this reason, water is not withheld presurgically in swine except in cases in which it is absolutely essential for gastric procedures. Placement of food and water sources should be considered in relation to the dunging pattern of the swine in the cage.

Cages without bedding are best washed with a hose once or twice daily to eliminate odor. The animals should be removed from the cage during the hosing procedure to avoid being wetted and chilled. However, they readily accept baths and can be periodically washed with mild soap and warm water. They also develop dry skin in some housing conditions and can be rubbed with moisturizing oils or ointments to prevent scaling and flaking of the skin. If deep bedding is used, the cage can be spot-cleaned daily because of the dunging pattern, and the bedding changed once or twice weekly. Swine tend to keep cleaner in bedding than in cages that are hosed. Drains should be large and easily flushed. If bedding is used, then the drains should be covered with solid caps to avoid blockage. The main disadvantage of using bedding in surgical protocols is that swine will eat it when fasted (Fisher, 1993; Panepinto, 1986; Swindle et al., 1994).

If modular units are utilized, they may be taken apart and cleaned in a cage washer to sanitize the cage between uses by different animals or every 1–2 weeks with chronically housed animals. Pressure washers may be used to clean caging units in place.

The recommended temperature range for housing laboratory swine is 16–27°C (61–81°F) in the Public Health Service (1996) guide. The Committees to Revise the Guide for the Care and Use of Animals in Agricultural Research and Teaching (1999) provide preferred ranges of temperatures depending upon the age of the animal. Generally, their standards recommend 26–32°C (79–90°F) for animals of less than 15 kg, 18–26°C (64–79°F) for swine of 15–35 kg, and 10–25°C (50–77°F) for larger swine. Increased environmental temperatures are appropriate for postsurgical care and other stressful situations and may be provided by suspended heat lamps. Normal swine are capable of surviving temperatures outside this range, especially at the lower end of the scale; however, environmental control is an essential part of the research environment and should be provided.

Standard laboratory animal practice is to provide 10–15 air changes per hour with 100% fresh outside air. Relative humidity ranges of 30–70% are also standard. This type of ventilation greatly aids in reducing odor and minimizing ammonia levels, which can contribute to respiratory disease. The location of air ducts will depend upon the design of the facility; however, care should be taken to ensure that temperature is controlled at the floor level to prevent the pigs from becoming chilled (Public Health Service, 1996).

The photoperiod for swine is not as critical as for other species, and they may be provided with up to 16 h of light in the laboratory setting (Committees to Revise the Guide for the Care and Use of Animals in Agricultural Research and Teaching, 1999).

DISEASE PREVENTION

Vaccination of swine depends upon the source of the animals, the length of time they are housed, and the protocol. Most of the vaccinations are given to neonatal and weanling animals, except those in breeding programs. The attending veterinarian should use professional judgment to establish the vaccination protocol, taking into account the source of the swine and the diseases prevalent in the area. Vaccination injections are conventionally given in the neck. The agents against which prophylaxis may be provided include Erysipelothrix, Pasteurella, Bordetella, Escherichia, Clostridium, Parvovirus, and Rotavirus (Straw et al., 1999; Swindle et al., 2003, Laber et al., 2002).

Swine require the trimming of needle teeth during the first day of life to prevent damage to the nipples of the sow and to their siblings. Newborn animals also should have the umbilicus cleaned with iodine solution. An iron dextran injection is given to 3-d-old animals to protect against the physiological anemia that occurs in animals not housed on soil. Swine are susceptible to vitamin E and selenium deficiencies, and care must be taken to ensure that an adequate level is provided in the feed (Fisher, 1993; Straw et al., 1999; Swindle et al., 2003).

In agricultural settings, castration and hernia repair are performed on neonates. However, it is not usually routine for miniature swine from commercial producers. If these surgeries are performed in an agricultural setting, it is not unusual to see incisional infections. Observation of animals upon receipt from the supplier should include an inspection for problems related to these surgeries.

All animals should be examined for health problems by the attending veterinarian upon receipt. It is a good practice to isolate and quarantine animals upon arrival away from animals already on the premises. It is also a good practice to house animals from different suppliers in separate rooms. Animals purchased from auctions are probably from mixed sources and should be considered to have an increased health risk, similar to that of dogs from municipal pounds. When purchasing animals, it is best to limit suppliers to those who have been determined to have high standards of husbandry and disease control. Specific pathogen-free (SPF) is a specific proprietary term used in swine breeding (National SPF, 2000; Saffron and Gonder, 1997). This means that the herd of animals has been certified by veterinary and gross necropsy examinations to be free of the specific diseases of atrophic rhinitis, pneumonia, swine dysentery, lice, mange, pseudorabies, and brucellosis. Although this certification does not guarantee that swine will be free of all diseases, it is a gold standard among swine producers and provides the best assurance that swine will be of a suitable condition for surgical protocols. Higher standards are required for animals used in xenografic procedures (Swindle, 1996). Zoonotic diseases are discussed in Chapter 14. European standards are summarized in the appendix (Table A.54). Dosages of antimicrobial agents that have been utilized in laboratory swine are included in the appendix (Table A.55).

RESTRAINT AND HANDLING

Agricultural methods of restraining swine are inappropriate for laboratory settings. These methods include snout tying, hog tying, and suspending animals by their rear legs. Such methodologies are stressful and make chronically housed animals timid and potentially aggressive toward their handlers. These animals are easily trained and can be restrained in sling apparatuses, such as the Panepinto sling or modifications of the original design (Panepinto et al., 1983) (Figure 1.11 and Figure 1.12). Small animals can be supported in the handler's arms (Figure 1.13), as with other species such as the dog. Larger animals may be herded and restrained against the side of the cage with handheld panels (Figure 1.14). Agricultural squeeze chutes may be appropriate in some

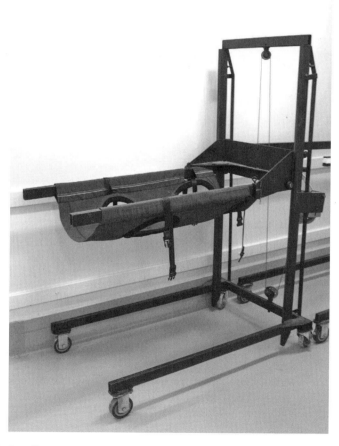

FIGURE 1.11 Restraint sling.

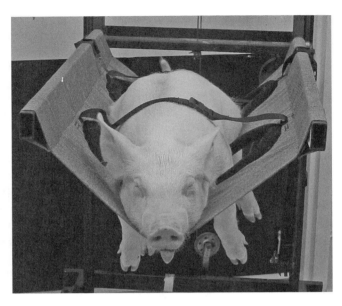

FIGURE 1.12 Pig resting in a humane restraint sling.

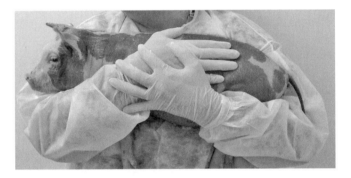

FIGURE 1.13 Manual restraint of a small pig.

circumstances for very large animals if care is taken to avoid trauma to the animal. Swine can also be trained to walk with a leash and harness (Houpt, 1986; Panepinto, 1986; Swindle et al., 1994).

Swine respond well to food treats for training, and food may be used to calm them during long-term restraint in slings. Foods that have been used successfully include dog biscuits, carrots, candy, doughnuts, and cookies.

If complete restraint is required, it is best to utilize short-term anesthetics and chemical restraint agents (Chapter 2). In addition, hydraulic lift devices may have to be utilized for ergonomic reasons; their use is depicted in Chapter 2.

ADMINISTRATION OF MEDICATIONS AND INJECTIONS

It should be noted that swine, which are in the human food chain, are restricted from receiving certain antibiotics (Table A.55). These are, generally speaking, antibiotics such as vancomycin, which are considered to be life-saving for humans. Judicious use of antibiotics in research animals is recommended, even though it is unlikely that they will become food for humans. Antibiotic resistance is a serious issue and veterinarians should take this factor into consideration when utilizing antimicrobial agents in research swine (Payne et al., 1999).

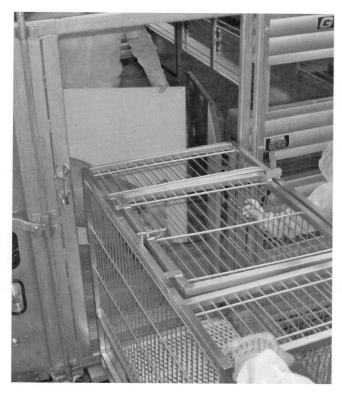

FIGURE 1.14 Herding a pig into a transport cart with a handheld panel.

Oral medications can be administered by multiple methods. The easiest method is to mix the medication with food. In the case of substances with a foul taste, they may be placed inside gelatin capsules. Medications can be mixed with chocolate syrup or canned cat food or dog food. Swine will consume these substances quickly and without substantial chewing; thus, breaking capsules and tablets is seldom necessary. Balling guns have been utilized in agricultural settings (Figure 1.15). If these devices are required, then it is best to restrain the animals in a sling and utilize equipment with flexible necks to avoid trauma to the pharynx and larynx. Swine can also be readily medicated using stomach tubes if the animal is restrained in a sling. Stomach tubes should be approximately the size of the trachea and have rounded tips (Figure 1.16). The tube should be lubricated and passed slowly through the side of the mouth. Medication should be administered quickly, and the tube removed. If precautions are not taken, swine may sever the tube with their incisors. Mouth gags may be utilized in smaller swine; however, larger swine are too powerful for the handler to hold the mandible closed around it (Swindle et al., 1994).

Intramuscular (i.m.) and subcutaneous (s.c.) injections may be given in the rear legs or neck. In the rear leg, the gluteal, semimembranosus, and semitendinosus muscles may be used (Figure 1.17). Care should be taken to avoid the sciatic nerve. The flank may be utilized for i.m. injections; however, s.c. injections require that the pigs be larger and have a layer of fat to separate the skin from the underlying muscles (Figure 1.18). Muscles on the sides of the neck or behind the ears may be utilized in small swine; however, injections given in this area in larger swine will be s.c. rather than i.m. because of the layers of fat that develop (Figure 1.19). Experience has shown that this does not present a problem for injectable anesthetics, and this area is preferred because larger-volume injections can be given with less pain to the animal than i.m. injections in the rear legs. Animals should be restrained in a sling or with panels when given injections with a hypodermic needle. It is seldom necessary to use a needle larger than 20 gauge (ga). A method that does not

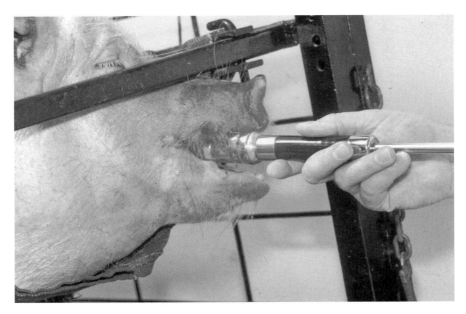

FIGURE 1.15 Administering a tablet to a pig in a sling, using a flexible tipped balling gun.

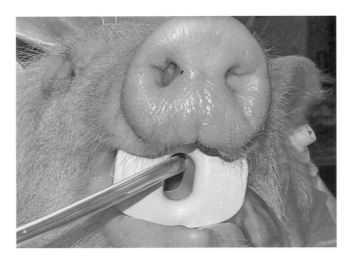

FIGURE 1.16 Administering medication with a stomach tube passed through a mouth gag.

require restraint is to use a slapping motion to instill a butterfly catheter into the side of the neck and allow the animal to recover from the insertion. The medication can then be administered through the butterfly catheter (Figure 1.20) while the animal is walking around the cage (Swindle et al., 1994; Swindle, 1983).

Intraperitoneal (i.p.) injections (Figure 1.21) may be given in the lower quadrants of the abdomen off the midline. However, they are rarely used except in neonates. Intrathoracic injections (Figure 1.22) should be given in the dorsocaudal intercostal spaces if they are required by the research protocol. Methodologies for giving injections and taking samples in the subarachnoid space and cisterna magna are discussed in Chapter 11.

Intravenous (i.v.) injections and venipuncture for sampling or implanting catheters can be performed in a variety of peripheral locations (Figure 1.23–Figure 1.32). Procedures for chronic catheterization and percutaneous catheterization for cardiovascular procedures are discussed in

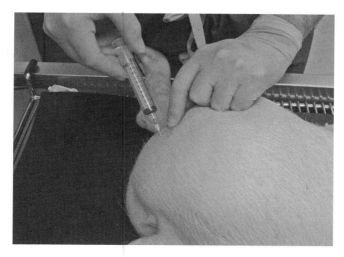

FIGURE 1.17 Intramuscular (i.m.) injection in the rear leg.

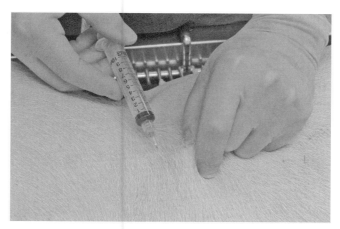

FIGURE 1.18 Subcutaneous (s.c.) injection in the flank.

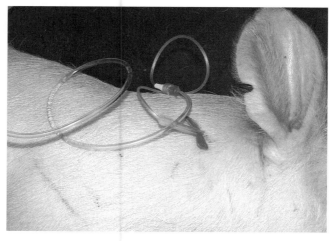

FIGURE 1.19 Subcutaneous (s.c.) injection in the neck. This is the preferred site and method of administering injections in swine.

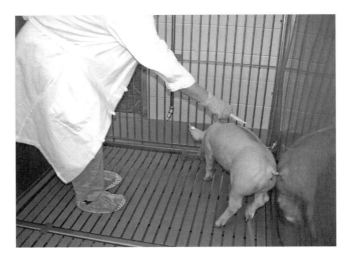

FIGURE 1.20 Administering a subcutaneous (s.c.) injection in the neck using a butterfly catheter and extension tube. Note that the animal is not physically restrained.

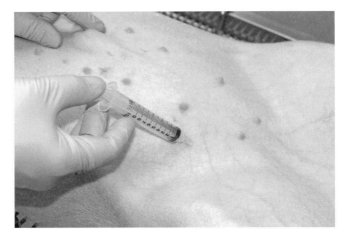

FIGURE 1.21 Intraperitoneal (i.p.) injection.

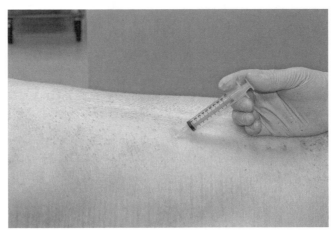

FIGURE 1.22 Intrathoracic (i.t.) injection.

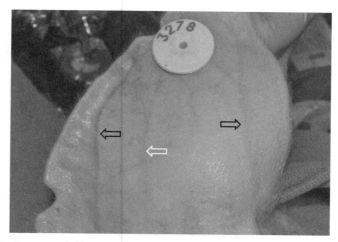

FIGURE 1.23 Auricular artery (white arrow) and auricular veins (black arrows).

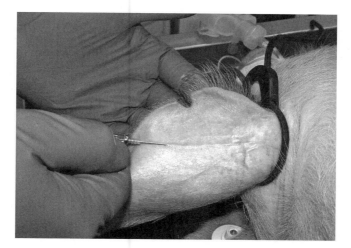

FIGURE 1.24 Intravenous (i.v.) injection in auricular (ear) vein.

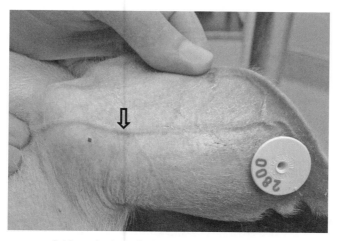

FIGURE 1.25 The anatomy of this auricular vein is conducive to using it to catheterize the external jugular vein from the ear.

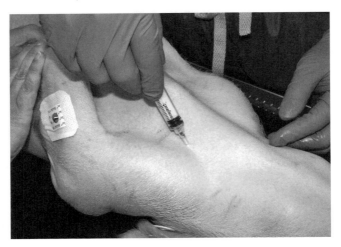

FIGURE 1.26 Venipuncture site for the external jugular vein.

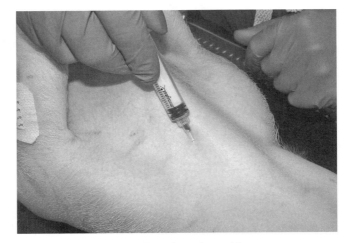

FIGURE 1.27 Access site for the internal jugular vein and carotid artery.

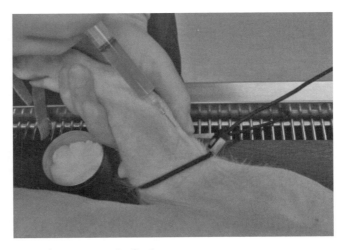

FIGURE 1.28 Cephalic venipuncture on the foreleg.

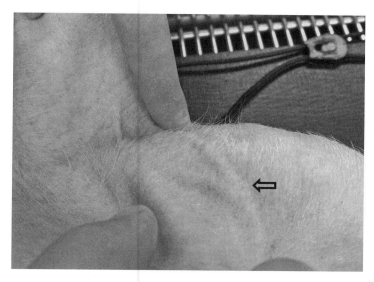

FIGURE 1.29 Cephalic vein (arrow) as it crosses the neck superficially at the thoracic inlet.

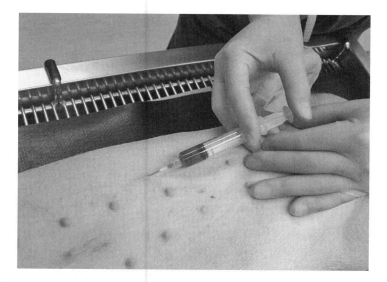

FIGURE 1.30 Venipuncture site for the superficial cranial epigastric vein.

Chapter 2, Chapter 9, and Chapter 12. Arterial pulse sites are illustrated in Chapter 2. The standard methodology for withdrawing blood samples in agricultural settings utilizes the precava (Figure 1.33). The use of large-gauge (14–16 ga) 3- to 5-in. "hog needles" is unnecessary except in large breeding stock. For swine less than 50 kg, the largest needle size that is required is 20 ga 1.5 in. Animals may be restrained in a sling or on their backs with the forelegs retracted caudally. In order to avoid injury to the vagus nerve, the needle is inserted into the right side of the neck, lateral to the manubrium sterni, and directed at an angle of 30 to 45° toward the left shoulder. A popping sensation will be felt when the needle enters the vein, and then blood can be readily withdrawn. This method can also be utilized for sequential venipuncture, but hematomas form in the area after the needle is withdrawn; therefore, it is best reserved for procedures that do not require withdrawal more often than weekly (Panepinto et al., 1983; Swindle, 1983; Swindle et al., 1994).

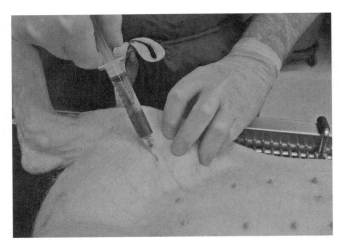

FIGURE 1.31 Access site for the femoral artery and vein.

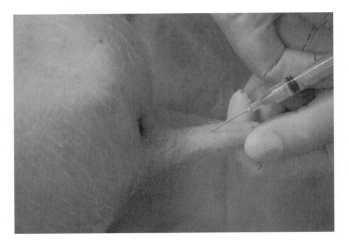

FIGURE 1.32 Venipuncture site for the coccygeal vein.

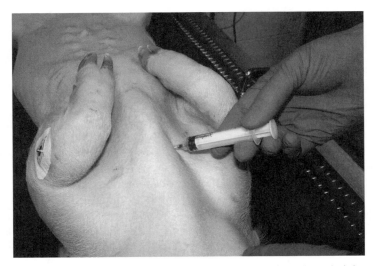

FIGURE 1.33 Venipuncture of the cranial vena cava at the right side of the thoracic inlet.

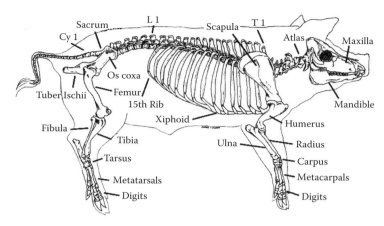

FIGURE 1.34 Skeleton of the pig.

GENERAL ANATOMY

Several textbooks describing the detailed anatomy of swine are available (Getty, 1975; Gilbert, 1966; Popesko, 1977; Sack, 1982). A recent review compares the anatomy and physiology of swine as it applies to their use as research animals (Swindle and Smith, 1998). This section provides an illustrated introductory overview of the gross anatomy of swine. Specific aspects of anatomy important to surgical procedures are included in the introduction to the various system chapters.

The vertebral formula is C7, T14–15, L6–7, S4, Cy20–23. Some miniature breeds may have one fewer of the thoracic or lumbar vertebrae or of both. There are seven sternal and seven asternal ribs. If a 15th rib is present, it is usually a floating rib rather than one attached to the cartilage of the costal arch. The clavicle is absent. In the forelimb, there are eight carpal bones, four metacarpal bones (2–5), and three phalanges; proximal and distal sesamoid bones are present. In the hind limb, there are eight tarsal bones, four metatarsal bones, and phalanges with sesamoid bones present (Figure 1.34).

The musculature of the pig is massive, as would be expected of an animal that has been bred predominantly for meat production (Figure 1.35).

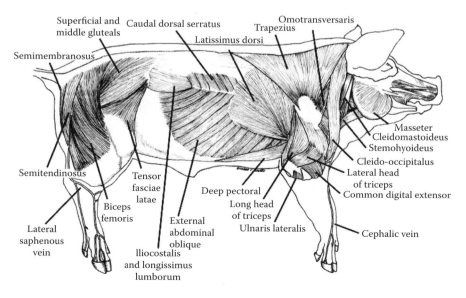

FIGURE 1.35 Superficial musculature of the pig.

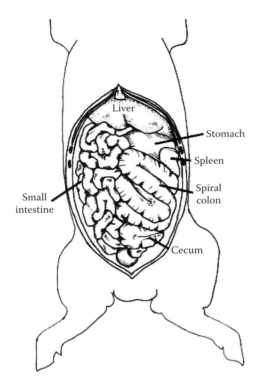

FIGURE 1.36 Ventral view of the abdominal viscera.

The unique features of the gastrointestinal tract include the torus pyloricus in the pyloric region of the stomach, the mesenteric vascular arcades, and the spiral colon. The torus pyloricus is a muscular and mucoid glandular structure adjacent to the pylorus, which is involved in the functional closure of the orifice. The small intestine is arranged in a series of coils from the stomach to the pelvis, dorsal and lateral to the spiral colon. The bile duct and pancreatic ducts enter the duodenum separately in the proximal portion in the right upper quadrant. The mesenteric vascular arcades form in the subserosa of the intestine rather than the mesentery, giving a fanlike appearance. The spiral colon contains the cecum, the ascending, transverse, and main portion of the descending colon arranged in a series of centrifugal and centripetal coils in the left upper quadrant of the abdomen, caudal to the stomach. The descending colon continues caudally on the left side to become the rectum (Figure 1.36–Figure 1.40).

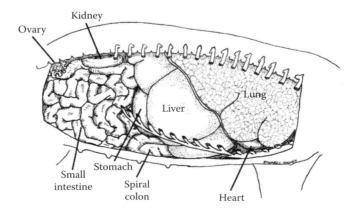

FIGURE 1.37 Right lateral view of the thoracic and abdominal viscera.

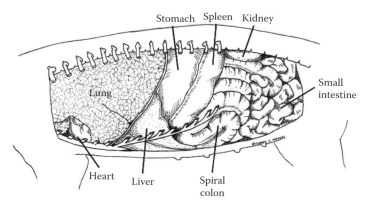

FIGURE 1.38 Left lateral view of the thoracic and abdominal viscera.

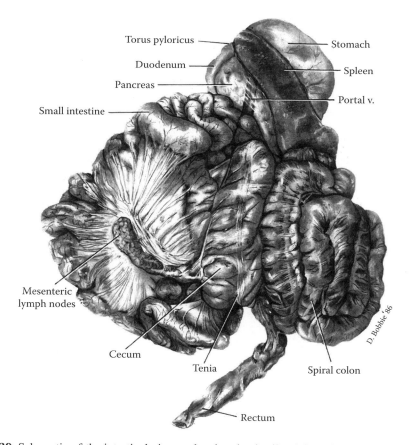

FIGURE 1.39 Schematic of the intestinal viscera showing the details of the spiral colon.

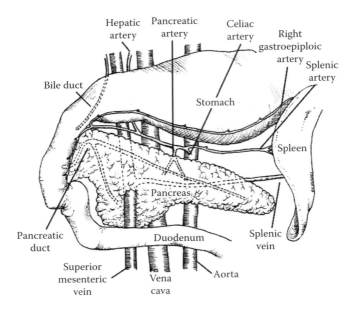

FIGURE 1.40 Schematic of the pancreatic blood supply and ductal system.

The kidneys are usually ventral to the transverse processes of the first four lumbar vertebrae with the left kidney usually more cranial than the right one. The adrenal glands are craniomedial to the hilus of the kidneys. The right gland is attached to the vena cava (Figure 1.41).

The male urogenital system contains large vesicular glands, a prostate, and bulbourethral glands, as accessory genital glands. The scrotum and testicles are ventral to the anus and more caudal than ventral on the perineum. The fibromuscular penis has a sigmoid flexure and terminates in a corkscrew-shaped tip in the preputial diverticulum, caudal to the umbilicus (Figure 1.42). The female urogenital tract has long, flexuous fallopian tubes and a bicornuate uterus with a small body. The urethra enters the vagina on the ventral floor within the pelvic cavity, cranial to the vestibule (Figure 1.43). There are usually 10–12 paired mammary glands on the ventral abdomen.

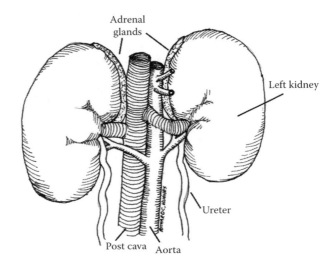

FIGURE 1.41 Ventral view of the kidneys and adrenal glands.

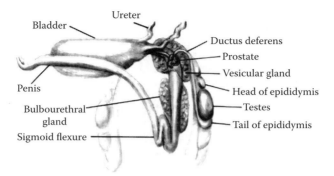

FIGURE 1.42 Left lateral view of the male urogenital system.

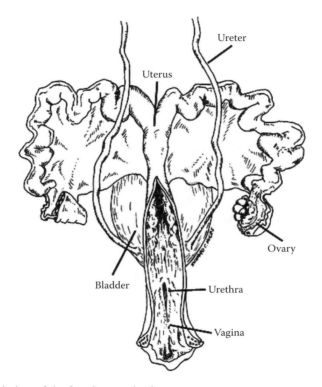

FIGURE 1.43 Dorsal view of the female reproductive tract.

The larynx is prominent with a large vestibule that narrows caudally because of internal compression of the cricoid cartilage. There are middle and lateral ventricles that have to be avoided during intubation (Chapter 2).

The thyroid gland is located on the ventral midline of the trachea at the level of the thoracic inlet. A pair of parathyroid glands can be found associated with the craniomedial portion of the thymus in the neck (Figure 1.44). The lymph nodes have an inversion of the cortex and medulla. Histologically, this presents a unique appearance with the more central location of the germinal centers (Figure 1.45).

The trachea extends from C4–5 to T5 where it bifurcates into the bronchi. At T3, it provides a bronchus to the apical lobe of the right lung. The lungs are composed of apical, middle, and

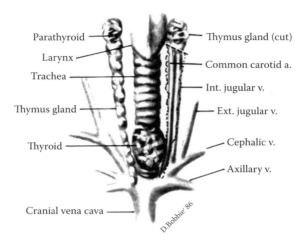

Parathyroid — Thymus gland (cut)
Larynx — Common carotid a.
Trachea — Int. jugular v.
Thymus gland — Ext. jugular v.
Thyroid — Cephalic v.
Axillary v.
Cranial vena cava — D.Bobbie '86

FIGURE 1.44 Schematic of the ventral aspect of the trachea and glandular structures of the neck.

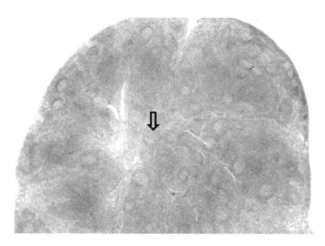

FIGURE 1.45 Cross section of a lymph node demonstrating the inversion of the cortex and medulla. A germinal center is illustrated with an arrow. H&E, ×100.

diaphragmatic lobes, with an accessory lobe to the right lung. The intralobular fissure is incomplete between the left apical and middle lobes.

The heart extends from T2 to T7 and has sternal contact over most of the caudal distance (Figure 1.46). The left azygous vein is the most unique feature of the external anatomy. It curves caudoventrally from the dorsal thorax across the dorsal surface of the heart to enter the right atrium in the coronary sinus.

Unique aspects of the vasculature and the other visceral organs are discussed in the various system chapters.

MODEL SELECTION

The principles for selecting swine as a model are similar to those of other species, and the references on symposia proceedings cited in the introduction to this chapter contain descriptions of many diverse biomedical models developed in this species. This textbook details many of the surgical procedures utilized in the development of induced porcine models.

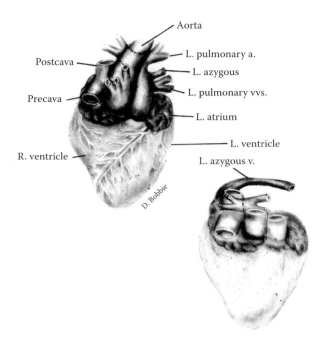

FIGURE 1.46 Gross anatomy of the heart.

One of the principal concerns when considering the use of swine is the age of the animal, because swine grow rapidly. If small domestic pigs are used as biological models, the physiological process being studied may be defined as that of a pediatric rather than an adult model. Therefore, the animal selected should be either a miniature pig or a larger domestic animal if maturity is a factor to be considered in the experiment.

Likewise, if a chronic experiment is planned, then the growth of the animal is a consideration, especially if biomaterials are implanted. As a general rule, the growth of sexually immature domestic swine over a 3-week period will be significant enough to have an impact on the physiological parameters of the study. Consequently, the use of miniature breeds should be considered for experiments in which growth could be a factor.

Also, as a general rule, miniature pigs are more mature at a given body weight than are domestic swine, and this should be considered if maturity of the system or wound healing characteristics are a factor in the experiment.

When comparing experiments between laboratories, animals should be matched for age, weight, gender, and breed. Because of the linebreeding that occurs in herds of commercial animals raised for food, there may even be differences between animals of the same breed from different herds. Animals bought from the same supplier may be siblings or otherwise closely related; therefore, the relatedness of the animals should be considered if it is a potential factor in the experiment. Consequently, if differences are noted in experiments between laboratories, the genetic factors should be considered.

Most of the porcine models are selected because of the close similarity of the physiology of the various systems to those of humans. In the literature, most of the models involve either the cardiovascular or the digestive system, a fact reflected in the disparity in the size of various system chapters of this textbook. The reasons for the selection of models of different body systems are discussed in those chapters.

A list of general references, which may be useful in providing information on the use of swine as animal models in biomedical research, is provided in the appendix.

REFERENCES

Boldrick, L., 1993, *Veterinary Care of Pot-Bellied Pet Pigs*, Orange, CA: All Publishing Co.

Bollen, P.J.A., Hansen, A.K., and Rasmussen, H.J., 2000, *The Laboratory Swine*, Boca Raton, FL: CRC Press.

Bollen, P.J.A., 2001, Nutrition of Göttingen Minipigs, Ph.D. thesis, University of Southern Denmark, Odense, DK.

Committees to Revise the Guide for the Care and Use of Animals in Agricultural Research and Teaching, 1999, Guide for the Care and Use of Agricultural Animals in Agricultural Research and Teaching, Savoy, IL: Federation of Animal Science Societies (FASS).

Council of Europe, 2006, European Convention for the protection of vertebrate animals used for experimental and other scientific purposes, ETS 123, Strasbourg, http://conventions.coe.int/Treaty/en/Treaties/Html/123.htm.

David, R.B., Blom, A.K., Harbitz, I., Framstad, T., and Sjaastad, O.V., 2002, Responses of plasma Epo and kidney and liver Epo mRNA to hemorrhage in perinatal pigs, *Domest. Anim. Endocrinol.*, 23(4): 507–516.

Feldman, B.F., Zinkl, J.G., and Jain, N.C., Eds., 2000, *Schalm's Veterinary Hematology*, Baltimore, MD: Lippincott, Williams and Wilkins.

Fisher, T.F., 1993, Miniature swine in biomedical research: applications and husbandry considerations, *Lab Anim.*, 22(5): 47–50.

Frandsson, R.D., 1981, *Anatomy and Physiology of Farm Animals*, 3rd ed., Philadelphia, PA: Lea and Febiger.

Getty, R., Ed., 1975, *Sisson and Grossman's the Anatomy of the Domestic Animals: Porcine*, Vol. 2., Philadelphia, PA: W.B. Saunders, pp. 1215–1422.

Gilbert, S.G., 1966, *Pictoral Anatomy of the Fetal Pig*, 2nd ed., Seattle, WA: University of Washington Press.

Houpt, T.R., 1986, The handling of swine in research, in Stanton, H.C. and Mersmann, H.J., Eds., *Swine in Cardiovascular Research*, Vol. 1, Boca Raton, FL: CRC Press, pp. 25–38.

Idris, A.H., Becker, L.B., Omato, J.P., Hedges, J., Chandra, N., Cummins, R.O., Ebmeyer, U., Halperin, H., Kerber, R., Kern, K., Safar, P., Steen, P., Swindle, M.M., Tsitlik, J., von Planta, I., von Planta, M., Wears, R., and Weil, M.H., 1996, Utstein-Style guidelines for uniform reporting of laboratory CPR research, *Circulation*, 94(9): 2324–2336, simultaneous publication in *Ann. Emergency Med. Resuscitation*, 33(1): 69–84.

Laber, K.E., Whary, M.T., Bingel, S.A., Goodrich, J.A., Smith, A.C., and Swindle, M.M., 2002, Biology and diseases of swine, in Fox, J.G., Anderson, L.C., Loew, F.M., and Quimby, F.W., Eds., *Laboratory Animal Medicine*, 2nd ed., New York: Academic Press, pp. 612–675.

Lindberg, J.E. and Ogle, B., Eds., 2001, *Digestive Physiology of Pigs*, New York: CABI Publishers.

National Research Council, 1998, *The Nutrient Requirements of Swine*, 10th ed., Washington, D.C.: National Academy Press.

National SPF Swine Accrediting Agency, 2000, Rules and Regulations, Conrad, IA: National SPF Swine Accrediting Agency, http://www.nationalspf.com/.

Panepinto, L.M., 1986, Character and management of miniature swine, in Stanton, H.C. and Mersmann, J.H., Eds., *Swine in Cardiovascular Research*, Vol. 1, Boca Raton, FL: CRC Press, pp. 11–24.

Panepinto, L.M., Phillips, R.W., Norden, S.W., Pryor, P.C., and Cox, R., 1983, A comfortable minimum stress method of restraint for Yucatan miniature swine, *Lab. Anim. Sci.*, 33(1): 95–97.

Payne, M.A., Baynes, R.E., Sundlof, S.F., Craigmill, A., Webb, A.I., and Riviere, J.E., 1999, Drugs prohibited from extralabel use in food animals, *J. Am. Vet. Med. Assoc.*, 215(1): 28–32.

Pond, W.G. and Mersmann, H.J., Eds., 2001, *Biology of the Domestic Pig*, Ithaca, NY: Comstock Publishing Associates.

Popesko, P., 1977, *Atlas of Topographical Anatomy of the Domestic Animals*, 2nd ed., Vol. 1, Philadelphia, PA: W.B. Saunders Company.

Public Health Service, 1996, *Guide for the Care and Use of Laboratory Animals*, Washington, D.C.: National Academy Press.

Reeves, D.E., 1993, *Care and Management of Miniature Pet Pigs*, Santa Barbara, CA: Veterinary Practice Publishing Co.

Sack, W.O., 1982, Essentials of pig anatomy, *Harowitz/Kramer Atlas of Musculoskeletal Anatomy of the Pig*, Ithaca, NY: Veterinary Textbooks.

Saffron, J. and Gonder, J.C., 1997, The SPF pig in research, *ILAR J.*, 38(1): 28–31.

Stanton, H.C. and Mersmann, H.J., 1986, *Swine in Cardiovascular Research*, Vol. 1 and 2, Boca Raton, FL: CRC Press.

Straw, B.E., D'Allaire, S., Mengeling, W.L., and Taylor, D.J., Eds., 1999, *Diseases of Swine*, 8th ed., Ames, IA: Iowa State University Press.

Swindle, M.M., 1983, *Basic Surgical Exercises Using Swine*, Philadelphia, PA: Praeger Press.

Swindle, M.M., 1992, *Swine as Models in Biomedical Research*, Ames, IA: Iowa State University Press.

Swindle, M.M., 1996, Considerations of specific pathogen free swine (SPF) in xeno-transplantation, *J. Invest. Surg.*, 9(3): 267–271.

Swindle, M.M., 1998, *Surgery, Anesthesia and Experimental Techniques in Swine*, Ames, IA: Iowa State University Press.

Swindle, M.M. and Smith, A.C., 1998, Comparative anatomy and physiology of the pig, *Scand. J. Lab. Anim. Sci.*, 25(Suppl. 1): 1–10.

Swindle, M.M., Smith, A.C., Laber-Laird, K., and Dungan, L., 1994, Swine in biomedical research: management and models, *ILAR News*, 36(1): 1–5.

Swindle, M.M., Laber, K., Smith, A.C., Goodrich, J.A., and Bingel, S.A., 2006, Biology and medicine of swine, in Reuter, J.D. and Suckow, M.A., Eds., *Laboratory Animal Medicine and Management*, Ithaca, NY: International Veterinary Information Service, http://www.ivis.org/library.asp.

Tumbleson, M.E., Ed., 1986, *Swine in Biomedical Research*, Vol. 1–3, New York: Plenum Press.

Tumbleson, M.E. and Schook, L.B., Eds., 1996, *Advances in Swine in Biomedical Research*, Vol. 1 and 2, New York: Plenum Press.

2 Anesthesia, Analgesia, and Perioperative Care

INTRODUCTION

The purpose of this chapter is to provide practical advice on anesthetic procedures in swine. An emphasis on the physiological effects of injectable anesthetics and cardiopulmonary bypass procedures is included in this publication. Recent veterinary publications (Riebold et al., 1995; Thurmon and Benson, 1996) provide an overview of anesthesia in swine with an emphasis on agricultural and pet pig procedures. Reviews of agents used in cardiovascular research (Thurmon and Tranquilli, 1986) and laboratory animal medicine (Flecknell, 1996; Hawk and Leary, 2005; Kohn et al., 1997; Swindle et al., 2002) are also available.

Anesthetic protocols for experimental procedures should be selected with consideration of the potential physiological complications on the experiment. For example, no anesthetic protocol has been developed that is without effects on cardiovascular hemodynamics; however, the effects may be minimized by judicious selection of the agents. This chapter discusses the most commonly used protocols in research and makes specific recommendations for their selection. Because most of the pharmaceuticals are not marketed as approved for swine, in our laboratories we use the human pediatric dosage as the trial dose when testing a new pharmaceutical agent. Physiological effects of the agents discussed in this chapter are dose dependent.

ANESTHETIC INDUCTION AND ANIMAL PREP ROOM ACTIVITIES

Animals may be induced under anesthesia in a prep room after transport from the housing area (Figure 2.1) or in their cage as described with the neck butterfly technique (Figure 2.2) in Chapter 1. For ergonomic protection of personnel, devices to minimize lifting should be utilized. Minimizing stressful manipulation of animals also aids in prevention of animal discomfort. If tranquilizers are to be used as part of the anesthetic protocol, it is best to administer them in the cage before the other anesthetic agents. Animals may be transported in transport carts (Figure 2.1) or lifted by personnel using a hammock (Figure 2.3). For larger swine, use of hydraulic lifting devices may be developed as illustrated in Figure 2.4–Figure 2.6. In those illustrations, a hydraulic engine lifter has been modified with a sling attachment to manipulate and transport large swine. The hydraulic lift table in the prep room also acts as a scale.

The prep room should be separate from the operating room, and preliminary aseptic preparation should be performed in that area. Animal prep room activities should include shaving, preliminary skin scrubbing, protection of the eyes with bland ophthalmic ointment (Figure 2.7), securing an intravenous (i.v.) catheter (Figure 2.8), placement of electrodes for electrocardiogram (ECG) monitoring (Figure 2.9), and endotracheal intubation (described in the following text). The techniques and theories for aseptic skin preparation in the operating room are discussed and illustrated in Chapter 3.

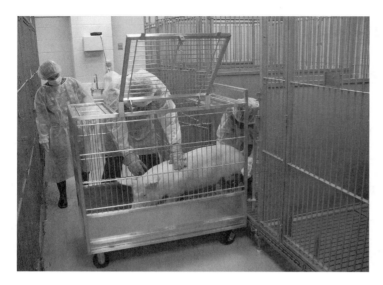

FIGURE 2.1 Pig being moved from a cage into a transport cart.

FIGURE 2.2 Subcutaneous injection in the neck using a butterfly catheter.

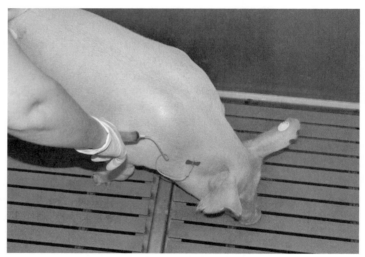

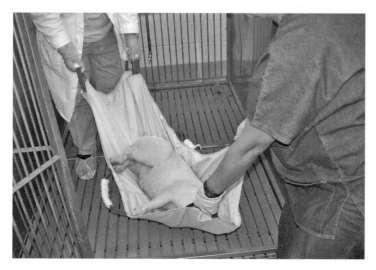

FIGURE 2.3 Anesthetized pig being moved with a transport hammock.

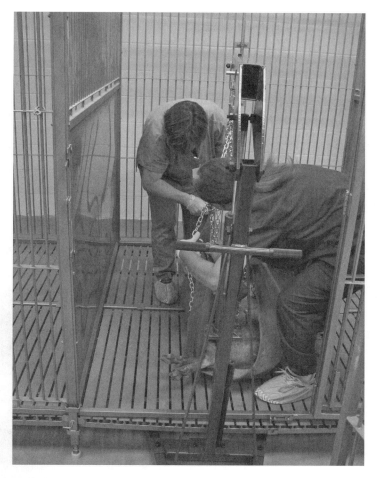

FIGURE 2.4 Large pig being hoisted with a hydraulic lift and hammock.

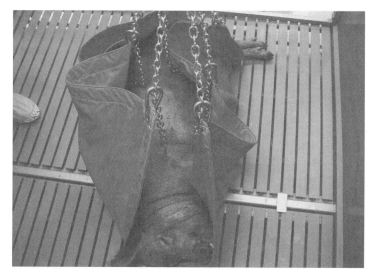

FIGURE 2.5 Close-up view of a large pig in the hammock.

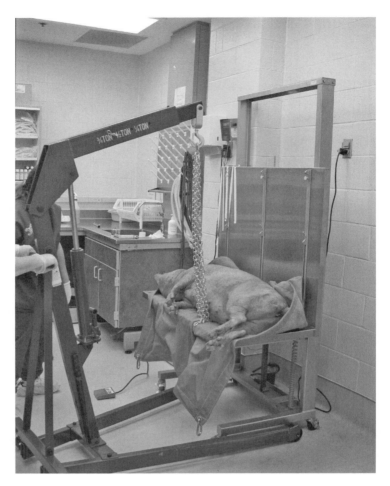

FIGURE 2.6 Transfer of a large pig from the hydraulic lift onto a hydraulic procedure table.

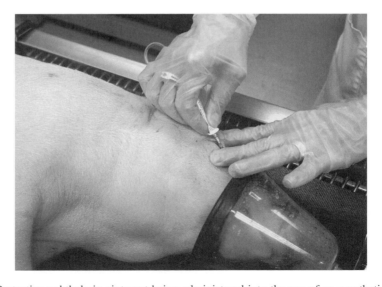

FIGURE 2.7 Protective ophthalmic ointment being administered into the eye of an anesthetized pig.

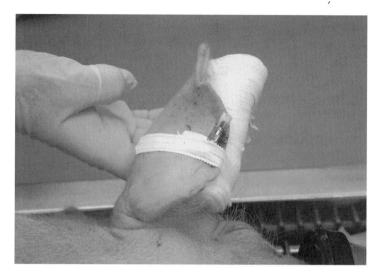

FIGURE 2.8 Ear vein catheter properly taped into place in the marginal ear vein.

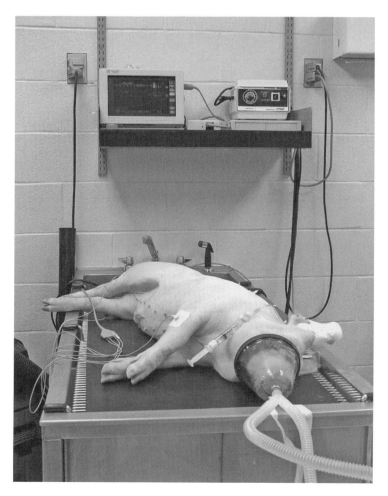

FIGURE 2.9 Anesthetized pig in the prep room with ECG electrodes attached.

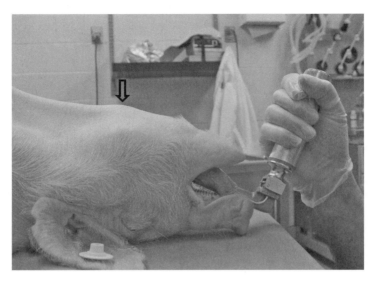

FIGURE 2.10 Correct position of the laryngoscope for intubation of a pig in dorsal recumbency.

ENDOTRACHEAL INTUBATION

Endotracheal intubation should be performed on all swine when they undergo general anesthesia. The procedure is easily performed when the species-specific anatomic considerations are understood. The laryngeal passage is narrow, and the vocal cords and blindfolds are easily traumatized if too large a tube or too much force is used during intubation. The lateral folds of the larynx can be easily ruptured and the tube passed into the subcutaneous tissues.

Swine may be intubated from any position. The most common positions are dorsal, lateral, and sternal recumbency. The dorsal recumbency position tends to be easier for swine less than 50 kg when personnel are used to human intubation. Straight laryngoscope blades with a curved tip are the best for swine. Standard laryngoscope blades, 195 mm or longer, are sufficient for swine less than 50 kg. For larger animals, modified blades with 3- to 5-cm extensions are optimal.

When intubating swine in dorsal recumbency, assistance with holding the jaws open is not necessary; a simplified atraumatic method of intubation has been published (Swindle, 1991). When the pig is placed in sternal recumbency, an assistant must hold the jaws open with gauze strips, or a mouth gag should be used. The method of unassisted intubation in dorsal recumbency is pictured (Figure 2.10 and Figure 2.11) and illustrated (Figure 2.12). The positioning for intubation in lateral recumbency is depicted in Figure 2.13.

After the laryngoscope is passed into the pharyngeal cavity, the tip is used to displace the epiglottis from the soft palate. After this procedure, the epiglottis and laryngeal aperture are easily seen, and the larynx is sprayed with a topical anesthetic, such as lidocaine, to prevent laryngospasm. The tip of the epiglottis is caught with the tip of the curved laryngoscope blade and displaced ventrally against the tongue. At this point, the vocal cords can be observed moving with each breath. The handle of the laryngoscope is tilted toward the operator at approximately a 45° angle. This will result in the larynx being flattened against the ventral surface of the neck; this can be seen readily from the outside. This maneuver will result in the laryngeal passage being straightened. The tip of the endotracheal tube is placed into the laryngeal cavity from the side of the oral cavity while watching the positioning of the tube along the laryngoscope blade. After the tip of the tube is in place, it is passed into the trachea while simultaneously rotating it in a screwlike fashion to facilitate passage through the aperture. Resistance should not be felt if the angle of the laryngoscope blade is correct and the size of the endotracheal tube is not too large.

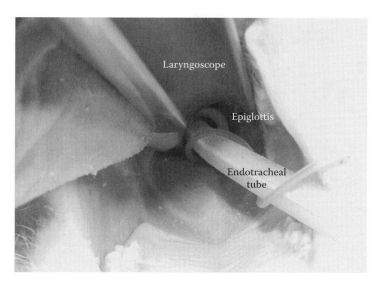

FIGURE 2.11 Oral view of the placement of a laryngoscopic tube in a pig in dorsal recumbency.

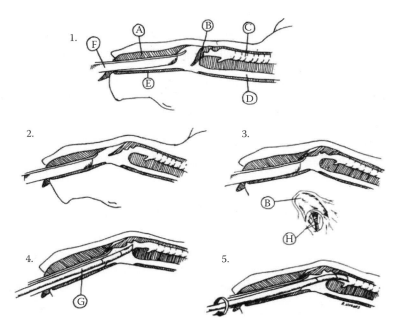

FIGURE 2.12 Schematic drawing of the steps involved in intubation of a pig. A — tongue, B — epiglottis, C — trachea, D — esophagus, E — hard palate, F — laryngoscope blade, G — endotracheal tube, H — vocal cords.

When using this method, the use of stylets or other assist devices is unnecessary. Endotracheal tubes ranging from 4.5 to 8.0 mm in outside dimension are sufficient for most swine used in biomedical research. The size of the tube required can be estimated by palpation of the trachea prior to intubation. As a general rule, most 20- to 30-kg swine can be intubated with 6.5- to 7.5-mm tubes.

With practice, small swine can be intubated without a laryngoscope. The technique involves placing the pig in dorsal recumbency and pinching the dorsum of the larynx between the thumb and forefinger of one hand. This pinching movement should elevate the larynx and close the

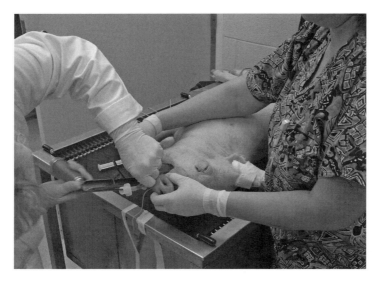

FIGURE 2.13 Correct position for intubating a pig in lateral recumbency.

esophageal passage. A popping will be felt when the epiglottis is displaced ventrally from the soft palate. The endotracheal tube is then passed blindly through the oral cavity with the other hand. This methodology can best be utilized in small swine in which the larynx can be easily manipulated from the outside.

Regardless of the methodology utilized, a free passage of air should be felt and heard when the pig is properly intubated. The two most common problems are inadvertent closure of the laryngeal opening with the laryngoscope and placement of the tube in the esophagus. With traumatic methodologies, the larynx may also either be ruptured through one of its membranes or traumatized sufficiently to produce laryngeal edema. Any gasping or cyanosis is a sign of improper tube or laryngoscope placement. Cyanosis can easily be observed in the snout or nipples of pigs with light-colored skin. The technique of tracheostomy is described in Chapter 9, should it be indicated.

SPECIAL PERIOPERATIVE CONSIDERATIONS

Consideration should be given to several issues concerning perioperative care and monitoring of swine while under anesthesia. These issues include methodologies to provide homeostasis and prevent other potentially fatal complications. The general principles of proper anesthesia and monitoring are applicable to swine, but some issues are species specific (Smith et al., 1997; Smith and Swindle, 1994).

PREOPERATIVE FASTING

Swine should be conditioned for 5–7 d in the facility prior to undergoing survival surgery. They tend to dehydrate and lose weight during shipping. Acute procedures may be performed on newly arrived animals, but i.v. fluids should be administered to maintain hydration. Swine have rapid intestinal transport times in the upper gastrointestinal (GI) tract and require only a few hours to empty the stomach. Consequently, a fast of solid food for 6–8 h preoperatively is sufficient for most surgical procedures. Water may be provided up until the time of surgery. Swine will readily consume most liquid diets and flavored drinks if they are required to prevent hypoglycemia from prolonged fasts, as for colonic procedures. Bedding should be removed from the cages of swine being fasted, because they will readily consume it if not provided food. Issues of fasting specifically applicable to GI procedures are discussed in Chapter 4.

INTRAVENOUS FLUID ADMINISTRATION

The sites for administration of i.v. fluids are discussed in Chapter 1. Once i.v. access is obtained, maintenance fluids should be administered for all anesthetic procedures requiring more than short-term chemical restraint. The rate of administration should be 5–10 ml kg^{-1}h^{-1} with isotonic solutions, unless a problem or specific indication for a different rate of administration is observed. A flow rate of approximately 3–5 ml/h is required to maintain patency of i.v. catheters.

THERMAL SUPPORT

The relatively hairless skin, the common use of alcohol in skin preparation for surgery, and administration of chemical restraint agents that induce peripheral vasodilation make swine more susceptible to hypothermia than most other animal species. Rectal temperature should be continuously monitored and not allowed to decrease below 36°C (normal, 38–39.5°C). The use of circulating hot water blankets and complete draping of the anesthetized animal are usually sufficient to prevent hypothermia. More intense methods, such as administration of warmed i.v. fluids and increasing the room temperature, may be necessary for some highly invasive procedures or if hypothermia occurs.

CARDIAC MONITORING AND ARRHYTHMIAS

Swine are susceptible to anesthetic-induced cardiac arrhythmias and, as a minimum requirement, should be monitored by ECG during anesthesia. For prolonged and invasive procedures, especially those involving the cardiothoracic system, blood pressure and blood gases should also be monitored. Pulse oximetry is useful, and finger cuffs can be placed either on the ears, tail, tongue, or the dewclaws (Figure 2.14–Figure 2.17). Peripheral blood pressure cuffs are most reliable for the coccygeal and median saphenous arteries. Palpation for a peripheral pulse is most reliable on the medial saphenous artery or the radial artery (Figure 2.18 and Figure 2.19). Peripheral arterial access in the median saphenous artery or using the methodologies described for arterial access in Chapter 9 and Chapter 12 can be utilized to implant catheters and measure blood gases.

Cardiac arrhythmias are more likely to be a problem during manipulation of the heart or central vessels or when using anesthetics such as xylazine and halothane, which have a proarrhythmic effect on the myocardium. Farm animals appear to be more susceptible than miniature breeds. Most

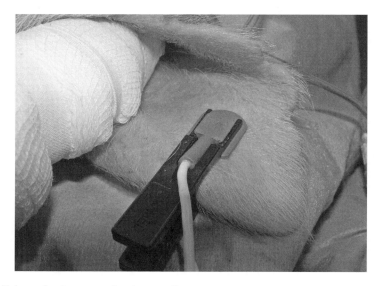

FIGURE 2.14 Pulse oximetry sensor in place on the ear.

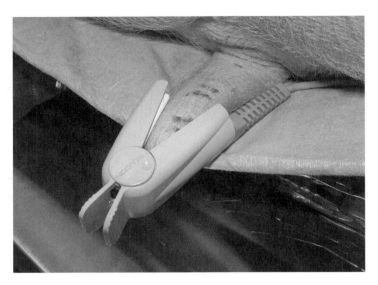

FIGURE 2.15 Pulse oximetry sensor in place on the tail.

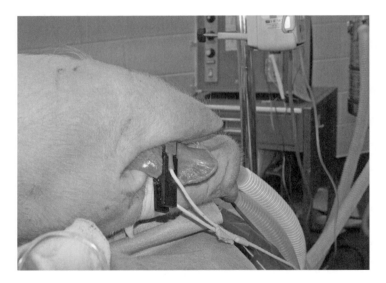

FIGURE 2.16 Pulse oximetry sensor in place on the tongue.

of the fatal instances of cardiac arrhythmias can be prevented by the administration of bretylium 3–5 mg/kg i.v. given by slow injection every 30 min during cardiac manipulation (Horneffer et al., 1986; Schumann et al., 1993). Bretylium is not currently being manufactured, and amiodarone 10–12 mg/kg i.v. followed by 0.5 mg kg^{-1}h^{-1} i.v. infusion has been utilized as a substitute for arrhythmia prevention. It is effective, but the infusion rate needs to be closely monitored because it can rapidly lead to hypotension in swine. Lidocaine (2–4 mg/kg i.v.) can be administered as a continuous i.v. infusion 0.3 mg kg^{-1}h^{-1} (50 μg kg^{-1}min^{-1}) as an antiectopic and antivasospasmotic agent. Other cardiovascular support agents can be administered as indicated; the dosages are included in Table 2.1.

If ventricular fibrillation occurs, then defibrillation should be attempted with 10-J countershock for internal paddles or 200 J for external paddles. The principles of treatment of this potentially fatal condition are the same as for other species.

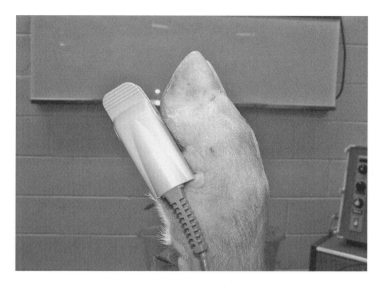

FIGURE 2.17 Pulse oximetry sensor in place on the dewclaw.

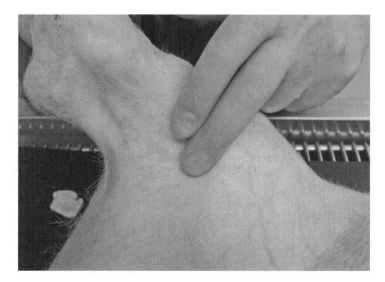

FIGURE 2.18 Palpation of the saphenous pulse on the medial aspect of the stifle (knee) joint.

SPECIALIZED INTRAOPERATIVE MONITORING

Bispectral index (BIS) monitoring, which is a processed electroencephalogram (EEG) index, has been evaluated in swine using various combinations of sevoflurane, isoflurane, propofol, fentanyl, and atacurium (Greene et al., 2004; Martin-Cancho et al., 2003; Martin-Cancho et al., 2004). BIS was determined to be reliable for identification of light vs. deep anesthesia but was not reliable for discrimination in the mid ranges of anesthesia with isoflurane. Misinterpretation of EEG burst suppression by the program in that anesthetic range is theorized to be a species-specific difference. Decrease in blood pressure and heart rate correlated with anesthetic depth with isoflurane (Greene et al., 2004) but not sevoflurane during BIS monitoring (Martin-Cancho et al., 2004). Without additional research to aid interpretation of results, BIS should be considered an adjunct research tool and not a replacement for monitoring of hemodynamics for depth of anesthesia in swine. A

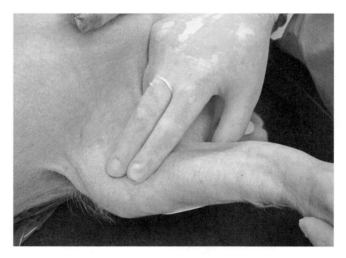

FIGURE 2.19 Palpation of the radial pulse on the medial aspect of the ulna.

TABLE 2.1
Cardiopulmonary Emergency Drugs

Agent	Dosage	Indication
Aminophylline	5.0 mg/kg i.v.	Produces bronchodilation
Amiodarone	10.0–12.0 mg/kg, followed by 0.5–3.5 mg $kg^{-1}h^{-1}$ i.v.	Antiarrhythmic
Atropine	0.05 mg/kg i.v.	Counteracts bradycardia, heart block
Bicarbonate Na	1.0 mEq/kg bolus, followed by 0.5–1.0 mEq $kg^{-1}h^{-1}$	Counteracts acidosis
Bretylium	3.0–5.0 mg/kg i.v.	Antiarrhythmic
Calcium chloride	5.0–7.0 mg/kg slow i.v. infusion	Increases contractility
Digoxin	0.01–0.04 mg/kg i.v.	Counteracts supraventricular arrhythmias; decreases conduction; increases contractility
Dopamine	2.0–20.0 µg $kg^{-1}min^{-1}$ i.v.	Counteracts hypotension, cardiogenic shock
Dobutamine	2.5–10.0 µg $kg^{-1}min^{-1}$ i.v.	Counteracts hypotension, cardiogenic shock
Epinephrine	0.5–2.0 ml of 1:10,000 solution i.v. or i.c. (30 µg/kg)	Counteracts asystole, decreased contractility
Isoproterenol	0.01 µg $kg^{-1}min^{-1}$ i.v.	Induces brochodilation; counteracts AV block, sinus bradycardia
Lidocaine	2.0–4.0 mg/kg bolus followed by 50 µg $kg^{-1}min^{-1}$ i.v.	Antiarrhythmic, antiectopic
Nitroprusside Na	0.5–0.8 µg $kg^{-1}min^{-1}$ i.v.	Reduces hypertension
Neosynepherine	0.5–1.0 mg/kg i.v.	Increases blood pressure by vasoconstriction
Propanolol	0.04–0.06 mg/kg i.v.	Counteracts tachycardia

similar form of monitoring, cerebral state index (CSI) has been developed, which uses a different algorithm to calculate a numerical value (Bollen et al., in press). Likewise, this particular technique is in development.

Similarly, auditory evoked potentials (AEP) have been used for monitoring depth of anesthesia with propofol, isoflurane, and sevoflurane (Bollen et al., 2004). The values obtained did not directly correlate with data from humans; consequently, AEP should also be considered to be an experimental adjunct until further research validates the methodology.

MALIGNANT HYPERTHERMIA

Malignant hyperthermia is a genetic condition in certain breeds of domestic swine, such as the Landrace, Yorkshire, and Pietrain. The condition is transmitted as an autosomal dominant gene (Hal genotype). The ryanodine receptor gene (ryr-1 locus) is the probable site (Geers et al., 1992; Houde et al., 1993). The condition has not been reported in miniature swine.

The condition is induced by stress, i.e., porcine stress syndrome (PSS), or by many anesthetic and paralytic agents. Susceptible animals can be screened genetically or by testing for abnormal creatine phosphokinase serum levels. The condition may also be prevented by the prophylactic intramuscular (i.m.) or i.v. administration of dantrolene 5 mg/kg (Anderson, 1976; Ehler et al., 1985; Smith et al., 1997).

If malignant hyperthermia is encountered, it is associated with elevated rectal temperatures and skeletal muscle rigidity. Elevated CO_2 levels and associated cardiovascular responses such as tachycardia occur rapidly at the onset. The condition is rapidly fatal in susceptible animals. If encountered, it may be treated by discontinuing the triggering agent, cooling of the animal, and administration of dantrolene; however, it is best to avoid sources of animals that have the condition rather than using screening methods or pharmaceutical interventions to prevent the disease.

There is another postoperative condition in swine in which hyperthermia occurs during the recovery period, which is apparently not the same condition as malignant hyperthermia. The symptoms are similar and rapidly elevating temperatures can lead to death if untreated with cooling interventions, such as ice and cold i.v. solutions. It is uncertain if dantrolene is effective as a treatment; however, methylprednisolone 1–5 mg/kg i.v. has some effectiveness for shock, and diazepam 0.5–1 mg/kg i.v. may be useful for the muscular tremors. The pathogenesis of the condition has not been described, but it has been associated with an increase in lactate levels (>2.5 mmol/l, normal = <2.2 mmol/l) and pH (Ayoub et al., 2003). It tends to occur in groups of farm animals that may be closely related. The incidence is sporadic and unpredictable. It is not related to changes in the anesthetic or surgical protocol and tends to disappear from the herd without any intervention on the part of the breeder. It may occur suddenly in a group of animals from a supplier who has been used for long periods of time without ever experiencing the condition before, and whose herd has not experienced PSS or malignant hyperthermia. If the condition is noted in a research facility, the best prevention is to request unrelated swine from the same or a different breeder, because anecdotal information suggests a genetic predisposition.

PARALYTIC AGENTS

Paralytic agents may be indicated for some procedures either to paralyze the diaphragm during cardiac surgery or to provide increased muscle relaxation. Paralytic agents should not be administered during surgery until it is established that surgical analgesia has been obtained and baseline hemodynamic measurements have been recorded. For example, the use of paralytic agents is helpful to paralyze the diaphragm during cardiac surgical manipulations. The thoracotomy can be performed without the administration of paralytic agents to ensure that analgesia levels are sufficient. As a minimum requirement, at least the skin incision should be performed before the paralytic agent is administered to observe the animal's reactions. It is unnecessary to administer these agents throughout the surgical procedure in most cases.

Paralyzed animals should be monitored for a sustained increase in heart rate or blood pressure as an indication of inadequate analgesia. The initial administration of pancuronium (0.02–0.15 mg/kg, 0.003–0.030 mg kg^{-1}h^{-1} i.v. infusion) is associated with a physiological increase in heart rate. Vercuronium (1 mg/kg) does not affect the heart rate (Smith et al., 1997). Rocuronium (1–1.5 mg/kg, 2.0–2.5 mg kg^{-1}h^{-1} i.v. infusion) may be preferred for some protocols.

SURGICAL PROCEDURE / ANESTHESIA MONITORING

INVESTIGATOR _____   AR # _____

SURGERY DATE _____   ANIMAL # _____   WEIGHT_____KG

DESCRIPTION OF PROCEDURE _____

_____

_____

COMPLICATIONS _____

SURGEON _____   ASSISTANT _____   ANESTHETIST _____

SURGERY START TIME _____   SURGERY END TIME _____

Time																		
Oxygen (Liters)																		
Nitrous Oxide (Liters)																		
Isoflurane (%)																		
Pulse (HR)																		
Oxygen saturation																		
Respiratory rate																		
Tidal vol. (cm water)																		
Blood Pressure																		
End tidal CO_2																		
Esophageal Temp																		
Rectal Temp																		
Lactated Ringers ml/hr																		
NaCl ml/hr																		
1% Nembutol ml/hr																		

SURGICAL NOTES

FIGURE 2.20 Sample anesthesia and surgical procedure monitoring form.

ANESTHETIC MONITORING

Anesthetic monitoring can be performed by monitoring heart rate and blood pressure as described in the preceding text (Figure 2.20). This methodology is more sensitive than the muscular or ocular reflexes that are commonly used in veterinary medicine. Ocular reflexes are difficult to observe in swine because of the depth of the orbit and the frequently used combinations of drugs in porcine anesthesia that can make meaningful observations obscure. Muscular reflexes can be induced by pinching at the coronary band of the hoof, the tip of the ear, or the tail, or by observing mandibular jaw tone. Jaw tone seems to be the most reliable and is the preferred method of observing muscular reflexes. Rigidity of the mandibular muscles should be taken as an indication that the anesthetic level is light (Swindle, 1983).

VENTILATION RATES

The pulmonary tissue of swine is sensitive to overventilation and may rupture and cause emphysematous bullae, pneumothorax, and pneumoperitoneum. Pneumatosis intestinalis may occur in severe cases. The ventilatory pressure for swine should be 18–22 cm H_2O. The tidal volume for swine is 5–10 ml/kg. End tidal CO_2 is generally adjusted to 40–50 mmHg. Positive end-expiratory pressure (PEEP) may be adjusted with the ventilator to ensure proper pulmonary pressure. The respiratory rate varies depending upon the anesthetic and individual animal characteristics. For swine 20–40 kg on inhalational anesthesia, a rate of 12–15 breaths per minute is usually sufficient; however, monitoring with pulse oximetry, arterial blood gases, or end tidal CO_2 should be performed to ensure proper ventilation (Smith et al., 1997; Swindle, 1983).

POSTOPERATIVE MONITORING

The postoperative period should include monitoring of temperature, pulse, and respiration at least every 15 min until extubation and recovery of the righting reflex. For major procedures, monitoring of ECG and pulse oximetry should be included (Figure 2.20 and Figure 2.21).

Procedures for continuous monitoring in an intensive care setting (Figure 2.22 and Figure 2.23) for up to 7 d have been described (Hanneman et al., 2004). In this setting, sedation, analgesia, and parenteral nutritional support, as well as continuous intensive monitoring for homeostasis and infection, are required.

Following recovery from anesthesia, monitoring should be performed at least once a day until the sutures are removed or the incision is healed. The monitoring should include state of the incision, attitude and behavior, urination, appetite, feces, water consumption, temperature, pulse, and respiration. Use of a pain score is also helpful in evaluation of the need for analgesic administration.

Administration of systemic analgesics on a preset schedule without evaluation of the individual's condition is not recommended. Professional judgment is essential in the decision on whether analgesics should be administered. It may be harmful to the animal's recovery to be administered pharmacological agents when they are not necessary. The following pain assessment score is an example of such an evaluation system.

PAIN ASSESSMENT

Use the following number designations, as appropriate, to reference no pain perception or reaction as if painful.

1. Deep palpation of the surgical site and immediate surrounding tissue does not provoke a response. (Remember that freshly opened tissue is susceptible to infection and palpation should be done with a gloved hand.)
2. Deep palpation of the surgical site and immediate surrounding tissue provokes a response, but a similar response can be seen on the contralateral side or limb, suggesting a hyperesthetic or hyperreflexive state.
3. Deep palpation of the surgical site and immediate surrounding tissue that provokes a response much greater than a similar stimulus on a nonsurgical part of the body. Probably indicative of some pain and appropriate analgesic should be administered.
4. Deep palpation of the surgical site and immediate surrounding tissue that provokes a response much greater than a similar stimulus on a nonsurgical part of the body and accompanied by vocalization in an otherwise quiet patient. Requires analgesia.

Long-term monitoring may have to be performed for animals in which debilitating conditions, such as heart failure, is produced. This can involve daily monitoring for homeostasis for months. In this situation, the protocol and potential complications should be examined in advance and an appropriate monitoring system with endpoints developed by the investigator in collaboration with the veterinary staff. Daily examination can be aided by providing food treats during the examination (Figure 2.24).

NONPHARMACOLOGICAL CONTROL OF PAIN AND DISTRESS

Pain and distress can be largely prevented by nonpharmacological preventive measures in surgical protocols. Included in this is provision of environment and husbandry practices conducive to an

MUSC Department of Laboratory Animal Resources
Post-Operative Observations for Lab Animals

Please check the following daily for each animal that has undergone surgery or an invasive procedure.
Space is available for 7 days of observations. Use Progress Note form for observations beyond 7 days.
(N = normal)

Species _____   Procedure _____   ARC # _____
Animal # _____   Date of Procedure _____   PI _____

DAY						
DAY	Incision		Urine		TPR	
1	Attitude		Eating		Pain score	
	Feces		Drinking		Initials/Time	
DAY	Incision		Urine		TPR	
2	Attitude		Eating		Pain score	
	Feces		Drinking		Initials/Time	
DAY	Incision		Urine		TPR	
3	Attitude		Eating		Pain score	
	Feces		Drinking		Initials/Time	
DAY	Incision		Urine		TPR	
4	Attitude		Eating		Pain score	
	Feces		Drinking		Initials/Time	
DAY	Incision		Urine		TPR	
5	Attitude		Eating		Pain score	
	Feces		Drinking		Initials/Time	
DAY	Incision		Urine		TPR	
6	Attitude		Eating		Pain score	
	Feces		Drinking		Initials/Time	
DAY	Incision		Urine		TPR	
7	Attitude		Eating		Pain score	
	Feces		Drinking		Initials/Time	

For animal emergencies, questions regarding animal health evaluation and/or post-op care, contact DLAR office.

Phone:
Pagers:

Pain Assessment:
Use the following number designations, as appropriate, to reference no pain perception or reaction as if painful.
1. Deep palpation of the surgical site and immediate surrounding tissue does not provoke a response. (Remember that freshly opened tissue is susceptible to infection and palpation should be done with a gloved hand).
2. Deep palpation of the surgical site and immediate surrounding tissue provokes a response but a similar response can be seen on the contra-lateral side or limb, suggesting a hyperesthetic and/or hyperreflexive state.
3. Deep palpation of the surgical site and immediate surrounding tissue that provokes a response much greater than a similar stimulus on a non-surgical part of the body. Probably indicative of some pain and appropriate analgesic should be administered.
4. Deep palpation of the surgical site and immediate surrounding tissue that provokes a response much greater than a similar stimulus on a non-surgical part of the body and accompanied by vocalization in an otherwise quiet patient. Requires analgesia.

FIGURE 2.21 Sample postoperative observation and pain scoring form.

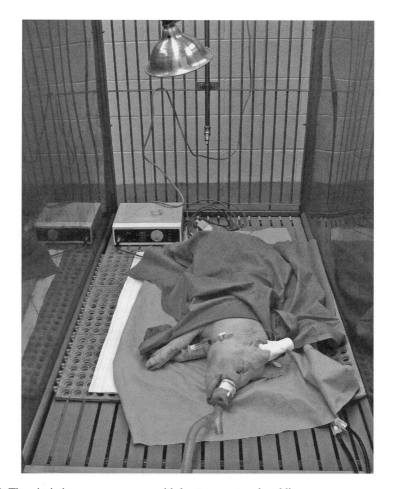

FIGURE 2.22 The pig is in a recovery cage with heat support and padding.

animal's well-being (Chapter 1). The skill of the surgeon is an important element in this equation. Attention to the basic principles of surgery (Chapter 3) and the species-specific requirements will be helpful in a shortened recovery period after surgery.

CHRONIC PAIN AND DISTRESS

Individual behavior variations may result in an animal that develops anxiety or chronic pain and distress on a protocol in which other individuals respond favorably. Some procedures, such as orthopedic surgery, may also produce chronic pain, which is significantly harder to control than soft tissue surgery.

Veterinary monitoring of the animals may identify these individuals by observation of hyperesthesia, hyperreflexia, pain facilitation, stereotypic behavior patterns, abnormal vocalizations, and attitude abnormalities.

In these cases, systemic analgesic administration may not be sufficient to correct the problem. Adjuncts to systemic analgesics, such as opioids, can include anxiolytic tranquilizers or sedatives, local nerve blocks, and anti-inflammatory agents.

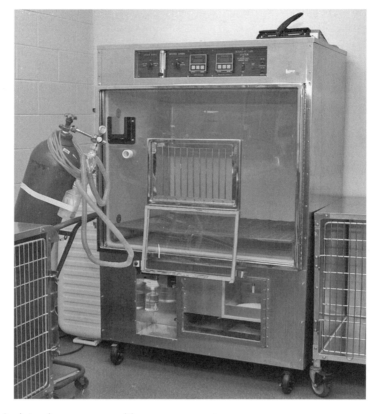

FIGURE 2.23 An intensive care cage with oxygen support.

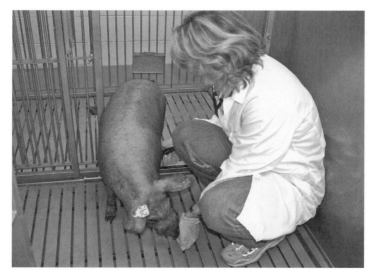

FIGURE 2.24 Socialization of a pig with a food treat during auscultation.

PREANESTHETIC AGENTS

Preanesthetic agents are useful to relieve anxiety, abolish the vagal reflex, decrease the amount of general anesthetic required, and facilitate handling. These agents fall into the categories of anticholinergics, sedatives, hypnotics, and tranquilizers. Giving these agents in the cage before inducing anesthesia may make the induction and transport of the animals less stressful and easier for the technical staff. For example, if the induction is to be performed with ketamine and acepromazine, administration of the acepromazine first calms the animal for the larger volume and more irritating injection with ketamine. The use of preoperative and intraoperative analgesics is discussed in the section on analgesics in this chapter.

ANTICHOLINERGICS

Atropine (0.05 mg/kg i.m., s.c. or 0.02 mg/kg i.v.) and glycopyrrolate (0.004–0.01 mg/kg i.m., s.c.) are used preoperatively to dry bronchiole secretions and abolish the vagal reflex during endotracheal intubation or suctioning. It is also useful to counter the bradycardia that is associated with the use of some anesthetic agents. Routine use of these agents is not required, and the physiological effects of tachycardia and vagal blockade should be considered when designing the protocol (Smith et al., 1997; Swindle, 1983).

TRANQUILIZERS AND SEDATIVES

The phenothiazine, benzodiazepine, and butyrophenone tranquilizers are the most commonly used agents for preanesthesia. All these agents have been combined with dissociative agents to induce anesthesia and are discussed in that context in the following text. Of the phenothiazines, acepro-mazine (1.1–2.2 mg/kg i.m., i.v., or s.c.) is the most commonly used agent. It is associated with peripheral vasodilation and α-adrenergic blockade in higher dosages. Its effects as a sole agent last for 8–12 h (Benson and Thurmon, 1979; Riebold et al., 1995; Swindle, 1983).

The two most commonly used benzodiazepine tranquilizers in porcine anesthesia are diazepam, which is fat soluble, and midazolam, which is water soluble. Diazepam (0.5–10 mg/kg s.c., 0.44–2 mg/kg i.v., 1 mg kg^{-1}h^{-1} i.v. infusion, or 2–10 mg/kg p.o.) provides good hypnosis and sedation for up to 6 h (Benson and Thurmon, 1979; Thurmon and Tranquilli, 1986). Midazolam (0.1–0.5 mg/kg i.m., s.c. or i.v., 0.6–1.5 mg kg^{-1}h^{-1} i.v. infusion) provides complete sedation for 20 min with minimal hemodynamic depression and can be used safely on a daily basis for prolonged periods of time (Ochs et al., 1987; Smith et al., 1991). However, the decrease in cardiovascular parameters at the higher dosage range (0.5 mg/kg i.m. or s.c.) is significant as compared to unsedated minipigs using peripheral cuff measurements (Goodrich et al., 2001). A combination of azaperone (4 mg/kg i.m. or s.c.) and midazolam (1 mg/kg i.m. or s.c.) has been used as a preanesthetic prior to propofol induction and inhalation anesthesia (Svendsen and Carter, 1997).

Butyrophenones are usually found in combination with other agents, except for azaperone (2–8 mg/kg i.m. or s.c.). It has minimal cardiovascular effects, but provides relatively short immobilization of about 20 min (Portier and Slusser, 1985; Riebold et al., 1995; Thurmon and Tranquilli, 1986).

INJECTABLE ANESTHETIC AGENTS

Injectable anesthetic agents used in swine include the dissociative anesthetics, barbiturates, opioids, and miscellaneous hypnotic agents. Most of these agents are used in combination with tranquilizers or other agents to provide surgical anesthesia. Experience in our laboratories has shown that these agents can be administered s.c. in the neck or flank to provide the same effect as i.m. injections, usually cited in the literature. The s.c. route is preferred because it is less traumatic and less painful for the animal when administering large volume or irritating substances. Unless these agents are meant to provide short-term chemical restraint, they should be administered as continuous i.v. infusions rather than repeated i.m. or i.v. injections in the research setting. Experience has shown that continuous i.v. infusions provide more stable hemodynamics than repeated injections. The i.v. dosages are variable depending upon the characteristics of the individual animal and the protocol. The dosages cited in this text are guidelines, and careful anesthetic monitoring should be used to determine if an adequate plane of anesthesia has been achieved. Agents commonly combined with dissociative agents, such as benzodiazepines, hypnotics, and α-2-adrenergic agonists are discussed with the dissociative agents, because they have little value as sole agents in swine.

DISSOCIATIVE AGENTS AND COMBINATIONS

Ketamine and the combination agent tiletamine/zolazepam (Telazol®, Ft. Dodge Animal Health (Wyeth), Overland Park, KS) are the two most common injectable anesthetic agents utilized in swine (Table 2.2). Usually, they are combined with other agents to produce surgical anesthesia and

TABLE 2.2
Ketamine Combinations

Drug	Dosage	Route of Administration
Ketamine	11–33 mg/kg	i.m., s.c.
	3–33 mg kg^{-1}h^{-1}	i.v. infusion
Ketamine	33 mg/kg	
Acetylpromazine	1.1 mg/kg	i.m., s.c.[a]
Ketamine	20 mg/kg	
Xylazine	2 mg/kg	i.m., s.c.
Ketamine	11 mg/kg	
Fentanyl-Droperidol		i.m., s.c.
(Innovar-Vet)	1 ml/14 kg	
Ketamine	2 mg/kg	i.v.
Xylazine	2 mg/kg	
Oxymorphone	0.075 mg/kg	(2X dose for i.m., s.c.)
Ketamine	15 mg/kg	
Azaperone	2 mg/kg	i.m., s.c.
Ketamine	20 mg/kg	
Diazepam	2 mg/kg	i.m., s.c.[a]
Ketamine	33 mg/kg	
Midazolam	500 µg/kg	i.m., s.c.
Ketamine	33 mg kg^{-1}h^{-1}	
Midazolam	1.5 mg kg^{-1}h^{-1}	Continuous i.v. infusion[a]
Ketamine	20 mg/kg	
Climazolam	0.5–1 mg/kg	i.m., s.c.
Ketamine	1 mg/ml	i.v. bolus followed by 1 ml kg^{-1}h^{-1a}
Xylazine	1 mg/ml	
Glyceryl guiaconate 5% in 5% dextrose	1 ml/kg	
Ketamine	1 mg/kg	i.m., s.c.[a]
Medetomidine	0.1 mg/kg	
	5 mg kg^{-1}h^{-1}	Continuous i.v. infusion[a]
	10 µg kg^{-1}h^{-1}	
Ketamine	9–19 mg kg^{-1}h^{-1}	
Pentobarbital	6.5–18 mg kg^{-1}h^{-1}	Continuous i.v. infusion[a]

[a] Most highly recommended agents and combinations.

only used as sole agents to provide up to 20 min of chemical restraint. They provide poor muscle relaxation but have minimal cardiovascular effects with a single i.m. injection in clinically normal animals (Benson and Thurmon, 1979; Cantor et al., 1981; Smith et al., 1997).

Ketamine (11–33 mg/kg i.m., 3–33 mg kg^{-1}h^{-1} i.v. infusion) does not provide visceral analgesia at any dose. It may be combined with other agents to provide muscle relaxation and analgesia for minor procedures (Benson and Thurmon, 1979; Boschert et al., 1996; Smith et al., 1997; Swindle, 1983). The most commonly used i.m. combinations in research are the following:

Ketamine 33 mg/kg and acepromazine 1.1 mg/kg
Ketamine 15 mg/kg and diazepam 2 mg/kg
Ketamine 10 mg/kg and flunitrazepam 0.2 mg/kg
Ketamine 33 mg/kg and midazolam 0.5 mg/kg
Ketamine 15 mg/kg and azaperone 2 mg/kg
Ketamine 20 mg/kg and xylazine 2 mg/kg
Ketamine 10 mg/kg and medetomidine 0.2 mg/kg

Only the combination with midazolam provides longer than 20–30 min of restraint; however, this combination is profoundly hypothermic. It may last 45–60 min and provide sufficient relaxation to perform intubation. Nevertheless, the side effects outweigh the advantages of this combination. The combination of ketamine and medetomidine has a wide range of dosages reported with the ketamine varying from 1 to 10 mg/kg and the medetomidine varying from 0.08 to 0.2 mg/kg. The dosage in the list in the preceding text is used by the author. In general, if you increase the ketamine, you decrease the medetomidine proportionately. Ketamine (5 mg kg^{-1}h^{-1})/medetomidine (10 µg kg^{-1}h^{-1}) infusions provide a stable plane of anesthesia.

The α-2-adrenergic agonists xylazine and medetomidine are commonly included as combinations with the dissociative agents. The combination with xylazine provides short-term analgesia (5 min) but prolonged cardiodepression and heart block, which may be reversed with anticholinergics. Medetomidine has less severe cardiodepression than xylazine (Flecknell, 1997). Other less commonly used agents in this class are romifidine, 80 µg/kg i.m. or s.c., and detomidine (2 µg/kg i.m. or s.c.).

The combinations with acepromazine, diazepam, and azaperone are similar in action but do not provide enough relaxation to perform intubation or to perform other than minor surgery. They all have the side effect of peripheral vasodilation but not as profoundly as the combinations with xylazine and midazolam. Atipamezole 1 mg/kg i.m., s.c., or i.v. is a specific antagonist to the α-2-adrenoreceptors (Flecknell, 1997).

Intravenous infusions of ketamine combined with other agents can provide visceral analgesia suitable for major surgical procedures. After induction with a loading dose of the agent, the following infusions can be used: ketamine (1 mg/ml) and xylazine (1 mg/ml) and glycerol guaiacolate (guaifenesin) (5%) mixed in 5% dextrose 1 ml/kg i.v. followed by 1 ml/kg/h of the mixture; ketamine 8–33 mg kg^{-1}h^{-1} and midazolam 0.5–1.5 mg kg^{-1}h^{-1}; or ketamine 5 mg kg^{-1}h^{-1} and medetomidine 10 µg kg^{-1}h^{-1}. Ketamine (9–19 mg kg^{-1}h^{-1} i.v.) and pentobarbital (6.5–18 mg kg^{-1}h^{-1}) as separate simultaneous infusions have been used for long-term 96-h shock studies (Goldmann et al., 1999). Following ketamine-azaperone sedation the i.v. infusion was started at the lower dosages and gradually had to be increased as tolerance developed. However, they were able to maintain a stable anesthetic plane as monitored by heart rate and mean arterial pressure.

All these agents as i.v. infusions can provide a stable plane of anesthesia. The ketamine/xylazine/glycerol guaiacolate (guaifenesin) solution, in particular, causes minimal cardiovascular depression and can be used as a substitute for α-chloralose infusions (Thurmon et al., 1986). Its main disadvantage is the need to mix the combination in the laboratory. The infusion combinations with medetomidine (Vainio et al., 1992) and midazolam are useful for cardiac catheterization protocols but do not provide good muscle relaxation.

The tiletamine/zolazepam (Telazol®, Ft. Dodge Labs, Ft. Dodge, IA) combination can provide 20 min of immobilization for minor surgery in the commercially available combination (2–8.8 mg/kg i.m.); however, the combination should not be used in animals with cardiovascular compromise because of cardiodepression and hypothermia. In agricultural and pet pig situations, Telazol is combined with xylazine or xylazine and ketamine (Ko et al., 1993; Ko et al., 1997). Single-dose administration of this agent to normal animals does not cause problems with homeostasis; however, it has been associated with problems with arrhythmias in manipulative cardiac surgical protocols. The combinations have also been shown to reduce insulin levels and be a potential complication in metabolic research (Heim et al., 2002). Telazol and its combinations are useful for large research swine >75 kg because of the lower volume of injection required to achieve sedation as compared to ketamine combinations.

All of the combinations are suitable for intubation and short-term anesthesia; however, hemodynamic data have not been published to prove the usefulness of the combinations in research settings. Clinical observation of animals under anesthesia with these combinations has included peripheral cyanosis, hypothermia, and death in animals with cardiovascular compromise. The i.m. combination dosages to provide 20–30 min of immobilization are the following:

Telazol 4.4 mg/kg and ketamine 2.2 mg/kg
Telazol 4.4 mg/kg, ketamine 2.2 mg/kg, and xylazine 2.2 mg/kg
Telazol 4.4 mg/kg and xylazine 2.2 mg/kg

Combinations useful for restraint of large swine are the following:

Ketamine (100 mg/ml) 0.1–0.15 ml/kg + diazepam (5.0 mg/ml) 0.2–0.3 ml/kg + medetomidine (1.0 mg/ml) 0.1 ml/kg + atropine (0.54 mg/ml); 2 ml/pig reversed with atipamezole (5.0 mg/ml) 1–2 ml/pig. Used for restraint of sexually mature minipigs (J.A. Goodrich, Medical University of South Carolina (MUSC), personal communication).
Tiletamine/zolazepam 125 mg each (one vial) + medetomidine 6.5 ml of 1 mg/ml solution + ketamine 1.25 ml of 100 mg/ml solution + butorphanol 2.5 ml of 10 mg/ml solution mixture. Give 0.67 ml/10 kg with atropine (K. Ravn, Novo Nordisk, personal communication).

BARBITURATES

Barbiturate anesthesia (Riebold et al., 1995; Smith et al., 1997; Swindle, 1983; Swindle, 1991; Thurmon and Tranquilli, 1986) must be administered i.v., usually after induction with one of the dissociative anesthetics to allow the anesthetist to insert an i.v. catheter (Table 2.3). The initial administration of these agents as a bolus will frequently induce apnea, which can be overcome by

---

TABLE 2.3
Barbiturates

Drug	Dosages	Route of Administration
Pentobarbital	20–40 mg/kg	i.v. infusion
	5–40 mg $kg^{-1}h^{-1}$	
Thiopental	6.6–25 mg/kg	i.v. infusion[a]
	3–30 mg $kg^{-1}h^{-1}$	
Thiamylal	6.6–25 mg/kg	i.v. infusion
	3–30 mg $kg^{-1}h^{-1}$	

[a] Most highly recommended.

the stimulation of endotracheal intubation. They have a dose-related cardiopulmonary depressant activity that increases over time with repeated i.v. boluses. The cardiovascular effects can be minimized by using thiobarbiturates, which have minimal hepatic metabolism as i.v. infusions. These agents are excreted by the kidneys and can be flushed out of the system with i.v. fluid administration. Pentobarbital is best reserved for nonsurvival procedures and should be administered as a continuous i.v. infusion. Dosages of barbiturates are guidelines and may be affected by other drugs and homeostatic factors. They should be given to effect with close monitoring of vital signs. The i.v. dosages of the most commonly used barbiturates are the following:

Thiopental 6.6–30 mg/kg, 3–30 mg $kg^{-1}h^{-1}$
Thiamylal 6.6–30 mg/kg, 3–30 mg $kg^{-1}h^{-1}$
Pentobarbital 20–40 mg/kg, 5–40 mg $kg^{-1}h^{-1}$

OPIOID INFUSIONS

Opioids can be used as i.v. infusions to provide the primary analgesia for cardiac surgery protocols; however, they have to be combined with other anesthetics, such as the inhalants, during the major manipulative procedures. In general, when isoflurane is used as an adjunct, a level of 0.5% is adequate. They can also be used as low-dose infusions during general surgery to provide balanced anesthesia and analgesia (Ehler et al., 1985; Lunn et al., 1979; Merin et al., 1982; Schumann et al., 1994; Smith et al., 1997; Swindle et al., 1986). The concept of analgesia with these agents is discussed in the section on analgesics in this chapter.

Opioid infusions have the advantages of not decreasing myocardial contractility and coronary blood flow. They produce a dose-related bradycardia that can be reversed with anticholinergics. They can also be used as stabile i.v. infusions for taking physiological measurements for cardiovascular protocols. Hypertension occurs in the higher dose ranges over time. In that situation, the adjunctive anesthetic agents can be eliminated after all the major surgical manipulations have been performed.

The most commonly used agents for these infusion procedures in swine are fentanyl (30–100 µg $kg^{-1}h^{-1}$) and sufentanil (7–30 µg $kg^{-1}h^{-1}$), although other agents in this class should be equally effective such as alfentanil (6 µg $kg^{-1}h^{-1}$) or remifentanil (30–60 µg $kg^{-1}h^{-1}$). They may be used for induction following placement of an i.v. catheter or following restraint with midazolam or ketamine. Starting the i.v. infusion prior to administering an i.v. bolus to induce anesthesia prevents the animals from exhibiting a sudden onset of bradycardia and muscle rigidity. These dosages are guidelines, and the i.v. infusion must be given to effect with constant monitoring of cardiovascular parameters. The i.v. dosages are as follows:

Fentanyl 0.050 mg/kg (50 µg) i.v. bolus, 0.030–0.100 mg $kg^{-1}h^{-1}$ i.v. infusion
Sufentanil 0.007 mg/kg (7 µg) i.v. bolus, 0.015–0.030 mg $kg^{-1}h^{-1}$ i.v. infusion
Remifentanil, 0.5–1 µg $kg^{-1}min^{-1}$ (0.030–0.060 mg $kg^{-1}h^{-1}$)
Alfentanil, 0.1 µg $kg^{-1}min^{-1}$ (0.006 mg $kg^{-1}h^{-1}$)

MISCELLANEOUS AGENTS (TABLE 2.4)

Propofol (4–20 mg/kg i.v.) is an i.v. hypnotic agent that can be used in combination with other agents to induce anesthesia. It has a relatively narrow therapeutic margin in swine and can produce severe hypotension and apnea. In lower dosages, cardiac output and coronary blood flow is minimally depressed; however, there is also poor analgesia. A continuous infusion rate of 12–20 mg $kg^{-1}h^{-1}$ can be used to provide stable general anesthesia (Foster et al., 1992; Raff and Harrison, 1989; Ramsey et al., 1993). Propofol (2.0–4.4 mg $kg^{-1}h^{-1}$) combined with fentanyl (0.003–0.005 mg $kg^{-1}h^{-1}$) and midazolam (0.4–0.7 mg $kg^{-1}h^{-1}$) have been described as effective for 6–7 h of

TABLE 2.4
Miscellaneous Drugs and Combinations

Drug	Dosages	Route of Administration
Alphaxolone/alphadolone	6–8 mg/kg followed by 2–3 mg/kg	i.m. i.v. infusion
α-Chloralose	55–100 mg/kg	i.v.
Atipamezole	0.24–1 mg/kg	i.v., i.m., s.c.
Atropine	0.02–0.05 mg/kg	i.m., s.c., i.v.
Azaperone	2–8 mg/kg	i.m., s.c.
Brontizolam	1–10 mg/kg	p.o.
Etorphine/acetylpromazine (Imobilon®)	0.245 mg/10kg	i.v.
Climazolam	0.5–1 mg/kg	i.m.
Diazepam	0.5–10 mg/kg 0.44–2 mg/kg	i.m., s.c., p.o. i.v.
Diprenorphine	0.3 mg/kg	i.v.
Etomidate	4–8 mg/kg	i.v.
Etomidate Azaperone	4–8 mg/kg 2 mg/kg	i.v., s.c., i.m.
Etomidate/ketamine	6 mg/kg followed by 10 mg kg^{-1}h^{-1}	i.v. followed by i.v. infusion
Flurazepam	2 mg/kg	i.v., p.o.
Glycopyrrolate	0.004–0.01 mg/kg	i.m., s.c., i.v.
Lorazepam	0.1 mg/kg	i.v.
Midazolam	100–500 μg/kg 0.6–1.5 mg kg^{-1}h^{-1}	i.m. or i.v., i.v. infusion[a]
Metomidate	4 mg/kg	i.v.
Nalbuphine	1–2 mg/kg	i.v.
Naloxone	0.5–2 mg/kg	i.v.
Pancuronium	0.02–0.15 mg/kg	i.v.
Propofol	0.83–1.66 mg/kg	i.v. followed by 14–20 mg kg^{-1}h^{-1} infusion
Propofol Midazolam Fentanyl	2.0–4.4 mg kg^{-1}h^{-1} 0.4–0.7 mg kg^{-1}h^{-1} 0.003–0.005 mg kg^{-1}h^{-1}	i.v. infusion after loading dose
Telazol® (Tiltamine:zolazepan)	2–8.8 mg/kg	i.m., s.c.
Telazol Xylazine	4.4 mg/kg 4.4 mg/kg	i.m., s.c.
Telazol Xylazine Butorphanol	4.4 mg/kg 2.2 mg/kg 0.22 mg/kg	i.m., s.c.
Telazol Xylazine Azaperone	4.4 mg/kg 2.2 mg/kg 0.88 mg/kg	i.m., s.c.

TABLE 2.4 *(Continued)*
Miscellaneous Drugs and Combinations

Drug	Dosages	Route of Administration
Vecuronium	1.0 mg/kg	i.v.
Xylazine	0.2 mg/kg	i.m., s.c.

[a] Most highly recommended.

anesthesia (Kaiser et al., 2003, 2006) following induction with ketamine/azaperone and an i.v. loading dose of the agents. Propofol (3.5 mg kg^{-1}h^{-1}) and fentanyl (17 μg kg^{-1}h^{-1}) have also been used to induce general anesthesia as an i.v. infusion (Bollen et al., in press).

Etomidate (4–8 mg/kg i.v.) is a hypnotic sedative that can be combined with other agents to produce analgesia. The combination of 0.6 mg/kg i.v. with a ketamine infusion of 10 mg kg^{-1}h^{-1} i.v. can be used for anesthesia (Holzchuh and Cremonesi, 1991; Worek et al., 1988).

The agent α-chloralose (55–86 mg/kg i.v.) has been used for nonsurvival surgery to record physiological measurements with minimal cardiovascular depression and minimal effects on the baroreceptors and chemoreceptors. It has questionable analgesic value except at the higher dose range, at which time the sparing effects on cardiovascular parameters are lost (Silverman and Muir, 1993; Thurmon and Tranquilli, 1986). It is best replaced by ketamine infusion protocols, opioid infusions, or inhalational anesthesia with isoflurane.

Prolonged i.v. anesthesia may be required for protocols that do not allow the use of inhalant anesthetics. Intravenous infusion with sufentanil, thiopental, ketamine/xylazine/glycerol guaiacolate, ketamine/midazolam, ketamine/pentobarbital, or propofol/fentanyl/midazolam as described in the preceding text are acceptable for these procedures.

No particular advantage to using these agents or older agents, such as alphaxalone, alphadolone, or etorphine, over other agents in this chapter have been published.

INHALANT ANESTHETICS

Inhalant anesthetics should be the primary agents considered for general anesthesia in swine (Smith et al., 1997). They provide a better control of the plane of anesthesia and analgesia and have a reduced recovery time over many of the injectable agents. When used in combination with intra-operative analgesics to provide balanced anesthesia, the anesthetist has the highest assurance that the animal is in an appropriate plane of anesthesia for major surgical procedures.

All these agents should be used in combination with gas scavenging and periodic monitoring of the gas anesthesia machines for leakage, because of the human health problems associated with chronic exposure to low levels of these agents. In particular, the exposure of personnel, especially pregnant women, to waste gases should be avoided with methoxyflurane, halothane, and nitrous oxide. The use of scavenging systems and absorbent filters in combination with closed or semiclosed anesthetic systems should be routine. The gas anesthetic machines should be modern in design and kept in good repair to provide the best assurance that the level of anesthesia indicated by the vaporizer is correct and to prevent personnel exposure to gases leaking from the equipment (Thurmon and Benson, 1996).

The agents that should be considered as the primary choices for use in porcine anesthesia are isoflurane, desflurane, and sevoflurane. Methoxyflurane is difficult to control because of its low potency, and the agent has the possibility of causing nephrotoxicity in humans. Consequently, it is recommended that its use be discontinued along with older agents such as ether. Halothane sensitizes the myocardium to catecholamine-induced arrhythmias and has more severe depressant effects upon the myocardium than the more recently developed agents. These physiological effects combined with the possibility of hepatotoxicity in humans should preclude its use as an anesthetic in swine.

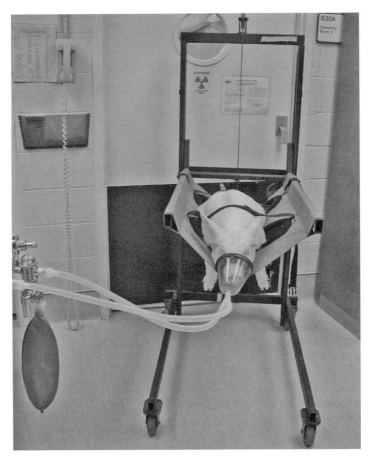

FIGURE 2.25 The pig is being induced with gas anesthesia in a humane restraint sling, using a face mask.

Enflurane is associated with seizure episodes in susceptible animals and does not offer any advantages over the use of other agents (Smith et al., 1997).

Isoflurane, desflurane, and sevoflurane all have similar physiological effects in swine and are relatively safe for personnel compared to the other inhalants (Weiskopf et al., 1992). The cost differential between isoflurane and the other two agents is significant. Because of the similar physiological effects of these three agents and the significant difference in cost, isoflurane is recommended as the primary inhalant anesthetic in swine at present (Smith et al., 1997).

Sevoflurane may be an appropriate choice for high-risk cases. Induction by face mask (Figure 2.25) followed by endotracheal intubation may be performed with isoflurane without nitrous oxide for protocols in which it is necessary to have a sole agent for anesthesia. The face mask should be free of leaks and the area adequately ventilated. This procedure carries minimal risk for personnel.

All the inhalant anesthetics increase cerebral blood flow and decrease coronary blood flow in a dose-dependent fashion. These effects are minimized with isoflurane, and it may increase coronary blood flow at some dosages. All produce a dose-related depression in myocardial contractility. Isoflurane, desflurane, and sevoflurane have significantly less deleterious effects on the myocardium than the other agents discussed in the preceding text (Smith et al., 1997; Weiskopf et al., 1992). Desflurane has also been shown to impair hepatic and small intestinal O_2 capacity, but not to cause sever tissue hypoxia (Armbruster et al., 1997).

The percentage of the inhalant used for anesthesia may be reduced by the administration of nitrous oxide. Nitrous oxide as a sole agent does not provide visceral analgesia in swine; however,

TABLE 2.5
Inhalant Anesthetics

Agent	Mean Alveolar Concentration (MAC) (%)
Isoflurane[a]	1.2–2.04
Desflurane	8.28–10.0
Halothane	0.91–1.25
Sevoflurane[a]	2.53
Enflurane	1.66
Nitrous oxide 1:1 or 2:1	195

[a] Most highly recommended agents.

it is effective as an adjunct agent when used in a 1:1 or 2:1 combination with oxygen to deliver the inhalant anesthetic. The combination of isoflurane with nitrous oxide and oxygen (2:1) provides the least myocardial depressant effects of any of the inhalant anesthetic agents and reduces the concentration of isoflurane required by approximately 50%. However, nitrous oxide has the potential of having adverse effects on the health of personnel, and adequate scavenging of waste gases should be assured (Smith et al., 1997).

The mean alveolar concentration (MAC) value is utilized as a measure of an inhalant anesthetic's potency and provides a guideline for the percentage of an anesthetic that should be required for general anesthesia (Table 2.5). The MAC value will vary with the age of the animal as well as other variables, such as the delivery system and protocol (Smith et al., 1997). The MAC values (volume %) of these agents in swine are nitrous oxide 195 (Tranquilli et al., 1985), halothane 0.91–1.25 (Eisele et al., 1985; Eisele et al., 1986; Tranquilli et al., 1983), isoflurane 1.2–2.04 (Eger et al., 1988; Eisele et al., 1985; Koblin et al., 1989; Lundeen et al., 1983), sevoflurane 2.53 (Thurmon and Benson, 1996), enflurane 1.66 (Thurmon and Benson, 1996), and desflurane 8.28–10 (Eger et al., 1988).

The flow rates for anesthetics will vary with the equipment and the procedure; however, a rate of 5–10 ml kg^{-1}min^{-1} is generally adequate. Anesthetic monitoring procedures described in the preceding text should be utilized to determine if the anesthetic level and oxygenation are adequate.

CARDIOPULMONARY BYPASS (CPB)

If performed as survival procedures, cardiopulmonary bypass (Figure 2.26) and extracorporeal membrane oxygenation (ECMO) (Figure 2.27) in swine are more difficult procedures to perform successfully than in most other species. Difficulties include friability of the atria, postperfusion pulmonary hypertension, cardiac arrhythmias, and edema of visceral tissues (Belanger et al., 2002; Cameron et al., 1992; Martens et al., 2004; Mohr et al., 1996; Myung et al., 2004; Pokela et al., 2002; Purohit et al., 1993; Qayumi et al., 1992; Smerup et al., 2004; Smith et al., 1997; Swan and Meaghar, 1971). The methodologies described in this section are derived mainly from the laboratory experiences described by Ehler and Swindle (Ehler et al., 1985; Smith et al., 1997; Swindle et al., 1986) with some recent modifications by Smerup et al. (2004). The use of a cooperative team approach among the perfusionist, surgeon, anesthetist, and veterinary staff is essential to the success of these protocols.

In its simplest form, blood is collected prior to entering the right side of the heart, circulated through the bypass system for oxygenation and filtering, and then returned to the arterial circulation without passing through the left side of the heart. Many variations to the surgical cannulation are performed depending upon the surgical protocol under investigation. The procedure may be performed with or without the induction of hypothermia and cardioplegia to stop electrical activity and lower myocardial metabolism. In general, the longer the procedure, the more the necessity for those procedures to protect the myocardium. CPB with aortic cross-clamp time of less than 30 min

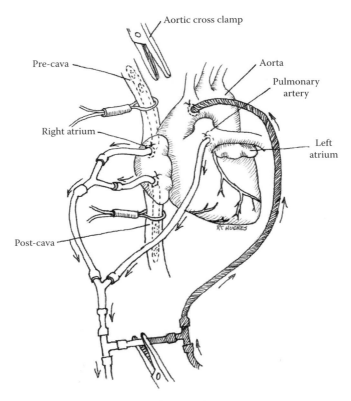

FIGURE 2.26 Catheterization circuit for cardiopulmonary bypass.

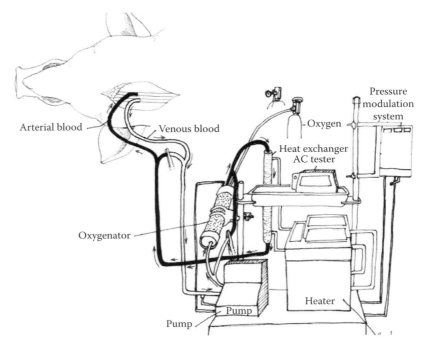

FIGURE 2.27 Extracorporeal membrane oxygenation circuit in swine. (Reprinted from Purohit, D.M. et al., 1993, *J. Invest. Surg.* 6, 503–508. With permission.)

is more likely to be uneventful in swine. Time spans of greater than 45 min are likely to involve more manipulations during weaning and recovery from CPB. Indomethacin suppositories (50 mg) administered to swine the night before surgery greatly reduces the incidence of postperfusion pulmonary hypertension due to the antiprostaglandin effect (Landis et al., 2001). In a recent publication (Smerup et al., 2004), methylprednisolone 500 mg i.v. has been demonstrated to also be protective against these complications if administered preoperatively.

CARDIOPULMONARY BYPASS EQUIPMENT

Membrane oxygenators are preferred for survival procedures. Generally, the bypass equipment should be a pediatric unit with adequate monitoring devices. Cardiopulmonary monitoring, including ECG, core temperature, arterial blood gases, blood pressure, and serum electrolytes, is essential. Monitoring of activated clotting time (ACT) is essential because of the necessity of systemic heparinization of the animal during the procedure. Monitoring of the hematocrit is also essential.

SURGERY

The surgical approach usually is via a median sternotomy (Chapter 9), and the heart is placed in a pericardial cradle. Femoral cutdown is performed for peripheral venous and arterial access during the procedure (Chapter 9). The animal is heparinized with 300 IU/kg. The pre- and postcava are cannulated after an atriotomy is performed in the right atrial appendage. The inserted cannulae are snared around the vessels with umbilical tape or elastic bands. This approach reduces the risk of tearing the friable right atria. Blood is returned to the arterial circulation by implanting a cannula in the aorta distal to the aortic valve and cross-clamping of the aorta between the valve and the cannula. Depending upon the procedure, insertion of a cannula to act as a pulmonary arterial vent may be required to provide drainage from the right ventricle and lungs and to manage postperfusion pulmonary hypertension (Horneffer et al., 1986). All the cannulae are held in place with purse-string sutures at their site of entrance into the cardiovascular system. After the cannulae are in place, the aorta may be cross-clamped, and cardioplegia solution containing potassium is injected into the aortic root. The surgical descriptions for thoracotomy and postoperative considerations discussed in Chapter 9 should be reviewed as they are applicable to CPB procedures.

MONITORING AND PERFUSIONIST PARAMETERS

The priming solution should be fresh donor blood to maintain the hematocrit above 25. Blood groups with weak blood group antigens occur in swine (16 types, A–P); however, cross matching is not usually necessary for a single procedure. Domestic swine may be used as donors for miniature pigs. It is preferred that the last unit of blood collected during terminal collection be discarded because of the potentially high level of catecholamines (Cameron et al., 1992). Crystalloid primes have been associated with visceral edema, and colloid solutions should be used if a supplement is required for the whole blood.

Heparinization of the animal should be initiated with 300 IU/kg and the ACT maintained at 180–300 sec with supplemental dosages in the 100–200 IU/kg range. An ACT of greater than 300 sec may be required with complex cardiac procedures and the lower range for procedures such as ECMO. These dosages of heparin are usually required approximately every 45 min if the higher ACT range is utilized. Unless absolutely essential, protamine should not be used to reverse heparinization at the end of the procedure because of the possibility of adverse reactions, which are common in swine. If it is required, it is given in a ratio of 1.3:1 (protamine:heparin). Control of hemorrhage should be a factor of careful attention to hemostasis by the surgeon rather than drugs.

Arterial pump flow rates are dependent upon the size of the animal and the core temperature. The smaller the animal, the higher the flow rate; and the cooler the temperature, the lower the flow rate. Flow rates for swine range from 60 to 100 ml kg^{-1}min^{-1} with an average of approximately 75 ml kg^{-1}min^{-1}. The mean arterial pressure is maintained at 50–60 mmHg with a central venous pressure of 0–5 mmHg during bypass. The systemic vascular resistance is maintained between 800 and 1400 dyn/sec/cm^{-5}. The core temperature is maintained between 15 and 37°C dependent upon the requirements of the protocol. Oxygen delivery is generally 2.2 l m^{2}min^{-1} or greater.

Neonatal piglets have been used in experimental protocols in which regional low-flow perfusion gave an improved neuorologic outcome with deep hypothermic circulatory arrest (18°C, 10 ml kg^{-1}min^{-1}) (Myung et al., 2004). CPB studies involving the injection of air vs. carbon dioxide at 1 ml/kg have demonstrated improved cerebral protection with carbon dioxide (Marten et al., 2004). Swine and other animals are intrinsically more resistant to air emboli than humans. Pigs subjected to hypothermic circulatory arrest at 20°C for >75 min develop an increase in intracranial pressure >17 mmHg which leads to brain infarction and other complications of increased intracranial pressure (Pokela et al., 2002).

Other parameters to be monitored by the perfusionist include blood gases and electrolytes. The approximate arterial blood gas parameters to be maintained include PaO$_2$ 100 mmHg, PaCO$_2$ 40 mmHg, pH 7.38–7.42, base excess 0 or less. Potassium should be maintained at 4.5–5.5 mmol/l. Venous O$_2$ saturation is usually 65–75.

Anesthesia

Most anesthetic regimens that have been utilized in swine have been tried during CPB. Isoflurane should be the primary agent of choice unless contraindicated by the protocol or the medical status of the patient. If the animal is in cardiovascular compromise or if malignant hyperthermia is a potential risk, the high-dose opioid infusion protocols described earlier should be the primary choice. The anesthetist will need to coordinate the procedures closely with the perfusionist. Adjunct agents that may be required include the usual list of emergency drugs listed in the appendix and antiarrhythmic agents such as bretylium. The procedures for administration of these anesthetics as described in the preceding text should be used.

Weaning from CPB

Most of the problems encountered in CPB in swine will occur within the first 2 h following termination of the procedure. Weaning from the procedure should be performed slowly and with careful monitoring of the parameters described in the preceding text. Measurement of central venous pressure (CVP) and pulmonary artery (PA) pressure should be performed with a Swan-Ganz catheter inserted from the femoral vein. Blood gas monitoring and ventilation adjustments to treat acidosis should be performed.

The right side of the heart is refilled by gradually occluding the venous return from the cannulae after releasing the snares from the caval vessels. The arterial cross-clamp is removed, and arterial perfusion is gradually stopped. Monitoring of CVP to return to values of 8–15 mmHg is performed. Mean arterial pressure is gradually returned to 90–110 mmHg. Donor whole blood is preferred to reinstitute adequate volume, but colloidal solutions may be administered if necessary. Rewarming should be gradual if hypothermia was used in the procedure.

Intravenous nitroglycerine and inhaled nitric oxide have been demonstrated to be useful in reducing central venous and left atrial pressures, thus attenuating pulmonary hypertension. Nitric oxide has the beneficial effect of also improving arterial oxygenation and pulmonary vasodilation without effects on systemic pressure; however, nitroglycerine reduces arterial blood pressure (Troncy et al., 1996, 1997).

Insulin-like growth factor 1 (1.2 mg/h i.v.) has been shown to significantly reduce oxygen consumption, increase cardiac output, and increase oxygen delivery with decreased oxygen extraction in neonatal piglets post hypothermic CPB. The improved oxygen transport may be beneficial to the survival of neonates following this procedure (Li et al., 2004).

Careful monitoring to return the animal to homeostasis using the parameters described in this section is essential, and demonstration of normative cardiac output should be determined prior to closing the surgical incisions. If the pig is not responding to the weaning procedures, CPB should be reinstituted and the procedure retried after 10–15 min. Pulmonary hypertension and acute right-sided heart failure or irreversible ventricular fibrillation are the two most common causes of failure during weaning procedures. Returning to CPB or PA venting should be instituted as an immediate step while controlling this condition. Pulmonary vasoconstriction or clumping of blood products may be involved and should be treated if necessary (Cameron et al., 1992).

Treatment of cardiac arrhythmias may be required, and the therapeutic protocols used are the same as for other species, with the exception of the species-specific considerations discussed in the section on arrhythmias. In our experience, prophylactic treatment with bretylium 5 mg/kg i.v. every 30 min or amiodarone 10–12 mg/kg i.v. followed by 0.5 mg kg^{-1}h^{-1} i.v. infusion during the cardiac manipulations prevents arrhythmias in most cases (Horneffer et al., 1986; Schumann et al., 1993; Swindle et al., 1986).

POSTOPERATIVE CONSIDERATIONS

The postoperative considerations discussed in other sections of this text and for thoracotomies in Chapter 9 are applicable to these procedures. Postoperative recovery and return to homeostasis should be gradual and require at least hourly, if not continuous, monitoring for the first 6–24 h. Close attention to thermoregulation and analgesia is as important as monitoring of the cardiovascular parameters. The use of intensive care cages with ECG, pulse oximetry, and blood pressure monitoring should be utilized. A team approach to recovery should include a veterinarian with experience in postoperative care for cardiothoracic procedures. Over time, the team members will be able to develop protocols for performing the procedures in their laboratories, and most of these procedures will become routine. Most swine that develop a righting reflex and can be extubated will recover and be able to eat the following day.

REGIONAL LOW-FLOW PERFUSION AND NEURAL PROTECTION

Regional low-flow perfusion is an alternative to deep hypothermia and circulatory arrest used in infants (Myung et al., 2004). In this technique in neonatal swine, an aortic or carotid cannula is advanced cranially and low-flow perfusion of 10 ml kg^{-1}min^{-1} is maintained in an effort to provide neurologic protection during CPB. Modifications of this technique may also be useful for prevention of spinal cord ischemia during aortic cross-clamping.

Increases in intracranial pressure and brain infarction can also be complications of CPB (Pokela et al., 2002). Air emboli may also be accidentally introduced in the pump circuit resulting in death or dysfunction (Martens et al., 2004). Use of CO_2 has been shown to be protective at 1–2 ml/kg as compared to air emboli at 1 ml/kg following catheterization of the carotid artery, which may indicate its use in cardiac surgery. Experiments from cardiopulmonary resuscitation experiments have shown that a combination of vasopressin 0.4–0.8 IU/kg combined with epinephrine 45 μg/kg as an i.v. infusion is protective following cardiac arrest (Stadlbauer et al., 2003).

ANALGESICS

The use of analgesics should be routine in porcine surgical protocols (Table 2.6–Table 2.8). Preoperative or intraoperative use of analgesics prevents the pain reflex from being stimulated and reduces the postoperative recovery time. Combinations of local anesthetics infiltrated along the incision line with parenteral opioid or nonsteroidal anti-inflammatory drug (NSAID) analgesics and general anesthesia provide the most comprehensive preemptive prophylaxis. Postoperatively, the opioids may be combined with NSAIDs in cases in which the musculoskeletal component of the surgery is extensive. If preemptive analgesic regimens are used, it may not be necessary to readminister

TABLE 2.6
Postoperative Analgesia

Drug	Dosages	Route/Frequency
Aspirin	10–20 mg/kg	p.o./qid
Butorphanol	0.1–0.3 mg/kg	i.m., s.c./bid or tid
Buprenorphine[a]	0.01–0.05 mg/kg	i.m., s.c./bid or tid
	0.5–10 $\mu g\ kg^{-1}h^{-1}$	i.v. infusion
Carprofen[a]	2 mg/kg	s.c./sid
	2–3 mg/kg	p.o./bid
Fentanyl	30–50 $\mu g\ kg^{-1}h^{-1}$	i.v. infusion
Fentanyl transdermal patches	5 $\mu g\ kg^{-1}h^{-1}$ (highly variable)	Topical
Flunixine[a]	1–4 mg/kg	s.c., i.m./sid or bid
Ketoprofen[a]	1–3 mg/kg	i.m., s.c., p.o./bid
Ketorolac[a]	1 mg/kg	p.o., i.m., s.c./bid
Medetomidine	2 $\mu g\ kg^{-1}h^{-1}$	i.v. infusion
Meloxicam[a]	0.4 mg/kg	s.c./sid
Meperidine	10 mg/kg	s.c./tid
Morphine epidural	0.1 mg/kg	Epidural
Oxymorphone	0.15 mg/kg	i.m., s.c./bid or tid
Phenylbutazone	5–20 mg/kg	p.o./bid
Piritramide	75 $\mu g\ kg^{-1}h^{-1}$	i.v. infusion
Sufentanil	10–15 $\mu g\ kg^{-1}h^{-1}$	i.v. infusion
Tramadol	1–4 mg/kg	p.o./tid

[a] Most highly recommended agents.

postoperative analgesia in cases of minor surgery and only for a few days with major surgical procedures (Jenkins, 1987; Smith and Swindle, 1994; Smith et al., 1997). Most of the physiological variables and complications associated with the administration of opioids and NSAIDS are associated with long-term use and not a short-term period of administration postsurgically.

OPIOIDS

Most of the opioid analgesics have relatively short half-lives in swine (Table 2.6 and Table 2.7), which limits their usefulness in postoperative protocols (Blum, 1988; Flecknell, 1997; Swindle, 1991). Agents that have half-lives of less than 4 h include fentanyl (0.05 mg/kg i.v., s.c., or i.m.), sufentanil (0.005–0.010 mg/kg i.m., s.c., or i.v.), meperidine (2–10 mg/kg s.c. or i.m.), oxymorphone (0.15 mg/kg s.c. or i.m.), morphine (2.2 mg/kg s.c. or i.m.), piritramide ($\mu g\ kg^{-1}h^{-1}$ i.v. infusion), and pentazocine (1.5–3.0 mg/kg s.c. or i.m.). Morphine has been reported to cause excitement and other adverse behavioral patterns in swine and has a short half-life (Risdahl et al., 1992). However, morphine epidural solution 0.1 mg/kg administered preoperatively is effective for preemptive analgesia for abdominal procedures.

If these agents are used in opioid infusion protocols as described in the preceding text, then they may be continued as the postoperative analgesic as a gradually decreasing infusion. During the withdrawal phase from opioid infusions, some excitement or muscle rigidity may be encountered, which can be reversed by administration of acepromazine (0.5 mg/kg s.c. or i.m.) or diazepam (2–5 mg/kg s.c. or i.m.).

Fentanyl patches have been tried for postoperative analgesia in swine; however, titration of the dosage may be difficult, and the patches must be secured to the skin with bandages to prevent their ingestion. Experience has demonstrated that transdermal fentanyl patches may be highly variable in their efficacy in swine. Variables include breed, age, site of application, presence of moisture or

TABLE 2.7
Potential Physiological Effects of Opioid Analgesics

Anatomic Region of System	Effects (+ or −)
Pulmonary	
Respiratory function	−
Cough reflex	−
Cardiovascular	
Vasodilation	+
Peripheral vascular resistance	−
Baroreceptor reflexes	−
CO_2 reflex vasoconstriction	−
Heart rate	−
Cardiac output	−
Gastrointestinal	
Gastric motility	−
Gastric emptying time	+
Intestinal secretions	−
Anal sphincter tone	+
Intestinal contraction amplitude	+
Gastric acid production	−
Increase GI tone	+
CNS	
Depression	+
Cognitive dysfunction	+
Locomotor activity	+
Increase vagal tone	+
Miosis	+
Cerebral blood flow	−
Hepatic	
Biliary secretions	−
Bile duct pressure	+
Spasm of bile duct and sphincter	+
Pancreas	
Pancreatic secretions	−
Spasm of pancreatic duct and sphincter	+
Urogenital	
Urinary voiding reflex	−
External bladder sphincter tone	+
Spasm of ureteral smooth muscle	+
Uterine tone	−
Immunologic/endocrine	
Natural killer (NK) cell activity	−
Immunoglobulin production	−
Phagocytic activity	−
Antidiuretic hormone (ADH) release	−
Protactin release	−
Somatotropin release	−
Luteinizing hormone	−
Histamine release	+

heat on the patch, and type of procedure. It is possible to overdose swine with these patches, especially if they ingest them. There is also an increased potential for drug abuse, compared to administering parenteral injections, by humans because they are topical patches.

In Yucatan miniature pigs 17–22 kg, 100 µg/h patches provided therapeutic levels which peaked at 42–48 h after application. Lower dosages (25–50 µg/h patches) may be required for farm breeds, which tend to be younger at the same body weight and have thinner skin than minipigs (Wilkinson, et al., 2001; Harvey-Clark et al., 2000). As a starting point, if the dosage is not known, a patch delivering approximately 5 µg $kg^{-1}h^{-1}$ should be applied to the side of the chest. Clinical monitoring for signs of overdosage is essential.

Fentanyl has also been associated with long-lasting hyperalgesia (pain facilitation) in other species. Mu-receptor stimulation by fentanyl produces N-methyl-D-aspartate (NMDA) receptor activation, which can be associated with increased sensitivity to pain (windup phenomenon). The higher the dosage of fentanyl, the more pain is facilitated. This effect can be blocked by administration of ketamine or dextromethorphan, which act as NMDA receptor antagonists. Thus, caution should be taken if fentanyl is being used as the preemptive analgesic (Celerier et al., 2000).

Butorphanol (0.1–0.3 mg/kg s.c. or i.m. qid) and high-dose buprenorphine (0.05–0.1 mg/kg s.c. or i.m. bid) are long acting and have few side effects in swine. Buprenorphine has been extensively used without significant respiratory depression noted in postoperative protocols, including thoracotomy. It should be considered as one of the primary opioid analgesics used in porcine protocols (Hawk et al., 2005; Hermansen et al., 1986; Swindle, 1991).

Some confusion exists concerning the wide dosage ranges of buprenorphine that have been reported in swine (0.001–0.1 mg/kg i.m., s.c., or i.v.). In our experience, lower dosages (<0.01 mg/kg) do not provide prolonged analgesia for major surgical interventions. The lower dose range may be useful for preemptive analgesia or in combination with other agents. A recent publication indicates that 0.01–0.02 mg/kg or higher dosages q 8–10 h provides postoperative analgesia for a significant number of pigs (Rodriguez et al., 2001). Buprenorphine may also be given as a continuous i.v. infusion at a rate of 0.5–10.0 µg $kg^{-1}h^{-1}$.

Nonsteroidal Anti-Inflammatory Drugs

Traditional NSAIDs can be used in combination with opioids for balanced analgesia protocols involving muscular or orthopedic surgery (Table 2.8). Some of the newer agents, however, are adequate for postoperative analgesia as sole agents. NSAIDs are associated with fewer platelets, renal function changes, and gastric ulceration. These effects are more pronounced with the older agents such as aspirin. Most of the side effects are related to chronic administration of these agents and not the short-term usage for postoperative analgesia. For example, it is unlikely that short-term administration of NSAIDs for a few days for postoperative analgesia will have significant effects on bone healing or cartilage metabolism in swine.

Phenylbutazone 5–20 mg/kg p.o. bid. and enteric-coated aspirin (10–20 mg/kg qid.) may be used as adjuncts. Aspirin is also used for anticoagulation in some protocols as a daily dosage. Aspirin should be enteric coated to prevent gastric ulceration with chronic usage.

Ketoprofen (1–3 mg/kg i.v., s.c., i.m., or p.o. bid or tid) and ketorolac (1 mg/kg i.m., s.c., or i.v. bid), flunixine (1–4 mg/kg s.c. or i.m., sid or bid), meloxicam (0.4 mg/kg s.c. sid), and carprofen (2–4 mg/kg p.o. bid or s.c. sid) are newer agents that may have some opioid-receptor activity. They provide adequate analgesia to be used as sole agents. Carprofen and meloxicam in particular have efficacy as preemptive analgesics. In our experience, they are equivalent to buprenorphine if used in this manner. They have the advantages of parenteral administration q 24 h and their not being controlled substances. Carprofen may be increased to bid administration if increased analgesia is required in the immediate postoperative period. Currently, carprofen is the primary analgesic used in our laboratories, and swine readily ingest the chewable tablets.

TABLE 2.8
Potential Physiological Effects of
NSAID Analgesics

Anatomic Region of System	Effects (+ or –)
GI ulceration	+
GI hemorrhage	+
Platelet aggregation	–
Renal papillary necrosis	+
Intestinal nephritis	+
Prostaglandin function	–
Kinin function	–
Cyclo-oxygenase (COX) enzymes	–
Liver necrosis	+
Uterine contractions	–
Fetal circulation	–
Fetal abnormalities	+
Cognitive dysfunction	+
Cartilage metabolism	–
Bone fracture healing	–
Bone blood flow	–
Bone and cartilage remodeling	–
Bone ingrowth into implants	–
Soft tissue healing to bone	–
Spinal fusion healing	–

REVERSAL AGENTS FOR INJECTABLE ANESTHETICS, SEDATIVES, AND ANALGESICS

There may be an indication for reversal of various agents. However, caution should be taken to avoid using reversal agents for major invasive procedures in which it might be beneficial to keep the pig sedated. Generally, reversal agents are utilized for emergencies and reversal of chemical restraint protocols (Branson and Gross, 2001; Gross, 2001; Smith et al., 1997).

Naloxone (0.005–0.02 mg/kg i.v., i.m., or s.c.) is an opioid reversal antagonist at mu and kappa receptors. Nalbuphine (1–2 mg/kg i.v.) antagonizes the effects of opioids as a mu agonist while maintaining an analgesic effect at kappa receptors.

Diprenorphine (0.3 mg/kg s.c.) is a nonspecific opioid antagonist with activity at kappa, delta, and mu receptors. It is the agent used to reverse etorphine when it is used in dart guns in the field.

Atipamezole (0.24 mg/kg i.v.–1.0 mg/kg i.m. or s.c.) is an α_2-receptor antagonist and is generally the preferred agent for this class of drugs. Others include yohimbine (1 mg/kg i.v.), tolazoline (1.5 mg/kg i.v.), and idazoxan (0.03 mg/kg i.v.).

Flumazenil is a competitive benzodiazepine antagonist when administered at 1 part to 13 parts of the benzodiazepine.

LOCAL AND REGIONAL ANALGESIA

It is possible to use the local anesthetics to provide local, regional, and spinal analgesia. These procedures are not recommended in the research setting as the sole analgesic unless it is part of the protocol. Rather, they should be used as adjuncts to systemic analgesia. Long-acting agents, such as bupivicaine, can be used as dorsal nerve root blocks (Figure 2.28) in the paravertebral region to provide analgesia for such vertical incisions as lateral thoracotomies. They can also be

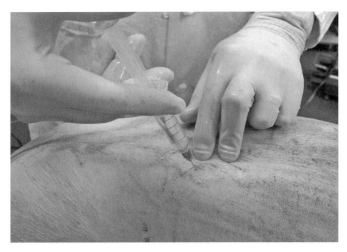

FIGURE 2.28 Dorsal nerve root block with a local anesthetic.

used to preemptively anesthetize the incision site locally or the peritoneum during general surgery in combination with parenteral agents.

The difficulties associated with performing epidural blocks in swine (Chapter 10) can be overcome with practice, and this procedure is effective as a preemptive analgesic for abdominal procedures. However, epidural morphine (0.1 mg/kg) is just as effective as local anesthetics for these procedures and does not produce the side effects that can be encountered with systemic administration of the opioid. Other epidural analgesics have been reported for use in the agricultural setting and may be useful for some research protocols. They include 2% lidocaine (1 ml/9 kg), xylazine (2 ml/kg diluted in saline), xylazine (1 mg/kg 10% solution) + lidocaine (10 ml 2% solution), and medetomidine (0.5 mg/kg diluted in saline) (Scarda, 1996; Ko et al., 1992, 1993; St-Jean et al., 1999). Precaution to prevent ascending flow of some of the agents to the brain should be taken to prevent seizures. This is usually not a problem with small volumes, and it has not been experienced with the standard human epidural preparation of morphine. The technique is illustrated in Chapter 10.

Topical anesthetic patches have been developed that anesthetize skin as well as mucous membranes. These patches help relieve the distress caused by repeated vascular access needle punctures (Smith et al., 1997; Thurmon and Benson, 1996). The transdermal applications contain lidocaine with or without prilocaine. The transdermal analgesics require 30–60 min to provide effective analgesia after application, and the analgesic effects may last up to 12 h, depending upon the product. Use of transdermal analgesic patches or creams or regional nerve blocks with local anesthetics may be desirable if the protocol requires repeated needle access to the port over a short period of time (Swindle et al., 2005).

COMMONLY RECOMMENDED PROTOCOLS

Some of the commonly recommended protocols that have been routinely used in particular research settings are tabulated in this section. Please refer to more complete information within the description of the surgical procedure and the discussion of the classes of anesthetic agents within this chapter.

NONSURVIVAL TEACHING PROTOCOLS

Induction: Ketamine 33 mg/kg i.m., acepromazine 1.1 mg/kg s.c., atropine 0.05 mg/kg s.c.
Maintenance: Thiopental 3–30 mg kg^{-1}h^{-1} i.v. infusion or pentobarbital 5–40 mg kg^{-1}h^{-1} i.v. infusion.

Comment: This protocol can be used for survival surgery if gas anesthesia is not available. Buprenorphine, meloxicam, or carprofen can be administered intraoperatively; however, analgesics will decrease the amount of barbiturate required by approximately 50%.

GENERAL SURGERY (WITHOUT PHYSIOLOGICAL MEASUREMENTS)

Induction: Ketamine 33 mg/kg s.c., acepromazine 1.1 mg/kg s.c., atropine 0.05 mg/kg s.c.
Maintenance: Isoflurane 1.5–2% in oxygen or 0.5–1.5% in nitrous oxide:oxygen, 2:1.
Comment: This protocol does not allow endotracheal intubation without administration of isoflurane via face mask during induction. Buprenorphine, meloxicam, or carprofen may be administered intraoperatively and may reduce the percentage of isoflurane required.

GENERAL SURGERY (WITH PHYSIOLOGICAL MEASUREMENTS)

Induction: Isoflurane 3–5% in oxygen via face mask.
Maintenance: Isoflurane 0.5–1.5% in nitrous oxide:oxygen, 2:1.
Comment: This is the simplest protocol that minimizes hemodynamic effects but provides sufficient analgesia and relaxation for major surgery. Following surgical manipulation and closure, it is possible to minimize the administration of the inhalant. Buprenorphine, meloxicam, or carprofen can be administered intraoperatively after the measurements are made.

CARDIOTHORACIC SURGERY (WITH CARDIOVASCULAR MANIPULATIONS)

Induction: Ketamine 33 mg/kg s.c., isoflurane 3–5% in oxygen via face mask.
Maintenance: Isoflurane 0.5–1.5% in nitrous oxide:oxygen, 2:1.
Adjunct agents: Bretylium 5 mg/kg i.v. by slow injection every 30 min before and during cardiac manipulation or amiodarone i.v. infusion 0.5 mg kg^{-1}h^{-1}.
Comment: An emergency kit for cardiopulmonary emergencies and a defibrillator should be available.

CARDIOTHORACIC SURGERY (WITH CARDIOVASCULAR COMPROMISE)

Induction: Start i.v. infusion with sufentanil 0.015 mg kg^{-1}h^{-1} (15 μg). Bolus 0.007 mg/kg (7 μg) i.v. 5 min after infusion is started. If relaxation is required to induce the i.v., then administer ketamine 11 mg/kg s.c. first.
Maintenance: Sufentanil 0.015–0.030 mg kg^{-1}h^{-1} (15–30 μg) i.v. infusion. Supplement with 0.5% isoflurane in oxygen if required for major surgical manipulations.
Adjunct agents: Atropine 0.02 mg/kg i.v. may be required for bradycardia, which can be profound during the induction. Bretylium 5 mg/kg i.v. every 30 min or amiodarone 0.5 mg kg^{-1}h^{-1} i.v. infusion during cardiac manipulation.
Comments: This protocol is useful for cardiopulmonary bypass procedures, especially if there is a predisposition for malignant hyperthermia. It is also useful as anesthesia for endoscopic thoracic surgery or coronary artery surgery in which bradycardia is required. The protocol minimizes the anesthetic effects on coronary blood flow and myocardial contractility. It has a protective antiarrhythmic effect during cardiovascular catheterization and electrophysiology studies. Acepromazine or diazepam may be required during the withdrawal phase of the protocol to counteract muscle tremors and rigidity. Other analgesics should not be administered until the i.v. infusion is decreased to less than 0.007 mg kg^{-1}h^{-1} (7 μg). A cardiopulmonary emergency drug kit should be available along with a defibrillator.

Coronary Artery Catheterization

Induction: Ketamine 33 mg/kg s.c. followed by mask induction with isoflurane 3–5%.

Maintenance: Isoflurane 0.5–1.5% in nitrous oxide:oxygen, 2:1.

Adjunct agents: During the last meal prior to induction of anesthesia animals are administered diltiazem 4 mg/kg and aspirin 10 mg/kg p.o. Bretylium 5 mg/kg i.v. or amiodarone 0.05 mg kg^{-1}h^{-1} and heparin 200 IU/kg are administered i.v. prior to introducing the catheter into the coronary artery. A slow 200-μg infusion of nitroglycerin is administered at the aortic root prior to introducing the catheter.

Comment: If stents are implanted, anticoagulant therapy may have to be administered postoperatively. This includes such agents as enteric coated aspirin, clopidogrel, or reviparin. Buprenorphine, meloxicam, or carprofen may be administered preemptively.

GENERAL PHYSIOLOGICAL EFFECTS OF ANESTHETICS

The general physiological effects of common anesthetic agents are summarized in the following text for reference when designing protocols for particular research projects (Table 2.9). Combining agents between classes may cause different effects. All effects are dose dependent and may vary among breeds (Benharkate et al., 1993). The information is summarized from Heavner (1994) and Smith et al. (1997). A complete discussion, by multiple authors, of the physiological effects of anesthetics and analgesics in all laboratory animals is available in Kohn et al. (1997).

Dissociative Agents

The physiological effects of these agents are bronchodilation, tachycardia, increased cardiac output, increased blood pressure, and increased circulating catecholamines.

1. Ketamine: Prolongs myocardial refractory period; peripheral and coronary vasodilation, increased pulmonary artery vascular resistance, increased cerebral blood flow, poor analgesia, and little muscle relaxation; it is an NMDA antagonist, and induces hepatic enzymes.
2. Tiletamine/zolazepam (Telazol): Mild myocardial depression, respiratory depression, and persistent hypothermia; contraindicated in renal disease and cardiovascular compromise; poor analgesia.

Barbiturates

1. Thiobarbiturates: Depressed cardiopulmonary function, decreased cerebral blood flow and intracranial pressure, decreased myocardial contractility, respiratory depression, minimal effects on peripheral vascular resistance, and short acting; redistribution from brain to visceral tissues occurs rapidly.
2. Pentobarbital: Respiratory depression, decreased myocardial contractility and cardiac output, increased peripheral vascular resistance, decreased cerebral blood flow, decreased hematocrit, and decreased rate of dissociation of gamma-aminobutyric acid (GABA) from its receptor; metabolized by liver.

Sedatives/Hypnotics

1. Phenothiazines (acepromazine): Hypotension, alpha adrenergic blockage, vasodilation, decreased systemic vascular resistance, and reduced sensitivity to circulating catecholamines; cardiac output and heart rate not significantly affected.

TABLE 2.9
Potential Physiological Effects of Intraoperative Drugs in Swine

	Cardiac Arrhythmias	Heart Rate	Cardiac Output	Myocardial Contractility	Blood Pressure	Right Atrial Pressure	Myocardial Oxygen Consumption	Cerebral Blood Flow
Atropine	Sinus tachycardia	↑	↑	↑	NC or ↑	→	↑	NC or ↑
Phenothiazine tranquilizers	Sinus tachycardia	↑	↑	→	→	→	NC or ↑	→
Dissociative agents	Sinus tachycardia	↑	↑	↑	↑	→	↑	→
Butyrophenones	Extrapyramidal activity	↑	NC or ↑	→	→	→	NC or ↑	→
α-2-Agonists	Sinus bradycardia, 2°–3° AV block, sinus arrest	→	→	NC or →	↑ then →	↑	↑	→
Benzodiazepines	Sinus bradycardia	NC	NC	NC	NC	NC	→	→
Barbiturates	Bradyarrhythmias, PVC, sinus tachycardia, ventricular arrhythmias	↑	→	→	→	→	NC or ↑	→
Etomidate, metomidate		NC or ↓	NC or ↓	NC or ↓	NC or ↓	NC or ↓	NC or ↑	→
Inhalant anesthetics	Sinus bradycardia, PVC, ventricular tachycardia, ventricular fibrillation	→	→	→	→	→	→	↑
Propofol	Sinus bradycardia, ventricular arrhythmias	NC or ↑	→	→	→	→	NC or ↑	→
Opioids	Sinus bradycardia, 1°–2° AV Block	→	→	NC or ↓	NC or ↓	NC	NC	→
Pancuronium		↑	↑	NC	↑	NC	↑	↑
Vercuronium		NC	NC	NC	NC	NC	NC	NC

Note: NC = no change.

2. Butyrophenones (azaperone, droperidol): Extrapyramidal activity due to GABA block-ade, hypotension, decreased cardiac output and heart rate, and some antiarrhythmic activity.
3. Benzodiazepines (zolazepam, diazepam, and midazolam): Decreased catecholamine release, increased coronary blood flow, slight cardiovascular effects unless combined with opioids (synergistic effect with severe cardiodepression), little effect on hepatic or renal function.
4. α_2-Adrenergic agonists (xylazine, medetomidine, and detomidine): Bradycardia, first- to third-degree heart block, decreased cardiac output, increased central venous pressure, hypotension, decreased myocardial contractility, decreased sympathetic tone, decreased coronary blood flow, increased susceptibility to catecholamines and arrhythmias, vaso-constriction, transient analgesia, reduced GI motility, increased urine production, and increased atrial natriuretic factor (ANF).
5. Propofol: Decreases cerebral blood flow and intracranial pressure; a cardiodepressant, it causes respiratory depression, but little analgesia.
6. Etomidate: Decreases cerebral blood flow and intracranial pressure, causes minimal cardiodepression, as well as adrenocortical suppression, has little effect on renal blood flow, and may induce seizures.

OPIOIDS

Decreased cerebral blood flow, respiratory depression, minimal cardiovascular effects, increased coronary blood flow, slight decrease in peripheral vascular resistance, depressed catecholamine response, bradycardia; some agents (morphine) may have stimulant effects; histamine release.

NONSTEROIDAL ANTI-INFLAMMATORY DRUGS (NSAIDS)

Effects vary widely between different classes of agents and are dependent upon dosage and length of administration. These are anti-inflammatory, and inhibit cyclooxygenase, lipoxygenase, kinins, and prostaglandins; cause gastrointestinal irritation, antiplatelet activity, renal and hepatic dysfunc-tion, and inhibition of bone healing.

INHALANT ANESTHETICS

All agents increase cerebral blood flow and cerebrospinal fluid, depress ventilation, depress oxygen consumption, produce hypercapnia, and induce bronchodilation.

1. Isoflurane: Decreased systemic vascular resistance, little effect on heart rate, unchanged coronary blood flow and cardiac output, little circulating catecholamine sensitivity, least effect on cardiac output, circulating catecholamines, best tissue perfusion.
2. Halothane: Decreased cardiac output, myocardial depression, depressed baroreceptor reflexes, peripheral vascular resistance unchanged, greatest effects on catecholamine sensitivity. It is not recommended because of human health hazard.
3. Enflurane: Associated with seizures, more cardiodepressant than halothane and isoflu-rane; decreases blood pressure, cardiac output, and systemic vascular resistance.
4. Methoxyflurane: Decreased cardiac output, blood pressure, and systemic vascular resis-tance; most metabolized effects, most renal effects, and most hepatic defluorination. Should not be used because of poor efficacy and human health hazard.
5. Nitrous oxide: Unacceptable as sole agent, slight cardiodepression.

EUTHANASIA

The 2000 Report of the American Veterinary Medical Association (AVMA) Panel on Euthanasia (AVMA Panel, 2001) is generally accepted as the standard for acceptable euthanasia criteria for swine and other species. The highest recommendation is euthanasia with an i.v. overdose of pentobarbital (>150 mg/kg). Larger animals may require sedation to facilitate i.v. access. Neonatal animals can be euthanized i.p. with pentobarbital. Commercially available euthanasia solutions used for pets can also be used. Other acceptable methods are the administration of KCl 2 mmol/kg i.v. or terminal exsanguination, both of which must be performed while the animal is under general anesthesia. Overdosage with an inhalant anesthetic as part of a terminal surgery should also be acceptable. In agricultural practice, CO_2 asphyxiation or captive bolt cerebral trauma are performed, mainly to prevent drug residues in meat products. These methods and other physical methods would generally not be used in research, and they would have to be approved on a scientific necessity basis by most institutional animal care and use committees (IACUCs).

REFERENCES

Anderson, I.L., 1976, Porcine malignant hyperthermia: effect of dantrolene sodium on *in-vitro* halothane-induced contracture of susceptible muscle, *Anesthesiology*, 44(1): 57–60.

Armbruster, K., Noldge-Schomburg, G.F., Dressler, I.M., Fittkau, A.J., Haberstroh, J., and Geiger, K., 1997, The effects of desflurane on splanchnic hemodynamics and oxygenation in the anesthetized pig, *Anesth. Analg.*, 84(2): 271–277.

AVMA Panel on Euthanasia, 2001, 2000 Report of the AVMA panel on euthanasia, *J. Am. Vet. Med. Assoc.*, 218(5): 669–696.

Ayoub, I.M., Kolarova, J.D., and Gazmuri, R.J., 2003, Hyperlactatemia in swine after stable surgical preparation, *Crit. Care Med.*, 31: A31.

Belanger, M., Wittnich, C., Torrance, S., and Juhasz, S., 2002, Model of normothermic long-term cardiopulmonary bypass in swine weighing more than eighty kilograms, *Comp. Med.*, 52(2): 117–121.

Benharkate, M., Zanini, V., Blanc, R., Boucheix, O., Coyez, F., Genevois, J.P., and Pairet, M., 1993, Hemodynamic parameters of anesthetized pigs: a comparative study of farm piglets and Göttingen and Yucatan miniature swine, *Lab. Anim. Sci.*, 43(1): 68–72.

Benson, G.J. and Thurmon, J.C., 1979, Anesthesia of swine under field conditions, *J. Am. Vet. Med. Assoc.*, 174(6): 594–596.

Blum, J.R., 1988, Laboratory animal anesthesia, in Swindle, M.M. and Adams, R.J., Eds., *Experimental Surgery and Physiology: Induced Animal Models of Human Disease*, Baltimore, MD: Williams and Wilkins, pp. 329–345.

Bollen, P.J.A., Nielsen, B.J. and Toft, P., in press, Propofol-fentanyl infusion in pigs with endotoxin induced sepsis requires smaller dosages as compared to healthy pigs at equal depth of anesthesia, *Lab Anim.*

Bollen, P., Schmidt, H., Lund, J., and Ritskes-Hoitinga, M., 2004, Auditory evoked potentials in pigs during isoflurane and sevoflurane anaesthesia, *Proc. 9th FELASA Symp.*, PS 4.7.

Boschert, K., Flecknell, P.A., Fosse, R.T., Framstad, T., Ganter, M., Sjstrand, U., Stevens, J., and Thurmon, J., 1996, Ketamine and its use in the pig, *Lab Anim.*, 30(2): 209–219.

Branson, K.R. and Gross, M.E., 2001, Opioid agonists and anatagonists, in Adams, H.R., Ed., *Veterinary Pharmacology and Therapeutics*, Ames, IA: Iowa State University Press, pp. 268–298.

Cameron, D.E., Tam, K.M., Cheng, W., and Braxton, M., 1992, Studies in the physiology of cardiopulmonary bypass using a swine model, in Swindle, M.M., Ed., *Swine as Models in Biomedical Research*, Ames, IA: Iowa State University Press, pp. 185–196.

Cantor, G.H, Brunson, D.B., and Reibold, T.W., 1981, A comparison of four short-acting anesthetic combinations for swine, *Vet. Med. Small Anim. Clin.*, 76(5): 715–720.

Celerier, E., Rivat, C., Jun, Y., Laulin, J.P., Larcher, A., Reynier, P., and Simonnet, G., 2000, Long-lasting hyperalgesia induced by fentanyl in rats: preventive effect of ketamine, *Anesthesiology*, 92(2): 465–472.

Eger, E., Johnson, B., Weiskopf, R., Holmes, M., Yasuda, N., Targ, A., and Rampil, I., 1988, Minimum alveolar concentration of I-653 and isoflurane in pigs: definition of a supramaximal stimulus, *Anesth. Analg.*, 67(12): 1174–1176.

Ehler, W.J., Mack, J.W., Brown, D.L., and David, R.F., 1985, Avoidance of malignant hyperthermia in a porcine model for experimental open heart surgery, *Lab. Anim. Sci.*, 35(2): 172–175.

Eisele, P.H., Talken, L., and Eisele, J.H., 1985, Potency of isoflurane and nitrous oxide in conventional swine, *Lab. Anim. Sci.*, 35(1): 76–78.

Eisele, P.H., Woodle, E.S., Hunter, G.C., Talken, L., and Ward, R.E., 1986, Anesthetic, preoperative and postoperative considerations for liver transplantation in swine, *Lab. Anim. Sci.*, 36(4): 402–405.

Flecknell, P.A., 1996, *Laboratory Animal Anaesthesia*, 2nd ed. New York: Academic Press.

Flecknell, P.J., 1997, Medetomidine and antipamezole: potential uses in laboratory animals, *Lab Anim.*, 26(2): 21–25.

Foster, P.S., Hopkinson, K.C., and Denborough, M.A., 1992, Propofol anaesthesia in malignant hyperpyrexia susceptible swine, *Clin. Exp. Pharmacol. Physiol.*, 19(3): 183–186.

Geers, R., Decanniere, C., Ville, H., Van Hecke, P., Goedseels, V., Bosschaerts, L., Deley, J., Janssens, S., and Nierynck, W., 1992, Identification of halothane gene carriers by use of an *in vivo* 3IP nuclear magnetic resonance spectroscopy in pigs, *Am. J. Vet. Res.*, 53(9): 1711–1714.

Goldmann, C., Ghofrani, A., Hafemann, B., Fuchs, P., Khorram-Seffat, R., Afify, M., Kupper, W., and Pallus, N., 1999, Combination anesthesia with ketamine and pentobarbital: a long-term porcine model, *Res. Exp. Med.*, 199(1): 35–50.

Goodrich, J.A., personal communication. Department of Comparative Medicine, Medical University of South Carolina, Charleston, SC.

Goodrich, J.A., Lackland, D.T., Del Signore, M.J., and Swindle, M.M., 2001, Non-invasive measurement of blood pressures in the Yucatan micropig, with and without midazolam-induced sedation, *Comp. Med.*, 51(1): 13–15.

Greene, S.A., Benson, G.J., Tranquilli, W.J., and Grimm, K.A., 2004, Effect of isoflurane, atacurium, fentanyl, and noxious stimulation on bispectral index in pigs, *Comp. Med.*, 54(4): 397–403.

Gross, M.E., 2001, Tranquilizers, α2 adrenergic agonists, and related agents, in Adams, H.R., Ed., *Veterinary Pharmacology and Therapeutics*, Ames, IA: Iowa State University Press, pp. 299–342.

Hanneman, S.K., Clubb, F.J., Jr., McKay, K., and Costas, G., 2004, Feasibility of a porcine adult intensive care model, *Comp. Med.*, 54(1): 36–43.

Harvey-Clark, C.J., Gillespie, K., and Riggs, K.W., 2000, Transdermal fentanyl compared with parenteral buprenorphine in post-surgical pain in swine: a case study, *Lab Anim.*, 34(4): 386–398.

Hawk, C.T., Leary, S.L., and Morris, T.H., 2005, *Formulary for Laboratory Animals*, 3rd ed., Ames, IA: Blackwell Publishing.

Heavner, J.E., 1994, Physiologic effects of anesthetic and analgesics, in Smith, A.C. and Swindle, M.M., Eds., *Research Animal Anesthesia, Analgesia, and Surgery*, Greenbelt, MD: Scientists Center for Animal Welfare, pp. 41–58.

Heim, K.E., Morrell, J.S., Ronan, A.M., and Tagliaferro, A.R., 2002, Effects of ketamine-xylazine and isoflurane on insulin sensitivity in dehydroepiandrosterone sulfate-treated minipigs, *Comp. Med.*, 52(3): 233–237.

Hermansen, K., Pedersen, L.E., and Olesen, H.O., 1986, The analgesic effect of buprenorphine, etorphine and pethidine in the pig: a randomized double blind crossover study, *Acta Pharmacol. Toxicol.*, 59(1): 27–35.

Holzchuh, M.P. and Cremonesi, E., 1991, Anaesthesia in pigs, Analysis of azaperone and etomidate effects separately and in associations, *Proc. 4th Int. Congr. Vet. Anaesth.*, Utrecht: The Netherlands, pp. 197–200.

Horneffer, P.J., Gott, V.J., and Gardner, T.J., 1986, Swine as a cardiac surgical model, in Tumbleson, M.E., Ed., *Swine in Biomedical Research*, Vol. 1., New York: Plenum Press, pp. 321–326.

Houde, A., Pomnier, S.A., and Roy, R., 1993, Detection of the Ryanodine receptor mutation associated with malignant hyperthermia in purebred swine populations, *J. Anim. Sci.*, 71(6): 1414–1418.

Jenkins, W.L., 1987, Pharmacologic aspects of analgesic drugs in animals: an overview, *J. Am. Vet. Med. Assoc.*, 191(10): 1231–1240.

Kaiser, G.M., Fruhauf, N.R., Zhang, H., Westermann, S., Bolle, I., Oldhafer, K.J., and Broelsch, C.E., 2003, Intravenous infusion anesthesia with propofol-midazolam-fentanyl for experimental surgery in swine, *J. Invest. Surg.*, 16(6): 353–357.

Kaiser, G.M., Heuer, M.M., Fruhauf, N.R., Kuhne, C.A., and Broelsch, C.E., 2006, General handling and anaesthesia for experimental surgery in pigs, *J. Surg. Res.*, 130(1): 73–79.

Ko, J.C.H., Thurmon, J.C., Benson, G.J., Gard, J., and Tranquilli, W.J.,1992, Evaluation of analgesia induced by epidural injection of detomidine or xylazine in swine, *J. Vet. Anesth.*, 19: 56–60.

Ko, J.C.H., Thurmon, J.C., Benson, G.J., Tranquilli, W.J., and Olson, W.A., 1993, A new drug combination for use in porcine cesarean sections, *Vet. Med. Food Anim. Pract.*, 88: 466–472.

Ko, J.C.H., Williams, B.L., McGrath, C.J., Short, C.E., and Rogers, E.R., 1997, Comparison of anesthetic effects of Telazol-xylazine-xylazine, Telazol-xylazine-butorphanol, and Telazol-xylazine-azaperone combinations in swine, *Contemp. Top. Lab. Anim. Sci.*, 35(5): 71–74.

Ko, J.C.H., Williams, B.L., Smith, V.L., McGrath, C.J., and Jacobson, J.D., 1993, Comparison of Telazol, Telazol-ketamine, Telazol-xylazine and Telazol-ketamine-xylazine as chemical restraint and anesthetic induction combination in swine, *Lab. Anim. Sci.*, 43(5): 476–480.

Koblin, D.D., Weiskopf, R.B., Holmes, M.A., Konopka, K., Rampil, I.J., Eger, E.I., and Waskell, L., 1989, Metabolism of I-653 and isoflurane in swine, *Anesth. Analg.*, 68(2): 147–149.

Kohn, D.H., Wixson, S.K., White, W.J., and Benson, G.J., Eds., 1997, *Anesthesia and Analgesia in Laboratory Animals*, New York: Academic Press, pp. 313–336.

Landis, P., Johnson, D., Kinter, L., Landis, A., Harling, E., and Cornacoff, J., 2001, A comparison of acute cardiovascular responses in swine and dogs, *Proc. Ellegaard Symp. Cardiovasc. Tech. Swine*.

Li, J., Stenbøg, E., Bush, A., Grofte, T., Redington, A.N., and Penny, D.J., 2004, Insulin-like growth factor 1 improves the relationship between systemic oxygen consumption and delivery in piglets after cardiopulmonary bypass, *J. Thorac. Cardiovasc. Surg.*, 127(5): 1436–1441.

Lundeen, G., Manohar, M., and Parks, C., 1983, Systemic distribution of blood flow in swine while awake and during 1.0 and 1.5 MAC isoflurane anesthesia with or without 50% nitrous oxide, *Anesth. Analg.*, 62(5): 499–512.

Lunn, J.K., Stanley, T.H., Eisele, J., Webster, L., and Woodard, A., 1979, High dose fentanyl anesthesia for coronary artery surgery: plasma fentanyl concentrations and influence of nitrous oxide on cardiovascular responses, *Anesth. Analg.*, 58(5): 390–395.

Martens, S., Theisen, A., Balzer, J.O., Dietrich, M., Graubitz, K., Scherer, M., Schmitz, C., Doss, M., and Moritz, A., 2004, Improved cerebral protection through replacement of residual intracavital air by carbon dioxide: a porcine model using diffusion-weighted magnetic resonance imaging, *J. Thorac. Cardiovasc. Surg.*, 127(1): 51–56.

Martin-Cancho, M.F., Carrasco-Jimenez, M.S., Lima, J.R., Ezquerra, L.J., Crisostomo, V., and Uson-Gargallo, J., 2004, Assessment of the relationship of bispectral index values, hemodynamic changes, and recovery times associated with sevoflurane or propofol anesthesia in pigs, *Am. J. Vet. Res.*, 65(4): 409–416.

Martin-Cancho, M.F., Lima, J.R., Crisostomo, V., Ezquerra, L.J., Carrasco, M.S., Uson-Gargallo, J., 2003, Bispectral index, spectral edge frequency 95%, and median frequency for various concentrations of isoflurane and sevoflurane in pigs, *Am. J. Vet. Res.*, 64(7): 866–873.

Merin, R.G., Verdouw, P.D., and deJong, J.W., 1982, Myocardial functional and metabolic responses to ischemia in swine during halothane and fentanyl anesthesia, *Anesthesiology*, 56(2): 84–92.

Mohr, M., Vicol, C., Mensing, B., Schunck, O., Baryalei, M., Dalichau, H., and Sonntag, H., 1996, A technique for extracorporeal circulation in the Gottingen minipig allowing recovery and long-term follow-up, *J. Exp. Anim. Sci.*, 38(2): 82–92.

Myung, R.J., Petko, M., Judkins, A.R., Schears, G., Ittenbach, R.R., Waibel, R.J., and DeCampli, W.M., 2004, Regional low-flow perfusion improves neurologic outcome compared with deep hypothermic circulatory arrest in neonatal piglets, *J. Thorac. Cardiovasc. Surg.*, 127(4): 1051–1057.

Ochs, H.R., Greenblatt, D.J., Eichelkraut, W., Bakker, C., Gobel, R., and Hahn, N., 1987, Hepatic vs. gastrointestinal presystemic extraction of oral midazolam and flurazepam, *J. Pharmacol. Exp. Ther.*, 243(3): 852–856.

Pokela, M., Romsi, P., Biancari, F., Kiviluoma, K., Vainionpaa, V., Heikkinen, J., Ronka, E., Kaakinen, T., Hirvonen, J., Rimpilainen, J., Anttila, V., Leo, E., and Juvonen, T., 2002, Increase of intracranial pressure after hypothermic circulatory arrest in a chronic porcine model, *Scand. Cardiovasc. J.*, 36(5): 302–307.

Portier, D.B. and Slusser, C.A., 1985, Azaperone: a review of a new neuroleptic agent for swine, *Vet. Med.*, 80(3): 88–92.

Purohit, D.M., Swindle, M.M., Smith, C.D., Othersen, H.B., Jr., and Kazanovicz, J.M., 1993, Hanford miniature swine model for extracoporeal membrane oxygenation (ECMO), *J. Invest. Surg.*, 6(6): 503–508.

Qayumi, A.K., Jamieson, W.R.E., Poostizadeh, A., German, E., and Gillespie, K.D., 1992, Comparison of new iron chelating agents in the prevention of ischemia/reperfusion injury: a swine model of heart-lung transplantation, *J. Invest. Surg.*, 5(2): 115–128.

Raff, M. and Harrison, G., 1989, The screening of propofol in MHS swine, *Anesth. Analg.*, 68(6): 750–751.

Ramsey, D.E., Aldred, N., and Power, J.M., 1993, A simplified approach to the anesthesia of porcine laparoscopic surgical subjects, *Lab. Anim. Sci.*, 43(4): 336–337.

Ravn, K., personal communication, Novo Nordisk A/S, Gentofte, Denmark.

Riebold, T.W., Geiser, D.R., and Goble, D.O., 1995, *Large Animal Anesthesia: Principles and Techniques*, 2nd ed., Ames, IA: Iowa State University Press.

Risdahl, J.M., Chao, C., Murtaugh, M.P., Peterson, P.K., and Molitor, T.W., 1992, Acute and chronic morphine administration in swine, *Pharmacol. Biochem. Behav.*, 43(3): 799–806.

Rodriguez, N.A., Cooper, D.M., and Risdahl, J.M., 2001, Antinociecptive activity of and clinical experience with buprenorphine in swine, *Contemp. Top. Lab. Anim. Sci.*, 40(3): 17–20.

Scarda, R.T., 1996, Local and regional anesthesia in ruminants and swine, anesthesia update, *Vet. Clin. N. Am.*, 12(3): 579–626.

Schumann, R.E., Harold, M., Gillette, P.C., Swindle, M.M., and Gaymes, C.H., 1993, Prophylactic treatment of swine with bretylium for experimental cardiac catheterization, *Lab. Anim. Sci.*, 43(3): 244–246.

Schumann, R.E., Swindle, M.M., Knick, B.J., Case, C.L., and Gillette, P.C., 1994, High dose narcotic anesthesia using sufentanil in swine for cardiac catheterization and electrophysiologic studies, *J. Invest. Surg.*, 7(3): 243–248.

Silverman, J, and Muir, W.W., III, 1993, A review of lab animal anesthesia with chloral hydrate and chloralose, *Lab. Anim. Sci.*, 43(3): 210–216.

Smerup, M., Pedersen, T.F., Nyboe, C., Funder, J.A., Christensen, T.D., Nielsen, S.L., Hjortdal, V., and Hasenkam, J.M., 2004, A long-term porcine model for evaluation of prosthetic heart valves, *Heart Surg. Forum*, 7(4): E259–264.

Smith, A.C. and Swindle, M.M., Eds., 1994, *Research Animal Anesthesia, Analgesia and Surgery*, Greenbelt, MD: Scientist's Center for Animal Welfare.

Smith, A.C., Zellner, J.L., Spinale, F.G., and Swindle, M.M., 1991, Sedative and cardiovascular effects of midazolam in swine, *Lab. Anim. Sci.*, 41(2): 157–161.

Smith, A.C., Ehler, W., and Swindle, M.M., 1997, Anesthesia and analgesia in swine, in Kohn, D.H., Wixson, S.K., White, W.J., and Benson, G.J., Eds., *Anesthesia and Analgesia in Laboratory Animals*, New York: Academic Press, pp. 313–336.

St-Jean, G. and Anderson, D.E., 1999, Anesthesia and surgical procedures in swine, in Straw, B.E., D'Allaire, S., Mengeling, W.L., and Taylor, D.J., Eds., *Diseases of Swine*, 8th ed., Ames, IA: Iowa State University Press, pp. 1133–1154.

Stadlbauer, K.W., Wagner-Berger, H.G., Wenzel, V., Voelckel, W.G., Krismer, A.C., Klima, G., Rheinberger, K., Pechlaner, S., Mayr, V.D., and Lindner, K.H., 2003, Survival with full neurologic recovery after prolonged cardiopulmonary resuscitation with a combination of vasopressin and epinephrine in pigs, *Anesth. Analg.*, 96(6): 1743–1749.

Svendsen, P. and Carter, A.M., 1997, Blood gas tensions, acid-base status and cardiovascular function in miniature swine anesthetized with halothane and methoxyflurane or intravenous metomidate hydrochloride, *Pharmacol. Toxicol.*, 64(1): 88–93.

Swan, H. and Meagher, D.M., 1971, Total body bypass in miniature pigs, *J. Thorac. Cardiovasc. Surg.*, 61(6): 956–967.

Swindle, M.M., 1983, *Basic Surgical Exercises Using Swine*, Philadelphia, PA: Praeger Press.

Swindle, M.M., 1991, *Anesthetic and Perioperative Techniques in Swine*, Andover, MA: Charles River Laboratories.

Swindle, M.M., Horneffer, P.J., Gardner, T.J., Gott, V.L., Hall, T.S., Stuart, R.S., Baumgartner, W.A., Borkon, A.M., Galloway, E., and Reitz, B.A., 1986, Anatomic and anesthetic considerations in experimental cardiopulmonary surgery in swine, *Lab. Anim. Sci.*, 36(4): 357–361.

Swindle, M.M., Vogler, G.A., Fulton, L.K., Marini, R.P., and Popilskis, S., 2002, Preanesthesia, anesthesia, analgesia, and euthanasia, in Fox, J.G., Anderson, L.C., Loew, F.M., and Quimby, F.W., Eds., *Laboratory Animal Medicine*, 2nd ed., New York: Academic Press, pp. 955–1005.

Swindle, M.M., Nolan, T., Jacobson, A., Wolf, P., Dalton, M.J., and Smith, A.C., 2005, Vascular access port (VAP) usage in large animal species, *Contemp. Top. Lab. Anim. Sci.*, 44(3): 7–17.

Thurmon, J.C., and Benson, G.J., Eds., 1996, *Lumb and Jones Veterinary Anesthesia*, 3rd ed., Baltimore, MD: Williams and Wilkins.

Thurmon, J.C. and Tranquilli, W.J., 1986, Anesthesia for cardiovascular research, in Stanton, H.C. and Mersmann, H.J., Eds., *Swine in Cardiovascular Research*, Vol. 1, Boca Raton, FL: CRC Press, pp. 39–59.

Thurmon, J.C., Tranquilli, W.J., and Benson, G.J., 1986, Cardiopulmonary responses of swine to intravenous infusion of guaifenesin, ketamine, and xylazine, *Am. J. Vet. Res.*, 47(10): 2138–2140.

Tranquilli, W.J., Thurmon, J.C., Benson, G.J., and Steffey, E.P., 1983, Halothane potency in pigs (Sus scrofa), *Am. J. Vet. Res.*, 44(6): 1106–1107.

Tranquilli, W.J., Thurman, J.C., and Benson, G.J., 1985, Anesthetic potency of nitrous oxide in young swine (Sus scrofa), *Am. J. Vet. Res.*, 46(1): 58–60.

Troncy, E., Jacob, E., da Silva, P., Ducruet, T., Collet, J.P., Salazkin, I., Charbonneau, M., and Blaise, G., 1996, Comparison of the effect of inhaled nitric oxide and intravenous nitroglycerine on hypoxia-induced pulmonary hypertension in pigs, *Eur. J. Anaesth.*, 13(5): 521–529.

Troncy, E., Francoeur, M., Salazkin, I., Yang, F., Charbonneau, M., Leclerc, G., Vinay, P., and Blaise, G., 1997, Extra-pulmonary effects of inhaled nitric oxide in swine with and without phenylephrine, *Br. J. Anaesth.*, 79(5): 631–640.

Vainio, O.M., Bloor, B.C., and Kim, C., 1992, Cardiovascular effects of a ketamine-medetomidine combination that produces deep sedation in Yucatan mini swine, *Lab. Anim. Sci.*, 42(6): 582–588.

Weiskopf, R.B., Holmes, M.A., Eger, E.I., II, Yasuda, N., Rampil, I.J., Johnson, B.H., Targ, A.G., Reid, I.A., and Keil, L.C., 1992, Use of swine in the study of anesthetics, in Swindle, M.M., Ed., *Swine as Models in Biomedical Research*, Ames, IA: Iowa State University Press, pp. 96–117.

Wilkinson, A.C., Thomas, M.L., III, and Morse, B.C., 2001, Evaluation of a transdermal fentanyl system in Yucatan miniature pigs, *Contemp. Top. Lab. Anim. Sci.*, 40(3): 12–16.

Worek, F.S, Blumel, G., Zeravik, J., Zimmerman, G.J., and Pfeiffer, U.J., 1988, Comparison of ketamine and pentobarbital anesthesia with the conscious state in a porcine model of Pseudomonas aeruginosa septicemia, *Acta Anaesthesiol. Scand.*, 32(7): 509–515.

3 Wound Closure and Integument

GENERAL PRINCIPLES AND SURGICAL PREPARATION

The pig is a relatively hairless animal with a fixed skin tightly attached to the subcutaneous tissues similar to that in humans. The cutaneous blood supply and sequence of events in wound healing are also similar to that in humans. However, the skin of the pig is thicker and less vascular overall than human skin. The thickness of the skin is especially pronounced in sexually mature animals on the dorsal surface of the neck and back, and in some breeds such as the Yucatan. There are also differences in the accessory tissues, such as the variations in sweat glands and the presence of an intrafollicular muscle in swine (Figure 3.1 and Figure 3.2). Pigs have sebaceous glands, which are relatively insignificant. There is a variation from humans in the number and function of the apocrine and eccrine sweat glands. Eccrine glands in pigs are limited to the snout and carpal glands, whereas in humans they are extensive and active in the sweating phenomenon. Apocrine sweat glands are more extensive in pigs but, as in humans, do not contribute to sweating or thermoregulatory functions to a high degree. Secretions on the skin may help to prevent fluid loss, but pigs in outdoors subjected to high temperatures thermoregulate by wallowing or seeking shade rather than actively sweating. There is a mental gland between the mandibles that contains tactile hairs and provides sebaceous and apocrine secretory functions (Argenzio and Monteiro-Riviere, 2001; Monteiro-Riviere, 1986, 2001).

The pig has been used extensively as a model for superficial and deep wound healing, including thermal injury, and plastic surgical techniques, and it has been developed as a model of dermal toxicity, percutaneous absorption, and phototoxicity (Bolton et al., 1988; Chvapil and Chvapil, 1992; Kerrigan et al., 1986; Mertz et al., 1986; Middelkoop et al., 2004; Monteiro-Riviere, 1986, 2001; Monteiro-Riviere and Riviere, 1996, 2005; Ordman and Gillman, 1966; Pietrzak et al., 2006; Riviere et al., 1986; Sullivan et al., 2001; Wang et al., 2001).

Any standard method of aseptic preparation of the skin for humans or other species may be applied to the pig. None of these methods, such as povidone-iodine and alcohol, ensures a completely sterile environment on the skin (Mertz et al., 1984) and, consequently, skin contact with other organs and tissues should be minimized when performing surgery in body cavities. The methodology preferred in the author's laboratories is described here (Figure 3.3–Figure 3.6).

Swine are cleaned of gross contamination from the total body in a separate surgical prep room for animals. The area of surgical intervention is clipped with electric clippers and in some cases is shaved. The skin is scrubbed three times with iodine surgical scrub and rinsed with alcohol. The animal is then transported to the operating room where a sterile preparation of iodine prep solution is applied using sponge forceps and sterile sponges. In most cases, the iodine solution is removed with alcohol, and the skin dried with sterile gauze sponges. A transparent iodine-impregnated adhesive drape is applied over the dry skin. If the iodine-impregnated drape is not used, as for some minor procedures, the last solution of iodine remains on the skin. The adhesive iodine-impregnated drapes work well on swine and provide protection against contamination of tissues

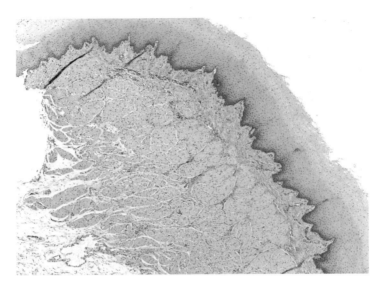

FIGURE 3.1 Histologic section of skin. H&E, ×10.

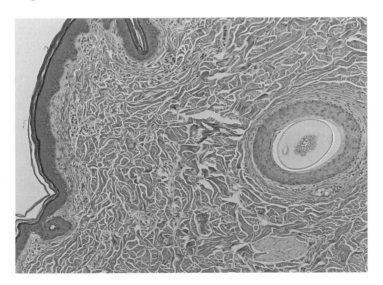

FIGURE 3.2 Histologic section of skin. H&E, ×40.

and organs from the skin after the incision is made, because they adhere to the edges of the incision if the skin preparation has been performed as described in the preceding text (Figure 3.7).

The principles of surgery are the same for swine as they are for other species. Careful attention to hemostasis, atraumatic handling of tissues, proper use of surgical instruments, closure of dead space, and aseptic technique will minimize complications associated with surgery (Ethicon, 1999; Swindle, 1983).

SUTURE SELECTION FOR WOUND CLOSURE

Selection of the appropriate size and type of suture material is important for the prevention of postoperative complications. In general, the suture material should not cause reactions that may impede healing and should be of the smallest appropriate size to provide appropriate wound closure.

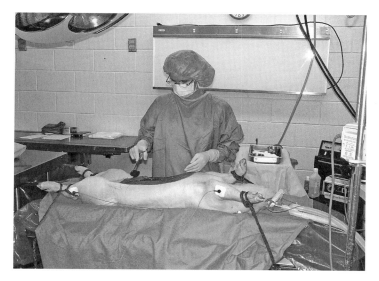

FIGURE 3.3 Sterile skin prep of a pig in the operating room.

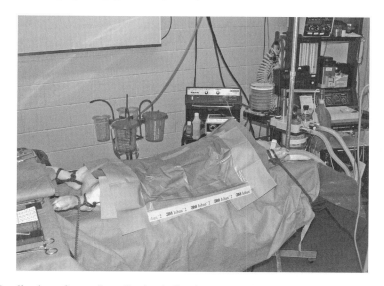

FIGURE 3.4 Application of a sterile, adhesive iodine-impregnated drape.

If too many sutures are placed or if the suture is much larger than necessary, it overloads the region with foreign material and may cause regional ischemia or create an inappropriate foreign body reaction. These generalities depend upon the region in which the suture is implanted and the type of suture material. It is beyond the purpose of this text to provide an instruction manual for beginning techniques in surgery or for a discussion of all of the aspects of suture selection. However, a technical training book is available detailing beginning surgical techniques in swine (Swindle, 1983), and a complete discussion of the principles of suture selection and wound healing are also available (Ethicon, 1999).

Selection of the appropriate-sized suture material is subjective and depends upon the experience of the surgeon. Several examples based upon experience may be of value in that selection and are listed here. When closing incisions in 25-kg swine, the selection of 2/0 suture for closure of the muscle layers and 3/0 suture for closure of the subcutaneous, subcuticular, or skin layers

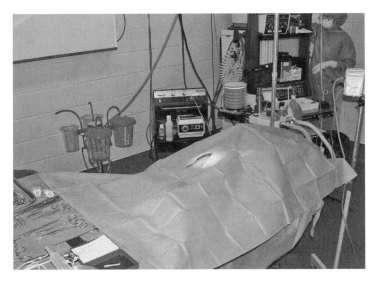

FIGURE 3.5 Application of a full-body sterile drape over the adhesive drape.

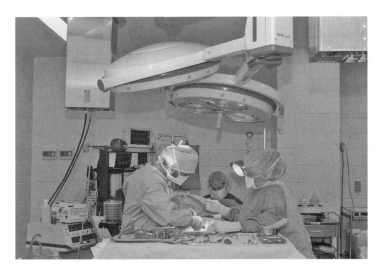

FIGURE 3.6 Surgical team in proper protective wear for sterile surgery.

works well. If closing the same incision in 50-kg swine, selection of 0 or 1 suture for the muscle layers, 2/0 suture for subcutaneous layers, and 3/0 suture for the subcuticular or skin layer would be appropriate.

One way of classifying suture material is whether the material is absorbable or nonabsorbable. Another classification would be whether the suture is manufactured from synthetic or natural materials. Other classifications based upon manufacturing techniques include braided or monofilament and coated or noncoated. Generally, sutures that are braided are manufactured to provide greater strength, and ones that are coated materials are to prevent reactions and to delay absorption. Selection of the type of material and the intended usage will also dictate the number of throws required in the surgical knot, with the coated or monofilament sutures usually requiring more than three throws (Ethicon, 1999).

Synthetic sutures of either absorbable or nonabsorbable material work well depending upon the surgical incision that is being closed. Silk, linen, cotton, and gut are natural materials that

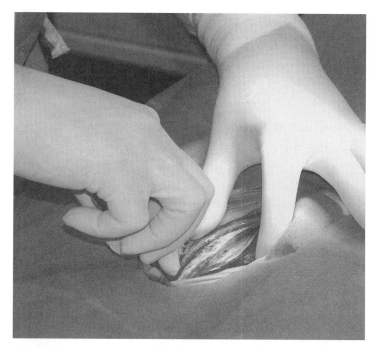

FIGURE 3.7 Making a skin and muscle incision with a scalpel through an adhesive drape.

should not be routinely used to close surgical wounds in swine. All these materials are reactive and may lead to inappropriate bodily responses, such as seromas, which may impede wound healing. Use of these materials should be reserved for a special circumstance dictated by the protocol.

Absorbable materials that have been routinely used without complications include the following synthetics: poliglecaprone 25, polydiaxonone, polyglycolic acid, polyglactin 910, polyglyconate, poliglecaprone 25, and lactomer 9-1. Nonabsorbable materials routinely used have included nylon, polyester, polypropylene, polyamide, polytetraflurethylene, polyglecaprone 25, and stainless steel. This list is not all inclusive, and, as a general rule, the synthetic manufactured materials developed in recent years have all proved to be safe and effective.

Both absorbable and nonabsorbable surgical staples have been developed, and staple surgical techniques greatly increase the speed of wound closure. These devices are essential in endoscopic surgical techniques. However, closure of the skin of animals with staples provides some opportunities for complications that are not as likely to occur with suture materials. Staples may be caught on cages and may hold contaminants, such as hair or feces, close to the skin incision more readily than some suturing techniques. These problems can be minimized by caging and bandaging procedures; however, the surgeon should be aware of their potential occurrence prior to selecting staples for skin closure. Absorbable staples (polylactic acid and polyglycolic acid) for subcutaneous closure of wounds have been recently developed (Insorb®, Incisive Surgical, Plymouth, MN), and this type of stapling technique may be useful for larger pigs (Figure 3.8 and Figure 3.9). In small fast-growing pigs, it is likely that the staple material will grow outward with the skin. At this time, 3-0 poliglecaprone 25 (Monocryl®, Ethicon, Sommerville, NJ), on a cutting needle is the preferred suture material for subcuticular closures in pigs <4 months of age in our laboratories. It is a synthetic monofilament, which is absorbed in approximately 3 weeks. Synthetics with a slower absorption rate (Dexon®, Vicryl®, PDS®, Ethicon, Sommerville, NJ) may grow outward with the epidermal layer onto the skin surface as the pig grows. This creates skin irritation and potential infection, even after the incision site is healed, but before the suture is completely absorbed. However, the longer absorption time may be needed for sexually mature pigs with slower healing times.

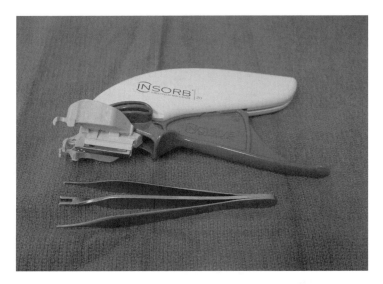

FIGURE 3.8 Subcutaneous stapling device and specialized tissue forceps for the device.

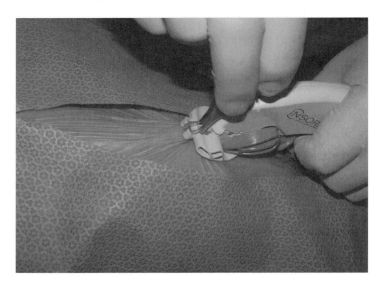

FIGURE 3.9 Using the subcutaneous stapling device in the abdomen.

WOUND CLOSURE AND BANDAGING TECHNIQUES

The same suture patterns and techniques that are used for wound closure for other species are applicable to the pig. Bandaging techniques are somewhat species specific and will be described in this section with a brief review of wound closure techniques (Smith and Swindle, 1994). Specific closures for areas, such as the abdomen or thorax, and suture techniques for visceral organs are discussed in the appropriate chapters of this text.

Closure of a wound should be performed in anatomically correct layers. Either simple interrupted or continuous sutures can be used on internal layers, such as peritoneum, muscle, and subcutaneous tissues (Figure 3.10 and Figure 3.11). Simple interrupted sutures provide more security but increase the foreign material load that is implanted and may provide uneven tension in a given layer because of variability between the individual sutures. Care must be taken when

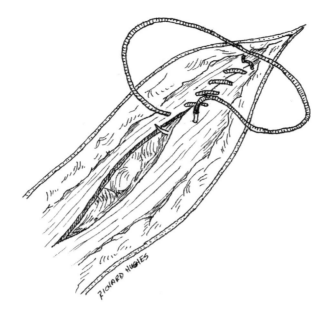

FIGURE 3.10 Closure of muscle layers for an abdominal incision.

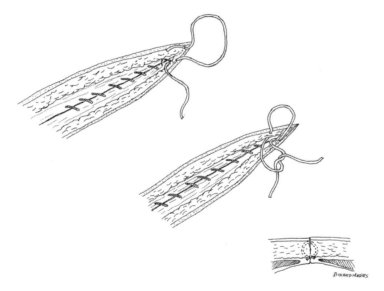

FIGURE 3.11 Simple continuous pattern in the subcutaneous tissues.

using continuous sutures to close these layers, because an improperly tied knot at either end of the suture line can lead to dehiscence of the wound. The distance between the suture insertions will depend upon the type of tissue, type of suture, and skill of the surgeon. Generally speaking, the suture placement should approximate the edges of the wound in an anatomically correct fashion without placing undue tension on the suture line and making sure that the closure does not leave dead space, which may lead to seromas or pockets of infection.

Thin muscle layers can be closed with a suture pattern that penetrates the full thickness of the muscle. Thick muscles can be closed with the external fascia only, as that is the layer that provides the strength for holding the sutures. Fat does not hold sutures and must be approximated with the

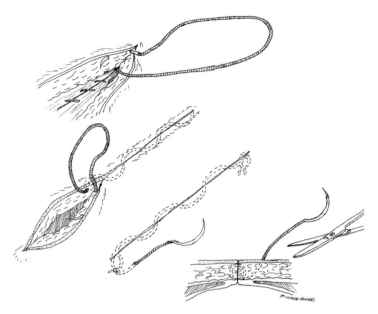

FIGURE 3.12 Subcuticular suture pattern with the knot buried at both ends.

subcutaneous layers. The subcutaneous layers are generally closed with a continuous suture pattern. In addition to closing dead space, this layer reduces the tension that must be applied to the skin sutures (Figure 3.10 and Figure 3.11).

Problems with closure of abdominal or subcutaneous incisions may be encountered in large swine because of excess fat deposition. Use of a rubber surgical retractor (surgical fish) to hold abdominal tissues *in situ* during closure of the peritoneal and initial muscle layers is recommended. These devices can be removed through the small opening when the last few sutures are ready to be placed. Fat deposition also makes the area greasy and suture materials difficult to tie. Horizontal mattress sutures may have to be placed in the muscle layers of large animals for tension relief on the suture line.

The skin must be approximated with a minimal amount of tension, because it swells during the healing process; too tight a closure will cause irritation and secondary cutting of the skin. The ideal closure for pigskin is subcuticular suture with buried knots using 3/0 absorbable synthetic suture (Figure 3.12). If the knot is buried at both ends, it provides a cosmetic closure with minimal complications. Simple interrupted sutures (Figure 3.13) may be used to close the skin using 3/0 synthetic nonabsorbable suture. As a general rule, simple interrupted sutures should be placed 5 mm from the skin edges with approximately 5–10 mm between sutures. Horizontal mattress sutures (Figure 3.14) may be used outside the suture line as tension-relief sutures on long incision lines but should not be used as the primary skin closure pattern. Vertical mattress sutures (Figure 3.15) can be used to give a secure cosmetic closure if an eversion pattern is desired. Skin staples can be problematic for the reasons described in the preceding text. Continuous suture patterns are best not used for routine closure of skin but may be acceptable in some situations related to the research (Figure 3.16).

If the skin closure is not anatomically correct and there is an eversion or outpouching of the skin at the end of the suture line due to uneven closure, corrective measures should be taken. Cutting through the outpouching at a 45° angle and placing a few simple interrupted sutures will usually correct most situations.

The suture line should not be placed over subcutaneously implanted devices. It is best to have the suture line either caudal or cranial to the device rather than dorsal or ventral. This prevents undue tension on the suture line from the weight or pressure of the device.

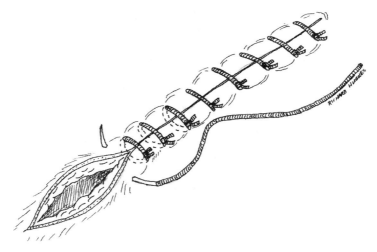

FIGURE 3.13 Simple interrupted skin suture pattern.

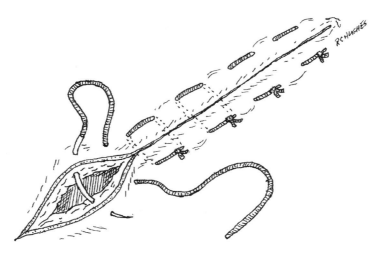

FIGURE 3.14 Horizontal mattress suture pattern in the skin.

Bandaging of the incision may be indicated in some situations, including large incisions under tension, implantation of subcutaneous devices, suture lines that are likely to be contaminated from urine or feces, and incisions that are placed in areas that the animal is likely to irritate. The use of topical spray bandages or tissue glues provide a short-term seal of the skin incision and is a good idea for most incisions. Bandages should be changed every 1–2 d, or earlier if they become contaminated with moisture, urine, or feces.

The pig should be bandaged in a circumferential fashion for incisions on the trunk and neck. Nonadhesive self-adhering bandage material can be used after placing sterile gauze pads to protect the suture line; however, these are easily removed by the animal after recovery. If they are used, the cranial and caudal ends of the bandage should be held in place with adhesive bandage material that includes the bare skin with the edge of the bandage material. Orthopedic stockinette can be used for a total body bandage after cutting out leg holes. This will provide a loose covering for wound-healing studies without directly applying pressure to the wound. Both the cranial and caudal ends of the stockinette should be secured with adhesive tape as described in the preceding text. Porous elastic adhesive tape in wide widths functions better than ordinary white bandage tape in

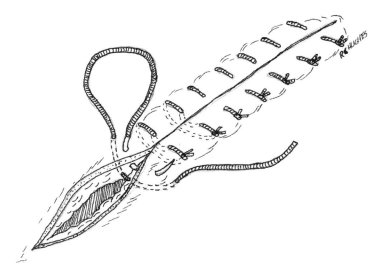

FIGURE 3.15 Vertical mattress suture pattern in the skin.

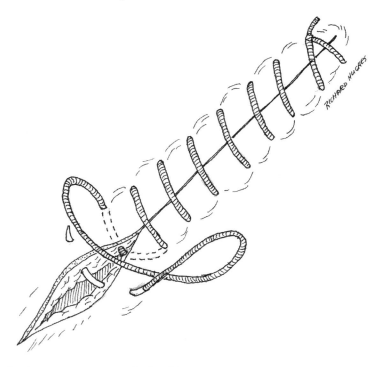

FIGURE 3.16 Continuous suture pattern in the skin.

swine because it provides a better contour fit and can be secured more tightly. Soft cloth surgical tape and clear self-adhering wound dressings are currently used in our laboratories for most applications (Figure 3.17).

Bandaging of the extremities and difficult areas, such as the perineum, requires some creativity. The same principles that apply to other animals apply to the pig. Use of skin adhesives may be necessary to provide additional security for the tape. Some of the plastic skin drape material used during surgery can be used for the short term; however, this material is nonporous and will keep

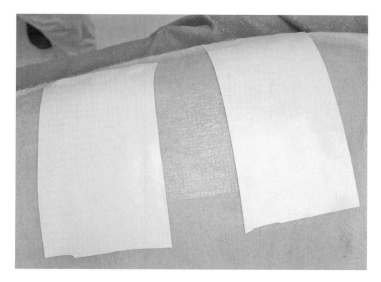

FIGURE 3.17 Soft cloth surgical tape and clear self-adhering bandage.

the wound moist and impair healing if used for long-term bandaging. Adhesive bandages that permit air transport are also useful for these areas.

Tether and harness systems can be designed to maintain chronic catheterization models (see Chapter 8, Figure 8.12). Jacket systems have also been designed for swine and are commercially available. Care must be taken to have different-sized jackets available for chronic models, because small swine will tend to outgrow them in a few weeks (Davies and Henning, 1986; Smith and Swindle, 1994; Swindle et al., 1996).

SKIN FLAPS AND GRAFTS

Swine have been important models in the study of skin flaps and grafts, and a technical manuscript reviewing the various types of flaps has been published (Figure 3.18) (Kerrigan et al., 1986). Swine have also been used for burn studies for both techniques and as a replacement for human skin, cutaneous pharmacology and toxicology, wound healing, and surgical techniques (Daniel et al., 1981; McGraft and Hundahl, 1982; Riviere et al., 1986; Sasaki and Pang, 1984; Shircliffe et al., 1974). The porcine skin has a cutaneous blood supply similar to humans because it is a fixed skin animal unlike most animal species (Forbes, 1969).

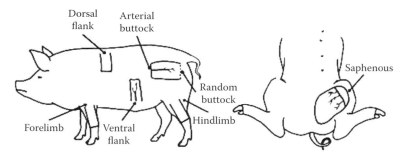

FIGURE 3.18 Location of the sites of various skin flaps and grafts. (Reprinted from Kerrigan et al., 1986, *Lab. Anim. Sci.*, 36: 408–412. With permission.)

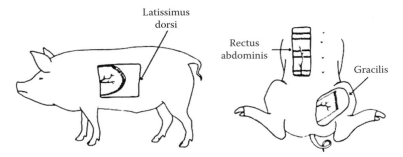

FIGURE 3.19 Location of myocutaneous flaps. (Reprinted from Kerrigan et al., 1986, *Lab. Anim. Sci.*, 36: 408–412. With permission.)

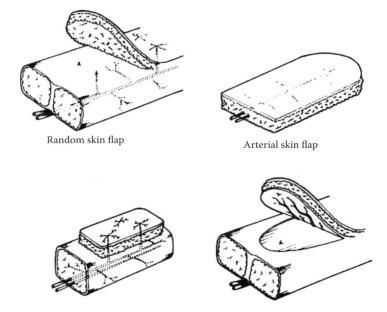

FIGURE 3.20 Location of fasciocutaneous flaps. (Reprinted from Kerrigan et al., 1986, *Lab. Anim. Sci.*, 36: 408–412. With permission.)

The classification of flaps described by Kerrigan et al. (1986) will be used here (Figure 3.19–Figure 3.21). Experimentally, the lengths of the flaps are longer than the described survival length to ensure a zone of necrosis. The zone of necrosis is the region generally studied for techniques and agents that enhance survival. If a zone of necrosis is not required, then the length of the flap is reduced to ensure that adequate blood supply to the flap remains intact.

RANDOM SKIN FLAPS

Random skin flaps include the dorsal flank flap, the random buttock flap, and the random limb flap. The dorsal flank flap is raised 4 cm ventral to the midline. The survival length of a 4-cm-wide flap is 6.75 cm. The full thickness flap is raised and elevated to its dorsal base. The length of the flap is varied depending upon the experimental parameters. Random buttock flaps are raised over the lateral thigh and will be free of panniculus carnosus, unlike the flank flap. Survival flaps are 10 cm in width and 4.6 cm in length. The flap is incised on three sides, raised to its dorsal margin, and sutured upon itself. The length of the flap is varied as required. Random skin flaps are used

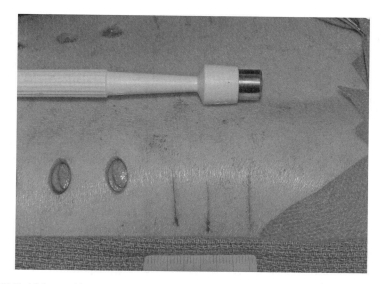

FIGURE 3.21 Full-thickness biopsy punch (1 cm) and scalpel incisional surgical wounds in the flank.

on both the forelimb and hind limb and are elevated in the subcutaneous tissues as before. Survival lengths for forelimb flaps are 7.2 cm and for hind limb are 6.7 cm.

ARTERIAL SKIN FLAPS

Arterial skin flaps include an arterial pedicle. The ventral flank flap is raised with the base 4 cm lateral to the nipple line and has a branch of the intercostal artery as its vascular branch. The survival length of a 4-cm-wide flap is 8.6 cm. A buttock arterial flap may be raised using the superficial circumflex iliac artery as the vascular pedicle. The 10-cm-wide flap is raised over the cranial dorsal iliac spine with a survival length of 13.3 cm. Because the lateral femoral cutaneous nerve is included in this flap, it also qualifies as a neurovascular pedicle. The saphenous flap uses the saphenous artery as its vascular pedicle and is located on the medial aspect of the hind limb. The location of the flap is its main disadvantage, and, because of the vascular supply, there is not a defined survival length.

MYOCUTANEOUS FLAPS

Myocutaneous flaps include the underlying muscle and a vascular supply. The latissimus dorsi flap is most commonly used and the large thoracodorsal artery provides predictable survival. A flap of 10 × 16 cm starting at the caudal border of the shoulder is predictably survivable. The latissimus dorsi muscle is dissected and isolated relatively easily compared to other models. The gracilis myocutaneous flap is raised on the medial hind limb and includes the deep femoral artery as its arterial pedicle. The flap usually measures 10 × 20 cm and is one of the few areas where a skin flap can be raised on the contralateral side for comparison. Its main disadvantage is its location and the relative difficulty in dissection. A rectus abdominus muscle may be raised on the ventral surface of the abdomen using the cranial epigastric artery. Flaps of two sizes are used: 5.5 cm and 6.5 × 18 cm. No predictable survivable flap size has been described. Besides location, there are differences in classification of the three muscles. The latissimus dorsi is a type V, the gracilis is a type II, and the rectus abdominus is a type III. Trapezius, pectoralis profundus ascendens, and biceps femoris myocutaneous flaps have found less usage and are not as well defined as these models because of the differences in conformation between swine and humans.

Fasciocutaneous flaps have been raised on the forelimb and hind limb to include the skin and deep fascia. The forelimb flap is raised 5 cm wide over the lateral condyle of the humerus at the juncture of the lateral head of the triceps and the extensor carpi radialis. The survival length of the flap is 8.2 cm. The hind limb flap is raised on the lateral aspect one half to two thirds of the distance between the major trochanter of the femur and the calcaneus. A 5-cm-wide flap has a survival length of 7.9 cm.

Skin flaps in swine can be problematic if multiple flaps are performed on the animal at the same time. If the suturing technique is adequate to prevent mobility of the flap, then problems of acute surgical pain can be largely avoided. If flaps are designed to have a zone of necrosis, then the animals should be monitored closely for signs of discomfort and infection. Use of stockinette bandages, as described in the preceding text, can protect the wound from contamination. The use of analgesics and antibiotics should be considered strongly unless they are contraindicated by the protocol.

WOUND-HEALING MODELS

The pig has been used for both superficial and deep-wound-healing studies (Bolton et al., 1988; Chvapil and Chvapil, 1992; Mertz et al., 1986; Ordman and Gillman, 1966). Epidermal and dermal repair models have been standardized in the pig and in many other protocols, such as those involving skin flaps, described in the preceding text; wound healing is a part of the protocol. Swine have also been used for cutaneous toxicological research (Riviere et al., 1986). Differences in rates of wound healing may be noted between breeds, possibly due to age and genetic differences when comparing animal studies (Chvapil and Chvapil, 1992). Consequently, use of mature miniature pigs rather than farm breeds is a good alternative for studying more chronic wounds. Using multiple wounds on the same animal provides the ability to have the animal serve as its own control and also to have different treatments represented on the same animal. A technique of implanting subdermal titanium wound chambers in which wound infections can be studied has been described (Steinstraesser et al., 2006). In this technique, multiple chambers can be implanted to study the effects of therapy on different organisms independently.

Pig skin is relatively thick compared to other species and is similar in blood flow to humans. In sexually mature pigs, the epidermal back thickness is approximately 52 μm with a stratum corneum thickness of 12 μm. In contrast, the skin of the abdomen is approximately 47 μm with a stratum corneum thickness of 15 μm. The blood flow in ml/min per 100 g varies between areas of the skin as well. Approximate measurements are as follows: buttocks, 3; ear, 12; humeroscapular joint, 7; thoracolumbar junction, 3; and ventral abdomen, 11 (Monteiro-Riviere and Riviere, 2005).

Epidermal wound healing is studied to evaluate pharmaceutical and bandaging interventions and their effects on epidermal regeneration. The pig has been evaluated both as a model of epidermal migration (Chvapil and Chvapil, 1992; Mertz et al., 1986) and as a model of epidermal proliferation (Winter, 1972). The method of wounding may vary slightly between studies but basically involves infliction of multiple epidermal wounds of the same size and depth bilaterally, using a keratome. A common configuration involves excision of 16–24 wounds 2.2 × 2.2 cm and 0.04 cm deep.

In contrast to the superficial wounds described in the preceding text, deep wounds heal by scarring rather than regeneration. Dermal wounds may involve the use of skin flaps, described previously, simple full-thickness incisions or excised full-thickness wounds. A size of 3 × 5 cm and 0.8–1.5 cm deep has been standardized for excision wounds in the miniature pig (Chvapil and Chvapil, 1992). Alternatively, circular full-thickness wounds with a diameter up to 2 cm can be created. Circular wounds generally show less, and more uniform, contraction, allowing for more time for wound evaluation until wound closure (Peter Glerup, personal communication). Our laboratories have used circular 1-cm biopsy punches for full-thickness excisional wounds for preclinical treatment evaluations (Figure 3.21).

In the case of both split-thickness and full-thickness wounds, the pig may experience postoperative discomfort. It is advisable to use the orthopedic stockinette bandaging technique described in the preceding text. The use of antibiotics and analgesics is strongly advised unless contraindicated by the research protocol. In our experience, epidural morphine administered preoperatively prevents most of the discomfort and shortens the period of time postoperatively required for analgesic administration when the wounds are made on the flank.

REFERENCES

Argenzio, R.A. and Monteiro-Riviere, N.A., 2001, Excretory system, in Pond, W.G. and Mersmann, H.J., Eds., *Biology of the Domestic Pig*, Ithaca, NY: Comstock Publishing, pp. 583–624.

Bolton, L.L., Pines, E., and Rovee, D.T., 1988, Wound healing and integumentary system, in Swindle, M.M. and Adams, R.J., Eds., *Experimental Surgery and Physiology: Induced Animal Models of Human Disease*, Baltimore, MD: Williams and Wilkins, pp. 1–9.

Chvapil, M. and Chvapil, T.A., 1992, Wound healing models in the miniature Yucatan pig, in Swindle, M.M., Ed., *Swine as Models in Biomedical Research*, Ames, IA: Iowa State University Press, pp. 265–288.

Daniel, R.K., Priest, D.L., and Wheatley, D.C., 1981, Etiological factors in pressure sores: an experimental model, *Arch. Phys. Med. Rehabil.*, 62(10): 492–498.

Davies, A.S. and Henning, M., 1986, Use of swine as a model of musculoskeletal growth in animals, in Tumbleson, M.E., Ed., *Swine in Biomedical Research*, Vol. 2, New York: Plenum Publishers, pp. 839–848.

Ethicon, 1999, *Wound Closure Manual*, Sommerville, NJ: Ethicon.

Forbes, P.D., 1969, Vascular supply of the skin and hair in swine, in Montagna, W. and Dobson, R.L., Eds., *Advances in Biology of the Skin*, New York: Pergamon.

Glerup, P., 2006, Personal communication, SCANTOX, Ejby, Denmark.

Kerrigan, C.L., Zelt, R.G., Thomson, J.G., and Diano, E., 1986, The pig as an experimental animal in plastic surgery research for the study of skin flaps, myocutaneous flaps and fasciocutaneous flaps, *Lab. Anim. Sci.*, 36(4): 408–412.

McGraft, M.H. and Hundahl, S.C., 1982, The spatial and temporal quantification of myofibroblasts, *Plast. Reconstr. Surg.*, 69(6): 975–983.

Mertz, P.M., Alvarez, O.M., Smerbeck, R.V., and Eaglstein, W.H., 1984, A new *in vivo* model for the evaluation of topical antiseptics on superficial wounds: the effect of 70% alcohol and povidone-iodine solution, *Arch. Dermatol.*, 120(1): 58–62.

Mertz, P.M., Hebda, P.A., and Eaglstein, W.H., 1986, A porcine model for evaluation of epidermal wound healing, in Tumbleson, M.E., Ed., *Swine in Biomedical Research*, Vol. 1, New York: Plenum Press, pp. 291–302.

Middelkoop, E., van den Bogaerdt, A.J., Lamme, E.N., Hoekstra, M.J., Brandsma, K. and Ulrich, M.M., 2004, Porcine wound models for skin substitution and burn treatment, *Biomaterials*, 25(9): 1559–1567.

Monteiro-Riviere, N.A., 1986, Ultrastructural evaluation of the porcine integument, in Tumbleson, M.E., Ed., *Swine in Biomedical Research*, Vol. 1, New York: Plenum Press, pp. 641–655.

Monteiro-Riviere, N.A., 2001, Integument, in Pond, W.G. and Mersmann, H.J., *Biology of the Domestic Pig*, Ithaca, New York: Comstock Publishing, pp. 625–652.

Monteiro-Riviere, N.A. and Riviere, J., 1996, The pig as a model for cutaneous pharmacology and toxicology research, in Tumbleson, M.E. and Schook, L.B., Eds., *Advances in Swine in Biomedical Research*, Vol. 2, NY: Plenum Press, pp. 425–458.

Monteiro-Riviere, N.A. and Riviere, J., 2005, The pig as a model for human skin research, *Proc. Swine Biomed. Res.: Update on Animal Models*, 56th AALAS Meeting.

Ordman, L.J. and Gillman, T., 1966, Studies in the healing of cutaneous wounds. III. A critical comparison in the pig of the healing of surgical incisions closed with sutures or adhesive tape based on tensile strength and clinical histological criteria, *Arch. Surg.*, 93(6): 911–928.

Pietrzak, W.S., An, Y.H., Kang, Q.K., Ehrens, K.L., Demos, H.A., 2006, Hemostatic potential of platelet-rich and platelet-poor plasma utilizing a partial thickness skin wound model, *Proc. Soc. Biomater.* (abstract).

Riviere, J.E., Bowman, K.F., and Monteiro-Riviere, N.A., 1986, The isolated perfused porcine skin flap: a novel animal model for cutaneous toxicologic research, in Tumbleson, M.E., Ed., *Swine in Biomedical Research*, Vol. 1, New York: Plenum Press, pp. 657–666.

Sasaki, G.H. and Pang, C.Y., 1984, Pathophysiology of skin flaps raised on expanded pig skin, *Plast. Reconstr. Surg.*, 74(1): 59–67.

Shircliffe, A.C., James, P.M., and Meredith, J.H., 1974, Technique for obtaining porcine heterografts for use on burned patients, *J. Trauma*, 14(2): 168–174.

Smith, A.C. and Swindle, M.M., 1994, Post surgical care, in Smith, A.C. and Swindle, M.M., Eds., *Research Animal Anesthesia, Analgesia and Surgery*, Greenbelt, MD: SCAW, pp. 167–170.

Steinstraesser, L., Vranckx, J.J., Mohammadi-Tabrisi, A., Jacobsen, F., Mittler, D., Lehnhardt, M., Langer, S., Kuhnen, C., Gatermann, S., Steinau, H.U., and Eriksson, E., 2006, A novel titanium wound chamber for the study of wound infections in pigs, *Comp. Med.*, 56(4): 279–285.

Sullivan, T.P., Eaglstein, W.H., Davis, S.C., and Mertz, P., 2001, The pig as a model for human wound healing, *Wound Repair Regeneration*, 9(2): 66–76.

Swindle, M.M., 1983, *Basic Surgical Exercises Using Swine*, New York: Praeger Publishers.

Swindle, M.M., Wiest, D.B., Garner, S.S., Smith, A.C., and Gillette, P.C., 1996, Pregnant Yucatan miniature swine as a model for investigating fetal drug therapy, in Tumbleson, M. and Schook, L., Eds., *Advances in Swine in Biomedical Research*, Vol. 2, New York: Plenum Press, pp. 629–635.

Wang, J.F., Olson, M.E., Reno, C.R., Wright, J.B., and Hart, D.A., 2001, The pig as a model for excisional skin wound healing: characterization of the molecular and cellular biology, and bacteriology of the healing process, *Comp. Med.*, 51(4): 341–348.

Winter, G.D., 1972, Epidermal regeneration in the domestic pig, in Maibach, H.I. and Rovee, D.T., Eds., *Epidermal Wound Healing*, Chicago, IL: Year Book, pp. 71–112.

4 Gastrointestinal Procedures

SURGICAL ANATOMY

The anatomy of the gastrointestinal system has been described in detail in the literature (Schantz et al., 1996; Yen, 2001) and in Chapter 1. The oral cavity is described in Chapter 10. In this section, the anatomy important to surgical procedures is discussed, and views of the intestinal viscera *in situ* are illustrated in Figure 4.1–Figure 4.3.

The esophagus originates from the pharynx at the second cervical vertebra and passes along the left side of the trachea. The muscularis mucosa is composed of inner circular and outer longitudinal layers which are composed of striated muscle fibers in the proximal 50% which progress to smooth muscle fibers. In humans, only the distal of the esophagus has smooth muscle cells. The mucosa is stratified squamous epithelium throughout the length. The esophageal diameter in domestic swine 10–50 kg ranges from 15 to 20 mm, and in Yucatan swine 45–50 kg, the range is 12–14 mm.

The stomach is divided into esophageal, cardiac, fundic, and pyloric regions with a diverticulum in the fundic region. The secretory functions and glandular mucosa of these gastric regions are similar to that of other mammals (Figure 4.4–Figure 4.6). The stomach in farm pigs after weaning is generally 5–9 g/kg body weight (BW) and gastrointestinal (GI) maturity at 12 weeks in swine is approximately equal to that of a 1-year-old human (Sangild, 2001). The stomach of an adult Yucatan weighing 47 kg has a fluid volume of approximately 1300 ml. Depending upon the bulk and particle size of the meal, the stomach is generally emptied in 2–8 h. Fasting before and feeding after administration of a test substance reliably empties the stomach in 2–4 h (Casteel et al., 1998). The muscular torus pyloricus must be considered in planning gastric surgical procedures because of its size and location near the pylorus.

The duodenum generally is located in the right cranial medial aspect of the abdominal cavity in the region of the 10th–12th intercostal spaces. It is tightly attached and relatively fixed in its position in its cranial aspect, and the pancreas is closely adherent to it. The bile duct enters the duodenum approximately 1.5–6 cm distal to the pylorus, and the separate pancreatic duct enters the duodenum 10–20 cm from the pylorus (Schantz et al., 1996; Yen, 2002). The distances increase depending upon the size of the pig; the smaller value represents weanlings, and the larger value represents adults. The duodenal portion of the small intestine courses medially and passes through the ligament of Treitz caudal to the stomach, after which it gradually develops into the jejunum. The duodenum is generally considered to be approximately the proximal 5% of the small intestinal mass. Small intestinal diameter in domestic swine of 25 kg is approximately 18–20 mm, and in 50-kg domestic swine, it is approximately 30 mm as compared to 50-kg Yucatan swine, in which it is approximately 20 mm.

The jejunum comprises approximately 90% of the small intestinal mass. Most of it is located in the right caudal ventral side of the abdominal cavity in tight coils. The gross differences between the jejunum and ileum are not distinct; however, the wall of the ileum is slightly thinner. The ileum is the distal 5% of the small intestine and generally originates in the middle of the abdominal cavity, in which it courses cranially to attach to the cecum in the spiral colon at the level of the left paralumbar fossa.

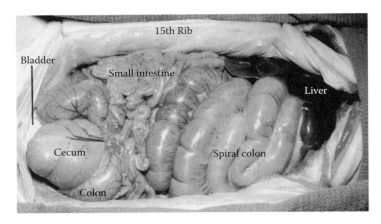

FIGURE 4.1 Ventral view of abdominal viscera.

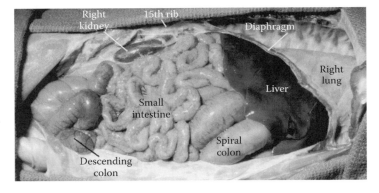

FIGURE 4.2 Right lateral view of abdominal viscera.

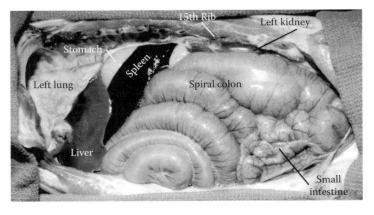

FIGURE 4.3 Left lateral view of abdominal viscera.

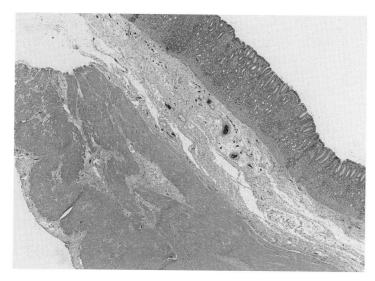

FIGURE 4.4 Histologic section of the esophageal region of the stomach. H&E, ×40.

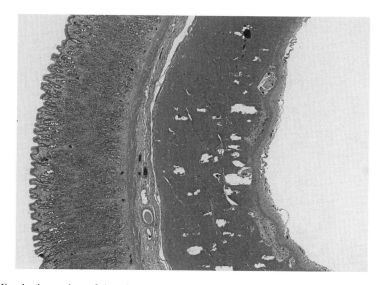

FIGURE 4.5 Histologic section of the glandular region of the stomach. H&E, ×40.

The mesentery of the small intestine is thin and friable with a unique fanlike pattern of mesenteric vessels with vascular arcades forming in the submucosa (Figure 4.7). Prominent lymph nodes are present in the root of the mesentery. The surgical modifications required for suturing the mesentery are discussed in the description of intestinal anastomosis in this chapter.

Generally, the small intestine comprises 20 to 40 times the length of the pig, approximately 4.5% of the body weight (7 to 8 g/kg BW) and requires 2 to 6 h for complete transport and emptying. GI transport is dependent upon the type of diet and age of the animal. In general, the length and width of the small and large intestine of a 30- to 40-kg pig equals that of an adult human (Schantz et al., 1996). A chart of the percentage of BW of various tissues and organs of the digestive system for 12-week-old pigs is given in the appendix (see Table A.31).

Histologically, the small intestine is composed of the mucosa, submucosa, muscularis, and serosa (Figure 4.8–Figure 4.10). The muscularis is composed of an inner circular layer and an outer

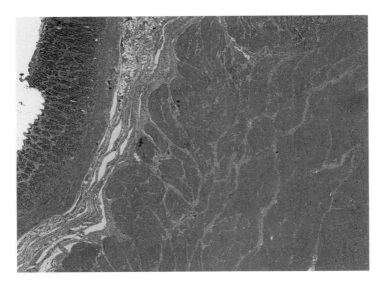

FIGURE 4.6 Histologic section of the pyloric region of the stomach. H&E, ×40.

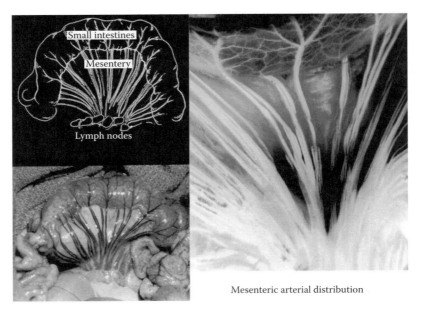

FIGURE 4.7 Small intestine showing the anatomy of the mesenteric vessels. The inset on the right is a negative image showing the arterial distribution in the intestinal wall.

longitudinal layer of smooth muscle. The mucosa is composed of columnar epithelium, lamina propria, and muscularis mucosa. The muscularis mucosa has the same two types of muscular layers, except that the longitudinal and circular layers are reversed in position from the muscularis. Peyer's patches (lymph nodules) are indistinct whitish oval nodules in the jejunum and ileum.

The spiral colon is located in the left upper quadrant of the abdomen and consists of the cecum, ascending, and proximal part of the transverse colon. Initially, the large intestine coils centripetally inward and then reverses after four coils to the centrifugal portion. The transverse colon exits the spiral colon cranially and then traverses caudally as the descending colon and rectum (Figure 4.11–Figure 4.13).

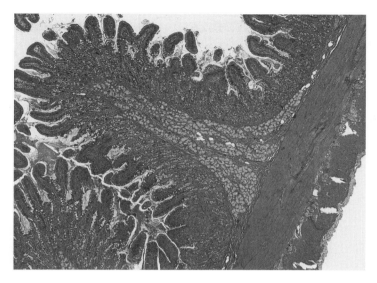

FIGURE 4.8 Histologic section of the duodenum. H&E, ×100.

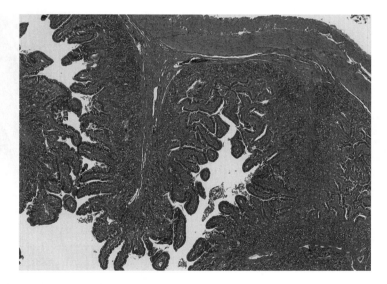

FIGURE 4.9 Histologic section of the jejunum. H&E, ×100.

The large intestine is generally about 25% the length of the small intestine but significantly slows the transit time of ingesta, requiring 24–48 h for complete emptying. It weighs 4.5–5.5 g/kg BW. The large intestinal diameter in 25-kg domestic swine is approximately 25 mm, in 50-kg domestic swine, approximately 55 mm, and in 50-kg Yucatan swine, 25 mm.

GENERAL PRINCIPLES OF ABDOMINAL SURGERY

Swine need to be fasted prior to surgery to facilitate the approach to the organs and to prevent vomiting, which rarely occurs. Unless a gastrotomy is to be performed, it is not necessary or advisable to withhold water because of their susceptibility to "salt poisoning" (Chapter 1). It is advisable to fast swine if the intestines are to be exteriorized for major abdominal surgery, because it decreases the edematous response. GI transit time varies with the breed, diet, and size of the pig;

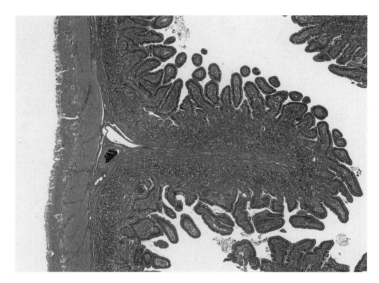

FIGURE 4.10 Histologic section of the ileum. H&E, ×100.

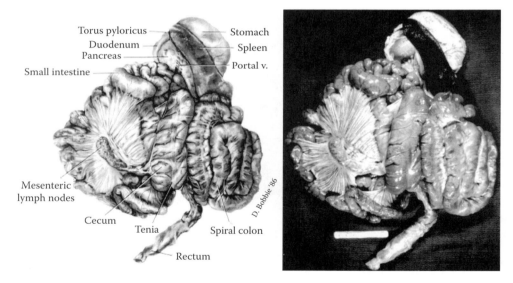

FIGURE 4.11 Gross anatomy of the spiral colon and large intestine.

however, the stomach and small intestine may generally be considered to be emptied by a 12-h fast. The large intestines, including the spiral colon and cecum, generally require 48 h to empty. Use of high-volume hypertonic osmotic purgative solutions will provide a more thoroughly cleansed intestinal tract; however, these solutions must be administered by stomach tube. Approximately 1 l/25 kg is required for purgation. The pills used for human colon cleansing (Visicol®, InKine Pharmaceuticals, Inc., Blue Bell, PA) are tolerated in feed and are effective. Use of enemas and stimulant purgatives is discouraged because of the difficulty of administration, discomfort to the animal, and the associated messiness of the procedure; however, they are effective. Bedding must be removed from the cages of fasted swine, because they will readily consume it, as well as any other foreign material that is available, in the absence of food. Pigs will readily consume commercially available glucose/electrolyte solutions (i.e., Gatorade®, Gatorade, Chicago, IL) or protein supplements (i.e., Ensure®, Abbott Labs, Abbott Park, IL). These can be given to pigs during the

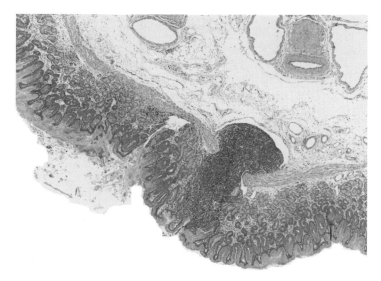

FIGURE 4.12 Histologic section of the large intestine from the spiral colon. H&E, ×40.

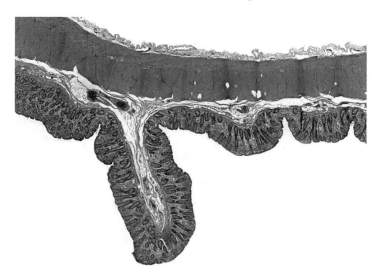

FIGURE 4.13 Histologic section of the colon. H&E, ×40.

prolonged 48-h fasts necessary for some procedures without increasing residue in the GI tract. It may also be useful in postoperative care situations in which the pig cannot be given solid food for a prolonged period of time. Prophylactic antibiotics preoperatively and intraoperatively are indicated if the intestines are to be entered surgically (Becker et al., 1992; Swindle, 1983). The pH of the stomach is generally <3.6 and is protective against microbes. Prior to surgically preparing the male pig for any type of abdominal surgery, the preputial diverticulum must be expressed as described for the urinary system in Chapter 7.

The laparotomy incision may be made in several locations depending upon the area of the small intestine to be approached. In general, the duodenum and root of the mesentery are best approached using a midline incision in the cranial abdomen. The bulk of the jejunum may be approached either by a midline, flank, or paramedian incision in the mid-to-caudal aspects of the abdomen. The ileum may be approached using a midline or flank incision in the cranial portion of the abdomen.

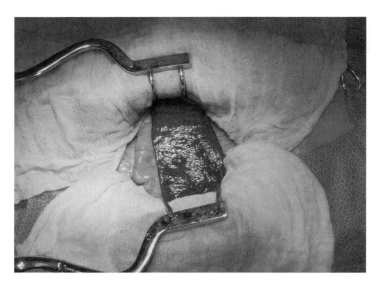

FIGURE 4.14 Laparotomy incision with edges of incision protected with wetted gauze sponges.

Following laparotomy, it is advisable to use saline-wetted laparotomy sponges to keep the tissue at the edges of the incision moist (Figure 4.14). Also, the use of sponges facilitates collection of the inadvertent spillage of GI contents to minimize contamination of the abdominal cavity during enterotomy. Gentle handling of the intestines with wetted sponges and atraumatic instrumentation is essential to minimize the complications associated with postoperative adhesions. The mesentery of the pig is very friable and prone to edema following prolonged manipulation. As for contaminated surgery in other species, it may be necessary to copiously flush the abdomen with isotonic solutions containing antibiotics, although this is not necessary as a routine. If only regional contamination occurs, then the flushing should only be performed in the area affected.

Closure of abdominal incisions is best accomplished in layers using synthetic absorbable sutures in either a simple interrupted or a continuous pattern. Closure of the peritoneum as an individual layer is not always possible in younger animals or in the caudal abdomen. In fact, closure of the peritoneum as a separate layer is unnecessary. Muscle fascia should be included in the sutures to bring the layers into proper apposition. Suturing of the skin is easily accomplished with subcuticular sutures, and this pattern is less likely to have localized wound inflammation than external suture patterns or staples (Chapter 3).

All GI procedures can be performed using staple surgery technologies, at least in part. Also, most of the procedures can be approached using laparoscopic or endoscopic surgical techniques rather than open surgical procedures. These techniques have been shown to be equivalent for wound-healing characteristics when compared to open techniques. For simplicity, the manual suturing techniques are described in this textbook (Kopchok et al., 1993; Noel et al., 1994; Olson et al., 1995). The unique anatomic features of the GI tract are outlined in Chapter 1. Photos of the abdominal viscera are included for reference when planning celiotomies (Figure 4.1–Figure 4.3, Figure 4.7, Figure 4.11). Methods of closing intestines and other hollow viscous organs are illustrated (Figure 4.15–Figure 4.18).

POSTOPERATIVE CARE

Postoperative recovery should be routine as for any other surgical procedure. However, some specific advice relevant when the intestinal tract is invaded surgically is provided in this section. Water may be provided immediately following recovery, and the animal may consume solid feed if only a

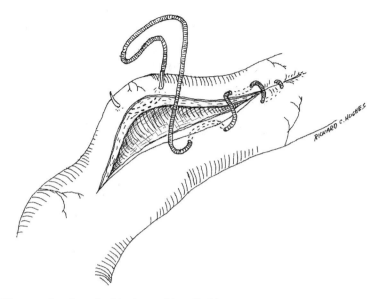

FIGURE 4.15 Closure of an intestinal incison with a Cushing pattern.

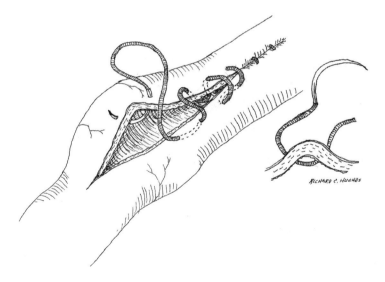

FIGURE 4.16 Closure of an intestinal incision with a Connell pattern (suture enters lumen).

catheter implantation was performed. Solid food should be withheld for the first day following surgery if an anastomosis was performed. Animals may be maintained on commercially available liquid diets such as Gatorade (glucose/electrolyte) or Ensure (protein/caloric). For a 20- to 25-kg pig, the calculated amount of diet is approximately 1 qt of the glucose/electrolyte solution and 2–3 cans of the protein/caloric supplement provided twice a day (bid). Postoperative analgesia should be provided, and the animal monitored for postoperative complications. Swine will readily eat canned pet food, chocolate syrup, pastry, or fruit, and oral medication may be hidden in these treats.

The most common complications that may occur are localized infection or peritonitis from an intestinal content leakage or intussusception. Animals should be monitored for fever and abdominal pain as well as the normal postural and behavioral characteristics. Treatment should be symptomatic; however, in a research setting animals generally are euthanized if such complications occur.

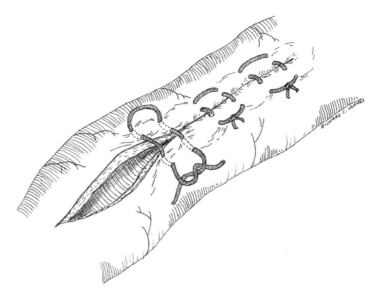

FIGURE 4.17 Closure of an intestinal incision with a Halsted pattern.

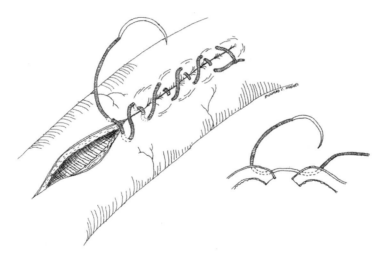

FIGURE 4.18 Closure of an intestinal incision with a Lembert pattern.

Intussusception is a rare occurrence, but it may be associated with telescoping of the intestine over the silicone cuff in intestinal catheter implantations, mesenteric rents, or adhesion formation. If the animal is exhibiting fever, inappetance, and abdominal pain, radiographs should be taken to observe the condition. Complications should be rare provided complete sterile techniques are utilized during the procedure.

GASTROTOMY AND GASTROSTOMY TECHNIQUES

The stomach is best approached from an upper midline incision from the xiphoid cartilage to the umbilicus. Following laparotomy, the stomach may be retracted gently out of the abdomen, and the edges of the incision are packed off with wetted laparotomy sponges. The gastrotomy incision is made in the avascular plane of the greater curvature after stabilization of the plane with Babcock

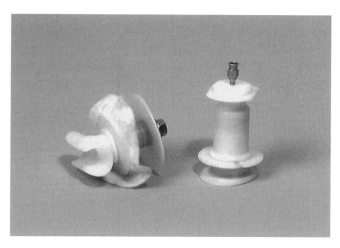

FIGURE 4.19 Cannulae for chronic fistulation of the colon (left) and the stomach (right).

forceps or stay sutures. Closure of the gastrotomy is performed with either staple surgical techniques or a two-layer inverting closure technique. The preferred suturing technique uses synthetic absorbable sutures in a Cushing pattern oversewn with a Lembert. The stomach should be thoroughly rinsed with saline prior to replacing it in the abdomen.

Gastrostomy tubes, ports, or cannulae may be sewn in place for gastric access using the same principles of surgery (Figure 4.19). Exteriorization of the devices is best performed on the lateral abdominal wall dorsal to the lateral border of the mammary glands or, preferably, on the dorsum of the flank. This prevents irritation of the exteriorized device when the pig is recumbent or rubs itself on the cage (Hennig et al., 1980; Pekas, 1983). A percutaneous method of placement of gastrostomy tubes using a modified Pezzar self-retaining mushroom catheter has been described (Gades and Mandrell, 2001). It involves passing of a trocar through the esophagus into the stomach and through the left abdominal wall followed by retrograde passage of the catheter. The procedure can be successful in small animals but has potential complications due to misdirection of the catheter. Surgical placement of pharyngostomy tubes caudal to the mandible is another option.

Heidenhein pouches (Figure 4.20) may be utilized in the pig in the same manner as originally described for other species to collect gastric secretions without gastric contents (Markowitz et al., 1964). For this procedure, a sleeve of the stomach is isolated from the body along the greater curvature while maintaining the blood supply of the gastroepiploic artery. The body of the stomach and the sleeve are sutured with a double row of inverting sutures. The isolated gastric pouch may be cannulated to the outside on the lower abdomen. In performing this procedure, the branches of the vagus nerve are sacrificed. A Pavlov pouch maintains the integrity between the cranial portion of the pouch with the body of the stomach, thus preserving innervation at that end. The distal end of the pouch is fistulated to the outside.

Gastrojejunostomy techniques may also be utilized in swine (Brenner et al., 2001). The jejunum is located by finding the root of the mesentery, which is caudal to the stomach and associated with the cranial mesenteric vessels. Care should be taken to ensure that there is no torsion of the mesentery and that the caudal direction of the peristalsis remains intact. A side-to-side surgical anastomosis is performed using standard techniques. Single-layer closure, using either interlocking or simple continuous sutures, is generally acceptable. Using two-layer inverting closure techniques may be necessary in large animals or in the case of existing pathology (Swindle, 1983).

A model of gastroesophageal reflux has been described (Schopf et al., 1997). This model is created by performing a longitudinal myectomy 3 cm proximal and distal to the gastroesophageal junction using a ventral midline incision from the xiphoid to the umbilicus. The approach and

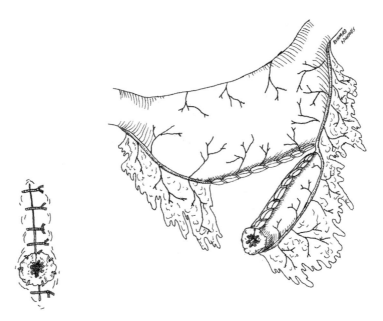

FIGURE 4.20 Creation of a Heidenhein pouch in the stomach.

dissection is similar to the one described for vagotomy in this chapter. The myectomy must be performed carefully to avoid incising the mucosal layer, similar to the dissection described for pyloroplasty in this chapter. However, the myectomy incision is not closed, and the animal should be kept on a liquid diet for 3 d postoperatively.

Otherwise, the abdominal incision is closed routinely, and postoperative care is routine. This procedure results in a chronic reflux esophagitis within days if the procedure is technically successful.

PYLOROPLASTY

The pylorus may be approached either through a midline or right paramedian incision. If the paramedian incision is used, it is made along the lateral aspect of the mammary glands from the last rib to the level of the umbilicus. The pylorus is identified by palpation and must be differentiated from the muscular torus pyloricus. The pylorus is exteriorized through the incision and stabilized by an assistant with wetted gauze sponges. A linear incision is made along the longitudinal plane of the stomach and duodenum in an avascular area. Repeated gentle incisions are made until all layers of the muscularis mucosa have been incised, and the submucosa bulges from the incision. At this point, the axis of the completed incision is changed at a right angle and the incision is closed using Lembert sutures. The net effect of the procedure is to enlarge the opening of the pylorus by incising the musculature and reversing the plane of the incision (Figure 4.21). Care should be taken not to incise the submucosa or mucosa; if this occurs, however, the closure of the incision described previously will repair the defect (Swindle, 1983).

ENTEROTOMY AND INTESTINAL FISTULATION

The small intestine (Figure 4.7) can be surgically entered using standard techniques (Anderson 2000; Swindle, 1983; Swindle et al., 1998). The duodenum can be approached by either a cranial midline incision, a right flank incision caudal to the ribs, or a right paramedian incision lateral to the mammary glands. The ileum is best approached through the cranial midline incision as for the proximal duodenum or close to the ileocecal junction through a right flank incision caudal to the

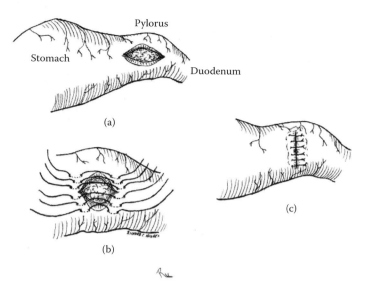

FIGURE 4.21 Closure of a pyloroplasty at right angles to the surgical incision.

last rib. The ileocecal junction is located in the dorsum of the abdominal cavity when using the flank incision. The majority of the small intestinal mass, including most of the jejunum, is in the right middle and caudal areas of the abdomen. It may be readily approached from the midline in females; however, a right paramedian incision in the caudal quadrant of the abdomen lateral to the mammary glands or a flank incision is preferable in males. This incision can be made through relatively thin abdominal musculature with minimal vasculature requiring ligation in this region.

Prior to enterotomy, the area of interest is brought out through the abdominal incision, and the area is packed off with wetted laparotomy sponges. A longitudinal incision is made along the antimesenteric border of the intestine in an avascular plane. If a catheter or other fistula device is to be inserted, then a stab incision may be made in the same plane with a no. 11 blade. It is not necessary to cross-clamp the intestine in most cases if the animal has been properly fasted. An assistant can preclude intestinal contents from entering the incision by pinching off the lumen at either end of the enterotomy incision. Following enterotomy, the incision may be closed using simple interrupted sutures with synthetic absorbable suture material.

For intestinal infusions, vascular access ports have been modified to function as intestinal access ports. A 7- to 9-Fr (French) silicone catheter with the end hole closed and four side slits approximately 1 cm in length has been found to be useful. The catheter has a bead preplaced 1 cm distal to a silicone flange that has been preplaced to provide an anchor for sutures to the intestinal serosa (Figure 4.22 and Figure 4.23). The access port may either be sutured to the skin on the outside or implanted subcutaneously in the flank or over the rib cage. The site of entrance into the intestine is closed between the bead and the flange with a purse-string suture. The flange is sutured to the intestine with two to four simple interrupted sutures (Figure 4.24). The specific procedures are described in detail in the next section. If a catheter is to be placed in the peritoneal cavity for infusion, the catheter must have multiple holes to prevent occlusion by the omentum (Figure 4.25).

The small intestine may also be fistulated as a Thiry fistula or Thiry-Vella loop (see later text). When either of these procedures is performed, then the fistula is best exteriorized on the lateral portion of the right flank to minimize tension on the isolated intestinal loop. Ileocutaneous bypass has also been described, which allows complete collection of ileal contents (Anderson et al., 2000). Ports may be placed at the site of the fistulation to minimize contamination and inflammation of the exit site. T cannulation has also been used for small intestinal fistulation (Wubben et al., 2001). In this type of procedure the tube is placed into the intestine and secured in place with a purse-

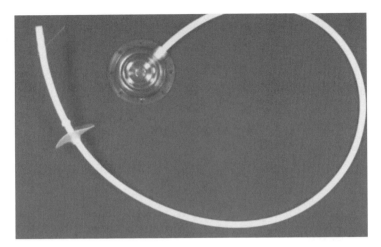

FIGURE 4.22 Intestinal access port for chronic infusion into the intestinal lumen. Note that the catheter has a bead for stability inside the lumen and a cuff for suturing to the serosa.

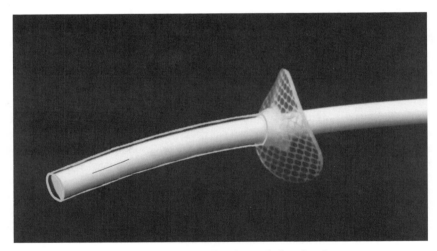

FIGURE 4.23 Tip of intestinal access port with a slit valve and closed end.

string suture using nonabsorbable suture material. The barrel of the tube is exteriorized through the flank. Tubes must be designed with threads and an exteriorized cap to allow adjustment of the length of the barrel as the animal grows. The barrel should also be designed such that a plug is included to prevent ingesta from entering the tube.

When fistulation is performed, the postoperative care should include local application of an antibiotic or zinc oxide ointment to prevent inflammation on the surface of the skin. Fistulas should not be accessed until the surrounding skin is thoroughly cleansed with an antibacterial soap. Depending upon the type of procedure performed, nutritional deficiencies, serum biochemical changes, or both may occur and potential corrective actions should be included in preoperative planning.

INTESTINAL INFUSION CATHETER IMPLANTATION

In pharmacological studies, it is frequently necessary to bypass the stomach and determine which area of the small intestine is responsible for absorption of the agent. This can be performed by implanting infusion catheters in various regions of the small intestine. Common sites would be the

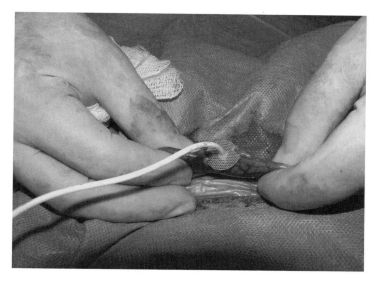

FIGURE 4.24 Intestinal access port catheter flange sutured to the serosa of the duodenum.

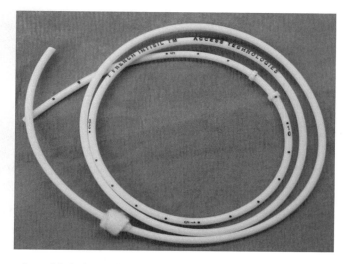

FIGURE 4.25 Intraperitoneal infusion catheter with multiple holes.

duodenum, jejunum, and ileum. Generally, duodenal catheters are implanted in the segment imme-diately caudal to the pancreatic duct. The proximal jejunum may be located at the root of the mesentery caudal to the stomach and midjejunum in the coils of the caudal abdomen. The ileum is best located by identifying the ileocecal junction and tracing the intestinal segment cranially.

Vascular access ports have been modified to be used as intestinal infusion ports and catheters (Swindle et al., 1996; Swindle et al., 2005). The port itself is of the same design but 7- to 9-Fr silicone catheters are modified for intestinal access. The tip of the catheter cannot be left open because it will rapidly become blocked with intestinal contents. The tip of the catheter is either constructed with a burp valve or four slits cut in the intraintestinal portion of the tip of the catheter. A suture retention bead is glued in place at the site of intraluminal placement and a silicone cuff is preplaced approximately 1 cm above the bead. Thus, there is an intraluminal segment with slits or a burp valve, a suture retention bead within the intestine at the site of enterotomy, and a silicone cuff for placing retention sutures on the serosa (Figure 4.22–Figure 4.25).

All the small intestinal sites can be accessed using a cranial to midabdominal midline incision. The procedures for isolating and packing the intestines are identical to that described earlier for anastomosis. A stab incision is made in the antimesenteric border of the intestine using a no. 11 blade, taking care to avoid direct penetration of a blood vessel. The catheter tip is inserted into the intestinal lumen in the direction of peristalsis. A purse-string suture using 3-0 PDS is placed in the serosa between the suture bead, which is in the lumen of the intestine, and the silicone cuff. The silicone cuff is tacked in place with 2–4 serosal sutures using 3-0 Ethibond or other soft nonabsorbable suture material (Figure 4.24).

An elliptical pocket for the port body is made on the lateral abdominal wall. The end of the catheter is tunneled through the wall of the abdomen into the port pocket. The end of the catheter is attached to the port, and the port and catheter are flushed copiously with sterile saline. The surgeon should be able to visualize the unobstructed passage of the fluid into the intestinal lumen without any leakage around the surgical site. The access port is sutured subcutaneously in place in the usual manner.

This procedure is repeated for every intestinal access catheter that is placed. The catheter length should be sufficient to allow for growth of the animal during the project period without putting undue tension on the intestine. Leaving too much extra catheter length in the abdomen may lead to torsion of the intestines. This technique is only useful for infusion of substances into the intestine. It is not possible to withdraw intestinal contents through the catheter. Catheters are maintained by keeping them filled with sterile saline. Access to the port site for injections should be performed under a sterile technique with skin preparation, sterile gloves, and sterile supplies.

INTESTINAL ANASTOMOSIS

The intestine may be approached surgically through any of the incisions described earlier for enterotomies (Swindle, 1983). The small intestine may be anastomosed by either end-to-end, end-to-side, or side-to-side techniques. The main variation between the pig and other species relates to the formation of the vascular arcades of the mesenteric vessels in the subserosa of the intestine rather than in the mesentery. The peculiar fanlike arrangement of the mesenteric vessels also necessitates a change in techniques to suture the mesentery (Schantz et al., 1996).

When performing an intestinal anastomosis, the vascular supply to the intestine that is to be removed is ligated at its base close to the root of the mesentery. The line of demarcation of the blood supply in the intestine should be closely observed to ensure that all infarcted nonviable intestine is removed. The intestine should be cross-clamped with intestinal forceps along the line of demarcation to ensure that the line of incision will be at the junction of viable and infarcted intestine. This line will be at an oblique angle to the long axis of the intestine. The angle will approximate the angle of the mesenteric arterial supply to the region. The section of intestine that has been ligated and its associated mesentery are excised after placing a second set of intestinal forceps at either end of the viable intestine to prevent contamination of the surgical site with reflux of intestinal contents. This pair of forceps should be applied atraumatically with the minimal amount of pressure required to prevent the movement of intestinal contents into the area of the incision. The intestinal forceps should be either linen or rubber shod to prevent cutting of the tissue by the metal forceps. Alternatively, an assistant may use digital pressure to pinch off the lumens of the viable intestine at either end of the incision. These proximal and distal clamps should be placed so that the excised ends of the remaining intestine are long enough for the edges to be sutured.

The intestinal anastomosis may be closed with simple interrupted sutures using synthetic absorbable sutures. This suture pattern enters the lumen and is pulled tightly enough when tying the knots to cut through the mucosa and become embedded in the intestinal wall. This is applicable to most small swine; however, in larger animals, either a continuous pattern or a two-layer closure of continuous sutures oversewn with inverting sutures may be required. Single-layer closure is usually indicated except in the case of larger animals or potential contamination that may impair

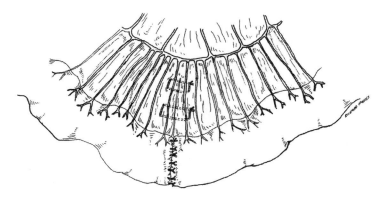

FIGURE 4.26 Closure of the mesentery with horizontal mattress sutures and an intestinal anastomosis closed with simple interrupted sutures.

healing. Regardless of which suturing technique is chosen, the sutures must be meticulously placed to provide for correct anatomic alignment and to provide a suture line without leakage. As a general rule, the sutures for this anastomosis should be approximately 5 mm from the edges of the incision and 5–10 mm between sutures. The remaining clamps should be removed and the incision line checked for leakage. In some cases, the intestinal lumen along the lines of excision may not be the same size, and it might require additional trimming of the tissue edges. Any leaks may be closed by the addition of simple interrupted or inverted sutures. Alternatively, the anastomosis may be performed using standard staple surgical devices.

The mesenteric incision will need to be sutured to prevent bowel torsion and stricture. In most cases, the edges of mesentery will retract to the adjacent mesenteric vessels and the mesenteric tissue adjacent to the incision will become edematous. If the edges of the mesentery are readily identifiable, then the incision may be closed with simple interrupted or continuous sutures using absorbable synthetic suture material. However, this will not be the case in most animals. In those animals in which the edges of the mesentery are not readily identifiable, a series of horizontal mattress sutures are placed on the proximal and distal sides of the first viable set of mesenteric vessels at either end of the excised intestines (Figure 4.26). This pattern will close the mesenteric rent without occluding the blood supply to the remaining intestine.

The anastomosed intestine should be rinsed copiously with isotonic saline solution, with or without antibiotics, prior to replacing it in the abdomen. If contamination is suspected, then rinsing of the abdomen with antibiotic-containing saline solution may be indicated.

INTESTINAL DIVERSION OR INTESTINAL BYPASS

Various techniques are used to perform small intestinal diversion or bypass in the experimental setting (Assimos et al., 1986; Fleming and Arce, 1986; Hand et al., 1981; Markowitz et al., 1964; Swindle et al., 1998; Turner and Mellwrath, 1982; Wubben et al., 2001). These would include such techniques as the Thiry fistula, Thiry-Vella fistula, T-tube cannulation, and jejunoileal bypass. The techniques for suturing the intestine are the same as those discussed for intestinal anastomosis. In this section, a review of some of the types of procedures that are possible in swine is provided. Examples of the specific porcine anatomic features that must be considered are provided.

The Thiry fistula (Figure 4.27) is performed by isolating a segment of small intestine with the vascular and nerve supply intact, closing one end by oversewing the stump, and exteriorizing the open end. The intestine from which the segment is isolated is closed using an end-to-end anastomosis. Peristalsis may either be directed into the abdomen or out of the fistulated abdominal wall depending upon the goals of the experiment. The Thiry-Vella loop (Figure 4.28) is isolated in the

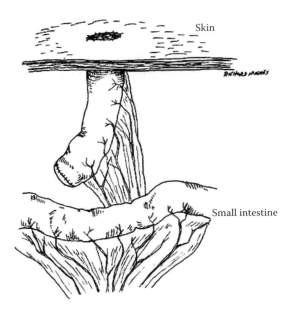

FIGURE 4.27 Thiry fistula.

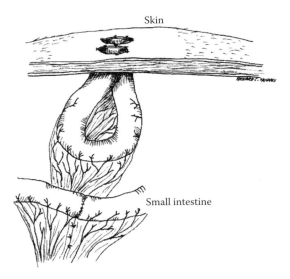

FIGURE 4.28 Thiry-Vella fistula.

same manner as the Thiry fistula, except that both ends of the intestine are exteriorized. When the intestinal segment is selected, it should be a section that will not have tension on the mesenteric attachment after isolation. The isolated segment should be flushed copiously with warm saline to minimize contamination of the abdomen and the exteriorization incision. Prophylactic antibiotics are indicated with this procedure (Markowitz et al., 1964).

The most appropriate place to exteriorize the intestine is on the right flank in a dependent portion. The thick musculature of the dorsal and lateral flank in larger swine will cause intestinal ischemia in the segment passing through the muscle. Toward the ventral portion of the abdominal wall, the muscle becomes much thinner. This problem is negated if the intestine is isolated in this area. The skin and muscle are incised, and the open end of the intestine is passed through the incision, care being taken to avoid spilling intestinal contents into the musculature. This can be facilitated by clamping the open end with atraumatic intestinal forceps. The end of the intestinal loop is sutured to the subcuticular layer of the skin using simple interrupted sutures with a monofilament nonabsorbable suture. Instead of exteriorizing the end of the intestine, it may be cannulated and left in the abdomen with only the prosthetic port exteriorized.

A model of jejunoileal bypass has been developed in swine to study nutritional complications associated with the procedure (Assimos et al., 1986). The intestine is divided caudal to the duodenum. The junction of the duodenum and jejunum is indistinct; however, it is generally considered to be caudal to the loop of the duodenum that passes cranially and then laterally from the caudal end of the body of the pancreas. The cranial end of the jejunum is oversewn and sutured to the cranial abdominal wall to prevent intussusception. The ileum is transected close to the ileocecal junction. The end of the duodenum is sutured in an end-to-end fashion to the distal end of the transected ileum. The transected proximal end of the ileum is sutured in an end-to-side technique to the ventrolateral portion of the spiral colon. This results in an almost complete bypass of the jejunum and ileum. Postoperatively, swine continue to maintain their weight with few gastrointestinal complications.

Potential methods of bypassing and fistulating the intestine are almost limitless. These more traditional procedures were chosen to illustrate specific surgical considerations in swine.

COLONIC ANASTOMOSIS AND FISTULATION

The procedures described for anastomosis and fistulation of the small intestine may be applied to the large intestine, after a consideration of the unique anatomy in the pig, especially the spiral colon (Eubanks et al., 2006; Harvey et al., 2001; Swindle, Harvey et al., 1998). The spiral colon, which contains the cecum and ascending colon, is approached through a cranial midline incision and, in larger animals, may have to be extended caudal to the umbilicus. The short transverse colon can be approached through the same incision. The descending colon may either be approached through a caudal midline incision in females or a left paramedian incision in males similar to the approach described earlier for the jejunum. A schematic diagram of the anatomy and direction of peristalsis is depicted in Figure 4.29.

Anastomosis of the descending colon may be performed in a similar manner as described for the small intestine; however, it is necessary to close the colon with two layers of sutures, preferably

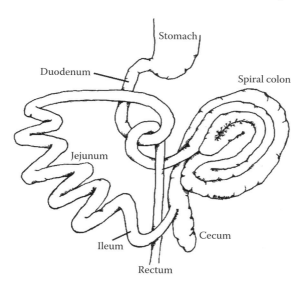

FIGURE 4.29 Schematic of the gastrointestinal (GI) tract illustrating the direction of peristalsis and the orientation of the spiral colon.

synthetic absorbables. The internal suture pattern should be continuous or simple interrupted. The outer layer should be closed with simple inverting Lembert sutures. It is essential to prevent contamination of the abdomen with colonic contents by careful packing of the colon prior to incising it and copious flushing of the finished incision.

The spiral colon is not amenable to anastomosis using standard techniques because of its unique anatomy (Figure 4.11 and Figure 4.29). In the research setting, anastomosis is not likely to be attempted. However, the use of fistulas for the study of colonic contents, transport mechanisms, or infusion of pharmacological agents may be indicated. In this case, the area of the colon to be fistulated may be readily identified by its gross anatomic characteristics. The spiral colon lies in the left upper quadrant of the abdomen and contains the cecum and the majority of the ascending colon in an outer centripetal coil and an inner centrifugal coil. The cecum is located in the caudal aspect and is joined by the ileum at the base of the spiral colon dorsally adjacent to the left kidney and pancreas. A vermiform appendix is not present. The outer coil continues ventrally in a clockwise pattern (from the dorsal perspective) to form the apex. The outer coil contains two tenia. The inner centrifugal coil does not contain tenia and progresses dorsally until it exits cranially at the base of the spiral colon. The transverse colon is short and quickly turns caudally to form the descending colon. A true sigmoid flexure, analogous to humans, is not present prior to its transformation into the rectum in the pelvic cavity (Schantz et al., 1996).

Fistulas and ports may also be created in the same manner as for the small intestine (Figure 4.19). For the cecum and large intestine, however, they need to be exteriorized on the left flank caudal to the last rib (Eubanks et al., 2006; Harvey et al., 2001; Swindle et al., 1998a). If functional ostomies, such as colostomies, are performed then they are best exteriorized on the thin-walled dependent portion of the abdomen to minimize skin contact with the excreta. Spiral colon bypass has been described to treat clinical stricture in a Vietnamese potbellied pig (Gallardo et al., 2003). In this case a fecal impaction was relieved by side-to-side anastomosis of the proximal centripetal loop to the distal straight centrifugal loop of the spiral colon. This type of procedure might be employed in a research setting for partial colonic bypass procedures.

TOTAL COLECTOMY

A total colectomy may be performed in the pig. In the experimental setting this would usually be performed to simulate the conditions of colectomy following necrotizing enterocolitis or trauma. The bowel prep should include hypertonic purgatives and antibiotics preoperatively. The ileum should be transected at the ileocecal junction and the spiral colon retracted caudally to expose the branches of the cranial mesenteric artery that provide blood supply to the structure. The dissection is continued caudally while ligating the arterial and venous branches supplying the mesocolon. The arterial branches are major subdivisions of the cranial and caudal mesenteric arteries, but the mesenteric veins have to be ligated separately. The transected ileum can be anastomosed, using an end-to-side or side-to-side anastomosis technique, to the rectum. Prior to transection of the large bowel, it should be ascertained that the ileum can be stretched to reach the area of transection.

The major postoperative complication will be diarrhea and nutritional deficiencies related to the shortened bowel. This surgery creates a similar condition as that which occurs with short-bowel syndrome in humans (Dudgeon et al., 1988). Spiral colon bypass with a side-to-side anastomosis of the proximal centripetal loop to the distal centrifugal loop has been described to clinically treat stricture in the spiral colon in geriatric potbellied pigs (Gallardo et al., 2003).

RECTAL PROLAPSE

Rectal prolapse is a clinical condition that may result secondarily to any condition that results in rectal straining such as diarrhea. It can also be produced experimentally by surgically prolapsing the rectum through the anus from a laparotomy.

Primary treatment should be targeted at reducing the swelling due to vascular congestion and edema, prior to replacement of the prolapsed segment into the pelvic cavity. If necrosis has already occurred, then the prolapsed segment must be amputated and a colonic resection performed. If the prolapsed segment is healthy, then swelling can be reduced by rinsing with hypertonic solutions such as 50% glucose. The segment should be lubricated with a water-soluble lubricant and replaced by gentle digital manipulation. A purse-string suture can be placed around the rectum temporarily to help prevent recurrence while the swelling is reduced and the condition is stabilized. A variety of prostheses have been developed to place into the rectum during this phase.

If the rectum must be amputated, then it is best accomplished with surgical staples. However, the prolapsed section of the rectum may be surgically amputated to the level of normal tissue and manually sutured, using an interlocking continuous suture with synthetic absorbable sutures. In young animals, prostheses may be placed in the rectum and rubber bands applied over the prostheses to cause necrosis of the prolapsed section of the rectum. This technique is employed in agricultural situations in the field and generally should not be used in laboratory settings in which there is availability of general anesthesia and surgical technologies (Kjar, 1976; St-Jean and Anderson, 1999; Turner and Mellwrath, 1982). Recurrence is likely if the primary cause of the prolapse is not treated.

INTESTINAL AND MULTIVISCERAL TRANSPLANTATION

Heterotopic and orthotopic transplantation of the small bowel has been described in swine. They have also been used as a model of multivisceral transplantation. Both models are performed from a ventral midline incision that may extend the complete length of the abdomen in a complex model, such as multivisceral *en bloc* transplantation (Alessiani et al., 1998; Podesta et al., 1994; Pritchard and Kirkman, 1988; Pritchard et al., 1986; Ricour et al., 1983).

An isolated loop of small intestine from the jejunum to the ileum is isolated and divided between intestinal clamps as described earlier for an intestinal anastomosis. The mesentery is divided, and the segment of the cranial mesenteric artery and vein supplying the graft are identified. In this region, the vessels will have the largest diameter. The donor is heparinized, and the segment of the artery and vein are divided. The graft is flushed with chilled heparinized crystalloid solution, and the donor is sacrificed.

Using a ventral midline incision, the recipient's infrarenal aorta and vena cava are isolated. The graft is placed transversely into the abdomen, and the cranial mesenteric artery and vein are sutured in turn in an end-to-side manner to the aorta and vena cava using Satinsky clamps. The transplanted graft is placed carefully to avoid torsion of the stump. The ends of the graft are isolated as stomas in the ventral abdomen as described earlier for Thiry-Vella loops (Figure 4.30).

For orthotopic transplant, the terminal ileum is used, allowing the surgeon to use the most accessible vessels supplying the graft. The segment of bowel is isolated as described earlier, except that only a branch of the mesenteric vessels supplying the segment is divided. Consequently, this may be done as a survival procedure for the donor, because the rest of the bowel is not devascularized as described for the heterotopic transplant. A reciprocal transplant may be performed with the recipient of this graft as well, if the experimental design allows it. The graft is sutured in an end-to-end pattern to the recipient's mesenteric vessels after a similar segment of small bowel has been extricated.

Multivisceral transplantation of the liver, stomach, duodenum, pancreas, small intestine, and a portion of the large intestine has been developed in swine (Figure 4.31). The donor is prepared in a standard fashion for a ventral midline incision from the xiphoid process to the pubis. The aorta and vena cava are isolated cranial to the liver and extending caudally to the kidneys, ensuring that the celiac, cranial mesenteric, and caudal mesenteric vessels are retained intact, but ligation of the lumbar branches is necessary. The esophagus is clamped and divided at its junction with the stomach, and the descending colon is divided distal to the major blood supply of the caudal

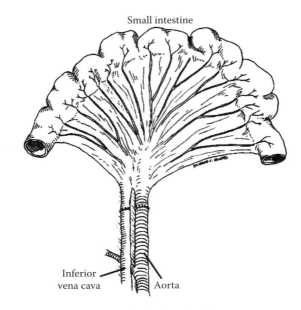

FIGURE 4.30 Segmental intestinal transplant with fistulated ends.

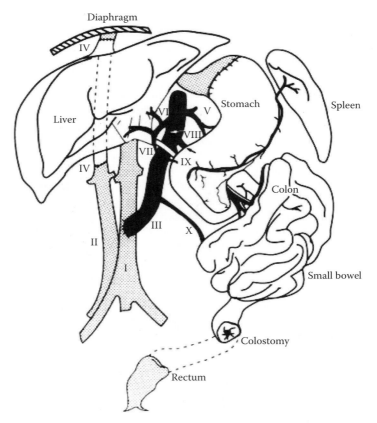

FIGURE 4.31 Diagram of multivisceral transplantation. (Reprinted from Podesta et al., 1994, in Cramer, D.V. et al., Eds., *Handbook of Animal Models in Transplantation Research*, Boca Raton, FL: CRC Press. With permission.)

mesenteric artery. The vessels supplying the kidneys, adrenals, and mesentery are sacrificed so that only the three major vessels listed earlier remain. The ligaments of the liver are divided so that all the *en bloc* viscera are mobilized.

Cannulae are placed in the proximal and terminal aorta, and cold perfusion is initiated after heparinization. The perfusate is removed using suction in the right atrium. After perfusion is under way, the remaining attachments are divided, and the block of viscera is transferred to a bowl of cold perfusate and preservation solution. The proximal end of the aorta is oversewn.

The recipient is prepared in a similar manner to the donor. A veno-veno bypass is prepared between the external jugular vein and the femoral vein. The colon and stomach are transected leaving a portion of the antrum of the stomach intact. The abdominal aorta is preserved in its entirety, including the kidneys. The vena cava remains intact, except for the portion that is intra-hepatic. The vessels are transected starting with the liver, and veno-veno bypass is initiated at the time that the celiac trunk and the cranial mesenteric artery are divided. This is the last step prior to removal of the organs.

The vessels of the donor organs are anastomosed into the recipient in the following order: suprahepatic vena cava, infrahepatic vena cava, and distal donor aorta to recipient infrarenal aorta in an end-to-side pattern. At this time, the aortic clamp is removed and the reperfusion process, including removal of the veno-veno bypass, is initiated. The intestinal tract continuity is reestab-lished in a standard fashion, by sewing the donor stomach to the recipient stomach cuff in an end-to-side pattern, and reanastomosing the colon in an end-to-end pattern.

Intraoperative monitoring and homeostasis control is a substantial task with this type of surgery, and hemodynamic control is of prime importance. Postoperative monitoring and reinitiation of oral nutrition is also a substantive issue. The list of complications to be considered in addition to the issues of graft vs. host disease and rejection include hemorrhage, ascites, thrombosis, infection, and malabsorption. This type of study should include a multidisciplinary team approach to these issues.

VAGOTOMY

The vagus nerve may be transected intra-abdominally as the branches of the nerve traverse along the esophagus cranial to the esophageal sphincter at the cardia of the stomach (Figure 4.32). Using a midline approach, the stomach can be retracted caudally and the liver, cranially to expose the caudal esophagus. The fascia over the esophagus is opened with scissors, and the branches of the vagus nerve can be observed along the ventral border on either side of the esophagus. The nerves can be transected with scissors and the fascia resutured. A section of the nerve can be removed to ensure that the transection remains permanent (Josephs et al., 1992; Swindle, 1983).

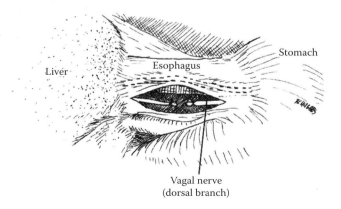

FIGURE 4.32 Technique of truncal vagotomy.

Selective vagotomy can be performed by tracing branches of the nerve, as they are associated with the blood vessels supplying the lesser curvature of the stomach. In a similar fashion to the truncal vagotomy described earlier, each nerve branch is isolated and severed. Manipulation of the vagus nerve has been associated with bradycardia and cardiac arrest in some cases. It is best to keep the animal atropinized during manipulation of the main branches of this nerve (Josephs et al., 1992).

INTRAPERITONEAL SEPSIS, SEPTIC SHOCK, AND HEMORRHAGIC SHOCK

Intraperitoneal sepsis leading to septic shock may be induced in swine by a variety of methods. Surgical incisions in various portions of the intestine leading to intestinal content leakage as well as infusion of lipopolysaccharides (LPSs) are standard methodologies in many species (Bathe et al., 1998; Greif and Forse, 1998; Hoban et al., 1992; Horstmann et al., 2002; Krones et al., 2005; Strate et al., 2003). Depending upon the clinical syndrome being investigated, perforations of the stomach, small intestine, and cecum will lead to development of a syndrome similar to the human situation. These procedures may be performed laparoscopically or endoscopically to avoid the complications of open abdominal incisional sepsis. Ischemia of the small bowel may also be induced by ligation of mesenteric vessels, or creation of pericardial tamponade by infusion of fluid into the pericardial sac, which leads to the development of decreased splancnic blood flow. Reversible intestinal ischemia may be accomplished by reversing the pericardial tamponade (cardiogenic shock) or by using clamps rather than ligatures to decrease mesenteric blood supply to the intestine (Bailey et al., 1986). LPS infusions at a rate of 1 µg/kg over a 30- to 60-min time frame will also induce the symptoms of septic shock. Alternatively, *Escherichia coli* strain B7 may be infused into the peritoneal cavity at a rate of 2×10^{10} cfu/kg to produce sepsis nonsurgically.

The porcine model has the advantage of being a large animal model with a cardiovascular systemic response similar to that of humans. Swine initially develop a hypodynamic state which progresses to a hyperdynamic state within 24 h, with increased cardiac output, pulmonary hypertension, and decreased systemic vascular resistance. Multiple systemic organ failure occurs with chronic models (Hoban et al., 1992).

Hemorrhagic shock models in swine have been reviewed (Hannon, 1992). In general, two types of models are employed: fixed pressure (Wiggers model) and fixed volume hemorrhage. Fixed volume hemorrhage is more clinically applicable and relevant to the condition that occurs with trauma patients. A predetermined amount of blood is removed via a catheter implanted in the carotid artery (Chapter 9). For awake models the catheter implantation procedure should be performed 1–2 weeks prior to the study, to allow wound healing to occur and platelet levels to return to normal. Porcine models respond to various levels of hemorrhage in a similar manner to humans.

Endotoxic and hemorrhagic shock models can be performed without anesthesia; however, precautions have to be taken to ensure that animal pain and distress are monitored and controlled. In general, infusions of opioids, such as sufentanil, will have the least effects on cardiovascular parameters during these procedures. If an anesthetized animal is used for the studies, then the selection process of the anesthetic regimen must include a determination of the agents that will have the least effects on the parameters being studied.

REFERENCES

Alessiani, M., Spada, M., Vaccarisi, S., Fayer, F., Puletti, G., Ruggiero, R., Bellinzona, G., Noli, S., Scandone, M., Maestri, M., Dionigi, P., and Zonata, A., 1998, Multivisceral transplantation in pigs: technical aspects, *Transplant. Proc.*, 30(6): 2627–2628.

Anderson, D.E., Kim, J.H., Hancock, J.D., and Han, I.K., 2000, Method and complications of ileocutaneous anastomosis for collection of ileal digesta in neonatal pigs, *Contemp. Top. Lab. Anim. Sci.*, 39(5): 26–28.

Assimos, D.G., Boyce, W.H., Lively, M., Weidner, N., Lewis, J.C., Howard, G., Furr, E., Sorrell, M., McCullough, D.L., Bullock, B.C., and Palmer, T.E., 1986, Porcine urologic models including jejunoileal bypass, in Tumbleson, M.E., Ed., *Swine in Biomedical Research*, Vol. 1, New York: Plenum Press, pp. 399–424.

Bailey, R.W., Oshima, A., O'Roark, W.A., and Bulkley, G.B., 1986, A reproducible, quantitatable and rapidly reversible model of cardiogenic shock in swine, in Tumbleson, M.E., Ed., *Swine in Biomedical Research*, Vol. 1, New York: Plenum Press, pp. 363–372.

Bathe, O.F., Rudston-Brown, B., Chow, A.W., and Phang, P.T., 1998, Liver as a focus of impaired oxygenation and cytokine production in a porcine model of endotoxicosis, *Crit. Care Med.*, 26(10): 1698–1706.

Becker, B.A., Niwano, Y., and Johnson, H.D., 1992, Physiologic and immune responses associated with 48-hour fast of pigs, *Lab. Anim. Sci.*, 42(1): 51–53.

Brenner, A., Marchesini, J.B., Bellaver, C., and Flores, R., 2001, Surgical stomach reduction in swine as a model of human obesity, in Lindberg, J.E. and Ogle, B., Eds., *Digestive Physiology of Pigs*, New York: CABI Publishing, pp. 360–365.

Casteel, S.W., Brown, L.D., Lattimer, J., and Dunsmore, M., 1998, Fasting and feeding effects on gastric emptying time in juvenile swine, *Contemp. Top. Lab. Anim. Sci.*, 37(3): 106–108.

Dudgeon, D.L., Gadacz, T.R., Gladen, H.E., Lillemoe, K.D., and Swindle, M.M., 1988, Alimentary tract and liver, in Swindle, M.M. and Adams, R.J., Eds., *Experimental Surgery and Physiology: Induced Animal Models of Human Disease*, Baltimore, MD: Williams and Wilkins, pp. 217–257.

Eubanks, D.L., Cooper, R., and Boring, J.G., 2006, Surgical technique for long-term cecal cannulation in the Yucatan minipig, *J. Am. Assoc. Lab. Anim. Sci.*, 45(1): 52–56.

Fleming, S.E. and Arce, D., 1986, Using the pig to study digestion and fermentation in the gut, in Tumbleson, M.E., Ed., *Swine in Biomedical Research*, Vol. 1, New York: Plenum Press, pp. 123–134.

Gades, N.M. and Mandrell, T.D., 2001, Nonendoscopic placement and use of percutaneous gastrostomy tubes in pigs, *Contemp. Top. Lab. Anim. Sci.*, 40(2): 37–39.

Gallardo, M.A., Lawhorn, D.B., Taylor, T.S., and Walker, M.A., 2003, Spiral colon bypass in a geriatric Vietnamese potbellied pig, *J. Am. Vet. Med. Assoc.*, 222(10): 1408–1412.

Greif, W.M. and Forse, R.A., 1998, Hemodynamic effects of the laparoscopic pneumoperitoneum during sepsis in a porcine endotoxic shock model, *Annal. Surg.*, 227(4): 474–480.

Hand, M.S., Phillips, R.W., Miller, C.W., Mason, R.A., and Lumb, W.V., 1981, A method for quantitation of hepatic, pancreatic and intestinal function in conscious Yucatan miniature swine, *Lab. Anim. Sci.*, 31(6): 728–731.

Hannon, J.P., 1992, Hemorrhage and hemorrhagic shock in swine: a review, in *Swine as Models in Biomedical Research*, Ames, IA: Iowa State University Press, pp. 197–245.

Harvey, R.B., Anderson, R.C., Young, C.R., Swindle, M.M., Genovese, K.J., Hume, M.E., Droleskey, R.E., Farrington, L.A., Ziprin, R.L., and Nisbet, D.J., 2001, Effects of feed withdrawal and transport on cecal environment and *Campylobacter* concentrations in a swine surgical model, *J. Food Prot.*, 64(5): 780–733.

Hennig, U., Idzior, B., Wunsche, J., and Bock, H.D., 1980, Fistulation technique for the digestive tract of swine for the examination of protein metabolism, *Arch. Exp. Veterinarmed.*, 34(3): 325–331.

Hoban, L.D., Paschall, J.A., Eckstein, J., Nadkarni, V., Lee, C.R., Williams, T.J., Reusch, D., Nevola, J.J., and Carcillo, J.A., 1992, Awake porcine model of intraperitoneal sepsis, in Swindle, M.M., Ed., *Swine as Models in Biomedical Research*, Ames, IA: Iowa State University Press, pp. 246–264.

Horstmann, R., Palmes, D., Rupp, D., Hohlbach, G., and Spiegel, H.U., 2002, Laparoscopic fluorometry: a new minimally invasive tool for investigation of the intestinal microcirculation, *J. Invest. Surg.*, 15(4): 343–350.

Josephs, L.G., Arnold, J.H., and Sawyers, J.L., 1992, Laparoscopic highly selective vagotomy, *J. Laparoendosc. Surg.*, 2(3): 151–153.

Kjar, H.A., 1976, Amputation of prolapsed rectum in young pigs, *J. Am. Vet. Med. Assoc.*, 168(3): 229–230.

Kopchok, G.E., Cavaye, D.M., Klein, S.R., Mueller, M.P., Lee, J.L., and White, R.A., 1993, Endoscopic surgery training: application of an in vitro trainer and in vivo swine model, *J. Invest. Surg.*, 6(4): 329–337.

Krones, C.J., Klosterhalfen, B., Butz, N., Hoelz, F., Junge, K., Stumpf, M., Peiper, C., Klinge, U., and Schumpelick, V., 2005, Effect of zinc pretreatment on pulmonary endothelial cells in vitro and pulmonary function in a porcine model of endotoxemia, *J. Surg. Res.*, 123(2): 251–256.

Markowitz, J., Archibald, J., and Downie, H.G., 1964, *Experimental Surgery*, 5th ed., Baltimore, MD: Williams and Wilkins.

Noel, P., Fagot, H., Fabre, J.M., Mann, C., Quenet, F., Guillon, F., Baumel, H., and Domergue, J., 1994, Resection anastomosis of the small intestine by celioscopy in swine: comparative experimental study between manual and mechanical anastomosis, *Ann. Chir.*, 48(10): 921–929.

Olson, K.H., Balcos, E.G., Lowe, M.C., and Bubrick, M.P., 1995, A comparative study of open, laparoscopic intracorporeal and laparoscopic assisted low anterior resection and anastomosis in pigs, *Am. Surgeon*, 61(3): 197–201.

Pekas, J.C., 1983, A method for direct gastric feeding and the effect on voluntary ingestion in young swine, *Appetite*, 4(1): 23–30.

Podesta, L., Cramer, D.V., Makowka, L., and Nores, M., 1994, Multivisceral transplantation in the pig, in Cramer, D.V., Podesta, L., and Makowka, L., Eds., *Handbook of Animal Models in Transplantation Research*, Boca Raton, FL: CRC Press, pp. 231–242.

Pritchard, T.J. and Kirkman, R.L., 1988, Transplantation of the gastrointestinal tract: small intestine, in Swindle, M.M. and Adams, R.J., Eds., *Experimental Surgery and Physiology: Induced Animal Models of Human Disease*, Baltimore, MD: Williams and Wilkins, pp. 291–293.

Pritchard, T.J., Kottun, W.A., and Kirkman, R.L., 1986, Technical aspects of small intestinal transplantation in young pigs, in Tumbleson, M.E., Ed., *Swine in Biomedical Research*, Vol. 1, New York: Plenum Press, pp. 391–398.

Ricour, C., Revillon, Y., Arnaud-Battandier, F., Ghnassia, D., Weyne, P., Lauffenburger, A., Jos, J., Fontaine, J.L., Gallix, P., and Vaiman, M., 1983, Successful small bowel allografts in piglets using cyclosporine, *Transplant. Proc.*, 15(Suppl. 1–2): 3019–3026.

Sangild, P.T., 2001, Transitions in the life of the gut at birth, in Lindberg, J.E. and Ogle, B., Eds., *Digestive Physiology of Pigs*, New York: CABI Publishing, pp. 3–16.

Schantz, L.D., Laber-Laird, K., Bingel, S., and Swindle, M., 1996, Pigs: applied anatomy of the gastrointestinal tract, in Jensen, S.L., Gregersen, H., Moody, F., and Shokouh-Amiri, M.H., Eds., *Essentials of Experimental Surgery: Gastroenterology*, New York: Harwood Academic Publishers, pp. 2611–2619.

Schopf, B.W., Blair, G., Dong, S., and Troger, K., 1997, A porcine model of gastrointestinal reflux, *J. Invest. Surg.*, 10(2): 105–114.

St-Jean, G. and Anderson, D.E., 1999, Surgical procedures in boars and sows, in Straw, B.E., D'Allaire, S., Mengeling, W.L., and Taylor, D.J., Eds., *Diseases of Swine*, 8th ed., Ames, IA: Iowa State University Press, pp. 1133–1155.

Strate, T., Schneider, C., Yekebas, E., Knoefel, W.T., Bloechle, C., and Izbicki, J.R., 2003, Systemic endotoxin and gastric mucosal pH are the best parameters to predict lethal outcome in a porcine model of abdominal sepsis according to multivariate analysis, *J. Invest. Surg.*, 16(1): 13–21.

Swindle, M.M., 1983, *Basic Surgical Exercises Using Swine*, Philadelphia, PA: Praeger Press.

Swindle, M.M., Harvey, R.B., Kasseri, E., and Buckley, S.A., 1998a, Chronic cecal cannulation in Yucatan miniature swine, *Contemp. Top. Lab. Anim. Sci.*, 37(6): 56–58.

Swindle, M.M., Smith, A.C., and Goodrich, J.G., 1998b, Chronic cannulation and fistulization techniques in swine: a review and recommendations, *J. Invest. Surg.*, 11(1): 4–14.

Swindle, M.M., Nolan, T., Jacobson, A., Wolf, P., Dalton, M.J., and Smith, A.C., 2005, Vascular access port (VAP) usage in large animal species, *Contemp. Top. Lab. Anim. Sci.*, 44(3): 7–17.

Turner, A.S. and Mellwrath, C.W., 1982, *Techniques in Large Animal Surgery*, Philadelphia, PA: Lea and Febiger, pp. 309–317.

Wubben, J.E., Smiricky, M.R., Albin, D.M., and Gabert, V.M., 2001, Improved procedure and cannula design for simple T cannulation at the distal ileum in growing pigs, *Contemp. Top. Lab. Anim. Sci.*, 40(6): 27–31.

Yen, J.T., 2001, Digestive system, in Pond, W.G. and Mersmann, H.J., Eds., *Biology of the Domestic Pig*, Ithaca, NY: Cornell University Press, pp. 399–453.

5 Liver and Biliary System

SURGICAL ANATOMY AND GENERAL PRINCIPLES OF SURGERY

From a surgical standpoint, the liver and gallbladder of the pig have relatively few differences from those of humans (Figure 5.1 and Figure 5.2). The bile duct of the pig enters the duodenum 2–5 cm from the pylorus, separately from the pancreatic duct. The sizes of the bile duct and sphincter of Oddi are variable depending upon the size and breed of the pig (Table 5.1). The diameter of the bile duct seems to vary substantially even in the same size and breed of pig; however, it readily dilates when catheterized. Normal pressure in the common bile duct is usually less than 10 cm H_2O.

The liver contains six lobes: the left lateral, the left medial, the quadrate, the right medial, the right lateral, and the caudate, which contains a caudate process partially surrounding the caudal vena cava. The gallbladder is located in a fossa formed by the left and right medial and quadrate lobes in the right upper quadrant of the abdomen. The liver decreases as a percentage of body weight (BW) with age, from 3% at birth to 1.5% at sexual maturity in farm pigs (Yen, 2001). The segmental anatomy of the liver has been studied extensively and has been found to be very similar to that of the human, in terms of the vascularity and biliary tree (Court et al., 2003; Farinon et al., 1981).

Bile production is variable, depending upon the weight and breed of the pig, frequency of feeding, and the composition of the diet, and normals must be established for each laboratory. As a general guideline, bile production in farm pigs is 0.6–1.1 ml $kg^{-1}h^{-1}$. This is extrapolated from studies of 24-h bile flow in instrumented farm pigs that had ranges of 45–60 kg BW and 24-h collections of 30–60 ml/kg bile (Yen, 2001), as well as from measurements made by the author on anesthetized animals. Composition of bile in swine (electrolytes, bile salts, phospholipids, cholesterol, mucus, pigments) is similar to that in most mammals, except that it has little cholic acid and a bile salt:phospholipid concentration of 9:1. Bile salts are reabsorbed from the small intestine and undergo enterohepatic recirculation, which helps to meet the metabolic demand (Yen, 2001).

The size and volume of the gallbladder is also variable, but, in a sexually mature pig, it measures approximately 3 cm wide by 5 cm long at the maximum points and contains about 25 ml of bile in a fasted animal at surgery. The hepatic bile duct exits the liver caudally dorsal to the gallbladder. It joins the cystic and common bile ducts shortly after entering the porta hepaticus. The bile duct is located in the porta hepaticus ventral to the portal vein and hepatic artery. It may be identified as a translucent tubular structure within the mesenteric attachments in this area, and it courses caudally to enter the duodenum as a separate duct from the pancreatic duct.

The hepatic artery and the portal vein enter the liver in close approximation to the common bile duct. Lymph nodes and fascia in the area make the dissection of these structures difficult. The liver of the pig is friable, but contains fibrous septations between lobules, which can be readily noted histologically (Figure 5.3) (Schantz et al., 1996).

The metabolic functions of the porcine liver are more similar to the human liver than even to those of most species of primates (Table 5.2). Consequently, interest in xenografic procedures has increased as immunosuppressive and transgenic technologies have improved (Institute of Medicine, 1996; Ryabinin, 1996). A porcine model of acute and chronic hepatic hemodynamics and metabolism of glucose, lactate, alanine, and glycerol was developed and validated because of its simi-

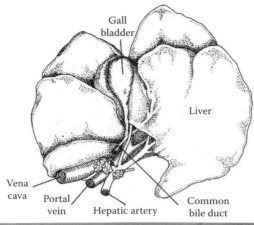

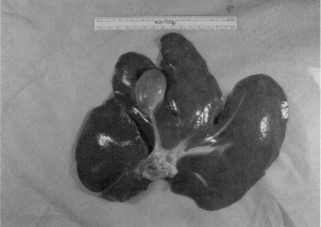

FIGURE 5.1 Visceral surface of the liver.

larities to human metabolism (Drougas et al., 1996). In a comprehensive study of hepatic hemo-dynamics (Drougas et al., 1996) in chronically catheterized conscious farm pigs 8–16 weeks of age (20–70 kg BW), total hepatic blood flow was found to be approximately 1100 ml/min, hepatic arterial pressure was equivalent to aortic pressure, portal vein pressure was approximately 8 mmHg, and hepatic vein pressure was approximately 4 mmHg (Table 5.3). There is an inverse relationship between hepatic arterial blood flow and portal vein blood flow, in that an increase in blood flow in one circuit leads to an increase in blood flow resistance in the other circuit. In general, approx-imately 25% of the cardiac output is included in total hepatic blood flow.

The cytochrome P450 system in swine has similar enzymatic activity to that in humans, except for the low level of CYP2C and the absence of CYP2D. Females have higher levels of some enzymes (CYP1A, CYP2E) than males (Skaanild and Friis, 1997; Skaanild and Friis, 1999). Bama miniature pigs have had their drug metabolizing activities compared with humans by using selective inhibitors of human CYP isozymes (Li et al., 2006). They found that the liver microsomes for metabolism of nifedipine and testosterone (CYP3A4) are similar to those in humans. Their results are summarized in Table 5.4. The oxidative biotransformation function of the liver is similar to that in humans; there is a high level of glucuronidation and acetylation, and low activity of sulfation (Skaanild and Friis, 1997). More information is available in Chapter 15.

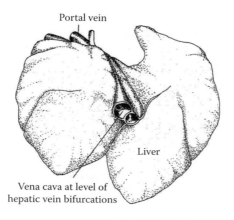

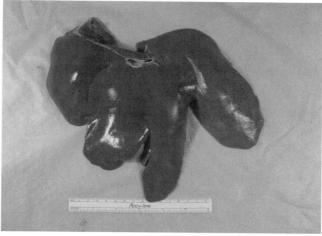

FIGURE 5.2 Diaphragmatic surface of the liver.

TABLE 5.1
Sample Sizes of Common Bile Duct Based upon Measurements

Breed	Weight (kg)	Bile Duct Diameter, ID[a] (mm)
Yucatan	29	3.0
	52	2.7–3.7
Yorkshire	16	3.0
	20	2.3
Landrace	47	2.7
	70	8–12

[a] ID = inside dimension.

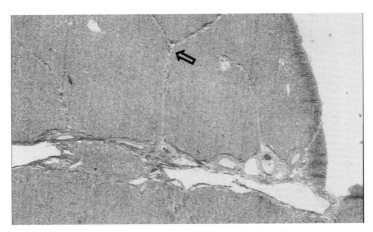

FIGURE 5.3 Histology of the liver illustrating fibrous septae (arrow). H&E, ×100.

TABLE 5.2
Hepatic, Gut, and Total Splanchnic Glucose Metabolic Data
(farm pigs, 3–4 months of age)

	Mean ± SEM			
Variable	Glucose	Lactate	Alanine	Glycerol
Arterial value (mm/l)	4.6 ± 0.3	0.53 ± 0.07	0.30 ± 0.07	0.12 ± 0.02
Hepatic fractional extraction rate (%)	—	24 ± 4	21 ± 7	22 ± 5
Net hepatic balance (μmol/kg per min)	9.9 ± 4.0	4.2 ± 0.4	2.3 ± 1.1	0.68 ± 0.22
Net gut balance (μmol/kg per min)	2.0 ± 2.5	1.1 ± 0.5	0.73 ± 0.18	0.69 ± 0.19
Net splanchnic balance (μmol/kg per min)	7.7 ± 1.9	3.1 ± 0.2	1.5 ± 1.1	1.4 ± 0.3

Source: Reprinted from Drougas et al., 1996, *Lab. Anim. Sci.* 46(6): 648–655. With permission.

CHOLECYSTECTOMY

The gallbladder can be approached with a right paramedian celiotomy incision lateral to the mammary glands, starting cranially at the caudal border of the last rib (Figure 5.4). The length of the incision will be variable, depending upon the size of the pig. Care should be taken to avoid the cranial epigastric vessels in the same area. The area of interest can be isolated with either laparotomy sponges or self-retaining retractors. The ventral tip of the gallbladder should be grasped with gallbladder forceps and gentle finger dissection can be used to separate it from the liver. The technique involves applying gentle pressure caudally with the forceps while making gentle side-to-side movements with the tip of the finger. Experience has shown that only in larger adult swine is it necessary to use other surgical instruments either to cut or cauterize during the dissection. Rupture of the gallbladder is rare if gentle handling and atraumatic forceps are used. The cystic duct is cross-clamped with two pairs of right-angle forceps and cut between them following the gallbladder dissection. A double ligature with synthetic absorbable sutures is applied to the stump of the duct. Hemostasis in the gallbladder fossa is usually achieved by packing the area with gauze sponges for 3–5 min. Oxycellulose sponges may be placed in the fossa for extra security against hemorrhage. Prior to closure of the incision, any bile that has leaked into the peritoneal cavity should be removed by flushing and suction. The peritoneum, muscle layers, and skin are closed routinely (Swindle, 1983).

TABLE 5.3
Hemodynamic Data (farm pig, 3–4 months of age)

Variable	Units	Intraoperative Mean	Final Mean	Steady State (d)	*P* Value
CO	l/min	4.46 ± 0.08	7.19 ± 0.15	2.4	0.002
CAP	mmHg	65 ± 3	101 ± 2	1.8	0.0001
PVP	mmHg	5.3 ± 0.9	7.8 ± 0.5	2.1	0.07
HVP	mmHg	2.0 ± 1.0	4.3 ± 0.4	1.3	0.12
PAP	mmHg	11.7 ± 1.2	21.4 ± 2.1	3.2	0.08
JVP	mmHg	2.9 ± 1.2	1.0 ± 0.3	1.8	0.10
HR	Beats/min	112 ± 4	116 ± 4	5	0.35
HABF	ml/min	262 ± 33	116 ± 24	7.5	0.04
PVBF	ml/min	631 ± 91	880 ± 130	7.5	0.09
THBF	ml/min	799 ± 133	1132 ± 187	7.5	0.19
HABF	%	35.0 ± 3.0	15.5 ± 2.7	7.5	0.001
PVBF	%	65.0 ± 3.0	84.5 ± 2.7	7.5	0.001

Note: Intraoperative values measured under isoflurane anesthesia. Final mean values were from awake, chronically catheterized pigs. CO = cardiac output, CAP = carotid artery pressure, PVP = portal vein pressure, HVP = hepatic vein pressure, PAP = pulmonary artery pressure, JVP = jugular vein pressure, HR = heart rate, HABF = hepatic artery blood flow, PVBF = portal vein blood flow, THBF = total hepatic blood flow.

Source: Reprinted from Drougas et al., 1996, *Lab. Anim. Sci.* 46(6): 648–655. With permission.

TABLE 5.4
Enzyme Activities (mean ± standard deviation) of Various Marker Reactions in Liver Microsomes from Chinese Bama Miniature Pigs and Humans

Substrate	Reaction	Activity[b] (mean ± standard deviation) Bama Miniature Pig (n = 6)	Human (n = 3)
Nifedipine	Oxidation	1414 ± 122	1360 ± 1102
Testosterone	6β-Hydroxylation	1140 ± 42	2065 ± 1380
Phenacetin	0-Deethylation	312 ± 49[a]	743 ± 236
Coumarin	7-Hydroxylation	30.8 ± 8.4[a]	392 ± 148
Dextromethorphan	0-Demethylation	2387 ± 264[a]	76 ± 59
Chlorzoxazone	6-Hydroxylation	278 ± 45[a]	538 ± 146

[a] $P < .05$ vs. value for human enzyme.
[b] Measured in pmol of product formed/min per mg microsomal protein.

Source: Reprinted from Li et al., 2006, *Comp. Med.*, 56(4): 286–290. With permission.

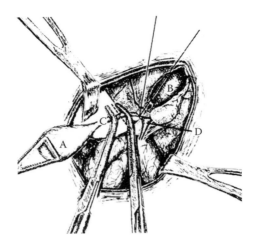

FIGURE 5.4 Cholecystectomy. A — gallbladder, B — fossa of gallbladder, C — cystic duct, D — common bile duct.

CANNULATION OR CONSTRICTION OF THE COMMON BILE DUCT

Reentrant cannulation of the common bile duct may be achieved with reasonable success if close attention is paid to the design of the cannula (Figure 5.5 and Figure 5.6). Generally, this procedure is performed simultaneously with a cholecystectomy to ensure that the bile sample collected is freshly produced by the liver and not stored in the gallbladder. The size of the bile duct will vary substantially, even at similar weights within the same breed. Typically, it is approximately 3 mm (inside dimension) in a 20–30 kg pig. However, most swine greater than 15 kg will accommodate at least a 5-French (Fr) catheter, and adult pigs can be cannulated with much larger catheters (Table 5.1).

Complete ligation of the common bile duct without cholecystectomy will result in great dilatation of the gallbladder and ductal system within a few hours. The common and cystic ducts will be impressively dilated with an accompanying increase in intraductal pressure. In spite of the amount of dilatation, the onset of clinical symptoms of biliary stricture is delayed and variable between breeds and sizes of swine. As a general rule, however, swine will become symptomatic 3–4 weeks following surgery. Cholecystectomy at the time of placing the stricture will result in a more rapid onset of symptoms.

Total ligation or constriction of the bile duct should be performed close to the sphincter of Oddi at the distal end of the duct. The ligature can be made to include a premeasured rod laid along the bile duct. After the ligature is placed, the rod can be removed to achieve a stricture instead of a total blockage.

If cannulation of the duct is to be performed, then it should be a reentry cannulation, unless the procedure is to be performed acutely or the animal supplemented orally with bile salts. The general principle of reentry cannulation involves placing a small catheter proximally into the common bile duct, exteriorizing it with a port or valve on the skin to collect samples, and then returning the bile via another catheter into the duodenum. There are insignificant differences between having the intestinal catheter enter through the sphincter of Oddi or another location in the proximal duodenum.

Reentry biliary catheters are commercially available or may be custom designed. Catheters within the abdomen are generally constructed of silicone for flexibility. Having a combination polyethylene catheter helps avoid kinking of the catheter. The tips of the catheter that are placed inside the duct are more readily placed if they are made of the sturdier polyethylene material. Having suture retention beads on the catheter helps to ensure retention within the duct. Reentry

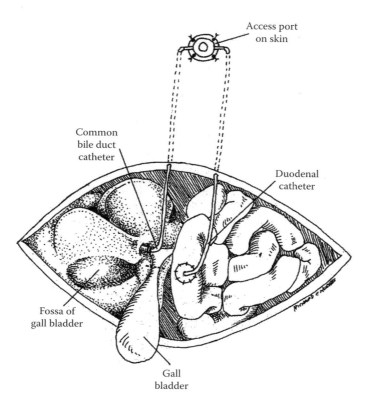

FIGURE 5.5 Reentrant cannulation of the bile duct.

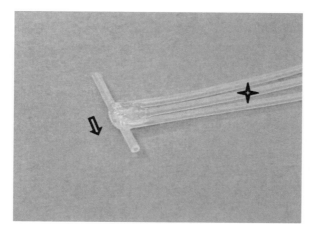

FIGURE 5.6 Reentrant cannula for bile duct and other continuous flow ducts (lymphatic, urinary). The arrow indicates the direction of normal bile flow. The star is on the catheter which inflates and deflates a balloon for occlusion of flow.

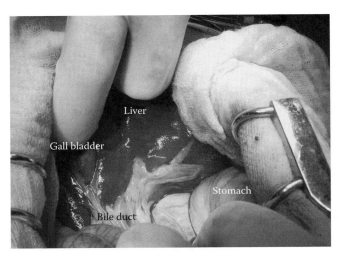

FIGURE 5.7 Surgical anatomy of the portal hiatus of the liver.

catheters typically cannulate both proximal and distal ends of the duct with a flow pathway from the hepatic side of the duct to a sampling port at the skin surface and then reflow into the duodenal side of the duct. Using this type of catheter, the flow of bile is interrupted for sampling by inflating a balloon in the catheter. Other types of catheters are inserted into the duct toward the liver with the distal end of the duct ligated. In this type of catheter, the flow of bile goes to a sampling port on the surface of the skin and then reflows into the duodenum through a catheter inserted into the duodenum. The reentrant catheter can be placed into the proximal duodenum, taking care not to disturb the pancreas or pancreatic duct. As per the description of the cannulae for an intestinal access port (Chapter 4), the catheter can be placed into the lumen of the duodenum after making a stab incision. The catheter should be open ended instead of slitlike according to the previous discussion of intestinal access ports. This modification is necessary because of the low pressure in the biliary system. In either design, the flow of bile from the liver to the duodenum is only interrupted during the sampling procedure.

A midline celiotomy is performed from the xiphoid process to the umbilicus. Self-retaining retractors and wetted laparotomy sponges are utilized to visualize the bile duct system in the right apical quadrant of the abdomen (Figure 5.7 and Figure 5.8). The gallbladder is visualized and squeezed lightly to illuminate the common bile duct with bile. The fascial tissue is dissected to expose the common duct. A wetted sponge is placed under the duct and an elastic vessel loop is preplaced cranial and caudal to the entry site for the catheter (Figure 5.9). After retraction, the duct is nicked with iris scissors. A vascular pick is utilized to open the lumen for catheterization (Figure 5.10). The catheter is inserted into the abdomen in the right cranial paramedian area of the abdominal wall, distant to the celiotomy incision.

When utilizing the T-tube catheter with an occlusal balloon, the tube is inserted cranially and then caudally in the common bile duct. Ligatures are placed around both ends of the catheter to keep it in place.

When utilizing the bypass catheter, the catheter with retention beads is placed retrograde into the duct. Ligatures are utilized cranially and caudally after insertion. The second duodenal catheter is inserted into the cranial duodenum with the retention bead inside the lumen. The catheter is held in place within the lumen with a purse-string suture and simple interrupted sutures through the cuff and the serosa.

If a cholecystectomy is to be performed, it is done at this time. The sampling port, which has been preplaced, is flushed with saline and a port pocket is made to place the device subcutaneously.

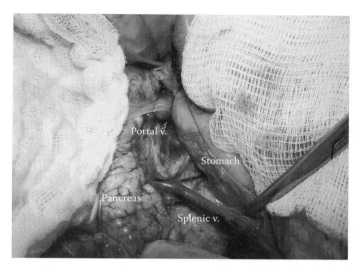

FIGURE 5.8 Surgical anatomy of the viscera and vasculature caudal to the portal hiatus.

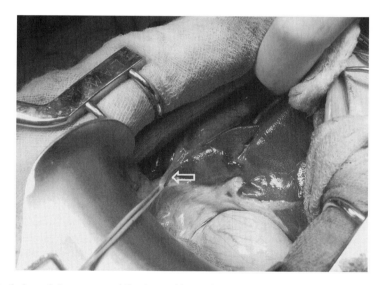

FIGURE 5.9 Isolation of the common bile duct with an elastic vessel loop.

For a procedure of only a few days, the sampling port may be sutured to the skin and protected with a circumferential bandage.

The abdomen is closed after sutures are placed in the peritoneum at the entrance of the two cannulae into the abdominal cavity to prevent a possible dehiscence. The midline incision is closed in a routine manner as described previously (Hand et al., 1981; Swindle, 1983; Terblanche and Van Horn-Hickman, 1978).

Patency of the catheter should be rechecked and biliary flow observed as soon as this procedure is finished. The device is flushed daily with saline if the reentry duodenal catheter is used. Flushing or filling the balloon device with hygroscopic or hypertonic solutions may result in the occlusal balloon closing spontaneously because of the infiltration of body fluids. These catheters may be maintained for months if the sampling ports are implanted subcutaneously and a meticulous aseptic technique is utilized. Ascending infections from the intestine to the biliary system and

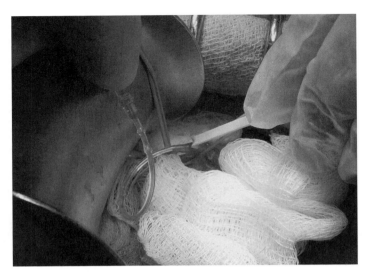

FIGURE 5.10 Use of a vascular pick to insert a catheter into the bile duct.

kinking of the catheter, resulting in biliary stasis and liver failure, are two potential complications of this procedure.

A porcine model of intraoperative radiation therapy combined with biliary-enteric bypass has been developed (Kaiser et al., 2005). Following resection of the gallbladder and common bile duct, pigs received 20–40 Gy of radiation. A Roux-en-Y hepaticojejunostomy is performed between the jejunum from the area of the ligament of Treitz and the residual extrahepatic biliary duct. In 20- to 25-kg Landrace pigs, an autologous jugular vein graft with a biodegradable endoluminal stent (6 mm in diameter) was used to repair defects in the bile duct. Animals were successfully followed for 6 months postoperatively (Heistermann et al., 2006).

PARTIAL HEPATECTOMY, LIVER BIOPSY, AND INTRAHEPATIC CANNULATION

Liver biopsies and partial lobectomies can be performed in swine using the same surgical techniques as for other species. The tip of a lobe can be removed by applying a suture ligature circumferentially around a small segment, referred to as the *guillotine technique*. Alternatively, a larger segment can be removed by cross-clamping with noncrushing intestinal clamps and placing overlapping mattress sutures or staples in the viable segment to provide hemostasis. Oxycellulose sponges may be applied to the cut edges to provide additional hemostasis. Percutaneous needle biopsies may be performed by using truecut biopsy needles passed caudomedially through either the 10th or 11th right intercostal spaces in the dorsal half of the lateral wall (Swindle, 1983).

Intrahepatic veins and ducts may be cannulated by modification of the procedure described earlier (Figure 5.11). After cross-clamping the left lobe of the liver, an incision is made from the edge into the parenchyma until a central vein is transected. The vein may be cannulated with an appropriate catheter. Biliary structures may also be cannulated. The incision is closed, as described previously, with suturing of oxycellulose sponges over the incision. The cannula can be externalized after surgical fixation in the abdominal cavity (Svendsen, 1997).

A model of segmental liver necrosis can be induced by hepatic artery embolization with biocompatible polyurethane (Maurer et al., 2000). Using a ventral midline abdominal incision, the hepatic artery to one lobe was dissected and cannulated. The polyurethane was infused at a rate of 1.5 mg/min. The liver hilus was checked for retrograde embolization, and recurrent arteries returning to the gallbladder, stomach, and GI tract were ligated. The technique led to sharp hepatic necrosis

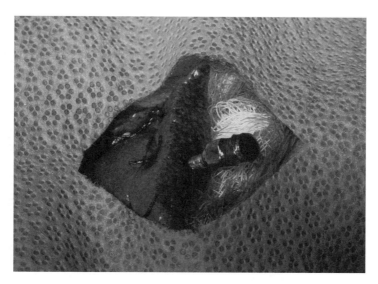

FIGURE 5.11 Cannulation of an intrahepatic vein.

without significant systemic effects due to occlusion of the arterial tree and concomitant portal vein occlusion. Ablation of hepatic parenchyma can be performed with radiofrequency catheter techniques, and some animals will develop portal vein thrombosis if the procedure is performed <5 mm of the intrahepatic portal vein (Frich et al., 2006).

Acute fulminent hepatic failure can be created by total hepatectomy or devascularization of the hepatic artery and vein with portocaval shunting (Fruhauf et al., 2004). From a midline abdominal approach, the infrahepatic vena cava and portal vein were isolated and circled by a tourniquet. Isolation and division of the hepatic artery and all accessory branches plus the common bile duct was performed. The vena cava is partially cross-clamped and an end-to-side anastomosis of the portal vein was performed to create a portocaval shunt. Animals will die in 12–21 h postprocedure with elevated serum liver enzymes, lactate, and ammonia levels. The total hepatectomy is performed in the same manner as for the donor liver in liver transplantation procedures (later text). A Y-shunting procedure between the two vena cava segments and the portal vein is performed. The models are useful for studying rescue methods using therapies such as bioartificial liver support system. Death is due to circulatory collapse.

Complete lobectomies may be performed by modification of the techniques described earlier for larger segments. The left lateral is the most easily removed lobe. Its excision is discussed in the following section (Camprodon et al., 1977; Kahn et al., 1994; Procaccini et al., 1994).

LIVER TRANSPLANTATION

Orthotopic, heterotopic, and xenografic transplantations have all been studied in this species. Hepatic transplantation in swine was developed because of the anatomic and physiological similarities of the porcine liver to human liver, notably because of its ability to withstand total portal vein occlusion up to 10 min, resistance to hepatic venous sphincter vasospasm, and its relative resistance to immunologic rejection posttransplantation. This last characteristic may be due to the use of related individuals from linebred herds of swine, rather than other characteristics of its immune system. Allografts, autografts, and segmental and auxiliary liver grafts have all been described in detail. Multivisceral transplantation including the liver has been previously described (see Chapter 4, Figure 4.31) (Calne et al., 1967; Dent et al., 1971; Flye, 1992; Gadacz, 1988; Hickman et al., 1971; Kahn et al., 1994; Mizrahi et al., 1996; Oldhafer et al., 1993; Pennington and Sarr, 1988; Procaccini et al., 1994; Ryabinin, 1996; Sika et al., 1996; Terblanche and Van Horn-Hickman, 1978; Terblanche et al., 1967).

For swine, in all phases of the surgery, the mean arterial pressure should be maintained at 60–70 mmHg, and swine should be kept normothermic by adequate perfusion with maintenance fluids. Animals need to be fasted from solids for 48 h to empty the bowel. Intestines may be packed off from the hepatic region with wetted laparotomy sponges or placed in a plastic bowel bag. Anesthesia, maintenance of homeostasis, and appropriate perioperative care are as essential to the success of this procedure as performing the surgery (Eisele et al., 1986; Mizrahi et al., 1996; Stump et al., 1986).

DONOR LIVER

Swine are anesthetized, and a midline celiotomy incision is made from the xiphoid process to the pubis. For the donor procedure, the sternum should be split for greater exposure. The falciform, left triangular, and gastrohepatic ligaments are divided. The porta hepatis is dissected free from the peritoneum to the level of the pancreas. This will expose the portal vein and hepatic artery. The caudal vena cava is dissected free of its peritoneal attachments from the level of the adrenal glands cranially through the diaphragm. Generous lengths of these vessels should be dissected to have adequate vessel length for reanastomoses during reimplantation. Consequently, their branches are ligated. At the time of harvest, the common bile duct, hepatic artery, portal vein, and vena cava are ligated and divided. The donor liver is cooled and flushed with a crystalloid solution or a preservation solution. The perfusion is performed through the portal vein during harvesting. Harvesting of the donor liver should be timed closely to coincide with the preparation of the recipient for transplantation. Prior to implantation, the excess tissue is trimmed from the liver. Blood from the donor pig should be collected by exsanguination and used postoperatively as required in the recipient pig.

ALLOGRAFT AND AUTOGRAFT IMPLANTATION

The recipient for whole-organ transplant is prepared in a manner similar to the preparation of the donor animal. An external jugular vein cutdown is performed to facilitate the bypass technique. A catheter is inserted into the splenic vein proximally in the heparinized recipient, and the primed catheter is placed into the external jugular vein to provide a passive bypass. If circulatory function is not adequate, then mechanical pumping may have to be provided. The same structures listed earlier for the donor organ are transected after initiation of the bypass and clamping of vessels with vascular clamps. Vascular suture in a continuous pattern is used to reanastomose the vessels in the following order: the prehepatic caudal vena cava, 90% of the infrahepatic vena cava, the portal vein, completion of the infrahepatic caudal vena cava, and the hepatic artery. After anastomosing the first two vessels, the liver is allowed to distend with blood by clamping the donor infrahepatic caudal vena cava prior to completing the anastomosis of the two segments of the vessel. Prior to tying the last knot of the anastomosis, the bypass segment is clamped, and the incomplete vascular connection is used as a vent and checked to ensure that air is not present, to remove 50–100 ml of waste blood after reperfusing the liver, and to see that the portal and vena caval circulations are restored. The hepatic artery is reanastomosed in a routine end-to-end manner; if a Carrell patch was taken during harvesting of the donor organ, it is reanastomosed to the aorta. The bile duct is the last connection and may be sutured using an intraluminal stent to guide the anastomosis (Figure 5.12).

An auxiliary liver transplant can also be performed by implanting the second liver into the right renal fossa of a recipient following excision of the kidney. The vascular anastomoses are hepatic artery or donor aorta to infrarenal aorta, hepatic vein or infrahepatic caudal vena cava to infrarenal caudal vena cava, oversewing of the suprahepatic vena cava, portal vein to superior mesenteric vein, and common bile duct to a Roux-en-Y limb of small bowel (Kahn et al., 1994).

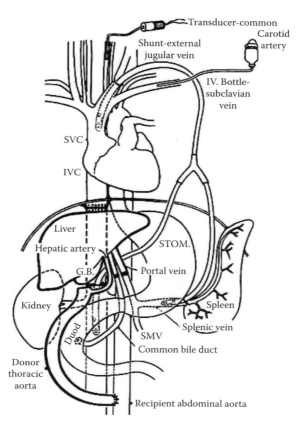

FIGURE 5.12 Orthotopic liver transplantation in the pig. During the anhepatic phase, venous blood is shunted from the portal system via the splenic vein and from the infrahepatic vena cava to the jugular vein. (Reprinted from Flye, M.W., 1992, in Swindle, M.M., Ed., *Swine as Models in Biomedical Research*, Ames, IA: Iowa State University Press, pp. 44–56. With permission.)

SEGMENTAL LIVER GRAFTS

A living donor may be used to transplant the left lateral lobe of the liver into a recipient. Approximately 10-g/kg body weight of liver tissue is necessary to provide normal metabolic functions. The segmental graft is harvested by incising the capsule and finger fracturing the parenchyma along the fissure of the lobe. The branches of the hepatic artery, hepatic vein, and portal vein are ligated, and the graft is treated as described earlier. The recipient liver is excised leaving the vena cava intact, and veno-veno bypass is instituted as described earlier. Reimplantation is made into the site of the excised liver by anastomosing the hepatic veins, followed by the portal vein, the hepatic artery, and the bile duct (Camprodon et al., 1977; Procaccini et al., 1994).

Postoperatively, care must be taken to provide adequate fluid therapy intravenously and to avoid solid food for 24–48 h. Aspirin may be given as an anticoagulant, depending upon the size of the vascular anastomoses. Systemic antibiotics are indicated. Immunosuppressive agents may be given depending upon the protocol.

HEPATIC XENOPERFUSION

Porcine liver has been utilized clinically as a bridge to transplantation in an effort to prevent fatal levels of ammonia and other toxic metabolites from accumulating in the patient, with minor success in the past (Norman et al., 1966). Devices containing porcine hepatocytes with filtration systems to prevent immunologic reactions to the cells have also been investigated. A renewed interest in the procedure has developed because of the possibility that transgenic manipulation of the donor swine will result in an increased success rate (Adham et al., 1996; Argibay et al., 1996; Collins et al., 1994; Mizrahi et al., 1996; Mora et al., 2002; Palmes et al., 2000; Pohlein et al., 1996; Terajima et al., 1996, 1997; Travis et al., 1996).

The liver may be harvested following the procedure for donor liver harvesting, discussed earlier in the section on liver transplantation. Female swine, 20–30 kg in body weight, are preferred for the procedure because of the size of the liver and vessels. If the system is to be used for clinical xenoperfusion, then the infectious disease precautions in Chapter 14 should be followed. Modifications to the dissection technique that may be applicable have been described by Mizrahi et al. (1996) and Travis et al. (1996). Dual cannulation of the portal vein and hepatic artery has been shown to be superior to vessel perfusion of the portal vein only (Mora et al., 2002).

The modifications of Mizrahi et al. (1996) include approaching the portal vein through the splenic vein for cannulation and not occluding the inflow or outflow vessels of the liver during cold perfusion. The technique also involves placing the gastrointestinal viscera in a sterile plastic bag to facilitate manipulation during the dissection.

Travis et al. (1996) also recommended adrenalectomy to prevent catecholamine production in the development of an isolated perfusion model for the study of pharmacological agents. Their system provides an *in situ* functioning liver (Figure 5.13).

When the system is to be used clinically for xenoperfusion, the isolated liver is kept in a sterile pan of iced saline and perfused through an extracorporeal system. The system involves shunting the human blood through the portal vein and suprahepatic vena cava to provide inflow and outflow lines. The hepatic artery is used for infusion in addition to the portal vein. Separate infusions with oxygenated blood are required. Using a two-pump system, the blood is circulated from the femoral vein of the patient through the liver and back into the venous system of the patient. The liver must be flushed with saline to exclude all porcine hematogenous products prior to connecting to the circuit. Hepatic hemodynamics in the isolated liver must be monitored during this procedure. Flow rates of approximately 1 ml/g of liver per minute have been recommended for the portal vein and approximately 25% of that rate for the hepatic artery (Terajima et al., 1997).

Liver function is monitored by measuring bile production, oxygen consumption, and by clinical observation of the organ for changes in color and consistency. Livers will develop progressive hypoalbuminemia and hypoproteinemia. These techniques are still experimental and will undoubtedly undergo further modification.

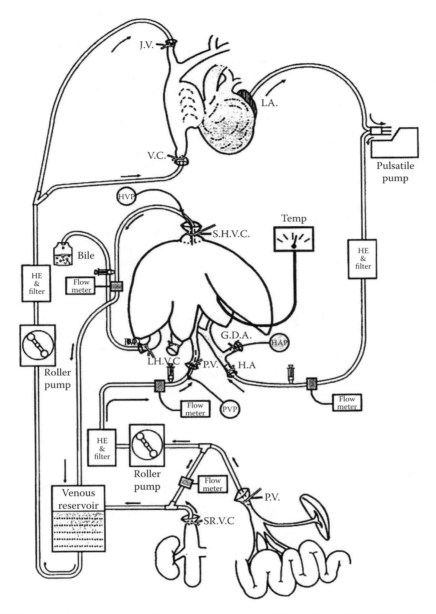

FIGURE 5.13 Isolated *in situ* liver perfusion system. (Reprinted from Travis, D.L., 1996, *J. Invest. Surg.*, 9(2): 131–147. With permission.)

REFERENCES

Adham, M., Peyrol, S., Vernet, M., Bonnefont, C., Barakat, C., Rigal, D., Chevallier, M., Berger, I., Raccurt, M., Ducerf, C., Baulieux, J., and Pouyet, M., 1996, Functional and immunological study of isolated liver xenoperfusion, *Transplant. Proc.*, 28(5): 2852–2853.

Argibay, P., Vazquez, J., Barros, P., Verge, D., Nunez, F., Garcia, H., Pekolj, J., and De Santibanes, E., 1996, Extracorporeal auxiliary xenoperfusion: animal model of support in fulminant liver failure, *Transplant. Proc.*, 28(2): 749–750.

Calne, R.Y., White, H.J.O., and Yoffa, D.E., 1967, Observations of orthotopic liver transplantation in the pig, *BMJ*, 2(1): 478.

Camprodon, R., Solsona, J., Guerrero, J.A., Mendoza, C.G., Segura, J., and Fabregat, J.M., 1977, Intrahepatic vascular division in the pig: basis for partial hepatectomies, *Arch. Surg.*, 112(1K0): 38–40.

Collins, B.H., Chari, R.S., Maggee, J.C., Harland, R.C., Lindman, B.J., Logan, J.S., Bollinger, R.R., Meyers, W.C., and Platt, J.L., 1994, Mechanisms of injury in porcine livers perfused with blood of patients with fulminant hepatic failure, *Transplantation*, 58(11): 1162–1171.

Court, F.G., Wermyss-Holden, S.A., Morrison, C.P., Teague, B.D., Laws, P.E., Kew, J., Dennison, A.R., and Maddern, G.J., 2003, Segmental nature of the porcine liver and its potential as a model for experimental partial Hepatectomy, *Br. J. Surg.*, 90(4): 440–444.

Dent, D.M., Hickman, R., Uys, C.J., Saunders, S., and Terblanche, J., 1971, Natural history of liver allo and auto transplantation in the pig, *Br. J. Surg.*, 58(6): 407–413.

Drougas, J.G., Barnard, S.E., Wright, J.K., Sika, M., Lopez, R.R., Stokes, K.A., Williams, P.E., and Pinson, C.W., 1996, A model for the extended studies of hepatic hemodynamics and metabolism in swine, *Lab. Anim. Sci.*, 46(6): 648–655.

Eisele, P.H., Woodle, E.S., Hunter, G.C., Talken, L., and Ward, R.E., 1986, Anesthetic, preoperative and postoperative considerations for liver transplantation in swine, *Lab. Anim. Sci.*, 36(4): 402–405.

Farinon, A.M., Zannoni, M., Lampugnani, R., DeLorenzis, G.F., and Freddi, M., 1981, Surgical anatomy of the liver and bile ducts in the most common experimental animals, *Chir. Patol. Sper.*, 29(5): 215–231.

Flye, M.W., 1992, Orthotopic liver transplantation in outbred and partially inbred swine, in Swindle, M.M., Ed., *Swine as Models in Biomedical Research*, Ames, IA: Iowa State University Press, pp. 44–56.

Frich, L., Hol, P.K., Roy, P.K., Mala, T., Edwin, B., Clausen, O.P.F., and Gladhaug, I.P., 2006, Experimental hepatic radiofrequency ablation using wet electrodes: electrode to vessel distance is a significant predictor for delayed portal vein thrombosis, *Eur. Radiol.*, 16(9): 1990–1999.

Fruhauf, N.R., Oldhafer, K.J., Westerman, S., Sotiropoulos, G.C., and Kaiser, G.M., 2004, Acute hepatic failure in swine: hepatectomy versus vascular occlusion, *J. Invest. Surg.*, 17(2): 163–171.

Gadacz, T.R., 1988, Portal hypertension, in Swindle, M.M. and Adams, R.J., Eds., *Experimental Surgery and Physiology: Induced Animal Models of Human Disease*, Baltimore, MD: Williams and Wilkins, pp. 250–253.

Hand, M.S., Phillips, R.W., Miller, C.W., Mason, R.A., and Lumb, W.V., 1981, A method for quantitation of hepatic, pancreatic and intestinal function in conscious Yucatan miniature swine, *Lab. Anim. Sci.*, 31(6): 728–731.

Heistermann, H.P., Palmes, D., Stratmann, U., Hohlback, G., Hierlemann, H., Langer, M., and Spiegel, H.U., 2006, A new technique for reconstruction of the common bile duct by an autologous vein graft and a biodegradable endoluminal stent, *J. Invest. Surg.*, 19(1): 57–60.

Hickman, R., van Hoorn, W.A., and Terblanche, J., 1971, Exchange transplantation of the liver in the pig, *Transplantation*, 24(2): 237.

Institute of Medicine, 1996, *Xenotransplantation: Swine, Ethics and Public Policy*, Washington, D.C.: National Academy Press.

Kahn, D., Hickman, R., Pienaar, H., and Terblanche, J., 1994, Liver transplantation in the pig, in Cramer, D.V., Podesta, L., and Makowka, L., Eds., *Handbook of Animal Models in Transplantation Research*, Boca Raton, FL: CRC Press, pp. 75–86.

Kaiser, G.M., Mueller, A.B., Sauerwein, W., Zhang, H.W., Westerman, S., Fruhauf, N.R., Kuehne, C.A., Stuschke, M., Oldhafer, K.J., and Broelsch, C.E., 2005, Biodigestive anastomosis after intraoperative irradiation in swine, *J. Invest. Surg.*, 18(3): 305–313.

Li, J., Liu, Y., Zhang, J.W., Wei, H., and Yang, L., 2006, Characterization of hepatic drug-metabolizing activities of Bama miniature pigs (Sus scrofa domestica): comparison with human enzyme analogs, *Comp. Med.*, 56(4): 286–290.

Maurer, C.A., Renzulli, P., Baer, H.U., Mettler, D., Uhlschmid, G., Neuenschwander, P., Suter, U.W., Triller, J., and Zimmermann, A., 2000, Hepatic artery embolization with a novel radiopaque polymer causes extended liver necrosis in pigs due to occlusion of the concomitant portal vein, *J. Hepatol.*, 32(2): 261–268.

Mizrahi, S.S., Jones, J.W., Jr., and Bentley, F.R., 1996, A facilitated technique for hepatectomy of porcine liver, *J. Invest. Surg.*, 9(3): 393–398.

Mora, N., Kaptanoglu, L., Ahang, Z., Niekrasz, M., Black, S., Ver Steeg, K., Wade, R., Siddall, V., Pao, W., Walsh, W., Ivancic, D., Kaufman, D., Abecassis, M., Stuart, F., Blei, A., Leventhal, J., and Fryer, J., 2002, Single vs. dual vessel procine extracorporeal liver perfusion, *J. Surg. Res.*, 103(2): 228–235.

Norman, J.C., Saravis, C.A., Brown, M.E., and McDermott, W.V., Jr., 1966, Immunochemical observations in clinical heterologous (xenogeneic) liver perfusions, *Surgery*, 60(1): 179–190.

Oldhafer, K.J., Hauss, J., Gubernatis, G., Pichlmayr, R., and Spiegel, H.U., 1993, Liver transplantation in pigs: a model for studying reperfusion injury, *J. Invest. Surg.*, 6(5): 439–450.

Palmes, D., Qayumi, A.K., and Spiegel, H.U., 2000, Liver bridging techniques in the treatment of acute liver failure, *J. Invest. Surg.*, 13: 299–311.

Pennington, L. and Sarr, M.G., 1988, Liver transplantation, in Swindle, M.M. and Adams, R.J., Eds., *Experimental Surgery and Physiology: Induced Animal Models of Human Disease*, Baltimore, MD: Williams and Wilkins, pp. 294–295.

Pohlein, C., Pascher, A., Bauman, P., Abendroth, D., Jochum, M., White, D.J., and Hammer, C., 1996, Transgenic porcine livers reduce liberation of humoral mediators during xenoperfusion with human blood, *Transplant. Proc.*, 28(2): 772–774.

Procaccini, E., Ruggiero, R., Rea, R., Boccia, G., Varletta, G., and Saccone, C., 1994, Segmental liver transplantation: experimental studies in swine, *Ann. Ital. Chir.*, 65(1): 125–129.

Ryabinin, V.E., 1996, Swine liver usage in extracorporeal detoxification, in Tumbleson, M.E. and Schook, L.B., Eds., *Advances in Swine in Biomedical Research*, Vol. 2, New York: Plenum Press, pp. 475–483.

Schantz, L.D., Laber-Laird, K., Bingel, S., and Swindle, M., 1996, Pigs: applied anatomy of the gastrointestinal tract, in Jensen, S.L., Gregersen, H., Moody, F., and Shokouh-Amiri, M.H., Eds., *Essentials of Experimental Surgery: Gastroenterology*, New York: Harwood Academic Publishers, pp. 2611–2619.

Sika, M., Drougas, J.G., Becker, Y.T., Chapman, W.C., Wright, J.K., Donovan, K.L., Striepe, V.J., Van Buren, D.B.H., Stokes, K.A., Barnard, S.E., Blair, K.T., Jabbour, K., Williams, P.E., and Pinion, C.W., 1996, Porcine model of orthotopic liver transplantation for chronic studies, in Tumbleson, M.E. and Schook, L.B., Eds., *Advances in Swine in Biomedical Research*, Vol. 1, New York: Plenum Press, pp. 171–187.

Skaanild, M.T. and Friis, C., 1997, Characterization of the P450 System in Göttingen minipigs, *Pharmacol. Toxicol.*, 80(Suppl. II): 28–33.

Skaanild, M.T. and Friis, C., 1999, Cytochrome P450 differences in minipigs and conventional pigs, *Pharmacol. Toxicol.*, 85(3): 174–180.

Stump, K.C., Pennington, L.R., Burdick, J.F., Hoshino, T., and Swindle, M.M., 1986, Practical anesthesia for orthotopic liver transplantation in swine, in Powers, D.L., Ed., *Proc. 2nd Annu. Meet. Acad. Surg. Res.*, Clemson, SC: Clemson University Press, pp. 10–12.

Svendsen, P., 1997, Anesthesia and basic experimental surgery of minipigs, *Pharmacol. Toxicol.*, 80(Suppl. II): 23–26.

Swindle, M.M., 1983, *Basic Surgical Exercises Using Swine*, Philadelphia, PA: Praeger Press.

Terajima, H., Shirakata, Y., Yagi, T., Mashima, S., Shinohara, H., Satoh, S., Arima, Y., Gomi, T., Hirose, T., Ikai, I., Morimoto, T., Inamoto, T., and Yamaoka, Y., 1996, Long-duration xenogeneic extracorporeal pig liver perfusion with human blood, *Transpl. Int.*, 9(Suppl. 1): S388–S391.

Terajima, H., Shirakata, Y., Yagi, T., Mashima, S., Shiohara, H., Satoh, S., Arima, Y., Gomi, T., Hirose, T., Takahashi, R., Ikai, I., Morimoto, T., Inamoto, T., Yamamoto, M., and Yamaoka, Y., 1997, Successful long-term xenoperfusion of the pig liver: continuous administration of prostaglandin E1 and insulin, *Transplantation*, 63(4): 507–512.

Terblanche, J. and Van Horn-Hickman, R., 1978, The prevention of gastric ulceration by highly selective vagotomy in a new peptic ulcer experimental model, the bile duct-ligated pig, *Surgery*, 84(2): 206–211.

Terblanche, J., Peacock, J.H., Hobbs, K.E., Hunt, A.C., Bowes, J., and Tierris, E.J., 1967, Orthotopic liver homotransplantation: experimental study in the unmodified pig, *S. Afr. Med. J.*, 42(20): 486–497.

Travis, D.L., Paulsen, A.W., and Genyk, Y., 1996, Development of an in situ isolated porcine liver perfusion model for tightly controlled physiologic and pharmacologic studies, *J. Invest. Surg.*, 9(2): 131–147.

Yen, J.T., 2001, Digestive system, in Pond, W.G. and Mersmann, H.J., Eds., *Biology of the Domestic Pig*, Ithaca, NY: Cornell University Press, pp. 399–453.

6 Pancreas and Spleen

SURGICAL ANATOMY AND GENERAL PRINCIPLES OF SURGERY

The pancreas of the pig is extensive, and the tail follows the lesser curvature of the stomach from the spleen and left kidney to a position along the proximal duodenum (Figure 6.1–Figure 6.5). The majority of the pancreas is retroperitoneal. The head of the pancreas gives rise to the body, tail, and an uncinate process. The pancreas encircles the portal and superior mesenteric veins and extends dorsally to the region of the left kidney. The pancreatic duct is composed of two separate ducts draining the tail and body. They anastomose to form the common pancreatic duct (accessory duct) immediately prior to the pancreatic sphincter. The pancreatic duct enters the duodenum caudal to and separate from the bile duct in the proximal duodenum approximately 20–25 cm distal to the pylorus (Figure 6.2–Figure 6.5). Surgically, it may be readily identified as a firm, whitish structure along the caudal third of the portion of the pancreas that is associated with the duodenum. There is usually a single pancreatic artery supplying the tail of the pancreas as a branch of the splenic or common hepatic (gastrohepatic) artery. The pancreatoduodenal artery courses between the duodenum and the pancreas along its joint border and supplies both from a series of small branches (Figure 6.4). Venous drainage is through the splenic vein. The pig pancreas has a high level of cholinergic control as in the human. Both exocrine and endocrine functions of the pancreas are negatively affected by anesthetics (Laber-Laird et al., 1992; Radberg et al., 1999). The pancreas accounts for approximately 0.1–0.29% of the body weight (BW) and increases in size with age and consumption of solid food.

Histologically (Figure 6.6), the pancreatic islet cells are relatively indistinct, but functionally similar to those in humans (Elowsson et al., 1997; Hand et al., 1981; Koyama et al., 1986; Niebergall-Roth, et al., 1997; Schantz et al., 1996; Stump et al., 1988; Yen, 2001).

The spleen is a pedunculated organ that is elongated in shape and located in close apposition to the greater curvature of the stomach in the left upper quadrant of the abdomen (Figure 6.7 and Figure 6.8). It extends from the left kidney ventrally to the midline. There are three main vascular supplies to the organ. These are located in the splenic ligament and are the left gastroepiploic, the splenic, and the short gastric arteries and veins. The vascular supply enters the organ from the head to one half the distance to the tail of the spleen (Getty, 1975; Swindle, 1983).

PANCREATECTOMY, ISLET CELL ABLATION, AND DIABETES

A total pancreatectomy can be performed without compromise or removal of the duodenum (Stump et al., 1988). With the pig in dorsal recumbency, a midline incision is made from the xiphoid cartilage to at least the umbilicus. In larger animals, the incision may have to be extended caudally. Balfour retractors and laparotomy sponges are utilized to pack off the spiral colon and small intestinal mass to see the tail of the pancreas. In larger animals, solid food should be withheld for 48 h to empty the spiral colon.

Using gentle dissection, the retroperitoneal portion of the pancreatic tail is dissected free, and, using gentle retraction, the dissection is continued until the pancreatic artery is encountered. After ligation and transection of the artery, the pancreas is dissected to the level of the pylorus. At this point, the dissection turns caudally, and the branches of the pancreatoduodenal artery supplying

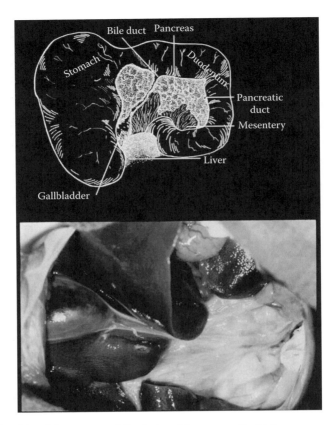

FIGURE 6.1 Relationship of the common bile duct and the pancreatic duct.

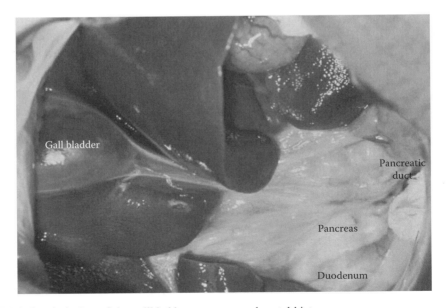

FIGURE 6.2 Surgical view of the gallbladder, pancreas, and portal hiatus.

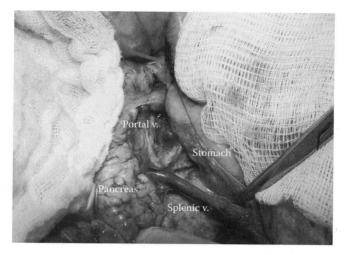

FIGURE 6.3 Relationship of the pancreas to the splenic and portal veins.

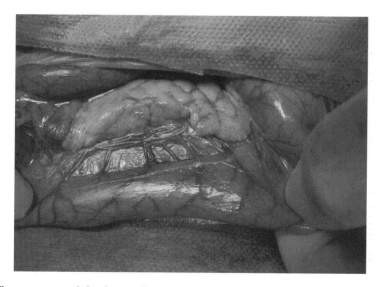

FIGURE 6.4 The pancreas and duodenum showing the pancreatoduodenal arterial supply.

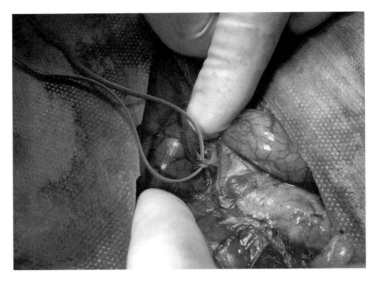

FIGURE 6.5 Pancreatic duct isolated with an elastic vessel loop.

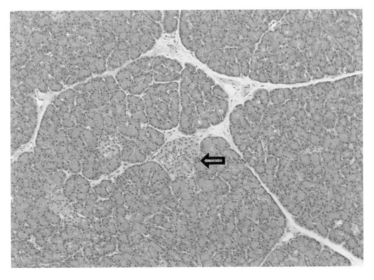

FIGURE 6.6 Islets of Langerhans (arrow) in the pancreas. H&E, ×100.

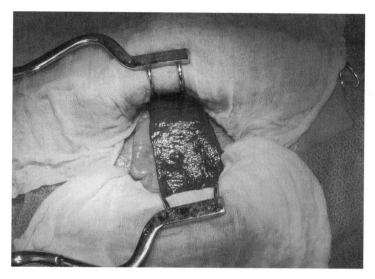

FIGURE 6.7 Midline abdominal incision showing the spleen in its normal position.

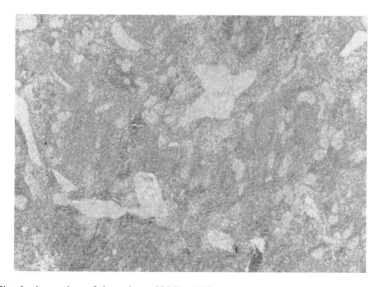

FIGURE 6.8 Histologic section of the spleen. H&E, ×100.

the pancreas are ligated as they are encountered. This dissection is more easily performed in the pig than in many other species because of the relatively loose connection between this artery and the pancreatic body. When the pancreatic duct is encountered, it is also ligated.

At this point, the dissection becomes more difficult. The major portion of the pancreatic body is deep and surrounds the portal vein and cranial mesenteric vessels. To perform this dissection, an assistant is required to provide additional retraction with handheld ribbon retractors. It is best to continue the dissection dorsally from the duodenum. The pancreas has to be split in order to dissect it from the portal vein. Care should be taken to minimize spillage of pancreatic enzymes, and the area should be flushed with saline following removal of the pancreas. The abdomen is closed in a routine manner.

A chemical ablation of the islet cells may be performed by injecting alloxan, 100–200 mg/kg i.v. or streptozotocin, 140–150 mg/kg, as an i.v. infusion over 5 min (Dixon et al., 1999; Larsen, et al., 2003; Mullen et al., 1992). A 24-h fast is required before either treatment, and the drugs are dissolved in saline, which might have to be acidified with citrate to properly dissolve the agent. There is a difference in reaction between breeds of swine and between age groups within the same breed with either chemical agent. Toxic reactions resulting in renal or hepatic failure are possibilities. It is best to start with a low dose and repeat in a week if signs of beta cell regeneration occur. With either agent it is best to provide i.v. access and fluid loading during and following drug administration. Beta cell lysis may initially result in high levels of insulin release leading to fatal hypoglycemia. Hyperglycemia will occur if the chemical ablation was successful, and the pigs need to be maintained on insulin.

Diet and insulin control of glucose levels is difficult in swine. An amount of feed equivalent to 4% of the body weight of the pig is provided as a starter ration. If pancreatectomy is complete, then oral pancreatic exocrine enzymes should be added to the food. Approximately 7 g of enzyme (Viokase-V®, Ft. Dodge Labs, Ft. Dodge, IA) is sufficient to digest 712 g of protein, 500 g of fat, and 1067 g of carbohydrate (Stump et al., 1988). In this species, as a general rule, elevations in blood glucose and glucosuria are moderate, and ketonuria and acidosis are not encountered as a major problem. Swine die within 10 d if not treated with insulin.

The goal of an experimental study requiring pancreatectomy is likely to be either treatment with various insulin protocols or islet cell transplantation. A detailed discussion of the monitoring and treatment of hyperglycemia is available (Mullen et al., 1992; Stump et al., 1988). Starting dosages for various types of insulin in swine 15–20 kg are as follows: regular insulin 4–5 U (4-h duration), Lente insulin 10 U (12-h duration), Ultralente 20 U (24-h duration). The regular and Lente insulin injections are given together in the morning and the Ultralente in the afternoon. Another method is to calculate approximately 1.6 total units of insulin/kg for maintenance. Blood glucose levels should be maintained at approximately 200–300 mg/dl depending upon the goal of the study. Normals for insulin levels and protocols for conducting both oral and intravenous glucose tolerance tests have been published (Laber-Laird et al., 1992; Mullen et al., 1992; Stump et al., 1988). There are variations among breeds and ages within the breed; consequently, it is appropriate to establish normals for each laboratory experiment (Larsen et al., 2001). As a generality, fasting swine have insulin levels of 5–10 µU/ml which will increase 2–3 times that amount following a meal. Blood glucose levels can be determined twice daily with microcapillary tube samples from the auricular vein. Swine can be trained to accept this blood sampling procedure with gentle handling and a noncomplicating food treat (carrots, dog biscuits).

Generally, swine may be monitored for weight loss and glucose for several days, prior to initiating insulin replacement. When they are treated with insulin, the total amount may be reduced after the dosage has stabilized for 3–4 weeks. Hypoglycemia can be treated by glucose infusion. As a guideline for glucose administration, intravenous glucose tolerance tests (IVGTT) require 0.5 g/kg of a 50% glucose solution, and oral GTT require 1.75–2 g/kg of the same glucose solution (Dixon et al., 1999; Laber-Laird et al., 1992; Mullen et al., 1992; Sasiki et al., 1984; Stump et al., 1988).

When monitoring glucose and insulin levels, the effects of anesthesia and sedation must be considered (Heim et al., 2002; Laber-Laird et al., 1992; Radberg et al., 1999; Vore et al., 2001). Induction of anesthesia and many sedatives may cause hyperglycemia and depressed insulin levels in most species. Included in these agents are inhalants (isoflurane, enflurane, nitrous oxide), benzodiazepines (midazolam), barbiturates, ketamine, and xylazine. Depressive effects may resolve with time; however, it is best to use chronically catheterized blood vessels for large samples, or microcapillary tubes filled after lancet pricks on the ear, as described earlier.

Atherosclerotic complications of diabetes are a possibility in this species, because they develop both spontaneous and experimental atherosclerosis. Currently, much of the development of porcine models of diabetes, complications of diabetes, and metabolic syndrome is being performed by Michael Sturek and his group, who have developed a line of wild-caught Ossabaw swine with a predisposition to the metabolic syndrome of obesity and diabetes (Dyson et al., 2006). Females of this breed have been developed as a model of the metabolic syndrome by feeding the thrifty genotype a diet with 45% kcal fat and 2% cholesterol. These animals develop obesity, insulin resistance, hypertension, and neointimal hyperplasia of the coronary arteries, and show increases in total cholesterol, triglycerides, and LDL/HDL.

Sturek has demonstrated that alloxan-induced diabetic dyslipidemia in Yucatan pigs fed an atherosclerotic diet leads to the development of some of the early signs of diabetic retinopathy, renal capillary basement membrane thickening, coronary artery atheroma, arterial fatty streaks, and arterial intimal thickening (Boullion et al., 2003; Hainsworth et al., 2002; Otis et al., 2003). Similar types of studies have been conducted in the smaller Göttingen minipig (Johansen et al., 2001; Larsen et al., 2001), which develop some of the metabolic characteristics of obese humans on a high-fat and high-energy diet. Serum leptin levels and widest-girth circumference have been described as means to noninvasively estimate body fat percentage in Yucatan swine. Normal leptin levels are approximately 2 ng/ml, and the normal value of the widest-girth circumference is approximately 92 cm in 60-kg male swine (Witczak et al., 2005).

Analgesics and i.v. infusions of fluids and nutritional solutions should be provided for 1–3 d postoperatively (Laber-Laird et al., 1992; Mullen et al., 1992; Sasiki et al., 1984; Stump et al., 1988).

SEGMENTAL PANCREATECTOMY, PANCREATIC TRANSPLANT, AND ISLET CELL ISOLATION

Most of the swine used in pancreatic transplantation are used for islet cell transplantation techniques after pancreatectomy, digestion of the organ for purification, and isolation of the beta cells (Nielsen et al., 2002). Much of the research in this area is directed toward preservation of the function of the cells and methods of delivery as xenografic transplants to humans. Fetal pancreases are frequently harvested and used in these procedures. Swine have also been employed as a model in segmental pancreatic transplant using the tail of the organ (Koyama et al., 1986; Mullen et al., 1992; Pennington and Sarr, 1988; Sasaki et al., 1984). Partial pancreatectomy has been demonstrated to result in pancreatic regeneration with hypertrophy and hyperplasia developing within 30 d (Morisset et al., 2001).

The same midline incision described for the total pancreatectomy (see earlier text) is used for this procedure. Starting at the tail and extending to the distal body near the duodenum, the organ is mobilized using gentle dissection. The tail is the ventral strip of the pancreas. It contains the main portion of the pancreatic duct and has a single arterial blood supply. It is this section of the pancreas that is harvested as a segmental donor organ (Figure 6.9). The short gastric and left gastric vessels are ligated, and the origin of the pancreatic blood supply is identified. It may branch off either the common hepatic artery or the splenic artery. The common hepatic artery and splenic artery are transected distal from the branch supplying the tail of the pancreas leave the celiac artery intact and to have ample distance to avoid damaging the pancreatic artery. The pancreatic

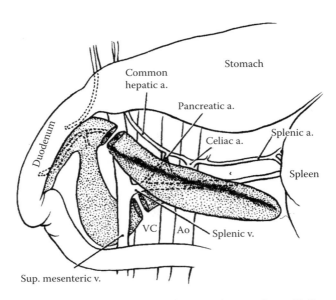

FIGURE 6.9 Harvesting the pancreas for a segmental pancreatic transplant with Roux-en-Y intestinal loop. (From Tumbleson, M.E., Ed., *Swine in Biomedical Research*, Vol. 1, New York: Plenum Press, pp. 385–389. With permission.)

vein is transected as it enters the splenic vein, and the tail of the organ is transected from the distal body of the pancreas at the level of the cranial mesenteric vein, which represents its narrowest section. The celiac artery is cannulated and transected, and the organ is perfused with cold perfusate and heparin.

The recipient animal has a left nephrectomy performed from a ventral midline celiotomy as described previously. End-to-end anastomosis is performed with the donor splenic vein to the renal vein, and the donor celiac artery to the renal artery. A Roux-en-Y loop is isolated in the recipient jejunum by transecting a section of the jejunum and performing an end-to-side anastomosis of the proximal segment to the distal segment (Figure 6.10). A 40-cm section of the loop is isolated and flushed free of intestinal contents. An invaginated section of the pancreas is anastomosed into the proximal end of the loop to provide exocrine duct entrance into the gastrointestinal tract without contamination by intestinal contents of the anastomotic site. The abdominal incision is closed in a routine manner.

Postoperative care should include systemic antibiotics, immunosuppressive therapy, and analgesics. Animals receive fluid and nutrition by a continuous i.v. infusion for 3 d prior to starting solid food.

Pancreatectomy is also performed to isolate islet cells for transplantation. Swine islet cells that retain physiological function are difficult to isolate in large numbers. The general methodology involves rapid removal of the pancreas following exsanguinations under anesthesia. The pancreas is washed, cooled on ice, and dissected free from adventitious tissue, the pancreatic artery or pancreatic duct is isolated for cannulation, and collagenase enzymatic solutions are infused. Islet cell yields increase with age, and more are located in the body and caudal portions of the pancreas. The pancreas undergoes digestion and isolation. Porcine islets are fragile because of a thin peri-insular connective tissue capsule. There are also differences in the amount and size of the islets and the collagen capsules between breeds of pigs. With a good technique, approximately 3000 islet equivalent number (IEQ)/g of islet cells can be isolated. A recent review of the techniques and refinement of the procedure using Liberase has been published (Kim et al., 2004; Nielsen et al., 2002).

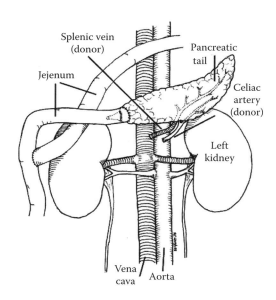

Splenic vein
(donor)

Pancreatic
tail

Jejenum

Celiac
artery
(donor)

Left
kidney

Vena
cava Aorta

FIGURE 6.10 Ligation of the vessels of the splenic hilus for splenectomy.

PANCREATIC DUCT ABLATION, CANNULATION, AND PANCREATITIS

It is more difficult to induce acute and chronic pancreatitis in swine than in other species. The pancreatic duct is readily identifiable at its entrance into the duodenum from the distal portion of the body. It is palpable as a firm tubular structure with a grayish white appearance. Its entrance into the duodenum is distal from that of the bile duct (Engelhardt et al., 1982; Sarr, 1988; Thorpe and Frey, 1971).

Acute pancreatitis has been produced by the injection, under pressure, of bile incubated with active trypsin. The lesions are much milder in the pig than in other species (Sarr, 1988; Thorpe and Frey, 1971). Modifications of the procedure by infusion of the pancreatic duct with taurocholic acid results in severe acute pancreatitis, which results in significantly impaired pancreatic oxygenation (Kinnala et al., 2001). Saline infusion in the same model results in a much milder form of pancreatitis with increased pancreatic oxygenation. Signs of pancreatitis are macroscopically detectable within minutes of performing the perfusions.

A model of chronic pancreatitis can be produced by ligation of the duct and creation of ischemia by ligating the branches of the pancreatoduodenal artery supplying the body of the pancreas. The blood supply to the tail is left intact. Lesions of chronic inflammation and fibrosis appear within weeks of the ductal ablation. Pseudocysts may also be present. There is exocrine deficiency with weight loss and gastrointestinal signs, but no signs of diabetes (Pitkaranta et al., 1989).

The pancreatic duct can be cannulated for short-term collection of pancreatic enzymes; however, animals will die of electrolyte imbalances and inability to digest nutrients in approximately a week. These problems can be alleviated by using reentry cannulation of the duodenum after exteriorizing the catheter on the abdominal wall to partially return pancreatic secretions. The catheter is passed into the main pancreatic duct and ligated in place. The catheter is exited through the ventral abdominal wall to the collection device and then reentered into the abdomen and the proximal duodenum. Suture retention beads should be used inside the pancreatic duct and the duodenum to avoid dislodgement. Alternatively, side entrance catheters can be used in the accessory duct or T-tubes in the main duct if only partial collection of the pancreatic secretions is desired (Niebergall-Roth et al., 1997; Swindle et al., 1998).

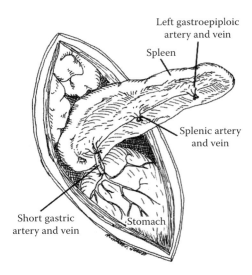

FIGURE 6.11 Splenectomy.

SPLENECTOMY, SPLENIC VASCULAR CATHETERIZATION, AND SPLENIC TRANSPLANTATION

The spleen is approached using a paracostal incision with the pig in dorsal recumbency. The incision starts from the lateral margin of the mammary glands at the halfway point between the first and second nipple on the left side. The incision parallels the caudal margin of the caudal edge of the rib line and extends caudolaterally to approximately the level of the third nipple. The splenectomy may also be performed from a midline incision; however, dissection of the short gastric vessels is more difficult (Swindle, 1983).

After celiotomy, the tail of the spleen is retracted out of the abdomen. The vessels supplying the splenic hilus are clamped, transected, and ligated in the following order: left gastroepiploic, splenic, and short gastric artery and veins. The arteries and veins may be ligated together. The short gastric vessels are deep in the abdomen and in close proximity to the stomach. They generally are ligated *in situ* and then transected. While dissecting this vessel, the surgeon should take care to avoid damage to the underlying pancreas (Figure 6.11).

The splenic vessels may also be used to catheterize the portal system with or without splenectomy (Figure 6.3). The surgical exposure for this procedure is easier than the exposure described for the portal vein catheterization in Chapter 9; however, the location of the tip of the catheter is not as readily discernable, and catheters made of nonflexible materials may penetrate into the abdomen at the entrance of the vessel into the portal vein. Sacrifice of a single vessel or pair of vessels in the spleen for this procedure does not cause a problem because of the extensive collateral circulation.

Splenic transplantation has been performed to study the immunologic effects in miniature swine as defined by major histocompatibility complex (MHC) (Dor et al., 2004; Gollackner et al., 2003). The technique involved excision of the spleen with its aortic and portal venous vascular pedicles which also necessitates dissection of the pancreas. Using a Carrel patch technique, the aorta and portal vein stumps were anastomosed to the abdominal aorta and caudal vena cava of a splenecto-mized recipient. Following transplantation, the spleen is positioned in the flank superficial to the bowel. Hematopoietic cell chimerism was detectable and rejection could be prevented by immun-osuppression with cyclosporine (10–30 mg/kg, trough level 400–800 *n*g/ml) or thymic irradiation (700 cGy) and/or total body irradiation (100 cGy). Posttransplant lymphoproliferative disease is a possible complication.

The anatomy of the lymphatic system and its drainage is depicted in Figure 6.12–Figure 6.15.

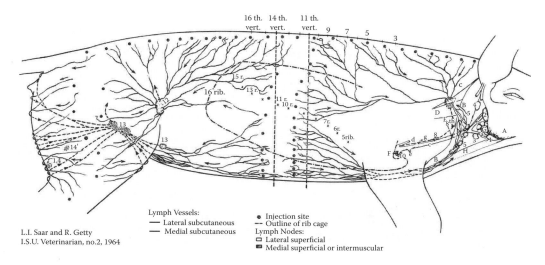

FIGURE 6.12 Superficial lymphatic system. (Reprinted from Sarr, L. and Getty, R., *I.S.U. Veterinarian*, No. 2, 1964. With permission.)

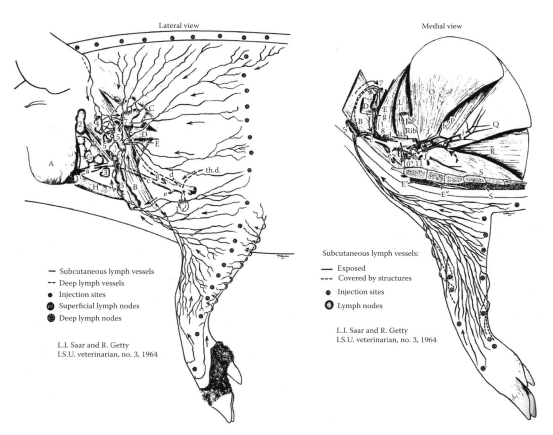

FIGURE 6.13 Lateral and medial views of the lymphatics of the foreleg. (Reprinted from Sarr, L. and Getty, R., *I.S.U. Veterinarian*, No. 2, 1964. With permission.)

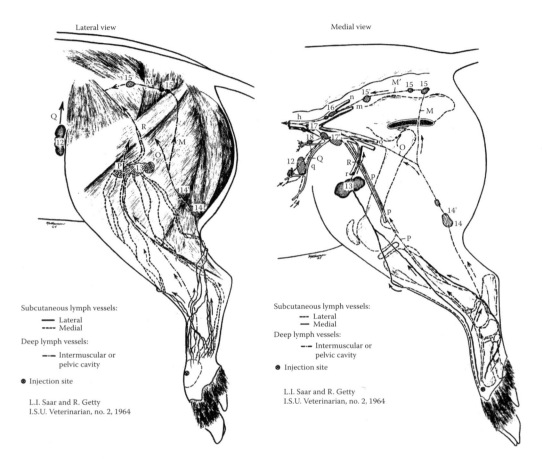

FIGURE 6.14 Lateral and medial views of the lymphatics of the hind limb. (Reprinted from Sarr, L. and Getty, R., *I.S.U. Veterinarian*, No. 2, 1964. With permission.)

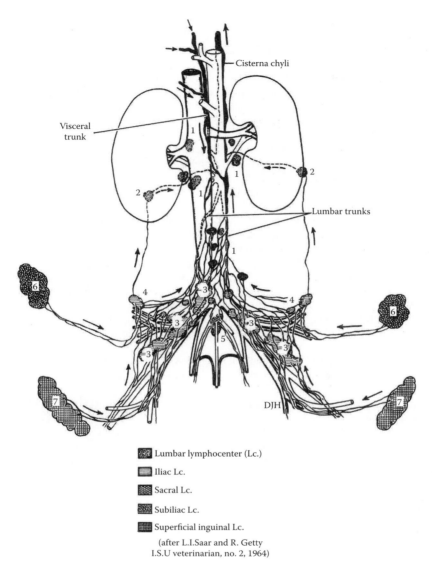

Cisterna chyli

Visceral
trunk

Lumbar trunks

DJH

Lumbar lymphocenter (Lc.)

Iliac Lc.

Sacral Lc.

Subiliac Lc.

Superficial inguinal Lc.

(after L.I.Saar and R. Getty
I.S.U veterinarian, no. 2, 1964)

FIGURE 6.15 Intra-abdominal lymphatic system. (Reprinted from Sarr, L. and Getty, R., *I.S.U. Veterinarian*, No. 2, 1964. With permission.)

REFERENCES

Boullion, R.D., Mokelke, E.A., Wamhoff, B.R., Otis, C.R., Wenzel, J., Dixon, J.L., and Sturek, M., 2003, Porcine model of diabetic dyslipidemia: insulin and feed algorithms for mimicking diabetes mellitus in humans, *Comp. Med.*, 53(1): 42–52.

Caronna, R., Diana, L., Campedelli, P., Catinelli, S., Nofroni, I., Sibio, S., Sinibaldi, G., and Chirletti, P., 2003, Gabexate mesilate (FOY) inhibition of amylase and phospholipase A$_2$ activity in sow pancreatic juice, *J. Invest. Surg.*, 16: 345–351.

Dixon, J.L., Stoops, J.D., Parker, J.L., Laughlin, M.H., Weisman, G.A., and Sturek, M., 1999, Dyslipidemia and vascular dysfunction in diabetic pigs fed an atherogenic diet, *Arterioscler. Thromb. Vasc. Biol.*, 19: 2981–2992.

Dor, F.J.M.F., Doucette, K.E., Mueller, N.J., Wilkinson, R.A., Bajwa, J.A., McMorrow, I.M., Tseng, Y.L., Kuwaki, K., Houser, S.L., Fishman, J.A., Cooper, D.K.C., and Huang, C.A., 2004, Posttransplant lymphoproliferative disease after allogeneic transplantation of the spleen in miniature swine, *Transplantation*, 78(2): 286–291.

Dyson, M., Alloosh, M., Vuchetich, J.P., Mokelke, E.A., and Sturek, M., 2006, Components of metabolic syndrome and coronary artery disease in female Ossabaw swine fed excess atherogenic diet, *Comp. Med.*, 56(1): 35–45.

Elowsson, P. and Carlsten, J., 1997, Body composition of the 12 week old pig studied by dissection, *Lab. Anim. Sci.*, 47(2): 200–202.

Engelhardt, W., Schwille, P.O., Gebhardt, C., Stolte, M., and Zirngibl, H., 1982, Pancreatic tissue hormones and molar insulin glucagon ratio in portal and peripheral blood of the minipig's influence of pancreatic duct occlusion, *Eur. Surg. Res.*, 14(2): 97–100.

Getty, R., Ed., 1975, *Sisson and Grossman's the Anatomy of the Domestic Animals: Porcine*, Vol. 2, Philadelphia, PA: W.B. Saunders, pp. 1215–1422.

Gollackner, B., Dor, F.J., Knosalla, C., Buhler, L., Duggan, M., Huang, C.A., Houser, S.L., Sachs, D.H., Kawai, T., Ko, D.S., and Cooper, D.K., 2003, Spleen transplantation in miniature swine: surgical technique and results in major histocompatibility complex-matched donor and recipient pairs, *Transplantation*, 75(11): 1799–1806.

Hainsworth, D.P., Katz, M.L., Sanders, D.A., Sanders, D.N., Wright, E.J., and Sturek, M., 2002, Retinal capillary basement membrane thickening in a porcine model of diabetes mellitus, *Comp. Med.*, 52(6): 523–529.

Hand, M.S., Phillips, R.W., Miller, C.W., Mason, R.A., and Lumb, W.V., 1981, A method for quantitation of hepatic, pancreatic and intestinal function in conscious Yucatan miniature swine, *Lab. Anim. Sci.*, 31(6): 728–731.

Heim, K.E., Morrell, J.S., Ronan, A.M., and Tagliaferro, A.R., 2002, Effects of ketamine-xylazine and isoflurane on insulin sensitive dehydroepiandrosterone sulfate-treated minipigs, *Comp. Med.*, 52(3): 233–237.

Kim, S.C., Han, D.J., Kang, C.H., We, Y.M., Back, J.H., Kim, Y.H., and Lim, D.G., 2004, Experimental islet isolation in porcine pancreas with new enzyme Liberase, PI., *Transpl. Proc.*, 36(7): 2197–2199.

Kinnala, P.J., Kuttila, K.T., Gronroos, J.M., Havia, T.V., Nevalainen, T.J., and Niinikoski, J.H., 2001, Pancreatic tissue perfusion in experimental acute pancreatitis, *Eur. J. Surg.*, 167(9): 689–694.

Koyama, I., Pennington, L.R., Swindle, M.M., and Williams, G.M., 1986, Pancreatic allotransplantation with Roux-en-Y jejunal diversion in swine: its technical aspects, in Tumbleson, M.E., Ed., *Swine in Biomedical Research*, Vol. 1, New York: Plenum Press, pp. 385–390.

Laber-Laird, K., Smith, A.C., Swindle, M.M., and Colwell, J., 1992, Effects of isoflurane anesthesia on glucose clearance in Yucatan minipigs, *Lab. Anim. Sci.*, 42(6): 579–581.

Larsen, M.O., Rolin, B., Wilken, M., Carr, R.D., Svendsen, O., and Bollen, P., 2001, Parameters of glucose and lipid metabolism in the male Göttingen minipig: influence of age, body weight, and breeding family, *Comp. Med.*, 51(5): 436–442.

Larsen, M.O., Rolin, B., Wilken, M., Carr, R.D., and Godtfredsen, C.F., 2003, Measurements of insulin secretory capacity and glucose tolerance to predict pancreatic b-cell mass *in vivo* in the nicotinamide/streptozotocin Göttingen minipig, a model of moderate insulin deficiency and diabetes, *Diabetes*, 52(1): 118–123.

Morisset, J., Morisset, S., Lauzon, K., Cote, S., Laine, J., Bourassa, J., Lessard, M., and Echave, V., 2000, Pancreatic inflammation, apoptosis, and growth: sequential events after partial pancreatectomy in pigs, *Pancreas*, 21(3): 321–324.

Morisset, J., Morisset, S., Lauzon, K., Cote, S., Laine, J., Bourassa, J., Lessard, M., and Echave, V., 2001, The message underlying pig pancreas regeneration after partial pancreatectomy, in Lindberg, J.E. and Ogle, B., Eds., *Digestive Physiology of Pigs*, New York: CABI Publishing, pp. 51–53.

Mullen, Y., Taura, Y., Nagata, M., Miyazawa, K., and Stein, E., 1992, Swine as a model for pancreatic beta-cell transplantation, in Swindle, M.M., Ed., *Swine as Models in Biomedical Research*, Ames, IA: Iowa State University Press, pp. 16–34.

Niebergall-Roth, E., Teyssen, S., and Singer, M.V., 1997, Pancreatic exocrine studies in intact animals: historic and current methods, *Lab. Anim. Sci.*, 47(6): 606–616.

Nielsen, T.B., Yderstraede, K B., and Beck-Nielsen, H., 2002, Isolation, transplantation, and functional studies of adult porcine islets of Langerhans, *Comp. Med.*, 52(2): 127–135.

Otis, C.R., Wamhoff, B.R., and Sturek, M., 2003, Hyperglycemia-induced insulin resistance in diabetic dyslipidemic Yucatan swine, *Comp. Med.*, 53(1): 53–64.

Pennington, L. and Sarr, M.G., 1988, Pancreas transplantation, in Swindle, M.M. and Adams, R.J., Eds., *Experimental Surgery and Physiology: Induced Animal Models of Human Disease*, Baltimore, MD: Williams and Wilkins, pp. 296–297.

Pitkaranta, P., Kivisaari, L., Nordling, S., Saari, A., and Schroder, T., 1989, Experimental chronic pancreatitis in the pig, *Scand. J. Gastroenterol.*, 24(8): 987–992.

Rådberg, K., Botermans, J., Weström, B.R., and Pierzynowski, S.G., 1999, Depressive effects of anesthesia or sedation on exocrine pancreatic function in pigs, *Lab. Anim. Sci.*, 49(6): 662–664.

Sarr, M.G., 1988, Pancreas, in Swindle, M.M. and Adams, R.J., Eds., *Experimental Surgery and Physiology: Induced Animal Models of Human Disease*, Baltimore, MD: Williams and Wilkins, pp. 204–216.

Sasaki, N., Yoneda, K., Bigger, C., Brown, J., and Mullen, Y., 1984, Fetal pancreas transplantation in miniature swine: developmental characteristics of fetal pig pancreases, *Transplantation*, 38(4): 335–340.

Schantz, L.D., Laber-Laird, K., Bingel, S., and Swindle, M., 1996, Pigs: applied anatomy of the gastrointestinal tract, in Jensen, S.L., Gregersen, H., Moody, F., and Shokouh-Amiri, M.H., Eds., *Essentials of Experimental Surgery: Gastroenterology*, New York: Harwood Academic Publishers, pp. 2611–2619.

Stump, K.C., Swindle, M.M., Saudek, C.D., and Strandberg, J.D., 1988, Pancreatectomized swine as a model of diabetes mellitus, *Lab. Anim. Sci.*, 38(4): 439–443.

Swindle, M.M., 1983, *Basic Surgical Exercises Using Swine*, Philadelphia, PA: Praeger Press.

Swindle, M.M., Smith, A.C., and Goodrich, J.A., 1998, Chronic cannulation and fistulization procedures in swine: a review and recommendations, *J. Invest. Surg.*, 11(1): 1–8.

Thorpe, C.D. and Frey, C.F., 1971, Experimental pancreatitis in pigs, *Arch. Surg.*, 103(6): 720–723.

Vore, S.J., Aycock, E.D., Veldhuis, J.D., and Butler, P.C., 2001, Anesthesia rapidly suppresses insulin pulse mass but enhances the orderliness of insulin secretory process, *Am. J. Physiol. Endocriol. Metab.*, 281(1): E93–E99.

Witczak, C.A., Mokelke, E.A., Boullion, R., Wenzel, J., Keisler, D.H., and Sturek, M., 2005, Noninvasive measures of body fat percentage in male Yucatan swine, *Comp. Med.*, 55(5): 445–451.

Yen, J.T., 2001, Digestive system, in Pond, W.G. and Mersmann, H.J., Eds., *Biology of the Domestic Pig*, Ithaca, NY: Cornell University Press, pp. 399–453.

7 Urinary System and Adrenal Glands

GENERAL PRINCIPLES OF SURGERY AND SURGICAL ANATOMY

The urinary system of the pig is anatomically similar to that of most species. The kidney of a 70-kg pig is approximately the size of that of an adult human. In newborn pigs, the development of nephrons continues for approximately 3 weeks in contrast to the fully developed nephron system in humans at birth. The left kidney is more cranial than the right kidney and its cranial pole is located at approximately the 13th rib (L1–L4). The renal artery and vein divide into two branches close to the renal hilus. The blood supply is divided into cranial and caudal segments rather than into longitudinal halves as in other species. This means that the avascular plane of the kidney is transverse rather than longitudinal (Figure 7.1–Figure 7.3). There are some differences in anatomy and function between the pig and human (Table 7.1–Table7.4), even though the internal renal anatomy is very similar (Figure 7.4). The multirenculate, multipapillate kidney of the pig contains a greater proportion of juxtamedullary glomeruli, the loops of Henle are relatively longer, and creatinine is absorbed from the proximal tubule (Figure 7.4–Figure 7.6). Maximum urine concentration in the pig is 1080 mOsm/kg, which compares favorably to that of the human, which is 1160 mOsm/kg. The calyx contracts approximately 15 times/min and the renal pelvis 3–6 times/min in both the pig and human (Assimos et al., 1986; Swindle et al., 2000; Swindle and Olson, 1988; Terris, 1986).

The ureters extend caudoventrally to the dorsolateral aspect of the neck of the urinary bladder (Figure 7.7 and Figure 7.8). The urinary bladder is large and thin walled but typical in morphology. It receives its innervation from S2 to S4. The urethra courses along the pelvic floor into the penis. The tip of the penis is located on the ventral abdominal wall in a preputial diverticulum. The external opening of the preputial diverticulum is located immediately caudal to the umbilicus. The contents of this structure must always be expressed prior to performing abdominal surgery in male swine. The desquamated cells and urine in the preputial diverticulum are foul smelling and contaminated with bacteria. Gloves should be worn during the expression of this material (Hodson, 1986; Russell et al., 1981; Swindle, 1983; Swindle et al., 2000; Swindle and Olson, 1988; Terris, 1986).

Catheterization of the urinary bladder through the penis is difficult, even impossible, depending upon the size of the animal and the breed, because of the male anatomy. Consequently, the urinary bladder can be emptied by manual expression in small animals or via needle aspiration. Needle aspiration should be performed very carefully because the bladder is relatively thin walled and tears easily. The male urethra may be entered percutaneously with an intracath needle as it courses ventrally over the pubis in the perineum. It may be palpated on the midline. The pelvic urethra of a 25- to 30-kg pig is approximately the size of that of a human. This catheterization procedure can be readily performed with practice. The female urethra may be catheterized conventionally and may be entered on the floor of the vagina approximately one quarter to one third of the distance to the cervix. Pigs produce 5–40 ml/kg urine per day depending upon the age and water consumption (Swindle, 1983).

In studies of fetal and newborn pigs, development of storage and bladder function develops between the mid-second and early third trimesters of pregnancy. Similar to human infants, they

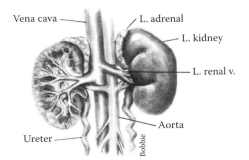

FIGURE 7.1 Anatomy of the kidneys and adrenal glands with the internal renal anatomy of the right kidney demonstrated.

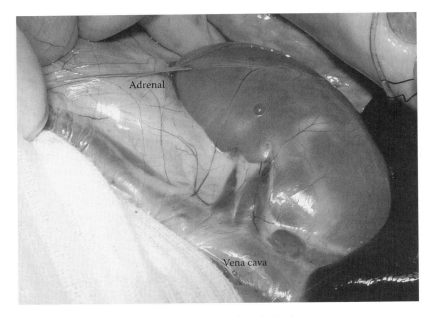

FIGURE 7.2 Surgical anatomy of the right kidney and adrenal gland.

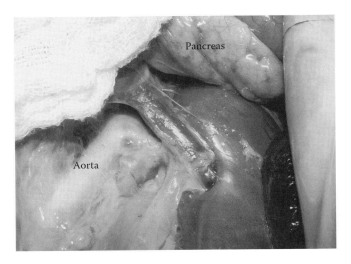

FIGURE 7.3 Surgical anatomy of the left kidney.

TABLE 7.1
Renal Function in Swine

	GFR			C_PAH			Tm_PAH			Tm_Glucose		
	$ml \times min^{-1} \times 1.73\ m^2$						$mg \times min^{-1} \times 1.73\ m^2$					
	Pig	Minipig	Man	Pig	Minipig	Man	Pig	Minipig	Man	Pig	Minipig	Man
Premature	—	—	16	—	—	39	—	—	14	—	—	93
Newborn	49	—	40	176	—	—	16	—	—	164	—	—
Young[a]	133	88	—	381	497	—	89	88	—	360	—	—
Adult	141	—	125	433	—	638	166	—	78	466	—	339

Note: GFR = glomerular filtration rate; C_{PAH} = renal plasma flow measure as clearance of para-aminohippurate; Tm_{PAH} = transport capacity of organic anions; $Tm_{Glucose}$ = capacity to reabsorb glucose from the urine.

[a] Minipigs: 4 months, domestic pigs: 2 months.

Source: Reprinted from Friis, C., 1998. *Scand. J. of Lab. Anim. Sci.,* Suppl. 1, p. 57, 1998. With permission.

TABLE 7.2
Urinalysis Results for Göttingen Minipigs

		Male			Female		
		N	Mean	SD	N	Mean	SD
pH		190	7.95	±0.64	192	8.11	±1.04
Osmolality	mmol/kg	106	543.491	±252.508	108	636.094	±241.578
Volume	ml/d	225	302	±221.5	228	290	±152.6

Note: Samples from 219 males 3.5 ± 0.6 months of age and 220 females 3.5 ± 0.7 months of age. N = number of pigs, SD = standard deviation.

Source: Courtesy of Ellegaard Göttingen Minipig ApS, Dalmose, Denmark.

TABLE 7.3
Urinalysis Results for Juvenile and Young Adult Hanford Miniature Swine

		Male				Female			
		Mean	SD	Min	Max	Mean	SD	Min	Max
pH		7.3	1.0	6.0	9.0	6.7	0.6	5.0	8.0
Specific gravity		1.0	0.0	1.0	1.0	1.0	0.0	1.0	1.0
Volume	ml/h	26.8	12.3	4.3	61.7	32.7	15.8	9.0	70.8

Note: N = 28 per gender group, age = ~4–8 months, SD = standard deviation.

Source: Courtesy of Sinclair Research Center, Auxvasse, MO.

TABLE 7.4
Urinalysis Results for Juvenile Sinclair Miniature Swine

		Male				Female			
		Mean	SD	Min	Max	Mean	SD	Min	Max
pH		6.9	1.0	5.0	9.0	6.7	0.8	5.0	9.0
Specific gravity		1.2	1.3	1.0	10.1	1.0	0.0	1.0	1.0
Urobilinogen	EU/dl	0	0.1	0	1	0	0.0	0	0
Volume	ml/h	14.6	9.9	4.3	58.8	13.0	7.3	3.4	30.4

Note: N = 51, age = ~3–4 months.

Source: Courtesy of Sinclair Research Center, Auxvasse, MO.

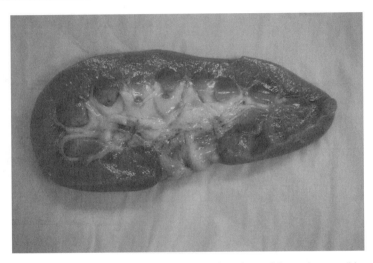

FIGURE 7.4 Longitudinal cross section of the kidney showing the multirenculate, multipapillate system.

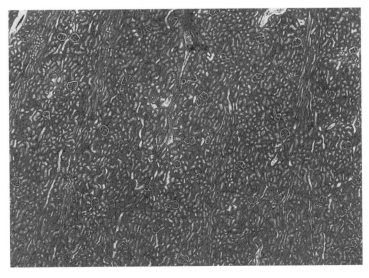

FIGURE 7.5 Histology of the renal glomerulus. H&E, ×100.

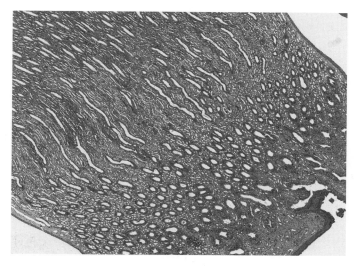

FIGURE 7.6 Histology of the renal pelvis. H&E, ×40.

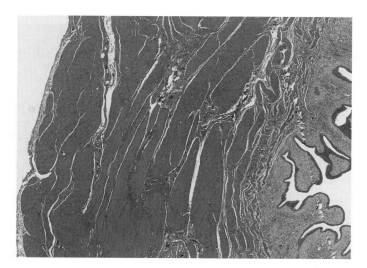

FIGURE 7.7 Histology of the urinary bladder. H&E, ×40.

have a dyscordinated voiding with staccato flow. Newborns void approximately 3.3 times per hour and fetuses 5.85 times per hour (Olsen et al., 2001, 2004; Peters, 2001).

The adrenal glands are associated with the medial surface toward the cranial pole of each kidney. The right adrenal gland is tightly adhered to the caudal vena cava. The arterial supply of the glands is from either the aorta or branches of the lumbar arteries, and the venous drainage is into either the vena cava or the renal veins (Figure 7.1–Figure 7.3) (Venzke, 1975; Swindle and Smith, 1998).

NEPHRECTOMY

Nephrectomy can be performed either through a ventral midline approach or a retroperitoneal approach through the flank (Figure 7.9 and Figure 7.10). The flank approach is the approach of choice if only one kidney is involved in the surgical procedure (Swindle, 1983; Webster et al., 1992).

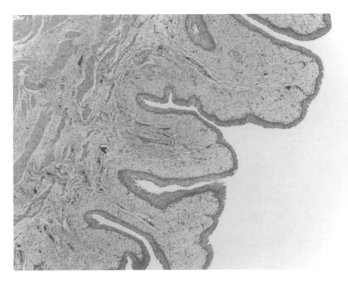

FIGURE 7.8 Histology of the bladder mucosal epithelium. H&E, ×100.

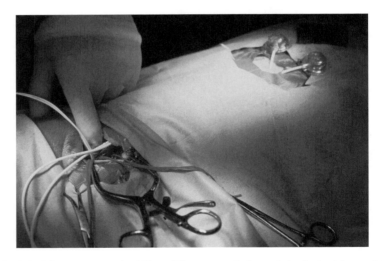

FIGURE 7.9 Flank incision to expose the kidney. The surgeon's finger is in the incision and the pig is in left lateral recumbency with the head to the right.

The flank approach is performed with the pig in ventral or lateral recumbency. A curved linear incision is made caudal to the last rib following its contour approximately one quarter to one third of the distance ventrally, from the lateral aspect of the vertebral wings to the midline. The muscle layers are either cut or bluntly divided and retracted until the peritoneum is exposed. Using manual manipulation, the peritoneum is retracted ventrally after peeling it from the dorsal aspect of the abdominal musculature and the kidney. When performed properly, the kidney is exposed without entering the abdominal cavity, thus avoiding interference with the abdominal viscera.

If bilateral renal procedures are to be performed or other abdominal procedures are involved in the protocol, then a ventral midline incision is the preferred approach. The spiral colon will interfere with observation of the kidneys, especially the left one, if it has not been emptied preoperatively. This may be performed either by a 48-h fast from solid foods or by administering hypertonic saline cathartics, as previously described. The ventral midline incision is initiated at the xiphoid process and extends caudally beyond the umbilicus. Balfour retractors and laparotomy

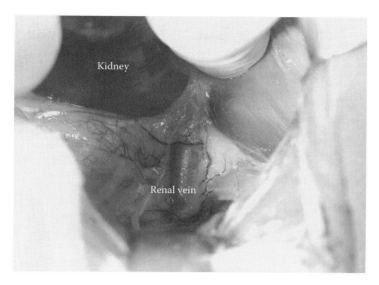

FIGURE 7.10 Close-up of the retroperitoneal approach to the kidney. The kidney is displaced dorsally to show the blood vessels.

sponges are required to retract the viscera for surgical exposure of the kidneys. The intestinal mass should not be exteriorized to enhance exposure because of the complications of edema and ischemia, to which the pig is highly susceptible.

The renal artery is bluntly dissected and ligated first. A branch of the suprarenal artery supplying the adrenals will have to be ligated in some cases, especially on the left kidney. This is followed by isolation and ligation of the renal vein and then the ureter. From the flank approach, it is helpful to make a sling of surgical gauze around the cranial and caudal poles of the kidney. This aids in the manipulation of the organ to enhance retraction and exposure. When dissecting in the midline region, the surgeon should take care to avoid damaging the lymphatics. They can usually be seen and should be ligated, if damaged, to avoid chyloperitoneum.

Following removal of the kidney, the incision is closed in a routine manner. When closing a flank incision, it is not necessary to suture the retracted peritoneum back in place. The muscle layers are closed in anatomically correct layers by suturing the fascia. The skin and subcutaneous tissues are closed in a routine fashion.

PARTIAL NEPHRECTOMY AND INTRARENAL SURGERY

The branches of the renal artery supplying the kidney divide the blood supply transversely rather than longitudinally. The avascular plane of the kidney may be readily demonstrated by temporarily occluding the blood supply of one of the branches of the renal artery in the hilus of the kidney (Russell et al., 1981; Swindle and Olson, 1988).

If a surgical approach to the renal pelvis is indicated, then this avascular plane forms the line of incision into the kidney parenchyma. The capsule of the kidney is incised with a scalpel, and the incision may be continued either with a scalpel or bluntly with a surgical spatula. The kidney is surgically repaired with mattress sutures of synthetic absorbable or nonabsorbable sutures, which occlude the edges of the incision and provide hemostasis. In heminephrectomy, this technique of closure will occlude most of the blood supply, but it may be necessary to provide additional hemostasis with oxycellulose sponges (Russell et al., 1981; Swindle and Olson, 1988).

The blood supply to the kidney may be reduced by surgical imbrication, inflatable circumferential cuffs (Figure 7.11), or Goldblatt clamp techniques that occlude the renal blood flow. This procedure is performed usually to produce a model of renal hypertension. To produce the model

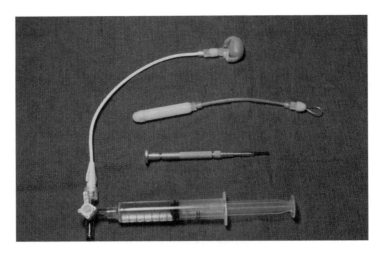

FIGURE 7.11 Inflatable cuffs to occlude the renal artery.

surgically, it is necessary to remove one kidney and significantly reduce the blood supply to the remaining kidney. The exception to this is the two-kidney deoxycorticosterone acetate (DOCA) salt model in Yucatan miniature swine (O'Hagan and Zambraski, 1986; Swindle and Olson, 1988).

To produce the model of hypertension, the left kidney is surgically removed as described previously. The right kidney, which has a longer artery than the left, is the kidney to which the blood supply is reduced. In our laboratories, a reduction of approximately 75% of the renal blood flow will produce chronic hypertension. An acute hypertensive episode may be initiated by challenge with 0.9% NaCl at a rate of 20 ml/kg i.v. as a bolus and maintenance infusion. An increase of 20% above baseline arterial pressure is considered significant.

Radiofrequency ablation has been used laparoscopically and percutaneously to study sequella associated with using the technique for ablation of renal tumors or other lesions (Gill et al., 2000; Wagner et al., 2005). The studies in swine have proved applicable to the postprocedural seqellae in humans. The renal tissue is dessicated, becomes necrotic, and undergoes autoamputation and resorption.

RENAL TRANSPLANT

The pig has been used in renal transplantation research to study organ preservation, rejection phenomena, and surgical procedures including allographic, xenografic, heterotopic, and orthotopic techniques. In addition to the anatomic characteristics of the kidneys described previously, it is important to use anesthetic and perioperative techniques that maintain adequate blood pressure to ensure tissue perfusion (>50 torr) and avoid vasospasm (Howard et al., 1994; Kirkman et al., 1979; Pennington, 1992; Sachs, 1992; Williams, 1988).

Selection of the donor and recipient breeds will be determined by the longevity of the experiment and the type of experiment being performed. For example, if the recipient is to be another pig and the experiment is meant to be longer than 3 weeks in length, then one of the miniature breeds should be considered because of the difficulty in maintaining large farm pigs postsurgically. Differences will be noted in the histocompatibility complex among breeds as well. Many sources of farm and miniature pigs will have closely related individuals in the herd even if they are not littermates.

The surgical approach to the kidneys and the general perioperative procedures, such as fasting, are the same as the ones noted for nephrectomy. The midline incision is preferred because of the increased surgical exposure. The flank approach may be preferred if the donor animal is expected to survive the experiment, especially if a future reimplantation procedure is anticipated using the midline approach.

In a nonsurvival donor procedure to harvest the kidneys, the aorta and vena cava are isolated cranial and caudal to the renal vessels, and the kidneys are harvested *en bloc*. This procedure will involve ligation of the dorsal lumbar branches of the aorta and careful dissection to avoid blood loss. The aorta and vena cava are ligated proximally and distally after heparinization of the animal. A sufficient length of ureter to ensure successful reimplantation without stretching should be simultaneously harvested.

In a survival procedure, a decision has to be made concerning which kidney is to be harvested. For the left kidney, the renal artery will be shorter and the renal vein longer. For the right kidney, the opposite is true, and the adrenal gland is closely associated with the junction of the renal vein and vena cava. If using a flank approach, the left kidney is generally the kidney of choice for removal. When a single kidney is harvested, it is best to use a Satinsky clamp to isolate the renal vessels and harvest them using a Carrel patch technique. Reimplantation of the renal vessels is greatly enhanced when such a patch is available. It also minimizes the manipulation of the renal artery, which is very prone to vasospasm. Care should be taken to avoid damaging the lymphatics in a survival procedure, because the accumulation of lymph in the abdominal cavity will result in a postoperative complication. They may either be ligated or cauterized. The donor kidney should be perfused with a cold preservation solution and kept in a chilled preservation solution or isotonic iced slurry until reimplantation.

The midline approach is preferred for reimplantation of the kidneys. A prolonged fast (24–48 h) ensures that the colon will be emptied, which aids both the surgical exposure and the prevention of edema postsurgically, following manipulation of the intestinal mass. The kidney is usually implanted into the distal aorta and vena cava or the iliac vessels to minimize the length of ureter that has to be reimplanted (Figure 7.12) and thus minimize the chances of ischemic necrosis of the structure. After heparinizing the recipient, a Satinsky clamp is applied to the artery and a longitudinal incision made. The cranial and caudal ends of the Carrel patch are sutured with 6/0 nonabsorbable

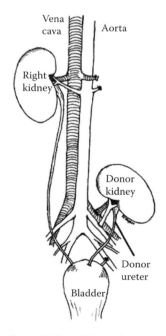

FIGURE 7.12 Implantation of a transplanted kidney (donor) into the iliac vessels.

cardiovascular suture, and the patch is anastomosed with a simple continuous pattern. The same procedure is performed for the renal vein, and blood reperfusion is allowed by removing first the venous and then the arterial clamps. The kidney is observed to return to a normal color following the resumption of blood flow through the vessels.

The ureter is trimmed to reach the dorsal surface of the bladder without stretching, and the end is spatulated. By opening the tip of the urethra longitudinally, the lumen of the anastomosed ureter is increased in size. A silicone tube or stent may be passed into the ureter to ensure that the lumen is not sutured closed. Simple interrupted sutures of 6/0 nonabsorbable cardiovascular suture are preplaced and the luminal tube removed prior to closure. A direct technique of uretero-neocystostomy has been described (Zonata et al., 2005). In this technique, an incision is made in both the ventral and dorsal portions of the bladder, and the ureter is threaded into the lumen through the small dorsal incision. The edges of the ureter are spatulated and sutured over the top of the mucosa.

Postimplantation, the animal should be flushed with i.v. fluid at a rate of 10–20 ml $kg^{-1}h^{-1}$ and an infusion of 50 ml of 50% mannitol or glucose. An i.v. injection of methylene blue may be used to check for leaks in the ureteral anastomosis. Closure of the surgical incision is routine, and the postoperative recovery procedures should be aimed toward maintenance of adequate fluid levels and normal body temperature. Use of postoperative analgesics, antibiotics, and other therapeutic agents depends upon the experimental protocol. Urine output is particularly important in these studies postoperatively and monitoring serum creatinine, and blood urea nitrogen (BUN) are standard techniques. Creatinine levels >6 mg/dl in association with clinical signs generally are prognostic for irreversible renal failure. Typically, these protocols are designed to test experimental renal preservation solutions or immunosuppressive regimens. One current recommendation is the use of tacrolimus 0.5 mg/kg bid and mycophenolate mofetil 250 mg bid (Zonata et al., 2005). Postoperative complications in addition to renal failure are mainly associated with stricture of the vascular or ureteral anastomosis.

CYSTOTOMY AND URETERAL DIVERSION

The bladder of the pig is thin walled and difficult to catheterize (see earlier text). Consequently, it may be desirable to suture a catheter in place during abdominal surgery in some experimental models. Atraumatic catheters have been designed for the bladder (Figure 7.13). In the pet pig population, urolithiasis is also a problem, and cystotomy may be part of the indicated treatment.

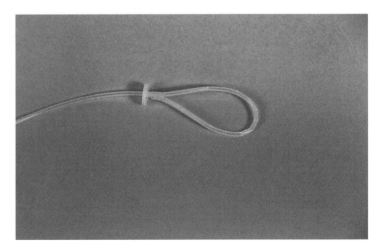

FIGURE 7.13 Urinary bladder catheter which is circular with multiple holes to prevent trauma to the mucosa.

The surgical approach is via a ventral midline incision in females and a paramedian incision lateral to the penis in the male. The bladder is usually drained carefully using a needle and syringe in the male because of the difficulty in catheterization. The surgical approach may be made in any avascular portion of the bladder after packing it away from the viscera with wetted gauze sponges.

Implantation of a Foley catheter may be used for urine collection after it is sutured in place with a purse-string suture in the perineum. If a cystotomy is performed to remove uroliths, the area is copiously flushed with saline prior to suturing the incision closed. The bladder is too thin walled for a double suture layer closure except in larger animals. Any type of suture pattern that achieves a waterproof seal is appropriate. These would include a two-layer pattern of Cushing oversewn with Lembert sutures, simple interrupted, or continuous patterns using synthetic nonabsorbable sutures. The abdominal incision may be closed using a standard technique (Swindle, 1983).

URINARY TRACT OBSTRUCTION, REFLUX NEPHROPATHY, AND HYDRONEPHROSIS

Swine are the preferred model for the study of lower and upper urinary tract obstruction and the resulting complications because of the similarities of their internal renal anatomy to that of humans. Models have been created in various ages of swine to study the different effects of maturity. Swine less than 1 month of age are similar to neonatal humans in development of the urinary tract and swine 5-6 months of age are similar to adults. Most of the pediatric models have been studied in 8- to 12-week-old pigs. Swine can have a spontaneous occurrence of both vesico-ureteral reflux and hydronephrosis and should be screened prior to surgery (Constantinou et al., 1986; Desai et al., 2005; Djurhuus et al., 1976; Jørgensen and Djurhuus, 1986; Jørgensen et al., 1983; Jørgensen et al., 1984a, 1984b; Melick et al., 1961).

A model of intrarenal reflux may be produced by surgically reimplanting the ureters. This is performed using the same ventral midline incision described for cystotomy. The intravesical ureteral roof is excised along with a small wedge of ipsilateral trigonal muscle. The ureteral roof is reimplanted at an angle to straighten the juxtavesicular portion of the ureter after performing a ventral cystotomy. The relaxation and changed angle of the ureteral orifice reliably produces vesico-ureteral reflux. This is an improvement over a previous model of cutting the lower 3–4 mm of the wall of the ureteric orifice following a cystotomy. Intrarenal reflux will not occur with this model unless there is a pressure increase secondary to lower urinary tract obstruction. This is performed by partially obstructing the ureter at the neck of the bladder with a wire or plastic ring. The amount of constriction is variable, depending upon the age and breed of the pig; however, reports range from 3- to 6-mm diameters for the rings. Reflux starts to occur at a bladder pressure of approximately 10 cm H_2O in operated animals, compared to a pressure of greater than 20 cm H_2O in nonoperated animals. Infection may be studied as a complication in either of these models. The progression of the syndrome depends upon the length of time of the extravesicular obstruction as well as the degree of constriction. This procedure may lead to renal failure (Jørgensen and Djurhuus, 1986; Jørgensen et al., 1984a, 1984b). Ureteral damage has been repaired with tubularized porcine small intestine submucosa (Duchene et al., 2004; Liatsikos et al., 2001; O'Connor et al., 2004; Smith et al., 2002) and biodegradable materials (Shalhav et al., 1999). The porcine submucosa induces ureteral ingrowth which remains functional with the characteristics of the normal ureter (Smith et al., 2002). Failures of these grafts are usually associated with inflammation and stricture.

Hydronephrosis and hydroureteronephrosis may also be produced surgically. The left ureter is primarily studied because of the increased incidence of left-sided involvement clinically in humans. The surgical approach is retroperitoneal through the flank, as described for nephrectomy (see earlier text). The ureter is identified as it progresses caudomedially to the caudal pole of the kidney in the retroperitoneal space. Complete obstruction is performed by ligating the ureter. This will lead to a

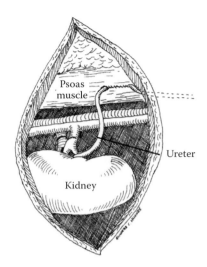

FIGURE 7.14 Suturing the urethra into the psoas muscle from a flank approach.

rapid dilation of the kidney within hours, after which the kidney then shrinks and develops a progressive nephropathy over months (Constantinou et al., 1986; Djurhuus et al., 1976).

Partial obstruction results in more progressive changes over a period of 3–4 months. Partial obstruction may be produced by partial occlusion with cuffs or sutures tied over a premeasured rod or catheter. However, a model of progressive chronic hydronephrosis can be consistently produced by implanting a 1- to 2-cm length of the ureter into the psoas muscle caudal to the kidney. For this model, the fascia of the psoas muscle is incised, and the muscle fibers are split in a curved fashion medially toward the midline in the body of the muscle. The ureter is gently placed into the psoas muscle without torsion or kinking (Figure 7.14). The sheath and ventral edge of the muscle are loosely approximated with simple interrupted sutures. This will lead to a progressive syndrome of chronic hydronephrosis secondary to obstruction within weeks. Percutaneous endopyeloplasty has been studied in a porcine model of partial obstruction created by laparoscopic ligation over a 5-French (Fr) catheter (Desai et al., 2005). Imaging of control and obstructed pigs are illustrated in studies by Thomas Dissing of Aarhus University Hospital (Figure 7.15–Figure 7.18).

The abdominal incision is closed in a routine manner.

PERINEAL URETHROSTOMY AND URINARY DIVERSION

In cases of urolithiasis or trauma in males, it may be necessary to permanently divert the urinary outlet to the perineum or ventral midline. In experimental models, it may be necessary to perform these procedures to facilitate chronic urine collection (Noordhuizen-Stassen and Wensing, 1983; Swindle, 1983; Tscholl, 1978).

The urethra may be palpated by using a rolling movement with the fingers on the brim of the pubis in the perineal region. If percutaneous catheterization (see earlier text) is not achieved or desired, then a perineal urethrostomy may be performed. A dorsal to ventral midline incision approximately 1–2 cm in length is made through the skin and subcutaneous tissue in the dependent portion of the perineum dorsal to the scrotum. The urethra and base of the penis can be identified between the crura and ischiocavernosus muscles and isolated in the subcutaneous tissue. The penis and urethra are ligated ventrally, and, using iris scissors, the urethra is split dorsally for a distance of at least 1 cm. Care should be taken to avoid trauma to this tissue by using atraumatic instruments, such as Debakey forceps, when handling the urethra. Complete hemostasis in the subcutaneous tissue is essential for the success of this procedure. After splitting the urethra, it is sutured to the

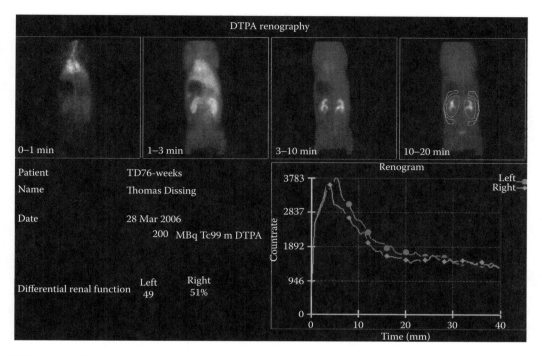

FIGURE 7.15 ^{99m}Tc-DTPA furosemide renography of a 4-week-old sham operated pig with normal kidneys. ^{99m}Tc-DTPA demonstrates glomerular function of the kidneys and urine transportation. The gamma rays emitted from the compound allows the gamma camera to obtain subsequent images displaying its distribution in the body. The resulting dynamic image recording is analyzed with regard to the kidneys filtration of ^{99m}Tc-DTPA and the clearance of the urine from the kidney. By administering furosemide diuresis is enhanced and the patency of the collecting system is demonstrated. The renogram shows the two kidneys both draining well and evenly. The differential renal function shows even function between the two kidneys. (Courtesy of Thomas Dissing, MD, Institute of Clinical Medicine, Aarhus University Hospital, Denmark.)

skin using a simple interrupted pattern with synthetic absorbable or monofilament nonabsorbable sutures. This will result in a dorsal oval-shaped entrance into the urethra with a ventral rectangular-shaped apron. The skin is closed with simple interrupted sutures (Figure 7.19).

If urine collection is the goal of this surgery, pediatric adhesive urine collection bags may be attached to the skin over the incision site. The skin must be prepped with alcohol to achieve adhesion with these bags, and stay sutures may be required. The main complication encountered postoperatively will be urine scalding, especially if the pig is uncastrated and the scrotum is prominent. This complication requires the use of topical anti-inflammatory and/or antibiotic ointments on a chronic basis if it occurs. Simultaneous castration may help relieve this complication by making the scrotum less prominent. Another complication to be considered is contamination with feces in this area. Alternatively, a Foley catheter may be placed into the incised urethra and directed caudally into the plastic adhesive pouch. In this case, the incision is closed with a purse-string suture.

If long-term maintenance of the animal is indicated, then it may be preferable to perform urinary diversion by performing an urethrostomy with the urethra directed ventrally cranial to the scrotum on the ventral midline.

PREPUTIAL DIVERTICULUM ABLATION

The preputial diverticulum may be surgically ablated to reduce the odor of male pigs and to relieve infection of the structure. The structure should be manually expressed and flushed with saline and

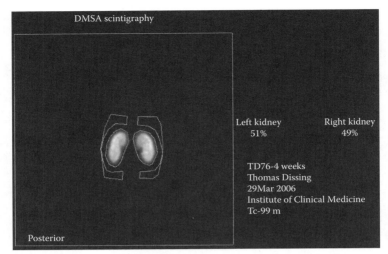

FIGURE 7.16 ^{99m}Tc-DMSA scintigraphy of the same pig (Figure 7.15) the following day. ^{99m}Tc-DMSA demonstrates renal tubular function. The compound is taken up by proximal tubular cells. The amount of uptake is in close relation to the amount of functioning renal mass. The following day after its administration the scintigraphy is performed. The image produced displays ^{99m}Tc-DMSA distributed in the body with the vast majority taken up by the kidneys. The functional distribution in this examination confirms even function of the two kidneys. (Courtesy of Thomas Dissing, MD, Institute of Clinical Medicine, Aarhus University Hospital, Denmark.)

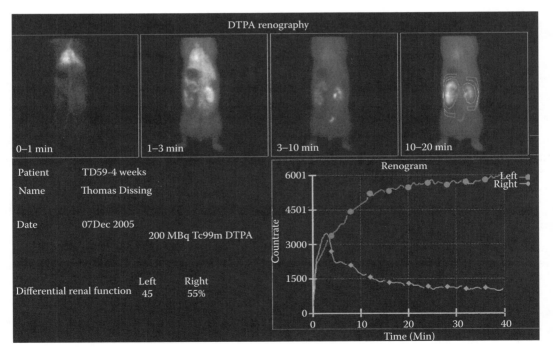

FIGURE 7.17 ^{99m}Tc-DTPA furosemide renography of a 4-week-old pig that was subjected to ureteric obstruction at the age of 2 d. The renogram shows severe hydronephrosis and impaired drainage of the left kidney. The differential renal function of the left kidney is slightly decreased, which could be interpreted as the onset of progressive kidney damage. (Courtesy of Thomas Dissing, MD, Institute of Clinical Medicine, Aarhus University Hospital, Denmark.)

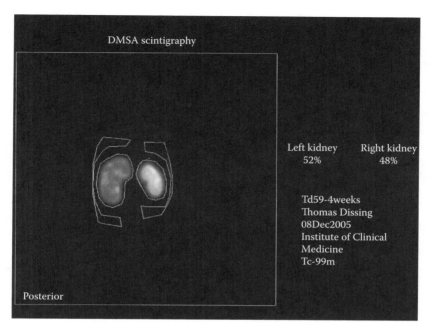

FIGURE 7.18 ^{99m}Tc-DMSA Scintigraphy of the 4-week-old pig (Figure 7.17). The left kidney has a slightly higher differential renal function. The suspicion of kidney damage raised by the renography is therefore not confirmed by the scintigraphy. Hence, the two investigations together do not demonstrate abnormal function of the obstructed kidney. (Courtesy of Thomas Dissing, MD, Institute of Clinical Medicine, Aarhus University Hospital, Denmark.)

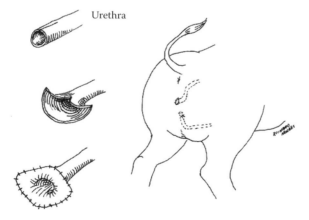

FIGURE 7.19 Perineal urethrostomy.

dilute Betadine solution prior to surgery. There are two lateral epithelial-lined pouches within the structure. These are exteriorized one at a time by inserting Allis or Babcock forceps into the preputial opening and directing them laterally. After grasping the lining of the structure with the forceps, the lining is steadily pulled out of the opening. This process is then repeated on the opposite side. Any visible blood vessels are cauterized or ligated, and the structure is excised. The resected pockets are packed with umbilical tape or gauze for 5–10 min to provide hemostasis. After the gauze is removed, the structure is examined for hemorrhage and repacked if necessary.

The surgery may also be performed by an open technique, in which the diverticular pouches are packed with umbilical tape or gauze to identify them, and a skin incision is made over each structure. The pouches are then dissected free from the subcutaneous tissue. The surgical wound is closed with subcuticular sutures (Bollwahn, 1992; Dutton et al., 1997; Kross et al., 1982; Lawhorn et al., 1994; St-Jean and Anderson, 1999).

ADRENALECTOMY

The surgical approaches to the adrenal gland are the same as for midline, flank, and retroperitoneal approaches to the kidney, described previously for nephrectomy. The surgical anatomy of the adrenal glands is depicted in Chapter 1, Figure 1.41 and Figure 7.1. Indications for adrenalectomy in swine will most likely involve the creation of a model of adrenal insufficiency and thus will probably be bilateral. If a unilateral adrenalectomy is indicated, the left adrenal gland is more readily removed (Dougherty, 1981).

Regardless of the surgical approach, the adrenal glands are readily mobilized by blunt dissection. In older animals, they will probably be covered with perirenal fat. After identification of the arterial branches, the branches are ligated and transected. Variations in the blood supply to both glands may be encountered, and care should be taken not to damage the renal vessels during the dissection. Careful dissection is required to separate the right adrenal gland from the wall of the caudal vena cava and to ligate the venous drainage. Removal of this gland may require repair of the vessel wall. After the adrenalectomy is performed, the abdominal incision is closed in a routine fashion.

Intraoperative and postoperative care is directed toward controlling the effects of glucocorticoid and mineralocorticoid insufficiency. In a bilateral procedure, these complications can rapidly lead to death from electrolyte imbalances. Unilateral procedures may induce adrenocortical insufficiency, which may require supplementation until the remaining adrenal gland hypertrophies and restores function. Monitoring of serum electrolytes, especially potassium, and glucose is essential. Fluid therapy and glucocorticoid administration, with such agents as prednisolone, will be necessary to restore imbalances. With a bilateral adrenalectomy, the exogenous maintenance therapy is permanent. Otherwise, postoperative care is routine for celiotomies and laparotomies.

REFERENCES

Assimos, D.G., Boyce, W.H., Lively, M., Weidner, N., Lewis, J.C., Howard, G., Furr, E., Sorrell, M., McCullough, D.L., Bullock, B.C., and Palmer, T.E., 1986, Porcine urologic models including jejunoileal bypass. In Tumbleson, M.E. (Ed.), *Swine in Biomedical Research,* Vol. 1, pp. 385–390.

Bollwahn, W., 1992, Surgical procedures in boars and sows, in Leman, A.D., Straw, B.E., Mengeling, W.L., D'Allaire, S., and Taylor, D.J., Eds., *Diseases of Swine,* 7th ed., Ames, IA: Iowa State University Press, pp. 782–793.

Constantinou, C.E., Djurhuus, J.C., Vercesi, L., Ford, A.J., and Meindl, J.D., 1986, Model for chronic obstruction and hydronephrosis, in Tumbleson, M.E., Ed., *Swine in Biomedical Research,* Vol. 3, New York: Plenum Press, pp. 1711–1724.

Dalmose, A.L., Hvistendahl, J.J., Olsen, L.H., Eskild-Jensen, A., Dhurhuus, J.C., and Swindle, M.M., 2000, Surgically induced urologic models in swine, *J. Invest. Surg.,* 13: 133–145.

Desai, M.M., Desai, R.M.R., and Gill, I.S., 2005, Percutaneous endopyeloplasty: current clinical status, *BJU Int.,* 95(Suppl. 2): 106–109.

Djurhuus, J.C., Nerstrom, B., Gyrd-Hansen, N., and Rask-Anderson, H., 1976, Experimental hydronephrosis, *Acta Chir. Scand.,* 472(Suppl.): 17–28.

Dougherty, R.W., 1981, *Experimental Surgery in Farm Animals,* Ames, IA: Iowa State University Press.

Duchene, D.A., Jacomides, L., Ogan, K., Lindberg, G., Johnson, D.B., Pearle, M.S., and Cadeddu, J.A., 2004, Ureteral replacement using small intestinal submucosa and a collagen inhibitor in a porcine model, *J. Endourol.,* 18(5): 507–511.

Dutton, D.M., Lawhorn, B., and Hooper, R.N., 1997, Ablation of the cranial portion of he preputial cavity in a pig, *J. Am. Vet. Med. Assoc.,* 211(5): 598–599.

Gill, I.S., Hsu, T.H.S., Fox, R.L., Matamoros, A., Miller, C.D., LeVeen, R.F., Grune, M.T., Sung, G.T., and Fidler, M.E., 2000, Laparoscopic and percutaneous radiofrequency ablation of the kidney: acute and chronic porcine study, *Urology*, 56(2): 197–200.

Hodson, C.J., 1986, The pig as a model for studying kidney disease in man, in Tumbleson, M.E., Ed., *Swine in Biomedical Research*, Vol. 3, New York: Plenum Press, pp. 1691–1704.

Howard, T., Cosenza, C.A., Cramer, D.V., and Makowka, L., 1994, Kidney transplantation in Yucatan miniature swine, in Cramer, D.V., Podesta, L., and Makowka, L., Eds., *Handbook of Animal Models in Transplantation Research*, Boca Raton, FL: CRC Press, pp. 19–28.

Jørgensen, T.M. and Djurhuus, J.C., 1986, Experimental vesicoureteric reflux in pigs, in Tumbleson, M.E., Ed., *Swine in Biomedical Research*, Vol. 3, New York: Plenum Press, pp. 1737–1751.

Jørgensen, T.M., Djurhuus, J.C., Jorgensen, H.S., and Sorensen, S.S., 1983, Experimental bladder hyperreflexia in pigs, *Urol. Res.*, 11(5): 239–240.

Jørgensen, T.M., Mortensen, J., Nielsen, K., and Djurhuus, J.C., 1984a, Pathogenetic factors in vesico-ureteral reflux: a longitudinal cystometrographic study in pigs, *Scand. J. Urol. Nephrol.*, 18(1): 43–48.

Jørgensen, T.M., Olsen, S., Djurhuus, J.C., and Norgaard, J.P., 1984b, Renal morphology in experimental vesicoureteral reflux in pigs, *Scand. J. Urol. Nephrol.*, 18(1): 49–58.

Kirkman, R.I., Colvin, R.B., Flye, M.W., Leight, G.S., Rosenberg, S.A., and Williams, G.M., 1979, Transplantation in miniature swine: VI. Factors influencing survival of renal allografts, *Transplantation*, 28(1): 18–23.

Kross, S.B., Ames, N.K., and Gibson, C., 1982, Extirpation of the preputial diverticulum in a boar, *Vet. Med. Small Anim. Clin.*, 77(4): 549–553.

Lawhorn, B., Jarrett, P.D., and Lackey, G.F., 1994, Removal of the preputial diverticulum in swine, *J. Am. Vet. Med. Assoc.*, 205: 92–96.

Liatsikos, E.N., Dinlenc, C.Z., Kapoor, R., Alexianu, M., Yohannes, P., and Anderson, A.E., 2001, Laparoscopic ureteral reconstruction with small intestinal submucosa, *J. Endourol.*, 15: 217.

Melick, W.F., Naryka, J.J., and Schmidt, J.H., 1961, Experimental studies of ureteral peristaltic patterns in the pig: similarity of pig and human ureter and bladder physiology, *J. Urol.*, 85(1): 145–148.

Noordhuizen-Stassen, E.N. and Wensing, C.J., 1983, The effect of transection of the main vascular and nervous supply of the testis on the development of spermatogenic epithelium in the pig, *J. Pediatr. Surg.*, 18(5): 601–606.

O'Connor, R.C., Hollowell, C.M., and Steinberg, G.D., 2002, Distal ureteral replacement with tubularized porcine small intestine submucosa, *Urology*, 60(4): 697.

O'Hagan, K.P. and Zambraski, E.J., 1986, Kidney function in deoxycorticosterone acetate (DOCA) treated hypertensive Yucatan miniature swine, in Tumbleson, M.E., Ed., *Swine in Biomedical Research*, Vol. 3, New York: Plenum Press, pp. 1779–1787.

Olsen, L.H., Dalmose, A.L., Swindle, M.M., Jørgensen, T.M., and Djurhuus, J.C., 2001, Male fetal pig lower urinary tract function in mid second and early third trimester of gestation, *J. Urol.*, 165(6 Pt. 2): 2331–2334.

Olsen, L.H., Dalmose, A.L., Swindle, M.M., Djurhuus, J.C., and Jørgensen, T.M., 2004, Male fetal pig lower urinary tract function. Part II: free voiding pattern close to term and in the newborn, *J. Urol.*, 171(6 Pt. 2): 2660–2663.

Pennington, L.R., 1992, Renal transplantation in swine, in Swindle, M.M., Ed., *Swine as Models in Biomedical Research*, Ames, IA: Iowa State University Press, pp. 35–43.

Peters, C.A., 2001, Animal models of fetal renal disease, *Prenatal Diagn.*, 21(11): 917–923.

Russell, J.M., Webb, R.T., and Boyce, W.H., 1981, Intrarenal surgery: animal model I. Invest, *Urology*, 19(2): 123–125.

Sachs, D.H., 1992, MHC-homozygous miniature swine, in Swindle, M.M., Ed., *Swine as Models in Biomedical Research*, Ames, IA: Iowa State University Press, pp. 3–15.

Shalhav, A.L., Elbahnasy, A.M., Bercowsky, E., Kovacs, G., Brewer, A., and Maxwell, K.L., 1999, Laparoscopic replacement of urinary tract segments using biodegradable materials in a large animal model, *J. Endourol.*, 13(4): 241–244.

Smith, T.G., Gettman, M., Lindberg, G., Napper, C., Pearle, M.S., and Caddedu, J.A., 2002, Ureteral replacement using porcine small intestine submucosa in a porcine model, *Urology*, 60: 931–934.

St-Jean, G. and Anderson, D.E., 1999, Anesthesia and surgical procedures in swine, in Straw, B.E., D'Allaire, S., Mengeling, W.L., Taylor, D.J., Eds., *Diseases of Swine*, 8th ed., Ames, IA: Iowa State University Press, pp. 1133–1154.

Swindle, M.M., 1983, *Basic Surgical Exercises Using Swine*, Philadelphia, PA: Praeger Press.

Swindle, M.M. and Olson, J., 1988, Urogenital system, in Swindle, M.M. and Adams, R.J., Eds., *Experimental Surgery and Physiology: Induced Animal Models of Human Disease*, Baltimore, MD: Williams and Wilkins, pp. 42–73.

Swindle, M.M. and Smith, A.C., 1998, Comparative anatomy and physiology of the pig, *Scand. J. Lab. Anim. Sci.*, 25(Suppl. 1): 1–10.

Terris, J.M., 1986, Swine as a model in renal physiology and nephrology: an overview, in Tumbleson, M.E., Ed., *Swine in Biomedical Research*, Vol. 2, New York: Plenum Press, pp. 1673–1690.

Tscholl, R., 1978, Urinary diversion, *Urol. Res.*, 6(1): 59–63.

Venzke, W.G., 1975, Porcine endocrinology, in Getty, R., Ed., *Sisson and Grossman's The Anatomy of the Domestic Animals: Porcine*, Vol. 2, Philadelphia, PA: WB Saunders, pp. 1304–1305.

Wagner, A.A., Solomon, S.B., and Su, L.M., 2005, Treatment of renal tumors with radiofrequency ablation, *J. Endourol.*, 19(6): 643–652.

Webster, S.K., Deleo, M.A., and Burhop, K.E., 1992, The anephric micropig as a model for peritoneal dialysis, in Swindle, M.M., Ed., *Swine as Models in Biomedical Research*, Ames, IA: Iowa State University Press, pp. 64–73.

Williams, G.M., 1988, Renal transplantation, in Swindle, M.M. and Adams, R.J., Eds., *Experimental Surgery and Physiology: Induced Animal Models of Human Disease*, Baltimore, MD: Williams and Wilkins, pp. 298–299.

Zonata, S., Lovisetto, F., Lorenzo, C., Abbiati, F., Alessiani, M., Dionigi, P., and Zonata, A., 2005, Ureteroneocystostomy in a swine model of kidney transplantation: a new technique, *J. Surg. Res.*, 124: 250–255.

8 The Reproductive System

GENERAL PRINCIPLES OF SURGERY

The reproductive tract of the female is typical of that of a bicornuate species that produces litters. The ovaries are located caudal to the kidneys and are only loosely attached by a thin ovarian ligament and suspended within the broad ligament of the uterus (mesometrium). The ovarian vessels are the last branches of the aorta and vena cava prior to the iliac bifurcation at approximately L5–L6. The fallopian tubes are long and tortuous and typically form coils in the caudal abdominal cavity (Chapter 1, Figure 1.43; Figure 8.1 and Figure 8.2). The fallopian tubes of an 80- to 100-kg pig approximate the diameter of those of an adult human (Rock et al., 1979). The uterine horns are long and curve cranially from the ovaries and then reverse direction to form the short body of the uterus at approximately the same region of the ovaries in the midsagittal plane. The cervix is thick, elongated, and has a curved cervical canal. The vagina extends caudally in the pelvic cavity and contains the urethral orifice on the ventral floor at approximately the level of the caudal edge of the pubic bone and has similar morphologic characteristics to humans (D'Cruz et al., 2005). The pig has a diffuse epitheliochorial placentation with drug transport and metabolic mechanisms similar to humans. This type of placenta does not invade the endometrium. The placental membranes include the yolk sac, amnion, allantois, and chorion, and the latter two membranes fuse at an early stage to form a chorioallantoic type of placenta. The chorioallentois is responsible for transplacental transport of nutrients from the sow (Bazer et al., 2001; Swindle and Bobbie, 1987; Swindle et al., 1996; Wiest et al., 1996).

Paired mammary glands are located on the ventral surface of the abdomen and may extend to the caudal thorax and caudal inguinal regions. The number of glands is highly variable with an average of 6–7 pairs. Generally, breeds that produce large litters have a greater number. The vasculature is located along the lateral edges of the row of glands. The pectoral and cranial abdominal glands receive their blood supply from branches of the internal thoracic artery, which continues along the glands on the abdomen as the cranial superficial epigastric artery. These mammary glands drain into the cranial superficial epigastric vein, which continues cranially as the internal thoracic vein. The caudal glands (2–3 pairs) receive their blood supply from the external pudendal arteries, and drainage is from the pudendal veins into the iliac system (Bazer et al., 2001).

The male reproductive system is typical of domestic animals in location; however, there are several variations in anatomy that are important surgically (see Chapter 1, Figure 1.42). The scrotum and testicles are located in the perineal region and may be of considerable size in adult males. The spermatic cord passes through each inguinal ring in the caudal abdomen. The spermatic vessels branch off the aorta and vena cava just cranial to the iliac bifurcation. Each ductus deferens enters the urethra independently on the dorsal surface at the neck of the bladder. The accessory sex glands are similar to those of humans except for the prominence of the various structures. The paired vesicular glands are large and located on either side along the neck of the bladder. The prostate is small and located on the dorsal surface of the urethra at the entrance of the ductus deferens. Paired bulbourethral glands extend along the dorsolateral surface of the urethra starting at the caudal brim of the pubis; these may extend along the entire length of the pubis in intact adults. The crus of the penis and the ischiocavernosus muscles form at the caudal surface of the pubis with the base of the penis. The penis extends ventrally and cranially forming a fibromuscular sigmoid flexure as it

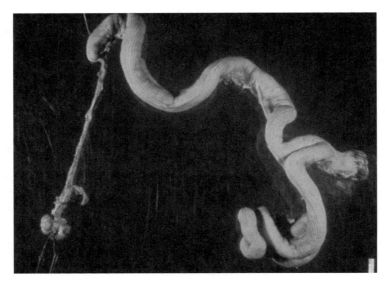

FIGURE 8.1 Anatomy of the female reproductive tract. The fallopian tube is fully extended on one horn.

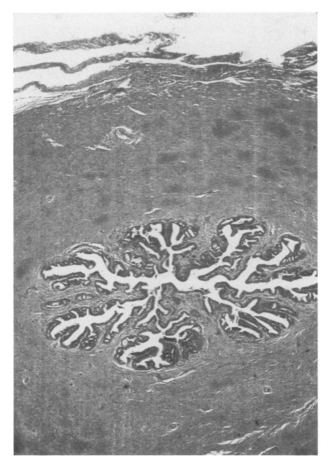

FIGURE 8.2 Histology of the fallopian tube. H&E, ×40.

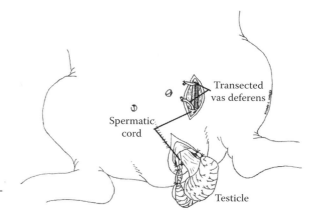

FIGURE 8.3 Castration and vasectomy surgical sites.

curves from the perineum to the ventral surface of the abdomen. The penis extends almost to the umbilicus before terminating in the preputial diverticulum in a corkscrew shape. The preputial diverticulum is described additionally with the urinary system; however, it is important to restate that it must be cleaned before surgically preparing the abdomen and that gloves should be worn to avoid contamination with the foul-smelling fluid contents. The tip of the penis is almost impossible to exteriorize without trauma (Swindle et al., 1988; Swindle and Bobbie, 1987).

CASTRATION (ORCHIECTOMY) AND VASECTOMY

Swine may be castrated either by scrotal, prescrotal, or ventral midline approaches. The most common approach in small swine is prescrotal, whereas the scrotal approach predominates in adult males. For either the prescrotal or the ventral midline approach, the testicle is manually manipulated cranially, and either a paramedian or midline incision is made over the testicle (Becker, 1992; Mayo and Becker 1982; McGlone and Hellman, 1988; St-Jean and Anderson, 1999; Swindle, 1983).

The skin and subcutaneous tissue are incised in the initial incision. The tunica vaginalis is incised without incising the testicular tissue. The testicle is exteriorized, and the spermatic cord is dissected away from the mesorchium. Clamps are placed across the scrotal ligament, and the spermatic cord and the testis are removed. The spermatic cord and the scrotal ligament are ligated with synthetic absorbable suture material. The incision is closed with continuous suture patterns in the tunica vaginalis and subcutaneous tissues. The skin is closed in a subcuticular pattern. It is unnecessary and undesirable to leave the castration incision open and draining as is done in the agricultural setting. If adequate hemostasis is achieved, seromas or hematomas will not be a problem.

If a vasectomy is to be performed, the spermatic cord is identified as it passes from the scrotum to the inguinal canal at approximately a 45° angle to the midline from the scrotum to the brim of the pubis. At approximately one half the distance between the scrotum and the inguinal canal, the spermatic cord can be palpated as a firm tubular structure. A skin incision is made over the spermatic cord, and the tunic is incised. The vas deferens can be identified as a firm whitish structure approximately 2–3 mm in diameter. The vas deferens is isolated, doubly ligated, and a segment removed. The tunic is closed with simple interrupted sutures, and the skin and subcutaneous tissues are closed in a routine manner (Figure 8.3).

OVARIOHYSTERECTOMY, HYSTERECTOMY, OVARIECTOMY, OR TUBAL LIGATION

The female reproductive tract is usually approached through a ventral midline incision except in the case of a cesarean section (see the following text). The incision extends from the brim of the

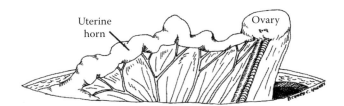

FIGURE 8.4 Exposure of the uterus and ovary.

pubis to approximately two thirds of the distance cranially to the umbilicus. Upon entering the abdomen, the fallopian tubes are likely to be the initial structures encountered in the nongravid system. They may be used to trace the origin of the ovaries and the horns of the uterus (Christenson et al., 1987; St-Jean and Anderson, 1999; Swindle, 1983).

The ovarian vessels are clamped, incised, and ligated proximally and distally. If only an ovariectomy is to be performed, then the fallopian tubes are divided surgically in the same manner, and the ovaries are removed. A tubal ligation may be performed by doubly ligating and dividing the structures or by placing occlusal devices on the structure for reversible sterilization (Rock et al., 1979).

If an ovariohysterectomy is to be performed, then it is necessary to dissect the horns of the uterus from the broad ligament of the uterus (Figure 8.4). This is performed by bluntly dissecting along the uterine vessels following the curvature of the uterine horns. The middle uterine vessels will have to be divided and ligated separately. The dissection is continued bilaterally to the level of the cervix.

At this point, the ovaries and uterine horns are retracted caudally, and the cervix is exteriorized. The blood vessels on the lateral sides of the vagina are individually ligated in place. The vagina proximal to the cervix is cross-clamped and divided. The vaginal stump is sutured with transfixing ligatures in the case of nulliparous animals. In sows, the stump may have to be divided using an inverting technique such as a Cushing oversewn with a Lembert pattern. In the case of a hysterectomy, the instructions for the ovariohysterectomy are followed except that the ovaries are left intact, and the initial surgical transection starts with the fallopian tubes (Figure 8.5).

The middle uterine artery may be surgically constricted to reduce blood flow to the fetuses dependent upon the blood supply to the uterus. If performed in the second trimester of pregnancy, it retards fetal and placental growth and development. It also reduces maternal estrogen blood levels (Molina et al., 1985).

Unlike many species of domestic animals, such as the dog and cat, swine rarely develop pyometritis, and the indications for these procedures are rarely clinical. Consequently, problems

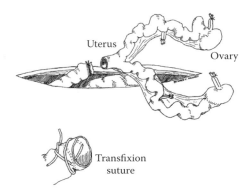

FIGURE 8.5 Ovariohysterectomy.

associated with removal of the gonads and retention of the uterus are rare. Rather, these procedures tend to be either research techniques or surgical sterilization procedures for the pet pig. In the case of pet pigs, the ovaries should be removed in order to avoid the behavioral problems associated with estrus.

CESAREAN SECTION (C-SECTION)

A c-section may be performed using a midline, paramedian, or flank surgical approach (St-Jean and Anderson, 1999; Swindle et al., 1996). The midline and paramedian incisions are made as described previously for ovariohysterectomy. If it is to be performed as a survival procedure with the pigs being allowed to nurse the sow, then it is best to avoid the midline approach. The midline will be constantly irritated by the pigs, and infection and refusal to nurse will be encountered as complications.

The paramedian incision is made along the dorsolateral margin of the mammary glands with the pig in lateral recumbency. The incision is made from the cranial margin of the retracted rear leg (approximately the brim of the pubis) to approximately the level of the umbilicus. In the pregnant sow, the muscle in this region will be thin and relatively avascular when cut; however, several branches of the caudal abdominal arteries (mainly external pudendal arterial branches) will have to be ligated or cauterized.

The flank approach is the most commonly employed approach for a c-section when the pigs are going to be allowed to nurse. A vertical incision is made from the level of the wings of the lumbar vertebrae ventrally to a point halfway to the mammary glands. The incision is located approximately one half of the distance between the cranial surface of the thigh to the last rib. After making the skin incision, the muscles may either be bluntly dissected or transected in layers until the abdominal cavity is exposed.

Depending upon the number of fetuses and the experimental purpose of the surgery, multiple incisions will probably have to be made along the uterine horn, rather than making a single incision in the body of the uterus and removing all the fetuses through it. If the uterus and fetuses are large, it may be possible to remove all the fetuses and membranes through an incision in the uterine horn. If fetuses have been manipulated experimentally, however, then an incision either over each fetus or between two fetuses may be required.

When the decision has been made to incise the uterus, the surgical site is packed off with warm saline-wetted laparotomy sponges. The uterotomy incision may be made using a scalpel; however, better hemostasis is achieved using absorbable GIA-60 3.8-mm staples (Figure 8.6). The device is inserted and fired after making a stab incision into the amniotic cavity. The fetus and membranes are extracted and handed to an assistant, who cleans and resuscitates the piglet after ligation of the umbilical vessels. The uterus will contract relatively rapidly following removal of a fetus, which hampers the effort to remove multiple fetuses from the same incision. Hemorrhage from removal of the fetal membranes is usually minimal, provided the c-section is performed at full-term gestation.

If a fetus is being removed before full-term gestation, then it is necessary to ligate and transect the umbilical vessels first. After this procedure, the membranes are bluntly separated from the uterine wall and extirpated. Gauze sponges may have to be used to provide hemostasis of the uterine wall following this procedure.

The uterotomy may be closed with a two-layer suture pattern of Cushing or Connell sutures oversewn with a Lembert suture pattern. It may also be closed with a staple surgical device, such as a TA-90 3.8 mm with absorbable staples, if staples were used to perform the uterotomy. In this case, the initial lines of staples are lifted together using Babcock forceps, and the TA device is closed distal to the suture line (Figure 8.7). After firing the device, a scalpel is used to trim the uterus between the device and the GIA staples. The line of TA staples is oversewn with a continuous Lembert pattern using absorbable sutures. The celiotomy incision is closed in a routine manner.

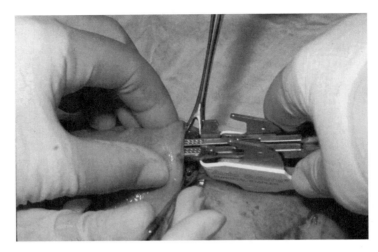

FIGURE 8.6 Uterotomy using a staple device. (Reprinted from Swindle et al., 1996, *Lab. Anim. Sci.* 46(1): 90–95. With permission.)

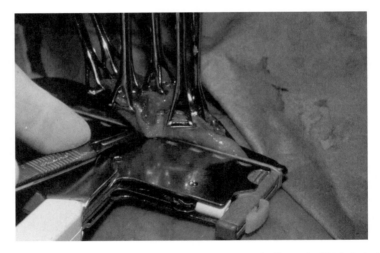

FIGURE 8.7 Closure of the uterus with staples. (Reprinted from Swindle et al., 1996, *Lab. Anim. Sci.* 46(1): 90–95. With permission.)

Fertility may be impaired following a c-section and this must be considered when making a clinical decision about performing the surgery as a survival procedure in the sow. Oxytocin may be given postoperatively if there is reason to believe that intrauterine hemorrhage may occur or that membranes remain in the uterus.

FETAL SURGERY AND FETAL CATHETERIZATION

The use of the pig as a fetal surgical model, described in the preceding sections, is increasing because of the metabolic and anatomic similarities to humans and the availability of miniature breeds. Miniature breeds should be used whenever possible, because of the ease of handling smaller animals, which makes them significantly safer for personnel. For instance, a pregnant Yucatan sow may weigh 45–60 kg in contrast to a pregnant domestic farm pig that will probably weigh in excess of 135 kg. In this section, only the general surgical principles and the fetal catheterization techniques will be described. Other models will be described in the systemic sections of this text (Care et al.,

TABLE 8.1
Relative Fetal Sizes for Various Breeds at Different Stages of Pregnancy

Breed	Gestation Day	Crown/Rump Length (cm)	Weight (g)
Yucatan	100	15.7–16.9	350–391.3
	90–92	15.8–17.5	318–403.5
Göttingen	111–112	13–16	305.3–370.4
Landrace	80	16.5–17.5	332.5–337

1986; Dungan et al., 1995; Jackson and Egdahl, 1960; Jones and Hudak, 1988; Kraeling et al., 1986; Randall, 1986; Rosenkrantz et al., 1968; Sims et al., 1997; Swindle et al., 1996; Wiest et al., 1996). The optimal embryonic age for harvesting of fetal tissues for transplantation have been outlined for the liver, pancreas, and lung (Eventov-Friedman et al., 2005). The embryonic age at which tissues are produced following subrenal capsular implant of macerated tissues in mice were as follows: liver (21- to 28-d gestation), pancreas (28- to 56-d gestation), lung (56- to 80-d gestation). Earlier implantation dates resulted in teratoma formation without functional adult tissue. Comparisons of embryonic development with humans and spontaneous congenital defects of minipigs are outlined in Table 8.2 and Table 8.3, respectively.

Timing of the surgery may make a difference in the selection of the breed because of size of the fetus. Each trimester of pregnancy is 38 d in a species with a 114-d gestation period. The last trimester of pregnancy (>78 d) is used for many procedures, because the size of the fetus makes it amenable to catheterization and device implantation. The consistency and volume of the amniotic fluid changes as gestation progresses. For the first two trimesters, the amniotic fluid has a watery consistency and occupies a relatively large volume of the amniotic sac. As parturition approaches, the amniotic fluid becomes relatively thick and yellowish in color from the passage of meconium. In the last few days of pregnancy, the fluid volume is substantially decreased. The fluid volume is highly variable between sows, and it is unclear whether replacement of the volume is necessary following fetal surgery. In our experience, the saline drip (described later) used during surgery is generally sufficient to replace the volume lost. Some relative sizes of the fetus at different stages of pregnancy for various breeds are given in Table 8.1.

Maintenance of normothermia and homeostasis of the sow is imperative in order to be successful with the procedures described here. This can be achieved by a combination of all or some of the following: (1) keeping the room temperature higher than 29°C, (2) use of circulating water blankets both below and above the sow's thorax, (3) use of heat lamps suspended near the surgical site, and (4) dripping saline of 37°C into the amniotic cavity during surgery. Use of the warmed saline drip allows lowering the room temperature and discontinuance of the heat lamps that can be desiccating to delicate fetal tissues.

Other perioperative procedures that contribute to the success of these procedures include restricting the fetus from breathing by keeping the head submerged in amniotic fluid, meticulous attention to asepsis, the prophylactic use of systemic antibiotics, delicate handling of tissues, and an anesthetic protocol that does not significantly depress the sow or fetus. Anesthesia is discussed in a separate chapter; however, analgesics and muscle relaxants may be delivered directly to the fetus if necessary. For example, pancuronium may be administered to restrict fetal breathing if the fetal head has to be removed from the uterus during surgery. Hemostasis is essential in any of the procedures performed because of the small blood volume of the fetus. Vessels should be ligated in advance of transection, if possible, and electrocautery on a low setting should be used. Use of microsurgical instruments and microsurgical cannonball and spear-shaped swabs are helpful in some procedures. All fetal tissue is extremely friable and can be readily traumatized by use of

TABLE 8.2
Embryonic Development in Göttingen Minipigs

	Minipigs		Humans	
Event	Gestation Day[a]	Length (mm)	Gestation Day[a]	Length (mm)
Two-cell stage	1		1	
Morula	3		2	
Blastula	5–6		4–5	
Somites appear	14–15	3.0	20–21	2–3
Optic vesicles form	16	3.5–4.5	24–25	3–4.5
Neural groove closes	16–18	4.5–5.5	24–27	3–5
Upper limb buds appear	18	5.5	26–27	3.5–5
Hind limb buds appear	20	8.5	28–30	4–6
Digital rays present	24	14–15	36–42	9–14
Nipples form	28	22.5	43–49	13–22
Eyelids form	35	30–35	43–49	13–22
Palate closes	35	30–35	56	21–31

[a] Fertilization day = 0.

Source: Reprinted from Jørgensen, K.D., 1998, *Scand. J. Lab. Anim. Sci.*, 25(Suppl. 1): 63–75; as modified from Glodek, P. and Oldigs, B., 1981, *Das Gottinger Miniatursch-wein*, Verlag Paul Parey-Berlin und Hamburg, pp. 130–142. With permission.

adult-sized surgical instruments. Ophthalmic and pediatric instruments are useful in cases in which the smaller microsurgical instruments are not required. All gauze should be wetted, and the fetus and membranes should be bathed regularly in saline warmed to 37–38°C. Monitoring the fetal heart rate is a very helpful indicator of fetal distress and hypothermia. In an 80- to 90-d-old fetus, the heart rate is approximately 180 beats per minute.

The paramedian surgical approach, as described for c-section, is preferred to avoid having undue pressure placed on the aorta when the sow is restrained in dorsal recumbency. This may lead to cardiovascular compromise, uteroplacental ischemia, or both. The line of incision is made in an avascular section along the antimesometrial border of the uterus. The uterotomy is best performed using staple surgical devices as described for c-sections (Figure 8.6). If the uterotomy is done using conventional surgical techniques, hemostasis becomes problematic for the fetal membranes. They are too friable for most hemostatic techniques, and electrocautery does not function well. Babcock forceps can be placed on the edges of the incision so as to provide occlusion of the hemorrhaging vessel. Use of surgical staples seems to help prevent the edematous reaction that occurs in the fetal membranes if conventional surgical methods are used.

The position of the fetus in the uterus can be determined prior to performing the uterotomy by careful palpation. The snout tends to be readily identifiable after the middle of the second trimester of pregnancy. Care should be taken to avoid damaging the membranes or the umbilical cord during the palpation and the surgical procedure. Hemorrhage in the membranes can lead to abortion, fetal mummification, or resorption. In the first trimester of pregnancy, pinching the membranes and the fetal head can be used as a technique to reduce the number of fetuses *in utero*.

The smallest incision possible should be used to expose the area of interest in the fetus. Following uterotomy, the fetal surgical site should be gently rotated into the incision with care, so that torsion of the umbilical vessels is avoided. An assistant can retain the fetal surgical site in the uterotomy exposure by applying gentle pressure beneath the fetus. The fetus can also be positioned by exposing a fetal leg and manually restraining it using a wetted gauze sponge. Loss of amniotic fluid is not

TABLE 8.3
Incidence of Congenital Anomalies in Göttingen Minipigs (2001–2005)

Description	Code	2005	2004	2003	2002	2001
Number of liveborn minipigs		4957	4957	3916	2887	3021
Male		2519	2569	2049	1490	1544
Female		2438	2388	1867	1397	1477
Stillborn	240303	230	298	305	212	216
Percentage of total pigs born		4.64	6.01	7.79	7.34	7.15
Cryptorchidism	241701	95	127	97	—	—
Percentage of male pigs born		3.77	4.94	4.73	—	—
Double cryptorchidism	241702	9	18	11	1	1
Percentage of male pigs born		0.36	0.70	0.54	0.07	0.06
Scrotal hernia	241703	101	172	157	—	—
Percentage of total pigs born		2.04	3.47	4.01	—	—
Inguinal hernia	411801	62	119	175	—	—
Percentage of total pigs born		1.25	2.40	4.47	—	—
Anal atresia	241801	1	1	3	0	1
Percentage of total pigs born		0.02	0.02	0.08	0.00	0.03
Defect in claw[a]	241901	2	0	0	0	0
Percentage of total pigs born		0.04	0.00	0.00	0.00	0.00
Polydactyly[b]	241902	84	154	223	66	42
Percentage of total pigs born		1.69	3.11	5.69	2.29	1.39
Syndactyly	410301	15	17	18	2	3
Percentage of total pigs born		0.30	0.34	0.46	0.07	0.10
Other deformity, leg[c]	410401	24	27	36	1	1
Percentage of total pigs born		0.48	0.54	0.92	0.03	0.03
Blind, one eye	410901	4	9	11	0	0
Percentage of total pigs born		0.08	0.18	0.28	0.00	0.00
Blind, both eyes	410902	0	2	1	1	0
Percentage of total pigs born		0.00	0.04	0.03	0.03	0.00
Defect in ears[d]	411201	5	9	8	21	0
Percentage of total pigs born		0.10	0.18	0.20	0.73	0.00
Other deformity, head[e]	411301	12	12	20	—	—
Percentage of total pigs born		0.24	0.24	0.51	—	—
Hermaphrodite	412101	0	0	0	0	0
Percentage of total pigs born		0.00	0.00	0.00	0.00	0.00
Defect in jaw[f]	411101	6	4	—	—	—
Percentage of total pigs born		0.12	0.08	—	—	—

Note: Dash (—) indicates items not registered.

[a] Process on claw, abnormal nail growth, etc.
[b] Includes front and rear legs.
[c] Stiff knee joint, crooked/gnarled leg, stiff leg aligned with body, etc. In all cases, both forelegs and hind legs, but most commonly forelegs. Can be one or more legs.
[d] Thick or very thick ear, part of ear missing, etc.
[e] Hole in skull, skull not closed, balloon-shaped skull, etc.
[f] Cleft palate, cleft lip and palate, deformed jaw, etc.

Source: Courtesy of Ellegard Göttingen Minipigs ApS, Dalmose, Denmark.

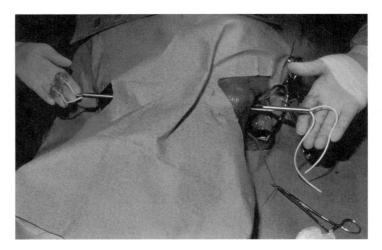

FIGURE 8.8 Trocar placement for catheterization of the neck vessels with the sow in lateral recumbency. (Reprinted from Swindle et al., 1996, *Lab. Anim. Sci.* 46(1): 90–95. With permission.)

harmful provided it is replaced with a similar volume of sterile saline. With continuous drip of warmed saline as the method of providing heat to the fetus, this volume is constantly replaced.

Once the fetal incision is made, the edges can be retained by clamping them to the edges of the uterotomy incision with Babcock forceps. Microsurgical or ophthalmic self-retaining retractors can also be applied into the incision and held by an assistant.

The site of the fetal surgical incision will depend upon the technique being performed; however, some general guidelines are useful. The area of the umbilicus and the cranial abdominal midline are problematic for incisions because of the possibility of damaging the umbilical vessels or causing vasospasm. It is best to use either lateral thoracotomies and paramedian or flank incisions to enter the thorax and abdomen rather than median sternotomies or midline celiotomy incisions. The flank region offers the most easily dissected subcutaneous tissue for implantation of devices.

Catheterization of the neck vessels can be done from either a ventral midline or preferably a paramedian incision made over the external jugular vein as described for the adult (Figure 8.8). The femoral vessels can be catheterized by externalizing the rear leg and performing the cutdown in the same manner as for adults. The axillary vessels are potentially useful, but difficult to access and catheterize because of the acute angles involved in catheter insertion. The umbilical vessels can be catheterized, but their tortuous course and friability frequently lead to extravasation, especially after they enter the abdomen and turn cranially. When manipulating the fetus without observing the umbilical vessels, as for these procedures, the surgeon must take care to avoid torsion of the umbilical vessels.

A variety of catheterization techniques have been described for fetal swine. The system of using vascular access ports has proved to be reliable and minimizes the opportunity for infection. The catheter system designed for use in our laboratory is a 4-Fr (French) catheter for the carotid artery and a 2-Fr catheter for the external and internal jugular veins and femoral vessels in a third-trimester fetus. These silicone catheters must be manufactured inside a larger 6-Fr catheter sheath to avoid kinking in the abdomen. The catheters are passed into the abdominal cavity using a trocar from the lateral wings of the lumbar vertebrae. The ports are either sutured to the dorsum of the pig or implanted subcutaneously. If externalized, they should be covered with a pouch or an adhesive plastic sheet (Figure 8.9). When threading the catheters into the blood vessels, it is essential to have a beveled tip and preplace a 2-French (Fr) wire catheter insertion aid into the lumen of the catheter. Polydiaxonone or other monofilament sutures are used to avoid vasospasm caused by braided sutures when tying the catheters in place. Catheter care should be the same as described for adults (Chapter 9).

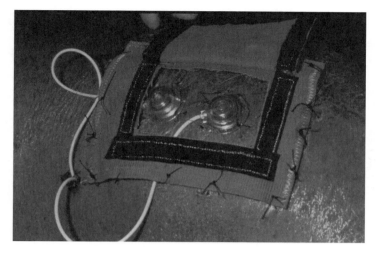

FIGURE 8.9 Canvas pouch sewn to the skin on the dorsum of the pig to protect externalized catheters. (Reprinted from Swindle et al., 1996, *Lab. Anim. Sci.* 46(1): 90–95. With permission.)

The closure of fetal incisions should be performed using an atraumatic technique and noninflammatory sutures. Continuous suture patterns are acceptable, and multiple muscle layers can be closed together depending upon the thickness of the layer. If subcuticular sutures are not used, then care should be taken to cut the suture ends close to the knot to avoid irritation of the fetal membranes.

Closure of the uterotomy and fetal membranes may be performed with staples as described earlier for c-section. A technique described by Randall (1986) for suturing the fetal and maternal membranes to reduce the possibility of conjoining the circulations should be used if staples are not available (Figure 8.10). The suture pattern consists of a continuous pattern in which the suture passes from the outside throughout the myometrium, endometrium, and allantochorion into the amniotic cavity. The suture then continues through both sides of the allantochorion passing across the incision in such a manner as to invert the edges of the membranes. The suture then passes

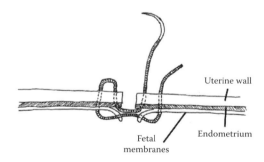

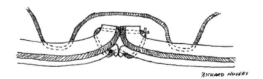

FIGURE 8.10 Manual suturing technique for fetal membranes.

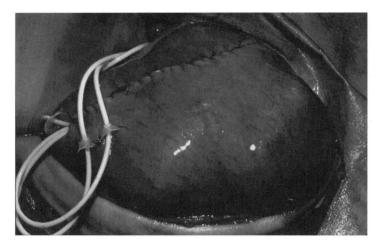

FIGURE 8.11 Lembert sutures oversewing the staple line and catheter flanges sewn to the uterine wall. (Reprinted from Swindle et al., 1996, *Lab. Anim. Sci.* 46(1): 90–95. With permission.)

completely through all three layers to the outside. The same suture is then reinserted through the myometrium and endometrium close to the edge of the incision, passed across the incision, and passed out through the endometrium and myometrium. After tying the suture, the effect from the outside is to have a vertical mattress-type pattern with inverted edges. This pattern is continuous along the entire edge of the incision. It is then oversewn with continuous or interrupted Lembert sutures. The suture used for these patterns should be a 2/0 or 3/0 synthetic absorbable material. If the goal of the project involves the necessity of preventing conjoinment of the maternal and fetal circulations, then the absence of gamma-globulins in the fetal plasma can be used as confirmation. Staple closures provide better hemostasis and a tighter seal and are more likely to prevent this phenomenon (Figure 8.7). They also greatly reduce operative time. Regardless of which uterine closure method is used, the final suture pattern is a Lembert to oversew the other layers, and catheter flanges are sutured to the uterine wall (Figure 8.11).

Complications of the surgery include sepsis, fetal death, and mummification, which may be followed by abortion. In our experience, the presence of a bloody vaginal discharge within 5 d postoperatively always leads to abortion. If this sign is noted, then an acute physiological experiment should be performed. Fetal death may lead to mummification without abortion. Fetal sepsis may lead to pyometritis and systemic sepsis, but more likely, to abortion. Factors that appear to lead to abortion include animals from herds susceptible to abortion, invasive procedures likely to be life threatening to the fetus, the presence of fetal distress at the time of surgery, and the presence of uterine contractions and other signs of uterine irritation. If abortion occurs as a complication, then the protocol should be reviewed for refinement, and progestins and agents that relax smooth-muscle contractions may be used for prophylaxis.

The progesterone agents include medroxyprogesterone (Depo-Provera®, Upjohn Co., Kalamazoo, MI), 15–50 mg i.m., 2 d before surgery, the day of surgery, and 2 d after surgery, or an oral progestin (ReguMate®, Hoechst Roussel, Philadelphia, PA), 0.1 mg kg^{-1} d^1 p.o., for the same time period. Nitroglycerine infusions or infusions with terbutalin may be used intraoperatively to prevent uterine contractions. Pancuronium, 0.02–0.15 mg/kg, is used as a muscle relaxant during surgery to increase exposure of the uterus; however, it is not effective in relaxing smooth muscle. Postoperative and intraoperative analgesia with buprenorphine prevents anxiety and straining by the sow. Nonsteroidal anti-inflammatory drug (NSAID) analgesics are contraindicated because they may induce parturition. Third-generation cephalosporins are useful as prophylaxis against infection, starting the day prior to surgery in order to allow the antibiotic to cross the fetal membranes. They

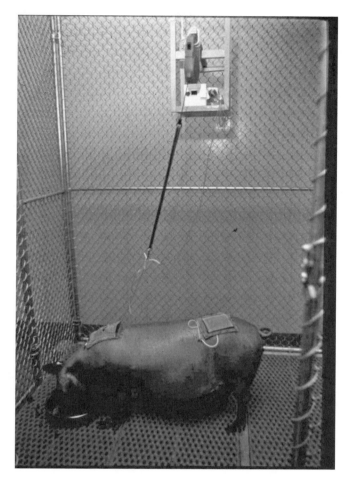

FIGURE 8.12 Harness and tether device for chronic infusion of vascular catheters in the sow and fetus. (Reprinted from Swindle et al., 1996, *Lab. Anim. Sci.* 46(1): 90–95. With permission.)

may also be used as a dilute flush in the amniotic sac prior to closing the incision. Tether and harness systems for providing chronic infusions have been developed (Figure 8.12).

Most fetal surgical models that have been applied in other species, notably the lamb, could be modified to be performed in swine. Other than fetal vascular catheterization (Figure 8.13), models that have been created include craniofacial defects, thoracotomy with pacemaker implantation (Figure 8.14), pulmonary arterial banding (Figure 8.15 and Figure 8.16), hydronephrosis, urinary function, and endocrine gland ablation (Care et al., 1986; Dalmose et al., 2000; Dungan et al., 1995; Jackson and Egdahl, 1960; Jones and Hudak, 1988; Kraeling et al., 1986; Olsen et al., 2001, 2004; Randall, 1986; Rosenkrantz et al., 1968; Schmidt et al., 1999; Sims et al., 1997; Swindle et al., 1996; Wiest et al., 1996).

PROLAPSE OF THE REPRODUCTIVE TRACT

Prolapse of the vagina, uterus, or both may occur during parturition or in the immediate peripartum period. Modifications of the techniques of St-Jean and Anderson (1999), Ladwig (1975), and Markham (1968) are described here. The prolapsed tissue should be examined to determine if it contains the urinary bladder, and a determination made whether fetuses are retained in the uterus.

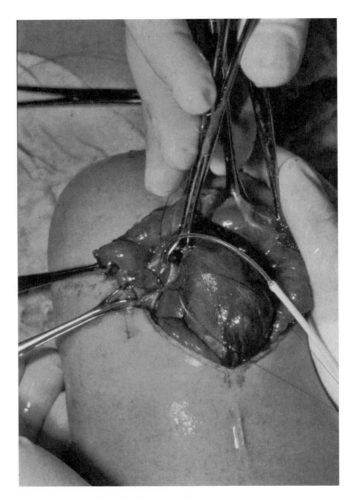

FIGURE 8.13 Catheter implantation into the fetal carotid artery.

Prolapse of the uterus and bladder or retention of additional fetuses requires a celiotomy. Any prolapsed tissue should be examined for necrosis and cleaned carefully with mild surgical soap solutions. Flushing the tissue with antibiotic solutions before reduction is also indicated.

If the vagina is prolapsed, it may be reduced by manual manipulation. The vagina is gently manipulated through the vulva after cleaning. This should not be done with sharp instruments or the extended fingers because the tissue will be friable and easily ruptured. If the prolapsed material can be manipulated into the vulva, it should be extended into the pelvic cavity. A deep subcutaneous purse-string suture should be placed to prevent recurrence, and the bladder should be catheterized.

If the uterus or bladder is involved, then a paramedian flank or midline abdominal incision is performed as previously described. The prolapsed structures are gently reduced, and any remaining fetuses are removed by c-section as described earlier. Oxytocin should be administered to promote uterine contraction. Use of the purse-string suture described previously for the vagina may help prevent recurrence. Use of a modified technique for primates may be useful, however, if the animal is to be retained for the long term (Adams et al., 1985). The technique involves suturing a loop of the ovarian ligament on both horns of the uterus to the abdominal wall on its corresponding side. This provides security against future prolapses by surgical fixation of the cranial poles of the uterus to the abdominal wall. The celiotomy incision is closed in a routine fashion, as previously described.

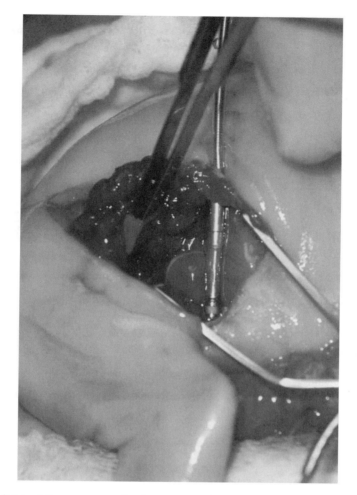

FIGURE 8.14 Left lateral thoracotomy to implant a pacemaker lead in a fetus.

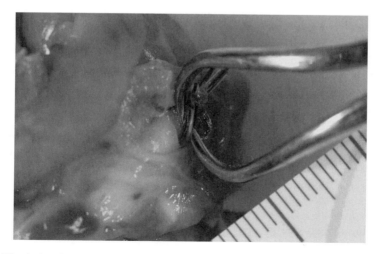

FIGURE 8.15 Silastic band on the pulmonary artery of a fetus.

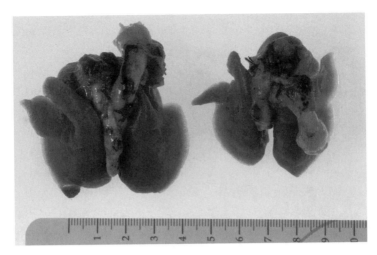

FIGURE 8.16 Heart and lung blocks from littermates at the end of gestation. The heart and lungs on the right have been retarded in growth from pulmonary artery banding in the third trimester.

If the tissue is necrotic, an amputation of the prolapsed stump may have to be performed. As described earlier, it should be ensured that the bladder or additional fetuses are not involved in the prolapse; a laparotomy should be performed if they are. The vaginal stump is best amputated using staple surgical techniques. If it is performed manually, then a V-shaped incision is made from the perineum to the tip of the viable tissue in the stump. The vessels are ligated, and the edges of the stump are oversewn with a continuous interlocking suture to ensure hemostasis and to provide a patent opening in the reproductive tract. Alternatively, an ovariohysterectomy may be indicated and performed as described previously.

If any of these conditions occur, restriction of future breeding or the use of c-section delivery of fetuses if breeding is necessary for research purposes should be considered.

ENDOMETRIOSIS

Endometriosis, characterized by the presence of endometrial glands and stroma outside the endometrial cavity, is a naturally occurring condition in humans and nonhuman primates. A model of endometriosis in pigs has been developed using laparoscopy techniques (Siegel and Kolata, 2003). Hormonal therapy is an essential element in the development of the model.

Using standard caudal abdominal laparotomy techniques, the uterine horn is exteriorized through a trocar, the abdomen is desufflated, and the trocar removed, which results in a portion of the uterus being exteriorized. This procedure can also be performed using open incision techniques.

After exteriorizing the uterus and holding it in place with Babcock clamps, a longitudinal incision is made in the uterus. Metzenbaum scissors are used to trim pieces of the endometrial lining. The endometrial pieces are minced with scissors and mixed with heparinized saline. After closure of the uterine incision and replacement in the abdomen, the solution of endometrial tissue is injected into the caudal abdomen using a 60-ml syringe attached to a catheter. The abdominal incision is closed in a routine manner.

The procedure was more effective in producing endometrial lesions in sexually mature Yucatan minipigs than in immature domestic swine. Hormonal injections were administered pre- and postoperatively. In minipigs, these were injections of estradiol cypionate 15 mg i.m. starting at 14 d preoperatively and administered every 7 d, including the day of surgery, followed by one injection 7 d postoperatively. Progesterone 100 mg i.m. was administered on the day of surgery, followed by one postoperative injection 7 d postoperatively. Similar injections of estradiol were given to the immature domestic swine, but progesterone was not administered because of concern that atrophy of the reproductive system may occur.

The lesions that were produced on the surface of the caudal abdominal viscera were generally foci of stroma, tubular glands, and fibrous tissue with inflammatory cells. Postoperative care also included the administration of analgesics. Pigs developed diarrhea, vomiting, and bloody vaginal discharge, which resolved within 4 d. The complications were mild and did not require treatment.

PELVIC ADHESIONS

Pelvic adhesion models to study prevention and treatment of the condition have been established (Christoforoni et al., 1996; Ferland et al., 2001; Montz et al., 1993). The basic technique requires a midline incision from the umbilicus to the pubis and causing an injury to the parietal or visceral peritoneum (or both). Some degree of damage may be caused by rubbing the visceral peritoneum with dry gauze sponges. However, the model of pelvic adhesion with uterine horn surgery creates a more reliable model (Ferland et al., 2001). In this model, the parietal peritoneum of the caudal pelvic wall opposed to the uterine horn is stripped in an area approximately 4×5 cm. The uterine horn is transected and reanastomosed with simple interrupted vicryl sutures. The abdomen is closed routinely. Pelvic adhesions will develop within 4–5 d, and the model can be completely evaluated for pelvic adhesions within 14 d.

ARTIFICIAL INSEMINATION AND EMBRYO TRANSFER

There is considerable interest in the development of transgenic and knockout swine for research purposes, agricultural methods of artificial insemination and semen collection and preservation; embryo collection, culture, and preservation are being modified for the purpose of maintaining genetically engineered lines of pigs (Abeydeera, 2001, 2002; Bazer et al., 2001; Beebe et al., 2005; Holker et al., 2005; Massip, 2001; Niemann and Rath, 2001; Prochazka et al., 2004; Sommer et al., 2002). There are many variables contributing to the success of these techniques, including breed, age, season, stress, and timing (Britt et al., 1999). The methodologies for most of these laboratory techniques are beyond the scope of this text; however, the surgical methods of collection and implantation will be described.

Synchronization of estrus and superovulation are essential techniques for these procedures. A simplified research technique for superovulation and artificial insemination has been described as a modification of common agricultural practice (Sommer et al., 2002). Briefly, gilts (150–160 d old) receive 1500 IU of pregnant mare serum gonadotropin (PMSG) i.m. followed by 500 IU of human chorionic gonadotropin (hCG) i.m. 72 h later. Gilts are inseminated at 42 and 47 h with thawed or fresh semen. This technique is less complicated than administering oral altrenogest followed by injections of PGF_{2a}, eCG, and hCG, the commonly used method (Bazer et al., 2001).

If natural estrus is used, the signs are swelling, reddening, and discharge of the vulva, as well as behavioral signs. The period of an estrous cycle is 17–25 d (average 21 d). During estrus, which lasts 1–3 d, the female is receptive to the male. Behavioral signs include vocalization, riding of other females and the standing reflex when exposed to pheromones from a boar, which generally occur within 24 h of ovulation. In the standing reflex, the female will stand rigidly when manually pressed on the lower back. Mating or artificial insemination is performed within 24 h after the onset of estrus, which occurs before ovulation. Ovulation is highly variable over 2–3 d, and it is generally best to mate or perform artificial insemination daily during estrus. A detailed discussion of breeding techniques in the agricultural setting has been published (Britt et al., 1999).

Using a porcine artificial insemination catheter, thawed sperm may be delivered into the cervix. The catheter is passed through the vulva and into the vagina at an upward angle to avoid entering the urethra. The catheter is screwed counterclockwise when resistance is encountered at the level of the cervix. By pulling with gentle pressure backward, you can determine if the catheter is locked in place in the cervix. The semen is gently injected into the cervix, and the catheter is screwed clockwise and removed.

Embryo transfer is performed by identifying the ovary and the infundibulum of the oviduct either surgically or laparoscopically (see the earlier section on ovariohysterectomy). Newer techniques have been developed using transcervical catheters and implantation in a retrograde fashion (Bazer et al., 2001; Hazeleger and Kemp, 2001; Li et al., 1996). The fertilized embryos are infused with gentle syringe or pipette pressure into the ampulla of both oviducts at 5–6 d of age. It is necessary to implant embryos in both oviducts to prevent resorption. Uterine implantation occurs approximately on day 13 or 14. Pregnancy can be reliably determined by ultrasound techniques in the middle of the first trimester of pregnancy (>20-d gestation). It is likely that embryo transfer and artificial insemination techniques will continue to evolve and improve because of the importance of the techniques to develop transgenic/knockout models.

MAMMECTOMY

Most sows have seven pairs of mammary glands on the abdomen; however, the number can vary substantially depending upon the breed. Surgical removal of a mammary gland may be indicated in chronic infection or trauma. Modifications of the techniques of St-Jean and Anderson (1999) and Mbiuki (1982) are described here. The vascular supply to the mammary glands is derived from branches of the internal thoracic, cranial epigastric, external pudendal arteries, and veins.

A paramedian skin incision is made over the center of the glandular structure to be excised. The skin is bluntly dissected to both edges of the gland. The vascular supply is identified, ligated, and transected before removal of the gland. The subcutaneous dissection is easily performed using Metzenbaum scissors. The vascularity of the gland increases substantially with lactation, and leakage of milk from adjacent glands should be prevented by taking care not to damage them during the dissection. After removal of the gland, the skin is trimmed and the nipple excised with the excised tissue. The subcutaneous pocket must be closed carefully to avoid a seroma. The skin is closed with subcuticular sutures. A circumferential bandage of the torso, including the surgical site, is indicated for the first 24 h to prevent seroma formation.

REFERENCES

Abeydeera, L.R., 2001, *In vitro* fertilization and embryo development in pigs, *Reproduction*, 58(Suppl.): 159–173.

Abeydeera, L.R., 2002, *In vitro* production of embryos in swine, *Theriogenology*, 57(1): 256–273.

Adams, R.J., Rock, J.A., Swindle, M.M., Garnett, N.L., and Porter, W.P., 1983, Surgical correction of cervical prolapse in three *Macaca mulatta, Lab. Anim. Sci.,* 33(5): 493–494.

Bazer, F.W., Ford, J.J., and Kensinger, R.S., 2001, Reproductive physiology, in Pond, W.G. and Mersmann, H.J., Eds., *Biology of the Domestic Pig*, Ithaca, NY: Cornell University Press, pp. 150–224.

Becker, H.N., 1992, Castration, vasectomy, hernia repair, and baby pig processing, in Leman, A.D., Straw, B.E., Mengeling, W.L., D'Allaire, S., and Taylor, D.J., Eds., *Diseases of Swine*, 7th ed., Ames, IA: Iowa State University Press, pp. 943–956.

Beebe, L.F., Cameron, R.D., Blackshaw, A.W., and Keates, H.L., 2005, Changes to blastocyst vitrification methods and improved litter size after transfer, *Theriogenology*, 64(4): 879–890.

Britt, J.H., Almond, G.W., and Flowers, W.L., 1999, Diseases of the reproductive system, in Straw, B.E., D'Allaire, S., Mengeling, W.L., and Taylor, D.J., Eds., *Diseases of Swine*, 8th ed., Ames, IA: Iowa State University Press, pp. 883–912.

Care, A.D., Caple, I.W., Singh, R., and Peddie, M., 1986, Studies on calcium homeostasis in the fetal Yucatan miniature pig, *Lab. Anim. Sci.*, 36(4): 389–392.

Christenson, R.K., Leymaster, K.A., and Young, L.D., 1987, Justification of unilateral hysterectomy-ovariectomy as a model to evaluate uterine capacity in swine, *J. Anim. Sci.*, 65(3): 738–744.

Dalmose, A.L., Hvistendahl, J.J., Olsen, L.H., Eskild-Jensen, A., Dhurhuus, J.C., and Swindle, M.M., 2000, Surgically induced urologic models in swine, *J. Invest. Surg.*, 13: 133–145.

D'Cruz, O.J., Erbeck, D., and Uckun, F.N., 2005, A study of the potential of the pig as a model for the vaginal irritancy of benzalkonium chloride in comparison to the nonirritant microbicide PHI-443 and the spermicide vanadocene dithiocarbamate, *Toxicol. Path.*, 33(4): 465–476.

Dungan, L.J., Wiest, D.B., Fyfe, D.A., Smith, A.C., and Swindle, M.M., 1995, Hematology, serology and serum protein electrophoresis in fetal miniature Yucatan swine: normal data, *Lab. Anim. Sci.*, 45(3): 285–289.

Eventov-Friedman, S., Katchman, H., Shezen, E., Aronovich, A., Tchorsh, D., Dekel, B., Freud, E., and Reisner, Y., 2005, Embryonic pig liver, pancreas, and lung as a source for transplantation: optimal organogenesis without teratoma depends on distinct time window, *Proc. Natl. Acad. Sci.*, 102(8): 2928–2933.

Glodek, P. and Oldigs, B., 1981, *Das Gottinger Miniaturschwein,* Verlag Paul Parey-Berlin und Hamburg, pp. 130–142.

Hazeleger, W. and Kemp, B., 2001, Recent developments in pig embryo transfer, *Theriogenology*, 56: 1321–1331.

Holker, M., Petersen, B., Hassel, P., Kues, W.A., Lemme, E., Lucas-Hahn, A., and Niemann, H., 2005, Duration of *in vitro* maturation of recipient oocytes affects blastocyst development of cloned porcine embryos, *Cloning Stem Cells*, 7(1): 35–44.

Jackson, B.T. and Egdahl, H., 1960, The performance of complex fetal operations in utero without amniotic fluid loss or other disturbances of fetal-maternal relationships, *Surgery*, 48: 564–570.

Jones, M.D. and Hudak, B.B., 1988, Fetal and neonatal surgery, in Swindle, M.M. and Adams, R.J., Eds., *Experimental Surgery and Physiology: Induced Animal Models of Human Disease*, Baltimore, MD: Williams and Wilkins, pp. 300–308.

Kraeling, R.R., Barb, C.R., and Rampacek, G.B., 1986, Hypophysectomy and hypophysial stalk transection in the pig: technique and application to studies of ovarian follicular development, in Tumbleson, M.E., Ed., *Swine in Biomedical Research*, Vol. 1, New York: Plenum Press, pp. 425–436.

Ladwig, V.D., 1975, Surgical procedure to control hemorrhage of porcine vulva, *J. Am. Vet. Med. Assoc.*, 166(6): 598–599.

Li, J., Rieke, A., Day, B.N., and Prather, R.S., 1996, Technical note: porcine nonsurgical embryo transfer, *J. Anim. Sci.*, 74: 2263–2268.

Markham, L., 1968, Replacement of prolapsed uterus in a sow, *Vet. Rec.*, 82: 605–606.

Massip, A., 2001, Cryopreservation of embryos of farm animals, *Reprod. Domest. Anim.*, 36(2): 49–55.

Mayo, M.B. and Becker, H.N., 1982, Unilateral castration to correct a peritesticular hematoma in a boar, *Vet. Med. Small Anim. Clin.*, 77(3): 449–451.

Mbiuki, S.M., 1982, Mammectomy for treatment of chronic mastitis in sows, *Vet. Med. Small Anim. Clin.*, 77(10): 1516–1517.

McGlone, J.J. and Hellman, J.M., 1988, Local and general anesthetic effects on behavior and performance of two and seven week old castrated and uncastrated piglets, *J. Anim. Sci.*, 66(12): 3049–3058.

Molina, J.R., Musah, A.I., Hard, D.L., and Anderson, L.L., 1985, Conceptus development after vascular occlusion of the middle uterine artery in the pig, *J. Reprod. Fert.*, 75(5): 501–506.

Montz, F.J., Monk, B.J., Lacy, S.M., and Fowler, J.M., 1993, Ketorolac tromethamine, a nonsteroidal anti-inflammatory drug: ability to inhibit post-radical pelvic surgery adhesions in a porcine model, *Gynecologic Oncology*, 48(1): 76–79.

Niemann, H. and Rath, D., 2001, Progress in reproductive biotechnology in swine, *Theriogenology*, 56(8): 1291–1304.

Olsen, L.H., Dalmose, A.L., Swindle, M.M., Jørgensen, T.M., and Djurhuus, J.C., 2001, Male fetal pig lower urinary tract function in mid second and early third trimester of gestation, *J. Urol.*, 165(6 Pt. 2): 2331–2334.

Olsen, L.H., Dalmose, A.L., Swindle, M.M., Djurhuus, J.C., and Jørgensen, T.M., 2004, Male fetal pig lower urinary tract function. Part II: free voiding pattern close to term and in the newborn, *J. Urol.*, 171(6 Pt. 2): 2660–2663.

Prochazka, R., Vodicka, P., Zudova, D., Rybar, R., and Motlik, J., 2004, Development of *in vivo* derived diploid and tetraploid pig embryos in a modified medium NCSU 37, *Theriogenology*, 62(1–2): 155–164.

Randall, G.C.B., 1986, Chronic implantations of catheters and other surgical techniques in fetal pigs, in Tumbleson, M.E., Ed., *Swine in Biomedical Research*, Vol. 2, New York: Plenum Press, pp. 1179–1186.

Rock, J.A., Rosewaks, Z., and Adashi, E.Y., 1979, Microsurgery for tubal reconstruction following Falope-Ring sterilization in swine, *J. Microsurg.*, 1 (1): 61–64.

Rosenkrantz, J.G., Simon, R.C., and Carlisle, J.H., 1968, Fetal surgery in the pig with a review of other mammalian fetal techniques, *J. Pediatr. Surg.*, 3(3): 392–397.

Schmidt, M.R., Stenbøg, E.V., Kristiansen, S.B., Smith, A.C., Djurhuus, J.C., and Swindle, M.M., 1999, Banding of the pulmonary artery in fetal swine, *J. Invest. Surg.*, 12(4): 222.

Siegel, J. and Kolata, R., 2003, Endometriosis model development in swine, *Lab Anim.*, 32(4): 41–45.

Sims, C.D., Butler, P.E.M., Casanova, R., Randolph, M.A., and Yaremchuk, M.J., 1997, Prolonged general anesthesia for experimental craniofacial surgery in fetal swine, *J. Invest. Surg.*, 10(1): 53–57.

Sommer, J.R., Collins, E.B., Neiding, T., Rozeboom, K., Wong, F., and Petters, R.M., 2002, Conservation and regeneration of transgenic lines of swine by semen cryopreservation and artificial insemination, *Lab Anim.*, 31(1): 25–31.

St-Jean, G. and Anderson, D.E., 1999, Anesthesia and surgical procedures in swine, in Straw, B.E., D'Allaire, S., Mengeling, W.L., and Taylor, D.J., Eds., *Diseases of Swine*, 8th ed., Ames, IA: Iowa State University Press, pp. 1133–1154.

Swindle, M.M., 1983, *Basic Surgical Exercises Using Swine*, Philadelphia, PA: Praeger Press.

Swindle, M.M. and Bobbie, D.L., 1987, Comparative Anatomy of the Pig, Charles River Technical Bulletin, Charles River Laboratories 4(1): 1–4.

Swindle, M.M., Smith, A.C., and Hepburn, B.J.S., 1988, Swine as models in experimental surgery, *J. Invest. Surg.*, 1(1): 65–79.

Swindle, M.M., Wiest, D.B., Smith, A.C., Garner, S.S., Case, C.C., Thompson, R.P., Fyfe, D.A., and Gillette, P.C., 1996, Fetal surgical protocols in Yucatan miniature swine, *Lab. Anim. Sci.*, 46(1): 90–95.

Wiest, D.B., Swindle, M.M., Garner, S.S., Smith, A.C., and Gillette, P.C., 1996, Pregnant Yucatan miniature swine as a model for investigating fetal drug therapy, in Tumbleson, M.E. and Schook, L.B., Eds., *Advances in Swine in Biomedical Research*, Vol. 2., New York: Plenum Press, pp. 629–636.

9 Cardiothoracic and Vascular Surgery/Chronic Intravascular Catheterization

GENERAL PRINCIPLES OF CARDIOTHORACIC SURGERY AND SURGICAL ANATOMY

Swine share important characteristics with humans in anatomy and physiology of the cardiovascular and pulmonary systems, making them useful models in the study of human diseases (Corin et al., 1988; Gardner and Johnson, 1988; Gootman, 2001; Horneffer et al., 1986; Hughes, 1986; Lee, 1986; McKenzie, 1996; Smith et al., 1990, 1994; Stanton and Mersmann, 1986; Swindle, 1983, 1986, 1992; Swindle and Adams, 1988; Swindle and Bobbie, 1987; Swindle et al., 1986, 1988). Besides the size and morphologic characteristics, there are physiological similarities in the areas of coronary blood flow, growth of the cardiovascular system, and neonatal pulmonary development. The approximate distribution of the coronary arteries is as follows (Gootman, 2001):

Right coronary artery — 72% right ventricle, sinaoatrial node, and atrioventricular node, 25% left ventricle

Left anterior descending coronary artery — 28% right ventricle, 49% left ventricle

The coronary circulation of the pig has few subepicardial collateral anastomoses, similar to 90% of the human population. The circulation to the conduction system is predominantly right-side dominant from the posterior septal artery, in contrast to the dog. Consequently, the pig responds in a similar manner to humans with acute myocardial infarction (Bloor et al., 1986, 1992; Gardner and Johnson, 1988; Unger, 2001; Verdouw et al., 1998; White et al., 1986). Various anatomic views of the heart are shown in Figure 9.1–Figure 9.8.

There are some differences from humans in physiological composition of the conduction system. The pig endocardium and epicardium are activated simultaneously because of differences in distribution of the specialized conduction system in the ventricles (Brownlee et al., 1997; Gillette et al., 1991; Hughes and Bowman, 1986; Schumann et al., 1994; Smith et al., 1997; Tong et al., 1995, 1996; Verdouw and Hartog, 1986). Atherosclerotic and coronary occlusion models are readily induced in swine and are discussed in this section; there is also additional information in Chapter 12 (Gal and Isner, 1992; Mitchell et al., 1994; Murphy et al., 1992; Rogers et al., 1988; Rysavy et al., 1986; White et al., 1992). The aorta has a true vaso vasorum unlike many species of animals but similar to humans; this structure leads to a difference in reaction to aortic banding techniques. The growth of the cardiovascular system from fetus to sexually mature adult in swine parallels the growth and development of the cardiovascular system of humans into early sexual maturity (Brutel de la Riviere et al., 1983; Gootman, 2001; Pae et al., 1981). Histology of the heart, great vessels, and conduction system are illustrated in Figure 9.9–Figure 9.15.

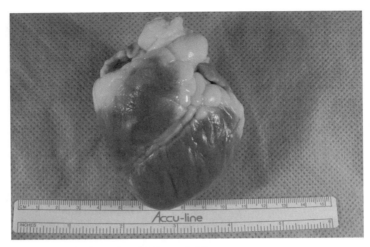

FIGURE 9.1 Ventral view of the heart in a 22-kg male Yucatan.

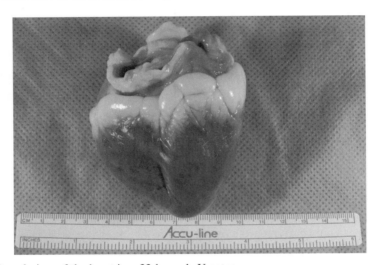

FIGURE 9.2 Dorsal view of the heart in a 22-kg male Yucatan.

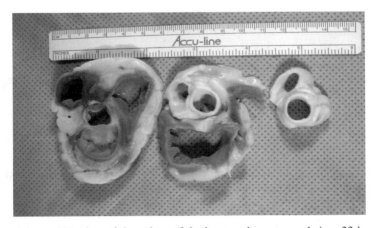

FIGURE 9.3 Cranial (topside) view of the valves of the heart and great vessels in a 22-kg male Yucatan.

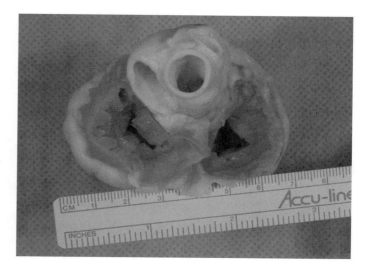

FIGURE 9.4 Cranial (topside) view of the cap of the heart and the valves in a 22-kg male Yucatan.

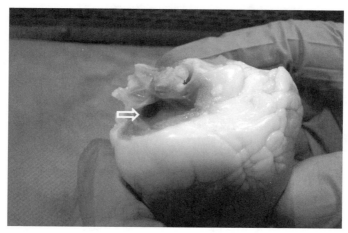

FIGURE 9.5 Coronary sinus (arrow) in the heart of a 22-kg male Yucatan.

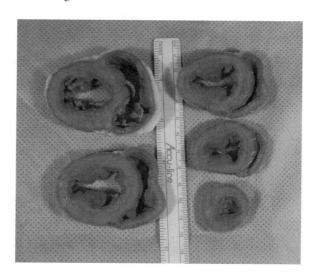

FIGURE 9.6 Serial cross sections of the heart of a 22-kg male Yucatan. The most dorsal (cranial) part of the heart is at the 11 o'clock position and the most caudal portion of the heart is at the 5 o'clock position.

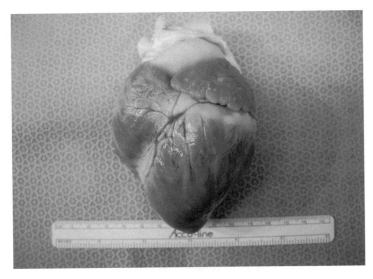

FIGURE 9.7 Ventral view of the heart in a 22-kg male Yorkshire farm pig for comparison to the Yucatan minipig.

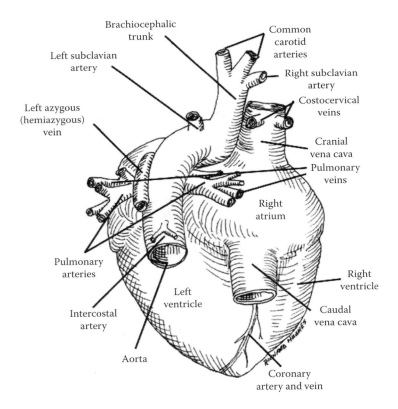

FIGURE 9.8 Dorsal view of the heart.

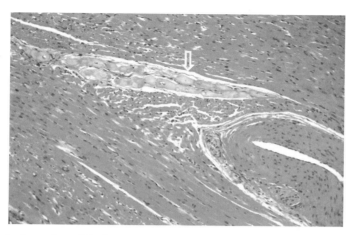

FIGURE 9.9 Histologic section of the heart. Purkinje cells are illustrated with the arrow. H&E, ×100.

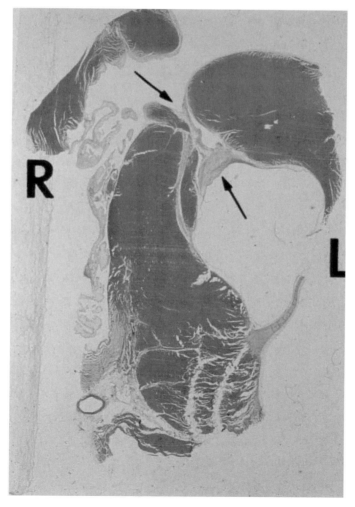

FIGURE 9.10 Subgross microscopy of the heart of a pig with a ventricular septal defect illustrating the close association with the conduction system (arrows). H&E, ×4.

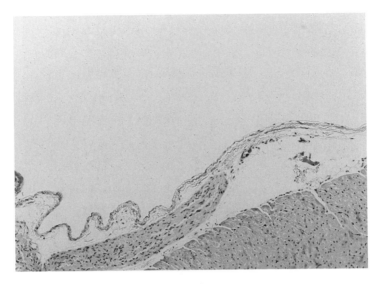

FIGURE 9.11 Histology of a cardiac valve. H&E, ×100.

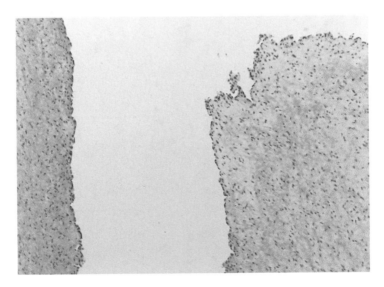

FIGURE 9.12 Histology of the atrium. H&E, ×100.

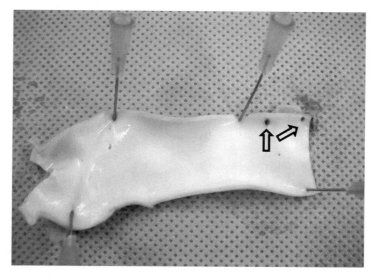

FIGURE 9.13 Aorta of the pig demonstrating vaso vasorum (arrows).

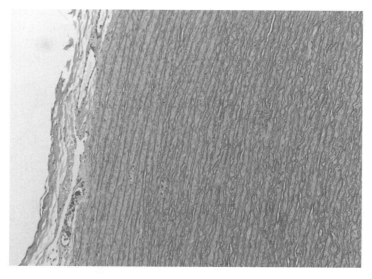

FIGURE 9.14 Histology of the aorta. H&E, ×100.

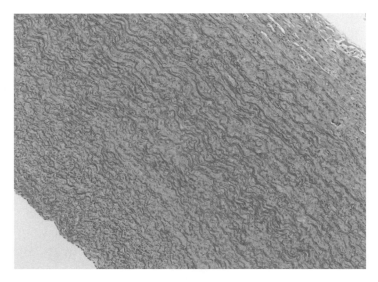

FIGURE 9.15 Histology of the pulmonary artery. H&E, ×100.

Pigs have been described as a translational model for arteriogenesis because of their reactions to stimuli inducing collateral growth of arteries (Hoefer et al., 2006). This is typically studied in a hind-limb model of femoral occlusion. Peripheral veins in the pigs have valves similar to humans, and this may be a problem with passage of catheters into the small vessels in the extremities.

The pulmonary tissues (Figure 9.16 and Figure 9.17) and pulmonary circulation have been studied from fetal life to 6 months of age and show similarities morphologically and functionally (Ackermann, 2001; Greenberg et al., 1981; Haworth and Hislop, 1981; Sparrow, 1996). Pulmonary function matures by 2 weeks of age, but growth and remodeling continue into adult life. The lungs have seven lobes: right and left cranial, middle and caudal, and an unpaired accessory intermediate lobe from the right side. The respiratory rate decreases with age, from approximately 40/min in the neonate to 15/min in the adult. The pulmonary tissues are friable and must be handled gently during thoracic surgery. Overinflation of the lungs with a respirator can cause alveolar rupture and

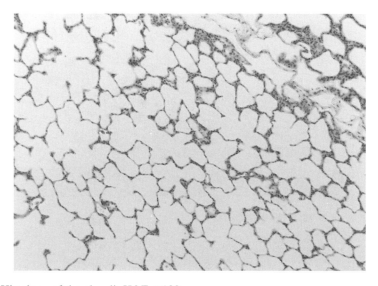

FIGURE 9.16 Histology of the alveoli. H&E, ×100.

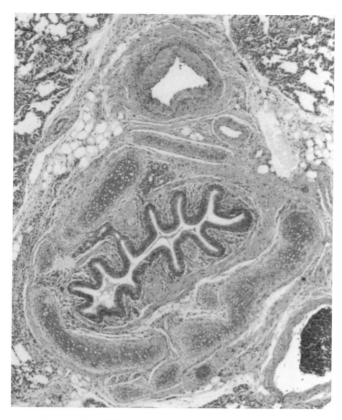

FIGURE 9.17 Histology of a bronchus. H&E, ×100.

emphysematous bullae. Air bubbles from this trauma can extend into the abdominal mesenteric tissues and create pneumotosis intestinalis. This is especially true of respirators without bellows, such as the Harvard pump. The tidal volume is approximately 10–15 ml/kg and the inflation pressure on a respiratory should not exceed 18–20 cm H_2O. Oxygen flow rates will differ between anesthetic machines, but 5–15 ml/kg/min is a general starting range (Swindle, 1983). Structures of the thorax with the lungs removed are illustrated in Figure 9.18 and Figure 9.19.

Lateral thoracotomies (Figure 9.20 and Figure 9.21) in the pig can be a challenge because of the width of the ribs and the narrowness of the intercostal spaces, which can result in minimal exposure of the structures of interest. Placing a rolled-up towel or sandbag under the thorax to make the operative side more convex will increase surgical exposure. Also, the incisions should be performed within the intercostal spaces parallel to the ribs. This means that lateral thoracotomy incisions will be oblique rather than vertical because of the anatomy of the ribs in swine. The pig usually has 15 pairs of ribs including the floating rib, and they can be counted to locate the appropriate intercostal space. Some miniature pigs may have one rib and one thoracic vertebra less than domestic swine (Swindle, 1983; Swindle et al., 1986). Swine have been developed as a model for induced hypothermia for emergency trauma surgery using a thoracotomy approach (Rhee et al., 2000).

Median sternotomy (Figure 9.22 and Figure 9.23) incisions can be performed successfully in swine as a survival procedure, unlike in many other animals. Pigs experience relatively little discomfort with the procedure, especially if the manubrium sterni is left intact, as it can be for many cardiac procedures. Care must be taken when performing this procedure, because the heart is in sternal contact between the fourth and seventh costal cartilages in most pigs. The sternum

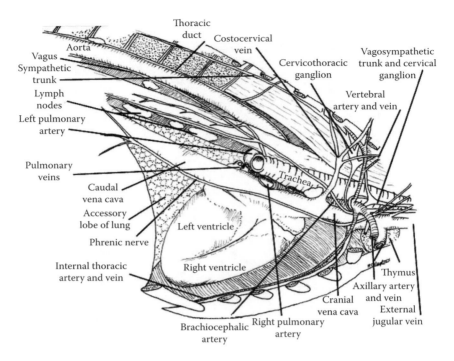

FIGURE 9.18 Right thorax with the right lung removed.

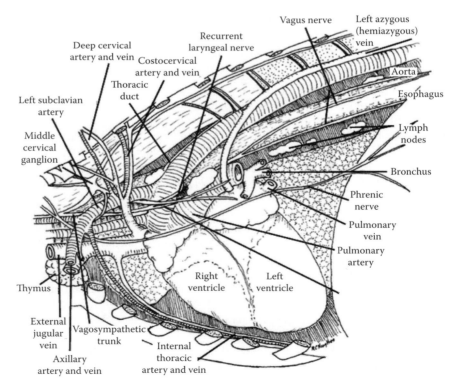

FIGURE 9.19 Left thorax with the left lung removed.

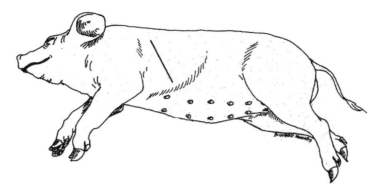

FIGURE 9.20 Position of the incision for a left lateral thoracotomy.

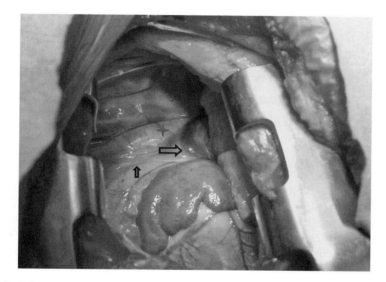

FIGURE 9.21 Left lateral thoracotomy through the fifth intercostal space. The large arrow points to the hemiazygous vein, the star is on the aorta, and the small arrow on the pulmonary trunk points to the phrenic nerve. The lungs have been packed out of the incision with wetted gauze pads.

may be bisected using a Stricker saw if a scalpel handle or straight ribbon retractor is held along the interior surface of the sternum to prevent cardiac trauma. It may also be bisected using sternal cutters of all the various configurations used for humans. The apex of the heart is in close apposition to the diaphragm at its most cranial attachment to the sternum at the level of the seventh costal cartilage. The heart will remain in a pericardial cradle after this procedure is performed because of the close attachment of the pericardium to the sternum (Swindle et al., 1986, 1988).

Cardiac and pulmonary tissue is very friable in swine, especially in the smaller farm pigs commonly used in research. This tissue friability decreases with maturity and, consequently, miniature pigs tend to be easier to manipulate surgically at the same weight as farm breeds because of their greater age at the same weight. Gentle handling of tissues using appropriate instrumentation is imperative to prevent complications, such as tearing of atrial tissue and rupture of pulmonary tissue, which may cause emphysematous bullae. Vessels are similar to those in humans except for the presence of the left azygous (hemiazygous) vein (Figure 9.8 and Figure 9.21) that crosses from the intercostal vessels ventral to the left hilum of the lung to drain into the coronary sinus (Swindle, 1983; Swindle and Bobbie, 1987; Swindle et al., 1986).

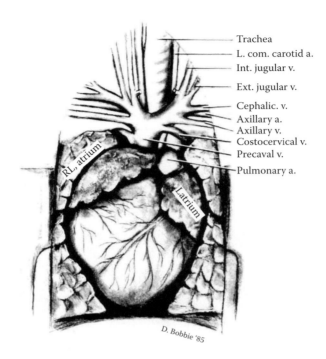

Trachea
L. com. carotid a.
Int. jugular v.
Ext. jugular v.
Cephalic. v.
Axillary a.
Axillary v.
Costocervical v.
Precaval v.
Pulmonary a.

RL, atrium

L atrium

D. Bobbie '85

FIGURE 9.22 Drawing of a median sternotomy.

The edges of thoracotomy incisions should by protected with wetted gauze laparotomy sponges when using retractors. The self-retaining retractors indicated for most swine need to be pediatric instruments with blunt blades to avoid injuring the underlying pulmonary tissue, likely with retraction blades that extend too deep into the thoracic cavity. The mediastinum is thin and easily ruptured in swine. Chest tubes or instruments will readily injure the structure and, as a practicality, the mediastinum should be considered incomplete, because it is likely that fluids or surgical hemorrhage from one side of the thoracic cavity will extend into the other side through inadvertent rents.

Closure of thoracic surgical incisions is comparable to other species. Lateral thoracotomies are closed with heavy-gauge (0–1) circumferential sutures that have been preplaced around the cranial and caudal ribs adjacent to the incision. Three to five sutures are usually required to close the incision adequately. Sutures may either be absorbable polydiaxonone or nonabsorbable materials. After preplacing all sutures, the central one in the incision is tied first, followed by the peripheral ones, with alternated tying of sutures in both directions. Rib-approximating forceps are helpful for tying the first suture. The latissimus dorsi always requires closure as a separate layer, even in the smallest pig. However, the decision whether or not to close the rest of the muscles in layers varies with the size of the pig. Muscle layers can be closed either with interrupted or continuous sutures of any of the synthetic absorbable materials. The subcutaneous tissues are also variable in thickness depending upon the size of the pig, but this layer is closed, if necessary, using synthetic absorbable materials. The skin layer is best closed with a subcuticular layer of 2/0 or 3/0 synthetic absorbable suture. Other types of closure may be used if preferred.

A median sternotomy is closed in a similar fashion to the lateral thoracotomy. Nonabsorbable heavy-gauge (0–2) wire, braided nonabsorbable sutures, or plastic lock ties are preplaced in the intercostal spaces from cranial to caudal. Care should be taken not to unnecessarily occlude the interior mammary artery with these sutures; however, it may be sacrificed if necessary. If the manubrium sterni was not transected, then the pig will have an easier recovery with less postoperative discomfort, and the surgical incision will be easier to close with proper alignment. If it was transected, then great care should be taken to ensure that closure of the sternotomy is performed

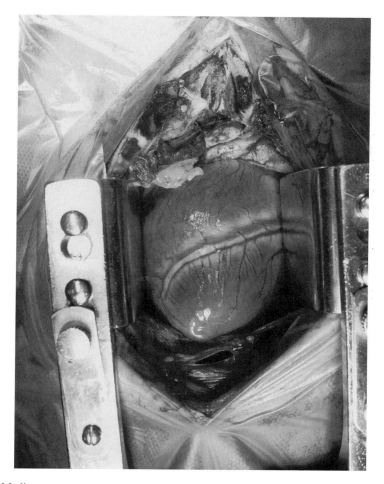

FIGURE 9.23 Median sternotomy.

in an anatomically correct fashion. The sutures are tied sequentially from cranial to caudal. The pericardium does not need to be sutured as a separate layer. A single-layer closure of muscle and subcutaneous suture using 2/0–3/0 synthetic absorbable suture should be placed next. The skin is closed in the same fashion as for the lateral thoracotomy.

Evacuation of air from the chest can be performed by a variety of methods (Figure 9.24). The lungs should be expanded to their maximum capacity to reduce the air volume of the thorax while closing the initial layer of the thoracotomy, whether it is a lateral or median incision. For simple procedures in which postoperative bleeding and leakage of air are not expected, the chest may be evacuated with a needle or preferably a small-gauge catheter and syringe with an attached three-way valve. The insertion is in the dorsocaudal area of the thoracic cavity, care being taken to avoid damage to the lung with the needle or catheter. This evacuation may be performed after closing the internal muscle layers so that a watertight seal exists. If a chest tube is to be placed, it is inserted while the incision is still open. It is placed in a dorsocaudal position at least two intercostal spaces caudal to the lateral thoracotomy. The tube is passed through the skin after a stab incision is made and then advanced into the thoracic cavity. For a median sternotomy, single or double chest tubes are placed on the ventrolateral aspects of the midthorax cranial to the attachment of the diaphragm. Tubes may either be the one-way valve Heimlich type for short- or mid-term usage, or the use of water-sealed systems may be required for more involved procedures that have the possibility of increased complications. Chest tubes are placed with purse-string sutures around them in the skin,

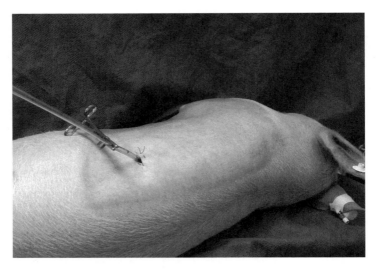

FIGURE 9.24 Chest tube placement in the left thorax.

and the chest tubes are removed and the purse-string sutures are tightened after it has been determined that pneumothorax or hemorrhage are no longer likely.

The major difficulties encountered in thoracic surgical procedures are likely to be cardiac arrhythmias and cardiodepression. Methods of preventing these common complications are detailed in Chapter 2. Likewise, procedures such as graft implantation, which are likely to induce thrombosis, can be effectively prevented with anticoagulant therapy as discussed in Chapter 2 and Chapter 12. Inherent in the design of these surgical protocols is the necessity of designing an appropriate anesthetic and analgesic protocol for the procedure being performed. Good surgical technique alone is not sufficient to have a successful outcome for thoracic surgery. Intraoperative and postoperative monitoring of heart rate, electrocardiogram, blood pressures, and blood gases are essential in these cases if survival is expected.

General principles of vascular surgery are discussed later in the sections on vascular cannulation and anastomosis. Some comparative cardiovascular measurements and hemodynamic values are included in Table 9.1–Table 9.4. Additional measurements and weights are given in the tables in Chapter 12 and in the appendix.

TABLE 9.1
Heart Weight to Body Weight of Various Pig Breeds

Breed	Body Weight (kg)	HW/BW (%)
Farm	25	0.49
	112	0.4[a]
Hanford	26	0.46
Sinclair	26	0.47
Yucatan	26	0.57
Yucatan Micro	26	0.55
Göttingen	11–13	0.46–0.49

[a] The heart weight (HW) decreases as a percentage of body weight (BW) in swine as they grow.

TABLE 9.2
Vessel Luminal Diameters (ID) in Various Breeds of Swine

Breed	Body Weight (kg)	Coronary Artery (mm)	Thoracic Aorta (mm)	Postrenal Abdominal Aorta (mm)	Carotid Artery (mm)	External Iliac Artery (mm)	Internal Iliac Artery (mm)	Posterior Vena Cava (mm)	Femoral Artery (mm)	Portal Vein (mm)	Renal Artery (mm)
Hanford[a]	15	2.0–2.5									
Hanford[b]	30–35	1–1.5									
Hanford[b]	44		13	5		3	2	14			
Yucatan[a]	10–20	2–3.5				2.5–4		20			
Yucatan[b]	29		12	6		2	1				
Yucatan[b]	48		11		4						4
Yucatan[b]	109		11	6		4	3				2
Yucatan Micro[a]	14–33		12	6		5	1–2		3.5		
Yucatan Micro[b]	55–60		9–16	5–7	3–4	2				10	
Sinclair[a]	45					4.8	3.5		4		
Göttingen[b,d]	20–40	1.5–2.0	14–16		3						
Göttingen[b]	37–50						3–5				
Farm[a,c]	30–39					5.3	3.4		4.8		
Farm[a,c]	40–49					5.8	3.7		4.9		
Farm[a,c]	50–59					5.9	4.5		4.6		
Farm[a,c]	60–69					6.1	4.2		5.6		
Farm[a]	55			12		6					
Farm[b]	70	3	12	5	3.5						
Farm[a]	16	3	13	8.5	4	4	2.1		4		2.5
Farm[b]	25		21	10	5	6	3	12		16	4
Farm[b]	47	3	22	15	5	6	4	18	4		5

[a] *In vivo* measurement using fluoroscopy and contrast material.
[b] *In vitro* necropsy measurement.
[c] Courtesy of Dagan Harris, MindGuard, Israel.
[d] Courtesy of Prof. Rainer Schulz.

TABLE 9.3
Cardiac Measurements at Necropsy

Breed	Body Weight (kg)	Heart Length (mm)	Heart Circumference (mm)	Left-Ventricular Chamber Length (mm)	Right-Ventricular Chamber Length (mm)	Mitral Valve Diameter (mm)	Tricispid Valve Diameter (mm)	Aortic Valve Diameter (mm)	Pulmonary Valve Diameter (mm)	Left-Ventricular Freewall (mm)	Right-Ventricular Freewall (mm)	Intraventricular Septum (mm)
Yucatan	47.6	95	230	48	75	63	65	11	11	16	7	15
Farm	47.5	120	190			25	27	22	22	20	6	16
Farm	25	82				20	23	21	21	12	7	7

TABLE 9.4
Cardiovascular and Hormonal Values of
Conscious Swine

Heart rate, beats/min	101 ± 2
Right atrial pressure, mmHg	0.8 ± 0.7
Pulmonary capillary "wedge" pressure, mmHg	5.1 ± 0.8
Mean aortic blood pressure, mmHg	96 ± 2
Mean pulmonary arterial blood pressure, mmHg	13.8 ± 0.7
Cardiac output, ml min^{-1}kg^{-1}	210 ± 6
Systemic vascular resistance, mmHg kg min/l	464 ± 21
Pulmonary vascular resistance, mmHg kg min/l	40.4 ± 2.6
Plasma rennin activity, ng Al ml^{1}h^{-1}	0.88 ± 0.17
Plasma vasopressin concentration, pg/ml	2.0 ± 0.4
Temperature (pulmonary artery blood) °C	38.99 ± 0.14
Arterial pH, units	7.458 ± 0.003
Arterial PCO$_2$, mmHg	44.5 ± 0.7
Arterial PO$_2$, mmHg	96.2 ± 2.2

Source: Reprinted from Weiskopf, R.B. et al., 1992. Use of swine in the study of anesthetics, in Swindle, M.M. Ed., *Swine as Models in Biomedical Research*, Ames: Iowa State University Press. With permission.

PULMONARY SYSTEM

TRACHEOSTOMY AND TRACHEOTOMY

Tracheostomy can be performed in the pig as a survival procedure either following an emergency or as part of a planned experiment. With the pig in dorsal recumbency, the cricothyroid cartilage can be palpated easily, even in large swine. The caudal end of the cartilage has a blunted tip similar to a bird's beak. The cricothyroid membrane is immediately caudal to this structure and is the preferred location for a tracheostomy (Swindle, 1983).

A 1- to 2-cm incision is made over the membrane on the ventral midline. The cutaneous coli and sternohyoideus muscles are separated longitudinally, and the membrane is identified. This procedure can be performed bloodlessly in seconds in an emergency. The cricothyroid membrane is incised, and either a tracheostomy tube or an endotracheal tube of the appropriate size can be inserted (Figure 9.25). The larynx may be held between the thumb and forefinger of the surgeons hand for countertraction to aid this procedure. As an option, the membrane between the first and second tracheal rings can be incised and used for this procedure. For a survival procedure, however, this transection does not heal as readily as an incision in the cricothyroid membrane. The larynx of swine is large, and the tracheal rings will be somewhat obscured by this structure, necessitating a longer incision.

The cricothyroid membrane can be sutured with a continuous pattern using synthetic absorbable sutures. Problems have not been noted with the suture material entering the lumen of the larynx; however, some surgeons may wish to use a continuous Lembert pattern instead. The sternohyoideus muscle is closed with a continuous suture pattern and the skin, with a subcuticular pattern, using synthetic absorbable material.

Chronic ostomies can also be maintained by suturing a standard tracheostomy tube to the skin after closing the muscular and subcutaneous tissues around the device. By making the incision in the cricothyroid membrane, complications associated with the vocal cords can be avoided as long as the surgeon passes the tracheostomy device caudally. An ostomy can also be formed by suturing

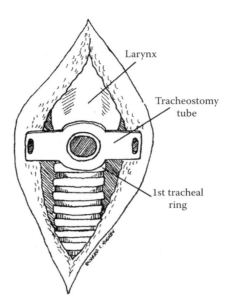

Larynx

Tracheostomy
tube

1st tracheal
ring

FIGURE 9.25 Tracheostomy.

the edges of a tracheal window to the skin. A tracheal window can be formed by resecting a rectangular section from the first few tracheal rings on the ventral surface. The trachea is too deep in the musculature of the neck to use this procedure beyond the area immediately caudal to the larynx.

PNEUMONECTOMY AND LOBECTOMY

The hilum of either lung is surgically approached through the fourth intercostal space. A total pneumonectomy is more easily performed on the left side and is described here (Swindle, 1983; Swindle et al., 1986). With the pig in right lateral recumbency, the left foreleg is drawn cranially, and a sandbag is positioned under the thorax. The incision is made obliquely from the dorsal caudal border of the scapula ventrocaudally toward the first nipple. After making the skin incision, the ribs may be palpated; the fourth intercostal space is the most cranial one approachable with this skin incision. The muscle layers are successively divided, and the thoracodorsal artery and vein within the body of the latissimus dorsi muscle will be the only major blood vessels encountered. The muscles are easily divided, and the intercostal muscles may be divided along the cranial border of the fifth rib using Metzenbaum scissors. At the dorsal edge of the incision, the superior intercostal vessels may be encountered and at the distal margin of the incision, the internal thoracic vessels should be avoided. Care should be taken to enter the thorax without damaging the lungs. This can be facilitated by underinflating the lungs and cutting the last muscle layer with Metzenbaum scissors.

After placing self-retaining retractors, the pulmonary ligament is identified at the dorsocaudal aspect of the caudal lobe of the lung. This fibrous structure cannot be seen through the thoracotomy and must be cut blindly with Metzenbaum scissors while retracting the tip of the caudal lobe proximally with the fingers. The caudal and apical lobes of the lung can now be exteriorized to expose the hilum of the lung. The lobes of the lung are retracted dorsally using wetted gauze pads.

The hilum of the lung (Figure 9.26) is dissected, and the blood vessels are identified and surgically transected in this order: cranial ventral branch of the pulmonary vein, left pulmonary artery, apical branch of the pulmonary vein, and caudal diaphragmatic branch of the pulmonary vein. The first branch of the pulmonary vein has to be transected to adequately expose the pulmonary artery branch. If these transections are being performed manually, then it is best to use transfixion sutures in the pulmonary artery. During this dissection, the left azygous (hemiazygous) vein that

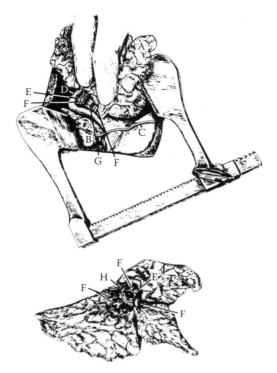

FIGURE 9.26 Hilum of the lung during left pneumonectomy. (Redrawn from Swindle, M.M. et al. 1986, *Lab. Anim. Sci.*, 36(4): 357–361. With permission.)

crosses ventrally to these vessels should not be damaged. However, it may be sacrificed, if necessary. The lung is then retracted ventrally to expose the bronchial artery on the dorsal aspect of the bronchus in order to transect it. If vagal stimulation resulting in bradycardia, cardiac standstill, or both is problematic during the deep dissection of the hilum, atropine should be administered.

After all the vessels have been ligated, then the bronchus is cleared of fascial tissue and transected. This transection is best performed with staples. However, if it must be performed manually, the bronchus is cross-clamped distally, and the bronchus is cut on the proximal end of the clamp a few millimeters at a time, while placing simple interrupted sutures using nonabsorbable suture material. As an alternative, a continuous horizontal mattress pattern can be used. This cut-and-suture technique is performed from the caudal end to the cranial end of the bronchus. The bronchus is checked for leaks with saline, and any leak noted is repaired with additional sutures. Leaks are most likely to occur at the middle of the bronchus where there is an indentation in the dorsal border. The leak can usually be repaired by placing a horizontal mattress suture in this area.

The right lung can be removed in a similar manner. However, the right cranial lobe bronchus branches directly from the trachea separate from the bronchus, which branches to supply the caudal and accessory lobes. Consequently, both bronchi have to be divided surgically. Access to the accessory lobe is difficult because of the location of the vena cava, which makes dissection of the pulmonary veins difficult.

Lobectomies and partial lobectomies of the lung in swine are technically feasible but difficult. Jangra et al. (2005) has described a thoracoscopic technique of partial lobectomies. In that model, platinum coils were implanted into the lung parenchyma to simulate cancerous nodules, which could be located using CT imaging. Division of the friable lung tissue always leads to leakage of air and, frequently, the formation of emphysematous bullae. The two best locations for attempting the procedure are the right cranial lobe followed by the left cranial lobe at the caudal interlobular fissure. These two locations provide the deepest fissure between lung tissue and have a single branch of the bronchus to transect.

The lung is divided using staples at the identified location. If staples are not available, manual suturing using a horizontal mattress suture pattern can be used; however, the pulmonary tissue frequently ruptures with this technique. The branches of the pulmonary artery and veins supplying the resected section are identified and surgically transected. The branch of the bronchus is then dissected free and transected with staples. The transected edge of the lung remaining in the animal will have to have the leaks sealed in the tissue following removal of the resected lobe. Various tissue glues and oxycellulose patches have been used to seal these leaks in the past with variable success. Tissue glues are probably more effective. The complication rate is high with this procedure because of the friability of the pulmonary tissue and the high potential for air leaks. Development of better methods of sealing the cut edges of the lung would help in this species.

The lateral thoracotomy is closed as described earlier.

PULMONARY TRANSPLANT

Swine have been used for single-lung transplantation and heart-and-lung transplantation (Baumgartner et al., 1988; Calne et al., 1976, 1978; Hall et al., 1986; Harjula and Baldwin, 1987; Hillinger, et al., 2000; Qayumi et al., 1990, 1991, 1993; Saito and Waters, 1994; Salminen, et al., 2000; Swindle et al., 1986). A left single-lung transplant is more applicable than a right-lung transplant because of the presence of the right cranial bronchus, which makes it substantially different from humans. Consequently, a left single-lung transplant is described here. Pulmonary denervation can lead to respiratory insufficiency, which can be a problem for long-term studies. This model develops obliterative lesions in small airways during chronic rejection, similar to humans (Salminen et al., 2000).

The donor is prepared for a complete median sternotomy. The left lung is removed following heparinization and subsequent transection of the following structures: left main bronchus, pulmonary artery, and atrial cuff containing the pulmonary veins. All structures should be transected so that the longest possible segment remains attached to the donor lung. It is perfused with cold preservation solution through the pulmonary artery while awaiting transplantation.

The recipient is prepared in a similar manner. The donor lung is sutured in place in the following order: atrial cuff with pulmonary veins, pulmonary artery, and bronchus. Suture selection depends upon the size of the animal and the experience of the surgeon. However, continuous suture pattern with nonabsorbable suture is the most common technique.

Immunosuppressive therapy typically includes such pharmaceuticals as methylprednisolone 2–20 mg kg^{-1}d^{1}, cyclosporine 10 mg kg^{-1}d^{1}, azathiprine 2 mg kg^{-1}d^{1}, and SDZ RAD 1.5 mg kg^{-1}d^{1}, all administered p.o. following an i.v. loading dose at surgery. In many instances, the goal of the research is to study immunosuppressive therapies, and the new compounds are studied with combinations of the standard immunosuppressive therapies. Preventive therapies with compounds such as prostaglandin E$_1$ 250 mg i.v. are also typically used. Postoperative complications include increased extravascular lung water due to reperfusion injury and obliterative bronchitis (Hillinger et al., 2000; Salminen et al., 2000).

Heart and heart-lung transplantations are discussed and illustrated in the following text.

CARDIOVASCULAR SYSTEM

PERIPHERAL VASCULAR CANNULATION AND CHRONIC CATHETERIZATION TECHNIQUES

General Principles

The most common sites of peripheral intravascular catherization in swine are auricular artery and vein, external and interior jugular vein, carotid artery, cephalic vein, femoral artery and vein, and medial saphenous artery. Internal sites include pulmonary artery, vena cava, hepatic artery and vein, portal vein, renal artery and vein, aorta, and internal and external iliac artery and vein. Regardless of the site, it is important that the tip of the catheter be in a high-flow, turbulent area and that the tip not be in contact with a vessel wall to help prevent thrombosis.

Except for the carotid artery, these vessels may be ligated and sacrificed bilaterally instead of being surgically repaired, without significant postoperative complications. Both carotid arteries can be sacrificed with staged surgeries to allow collateral circulation to develop. Collateral circulation is sufficient with one intact carotid artery. One of either the external or internal jugular veins on each side of the neck should also be left intact, but this is not essential. Other vessels that are chronically cannulated for specific research purposes include portal vein, pulmonary artery, and aorta. These vessel approaches will be discussed in this section. Using these vessels as an example, many other blood vessels can be cannulated if indicated by the research protocol. Superficial access to some veins makes it possible to cannulate the central venous system either percutaneously or with minor skin incisions. These veins include the auricular vein, the cephalic vein at the level of the thoracic inlet, and the cranial epigastric vein on the ventral abdomen.

General Surgical Principles for Catheterization

The general principles of surgery apply to these procedures. They are asepsis, closure of dead space, hemostasis, gentle handling of tissues, careful approximation of the wound, avoiding wound tension, and minimizing foreign material. In addition, there are specific principles that apply to the implantation of catheters: immobilization of the catheter, an atraumatic tunneling pathway, securing the exit site, antibiotic prophylaxis at the time of surgery, and use of anticoagulant therapy. It is very important to immobilize the catheter at the site of insertion into the blood vessel and at the site of exit from the skin. This can be performed by leaving a coil of the catheter subcutaneously and putting an s.c. purse-string suture around the catheter before closing the skin. At the exit site, the catheter should have a cuff that allows tissue ingrowth or fibrosis around it to ensure a permanent seal against infection. Antibiotic prophylaxis is not a substitute for an aseptic technique. The blood level of antibiotic present at the time of skin incision is the most important dose if such therapy is indicated. Long-term administration is not necessary unless contamination has occurred.

Swine also have species-specific considerations: do not use silk or gut sutures, be aware of their behavioral characteristics, exteriorize catheters from the dorsum, and use protective devices to prevent damage to the exteriorized catheter. Silk and gut sutures tend to be inflammatory in swine and can lead to seromas and infection. Swine rub themselves against their cages and do not chew or scratch their incisions with their feet. Consequently, catheter exit sites should be on the dorsum of the body. Canvas or plastic coverings, protective vests, or both can be put on swine to prevent trauma to the catheters. Swine of the same breed and age tend to have the same measurement from the catheter insertion point to the site of interest for the tip of the catheter. Therefore, catheters can be manufactured in advance with suture retention beads fixed in place (Figure 9.27).

The technique of incising the vessel for insertion of the catheter depends upon the catheter design and the experience of the surgeon. Systems with needles and guidewires are reliable in swine (see Chapter 12). The vessel should be occluded with elastic vessel loops (Figure 9.28) cranial and caudal to the site of entry and the vessel allowed to fill with blood. The vessel may be entered with a no. 11 surgical blade, iris scissors, or a needle tip. The author prefers to use iris scissors, because they tend to be less traumatic in small vessels and serve to prevent vasospasm. Suture material for tying the catheters in place for chronic cannulation depends upon the length of time that the animal will survive. Polydiaxonone is a good first choice if 3–6 months of suture retention is sufficient. Other synthetic absorbable or nonabsorbable materials may be more appropriate for some projects. Silk and surgical gut should not be used because of their inflammatory characteristics in swine. Both arteries and veins may be repaired surgically following catheterization using 5/0–6/0 cardiovascular suture material in a simple interrupted pattern.

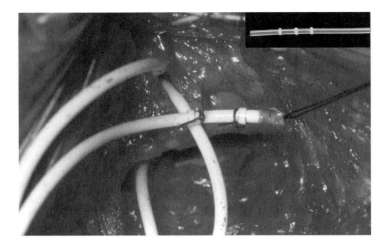

FIGURE 9.27 The insert shows three retention beads glued on the catheter. The surgical illustration demonstrates the proper method of suturing the catheter in place.

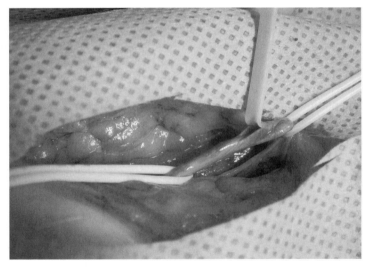

FIGURE 9.28 Elastic vessel loops are used to provide hemostasis during venotomy, in which a vessel pick is used to enlarge the lumen for catheter insertion.

Catheters for chronic implantation should have retention beads permanently fixed to the catheter at the site of vascular insertion (Figure 9.27). These can be simply beads of silicone glue instead of manufactured structures. When sutures are placed in between the beads, it provides some security that the catheter will not move after implantation. A loop of the catheter should also be coiled in the area of venous access to prevent tension on the catheter as a result of movement or growth. Retention beads or velcro cuffs may be necessary in the subcutaneous tissue to prevent the catheter from moving into and out of the skin causing contamination. Nylon velour cuffs or cuffs (Figure 9.29) of other porous material allow tissue ingrowth to form a barrier against contamination. When closing the skin around a catheter exit site, synthetic absorbable materials should be used in subcuticular purse-string fashion. Catheters for vascular access should never be exited through the surgical site, because of the stress on the suture line and the high probability of contamination. Monofilament sutures may be used on the surface of the skin for a tight closure. Tissue glues may be helpful for the purpose of sealing the exit site.

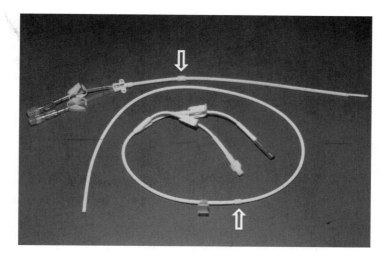

FIGURE 9.29 Hickman and Broviac catheters with cuffs (arrows) to allow tissue ingrowth.

Many of the vascular access sites in swine are relatively deep in the tissues. Venipuncture techniques have previously been described and the anatomic locations are illustrated in Chapter 1 (Bobbie and Swindle, 1986; Swindle, 1983). The Seldinger technique for vascular access for cardiac catheterization studies is discussed in Chapter 12 (Gaymes et al., 1995; Smith et al., 1989). A technique of using ultrasound guidance for vascular access has been described (Wallace et al., 2003). In this section, the surgical principles of vascular access to the main blood vessels will be described (Hand et al., 1981; Nicolau et al., 1996; Purohit et al., 1993; Smith et al., 1989; Swindle, 1983; Swindle et al., 1986, 1996, 1998, 2005).

Peripheral blood vessels of swine are prone to vasospasm and are relatively easy to rupture during catheterization techniques. Good surgical technique and gentle handling of tissues cannot be replaced by use of topical antispasmodic agents such as lidocaine or papaverine. When performing vascular access surgery, the division of muscular tissues should be performed in fascial planes between muscle bodies and not by dividing musculature. Blood vessels should be handled gently and suture material used around the blood vessels should not be abrasive; for example, silk should not be used. The use of elastic vessel loops, especially the rounded types, is the preferred method of isolating and occluding blood vessels during catheterizations. Experience has shown that they do not have the sawing action that braided suture materials have on vessels, which frequently leads to vasospasm. When using gauze, it should be wetted with warm saline to prevent hypothermic vasoconstriction. Gauze should be pressed and held on a bleeding site, never rubbed. The use of electrocautery for hemostasis and ablation of collateral branches works well, as long as the power settings are not high enough to cause collateral cauterization and vasoconstriction.

Catheters should be exteriorized on the dorsal surface of swine (Chapter 8, Figure 8.8 and Figure 8.12). Pigs do not scratch or bite at catheters because of their body conformation. Rather, they rub sites that irritate them. The cage design should be free of materials that a pig could reach by rubbing. Exteriorized catheters can be protected by pouches or covers sutured to the skin or secured with adhesives. Use of nylon jackets and vests designed for research purposes can also be used as well as tether and harness systems.

For continuous infusion catheters, such as those attached to portable infusion pumps, flow rates of 3–5 ml/h are generally high enough to prevent occlusion. Catheters should be filled with full-strength heparin (1:1000 solution) or other catheter lock solution at the time of surgery if they are static. The amount of heparin solution required to fill the catheter should be measured and recorded. Some prefer to add hypertonic solutions, such as 50% glucose, to the heparin solution to aid in prevention of thrombosis or antibiotic solutions to aid in the prevention of infection.

These are unnecessary if meticulous attention is paid to aseptic handling of the catheters during sampling and if the catheter solutions are withdrawn, flushed with sterile saline, and refilled with heparin two to three times a week. Closed systems, such as the vascular access ports, are more reliable in the prevention of complications than systems using three-way valves attached to the ends of open catheters (Swindle et al., 1998, 2005). Additional discussion of catheter lock solutions and postoperative maintenance techniques are discussed later in the subsection on catheter maintenance.

Catheter Design

Catheter selection is based on the technique and purpose of the experiment and the surgeon's preference and experience. Many laboratories manufacture their own catheters for cost savings; however, inappropriate designs and flaws can lead to problems more readily than if commercial catheters are used. Consequently, it is not recommended that investigators manufacture their own catheters for cost savings alone. There either should be an experimental reason to do so or the laboratory should be experienced in design and manufacture of catheters without sharp edges, surface flaws, or contaminants (Dougherty, 1981; Hand et al., 1981; Harvey and Jones, 1982; Swindle et al., 1988, 1998, 2005).

Many problems can be minimized by proper catheter design, which avoids traumatizing the vessel walls, thus initiating a thrombogenic response or erosion. For most procedures, biocompatible silicone or polyurethane catheters are appropriate, although other materials such as polyethelyne, teflon, or polyvinyl chloride may sometimes be indicated (Table 9.5 and Table 9.6). Silicone has the advantage of being soft, flexible, atraumatic, and autoclavable, although it is porous and is more difficult to insert than materials that are stiffer. Polyurethane is firm and easy to insert, but it is more traumatic to blood vessels and is not autoclavable. Trauma from this material on the vessel

TABLE 9.5
Comparison of Silicone vs. Polyurethane

Polyurethane		Silicone	
Benefits	**Disadvantages**	**Benefits**	**Disadvantages**
Material is stronger and less likely to tear	More difficult to modify than silicone	Softness renders it less traumatic to vessel	Less strong and thus more prone to tear
Because of its strength, thinner catheter walls are needed thereby yielding larger internal lumens and increased flow	Initial stiffness may be more damaging to the vessel	More easily modified because of reliable silicone adhesive	More difficult to insert and advance because of softness
Easier to insert and advance because of initial stiffness	Cannot be autoclaved	Smaller lumen yields less dead space, which is advantageous in certain applications	Difficult to coat with specialized coatings
Softens upon warming to body temperature, which may reduce vein trauma	Poor memory may result in loose-fitting connections over time	Can be autoclaved	
Can be coated with a variety of specialized coatings		Excellent memory may maintain tight-fitting connections	

Source: From Swindle, M.M. et al., *Contemp. Topics Lab. Anim. Sci.,* 44(3): 7–17, 2005. With permission.

TABLE 9.6
Catheter Sizes: Silicone and Polyurethane

| French Size | Approximate Gauge | Silicone Catheters | | | | Polyurethane Catheters | | | |
| | | Inner Diameter | | Outer Diameter | | Inner Diameter | | Outer Diameter | |
		in.	mm	in.	mm	in.	mm	in.	mm
1	27	0.007	0.2	0.016	0.4	0.008	0.2	0.017	0.4
2	23	0.012	0.33	0.025	0.6	0.012	0.3	0.025	0.66
3	20	0.020	0.5	0.037	0.9	0.023	0.6	0.037	0.9
4	18	0.025	0.6	0.047	1.2	0.025	0.6	0.044	1.1
5	16	0.030	0.7	0.065	1.7	0.040	1.0	0.065	1.7
7	13	0.050	1.3	0.095	2.4	0.058	1.5	0.095	2.4
9	11	0.062	1.6	0.125	3.2				

Source: From Swindle, M.M. et al., *Contemp. Topics Lab. Anim. Sci.,* 44(3): 7–17, 2005. With permission.

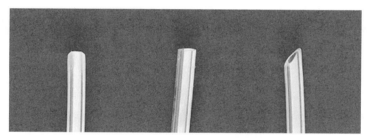

FIGURE 9.30 The catheter tip on the left is rounded and tends to be atraumatic to vessel walls as compared to cut (center) or beveled (right) tips. (Photo courtesy of Instech Solomon, Plymouth Meeting, PA.)

wall can lead to erosion or perforation of the vessel. Tips of the catheters should be tapered and have smooth, rounded edges (Figure 9.30). Part of the length of a silicone catheter can be partially covered with polyurethane to give stiffness to the body of the catheter and avoid kinking. This technique leaves only the length of rigid material exposed in the body cavity, with the softer silicone tip able to contact the vessel wall. Careful handling of silicone to prevent absorption of contaminants such as tissue glues, which can be toxic, should be ensured. A variety of implantable port devices (Figure 9.31) are available to avoid having to exteriorize the catheter from the skin (Swindle et al., 1998, 2005).

Hickman (Figure 9.29) and Broviac catheters are excellent catheters if large-bore or multiple-channel cannulae are required. Subcutaneously implantable catheters, referred to as *vascular access ports* (Figure 9.31), are manufactured by several companies (e.g., Access Technologies, Da Vinci, Instec-Soloman, Phamacia-Deltec, and Uno). There are a variety of designs for these ports, which need to be considered for the particular protocol for which they are being considered. These catheters may be modified or designed by the manufacturers to specifications for particular experimental purposes (Bailie et al., 1986; Swindle et al., 1986, 2005). These require special Huber point needles and placement techniques but have the advantage of reducing risk of infection to exit sites (Figure 9.31 and Figure 9.32). They may also be sutured onto the surface of the skin (Swindle et al., 2005). They offer an advantage of improved asepsis because of the closed nature of the design system. These catheters can also be procured with a tapered edge on the tip to help prevent vascular damage and thrombosis. Small catheters for short-term catheterization include the use of i.v. catheters available from any hospital supply.

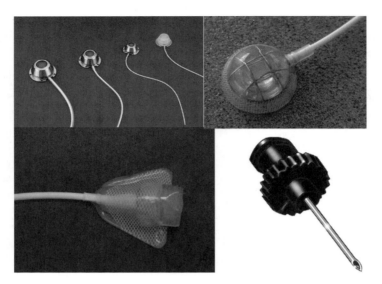

FIGURE 9.31 The composite shows a variety of designs of vascular access ports and a Huber point needle (lower right) for accessing them. (Photos courtesy of Access Technologies and Instech Solomon.)

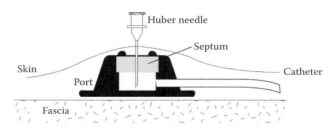

FIGURE 9.32 Schematic drawing of the use of a subcutaneously implanted vascular access port. (Photo courtesy of Access Technologies, Skokie, IL.)

Catheter Maintenance

Anticoagulant therapy is necessary to prevent blood from clotting within the catheter. Catheters used for continuous infusion do not need anticoagulation, but an infusion rate of 3–5 ml/h is necessary to prevent coagulation. Systemic coagulation is not required for intravascular catheters.

No consensus exists on a postoperative protocol for every type of intravascular catheterization. However, some principles utilized by our laboratories have proven effective for long-term catheter maintenance. It is essential to ensure complete asepsis with iodine preparation of the catheter and use of sterile gloves to handle an implanted catheter. At the time of implantation, the volume of the catheter should be determined, and the correct amount of 1:1000 heparin be injected into the catheter. Flushing of the catheter is necessary every time it is accessed or once or twice per week when not accessed for sample administration and collection. The procedure is to withdraw all the old heparin until blood is visualized, flush copiously with saline and then reinject the predetermined amount of heparin required to fill the catheter. Generally, 10–20% more than the predetermined fill amount of catheter lock solution is injected to ensure that the total catheter length is filled.

Other solutions that have been used include 10% heparinized saline, hypertonic 50% dextrose, enzymatic solutions, and antibiotics within the anticoagulant solution. The use of antibiotics is discouraged, and unnecessary, if a meticulous aseptic technique is used. Taurolidine citrate is an antimicrobial solution that has been developed as a substitute for antibiotics in catheter solutions. It has a wide range of activity against most types of infectious organisms, and the citrate provides

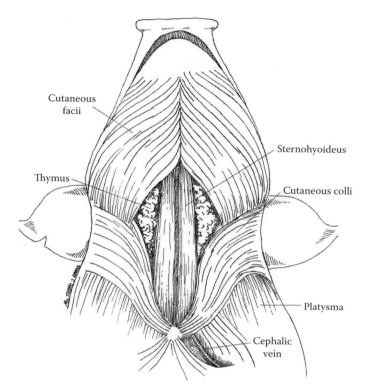

FIGURE 9.33 Superficial dissection of the neck (ventral aspect).

some anticoagulant activity (Betjes and van Agteren, 2004; Jurewitsch and Jeejeebhoy, 2005; Koldehoff and Zakrzewski, 2004; Swindle et al., 2005).

Neck Vessels: External and Internal Jugular Veins and Carotid Artery

The neck vessels can all be approached from an incision in the jugular furrow (Figure 9.33–Figure 9.35). By retracting one leg caudally with the pig in dorsal recumbency, the jugular furrow can be seen along a line drawn slightly medial from the point of the jaw to the point of the shoulder. An incision made in this plane will provide access to the external jugular vein, which is deep in the intermuscular plane between the brachiocephalic and sternocephalic muscles at the same level as the trachea. After incising the skin, subcutaneous tissue, and cutaneous coli muscle, the external jugular vein can be isolated by blunt dissection. From this incision, the two mandibular branches of the vein and the main trunk can be easily isolated.

The internal jugular vein, carotid artery, and vagus nerve can be isolated from this same incision (Figure 9.36), or they can be approached by a ventral midline or paramedian incision followed by dissection of the fascial plane parallel to the trachea. They are located at the same depth as the external jugular but are medial and lie along the ventral surface of the cervical vertebrae parallel to the trachea. They are exposed from the jugular furrow incision by dissecting the fascial plane on the dorsal surface of the sternocephalic muscle. After dissecting this fascia, the floor of the vertebrae and the carotid pulse can be palpated easily. The blood vessels can be retracted into the area of the external jugular vein with a right-angle forceps and isolated with vessel loops for cannulation.

From this location, all three vessels can be cannulated, and the catheters exteriorized if desired. Placement of the tip of the catheter in the correct location is important, and premeasurements in similar-sized pigs can be made to determine the length and premark the catheter with retention beads. Alternatively, the catheter placement can be checked radiographically, or pressure wave

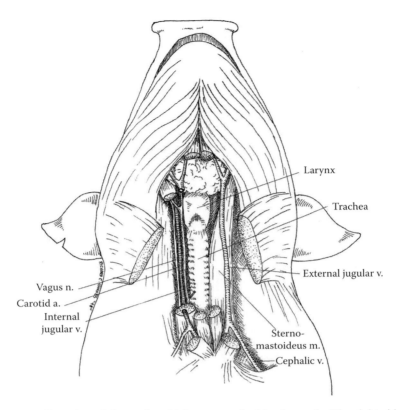

FIGURE 9.34 Deep dissection of the neck, which exposes the blood vessels. The right side has had the sternomastoideus muscle removed to expose the carotid sheath.

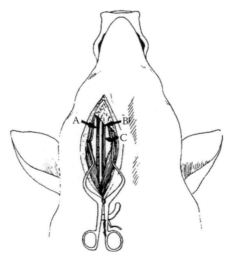

FIGURE 9.35 Surgical approach to the neck. A. External jugular vein. B. Common carotid artery. C. Internal jugular vein. (Reprinted from Smith, A.C. et al., 1989, *J. Invest. Surg.*, 2(2): 187–194. With permission.)

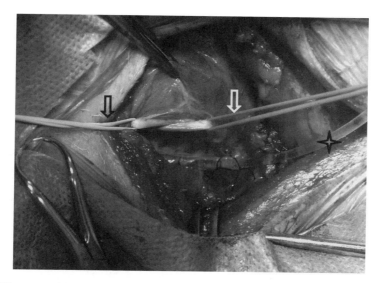

FIGURE 9.36 The external jugular vein has been catheterized (star). The internal jugular vein (black arrow) and the carotid artery (white arrow) have been retracted with elastic vessel loops after medial retraction of the sternothyrohyoideus muscle with dissection over its dorsal surface.

tracings can be used for confirmation. Generally, catheters in the jugular veins are meant for chronic infusion and sample withdrawal. Placement of the tip at the entrance of the precava to the right atrium (approximately at the second intercostal space) is optimal, because the turbulence and velocity of venous blood in this location helps prevent thrombosis. Placement into the atrium or ventricle can lead to cardiac arrhythmias, valvular damage, or atrial appendage thrombosis, rupture, or both.

Exteriorization of the catheters is best done on the dorsal surface of the caudal neck between the scapulas. To perform this surgery without repositioning the pig during surgery, the pig should be in lateral recumbency. The major neck vessels can all be isolated from the same incision, and the catheters passed through a rod tunneled through the subcutaneous tissues exiting the skin on the dorsum of the neck (see Chapter 8, Figure 8.8). If a subcutaneously implanted vascular access port is used, the tunneling rod is passed caudoventral to the axillary space to the lateral aspect of the thoracic wall. The port is implanted subcutaneously in the dorsal region of the chest wall. The port may also be implanted on the dorsum of the neck or the lateral aspect of the scapula. The subcutaneous pocket incision should be made either cranial or caudal to the site of the device implantation. The subcutaneous tissues are carefully dissected, and complete hemostasis must be ensured to prevent hematomas and seromas. The device should be anchored to the muscle fascia, and the dead space closed adequately with subcutaneous and subcuticular sutures. The suture line should not be under tension and should not overlap the device; this prevents the complications of suture line dehiscence and necrosis. Skin sutures are placed as required. The steps of implanting a vascular access port (VAP) are illustrated in Figure 9.37–Figure 9.43.

The neck incision is closed in three layers in most swine: muscles, subcutaneous tissues, and skin. In larger swine, dead space in the deep fascial plane of the incision may also have to be closed.

The cephalic vein can be percutaneously catheterized on the cranial aspect of the foreleg as well as the ventral surface of the neck at the thoracic inlet, as described in Chapter 1. The vein can be identified by applying digital pressure at the thoracic inlet and watching it fill with blood along its course from the leg through the neck. An incision over the vessel is made, and the dissection is continued through the skin, subcutaneous tissue, and thin body of the cutaneous coli muscle. The vein may be cannulated and the catheter tunneled subcutaneously as described for the other neck

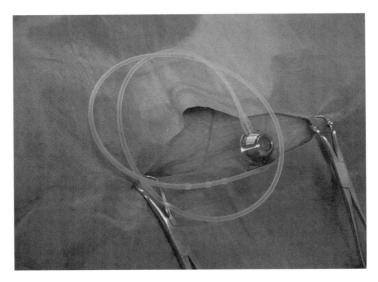

FIGURE 9.37 A vascular access port (VAP) with fixed vascular retention beads is sized to surgically produce an implantation pocket on the dorsolateral surface of the thoracic wall.

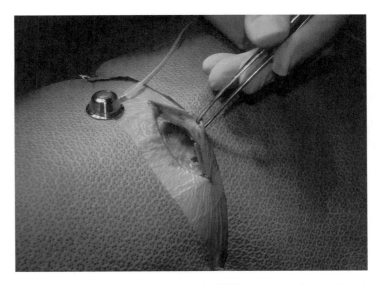

FIGURE 9.38 A curvilinear incision slightly larger than the VAP has been made into the subcutaneous tissues.

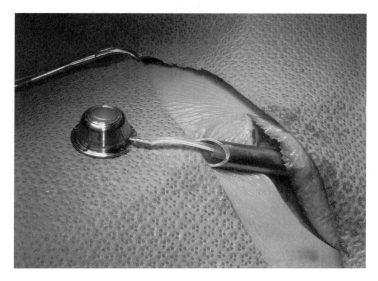

FIGURE 9.39 A trocar has been passed from the neck incision (see Figure 9.35) and the catheter has been passed through it.

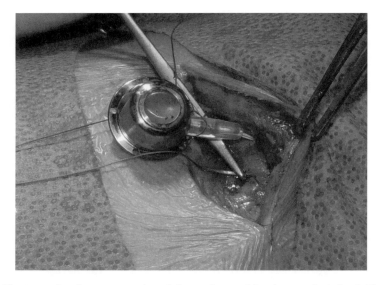

FIGURE 9.40 The trocar has been removed, and the neck vessel has been catheterized. The port has been filled with heparinized saline. Sutures are being placed through the suture holes of the port into the deep subcutaneous tissues. These sutures will ensure that the port does not migrate or flip in the pocket.

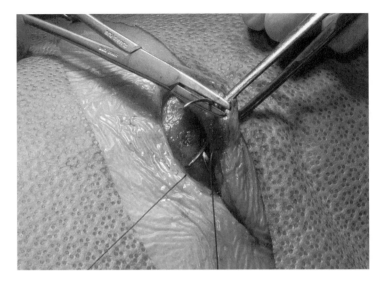

FIGURE 9.41 The vascular access port (VAP) has been anchored in the pocket, and a row of subcutaneous sutures is being placed to close the pocket and eliminate dead space.

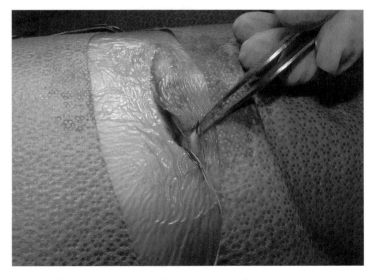

FIGURE 9.42 A subcuticular suture is used to close the port pocket.

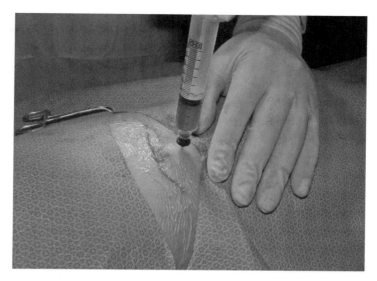

FIGURE 9.43 Fluid is withdrawn from the port using a syringe and Huber point needle. The catheter is flushed with saline and then filled with heparin.

vessels. For short-term catheterization, the exteriorization may be done on the ventrolateral aspect of the neck. The pig is likely to traumatize this site, however, unless it is protected with a bandage.

Leg Vessels

The femoral vessels and the medial saphenous vessel are all approached (Figure 9.44 and Figure 9.45) with the pig in dorsal recumbency and the rear leg retracted caudally. The pulse of the medial saphenous artery may be consistently palpated over the medial aspect of the stifle joint. This pulsation may be followed cranially to the level of the thigh, where the artery courses deeply into the musculature of the medial aspect of the leg. The division of the musculature where the arterial pulse disappears is the fascial division of the sartorius and gracilis muscles. The femoral artery, vein, and nerve are located below the edge of the body of the gracilis muscle.

The surgical incision for the medial saphenous artery may be made directly adjacent to the arterial pulse along the medial aspect of the stifle joint or tibia. The artery is superficial and may be isolated after dissection of the subcutaneous tissue. The vein is usually a plexus in this region

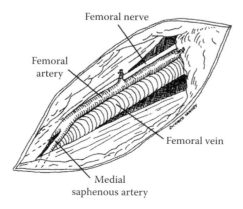

FIGURE 9.44 Surgical cutdown on the femoral and medial saphenous vessels.

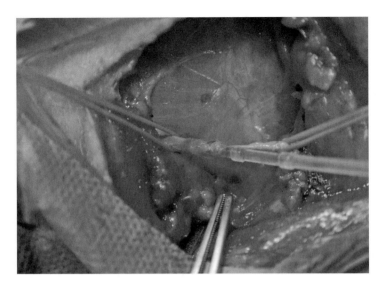

FIGURE 9.45 Catheterization of the femoral artery.

and not useful for cannulation. The artery may be cannulated as a superficial site for measuring arterial pressures and taking samples, or catheters may be passed into the femoral artery from the access site. Most small swine can accommodate 18- to 20-ga catheters in this vessel.

The femoral vessels may be approached by making either a longitudinal or a transverse incision over the fascial muscular division described previously on the medial aspect of the rear leg. There are lateral and deep branches of both the artery and vein that should be ligated or cauterized during the isolation of the vessels. Rupture of these branches usually leads to bleeding in the sheath of the vessels and vasoconstriction.

Portal Vein

The portal vein may be catheterized through a ventral midline incision from the xiphoid process to the umbilicus (also see Chapter 5). Access to the region is difficult, especially in large swine, and all the principles of abdominal surgery previously described should be followed. The liver needs to be retracted cranially and the stomach and duodenum, caudally. The intestinal mass will have to be excluded from the surgical area by packing them off with wetted laparotomy sponges. The portal vein can be identified at the hilum of the liver as it passes through the pancreas and dorsal to the duodenum (Figure 9.46; see also Chapter 5, Figure 5.7). The common bile duct runs on its ventral surface (Hand et al., 1981).

The portal vein may be carefully dissected around its dorsal surface above and below the area where the cannula is to be inserted. Elastic vessel loops are placed around the vessel to provide occlusion during the venotomy. The portal vein is thin walled, and extensive hemorrhage can occur if it is damaged. A preplaced purse-string suture is placed around the venotomy site. The best location for access is usually in the ventrocaudal portion close to the duodenum.

The portal vein is incised with either a no. 11 scalpel blade or iris scissors after cranial and caudal occlusion of the vessel with the vessel loops. A catheter with a retention bead is fed into the venotomy toward the liver (Figure 9.47). If the catheter actually passes into the liver, it is more likely to occlude. After placing the tip in the desired location, the purse-string suture is tightened so that a retention bead remains within the vessel. The cranial and then the caudal occlusion loops are loosened. The catheter should either be sutured to the side of the portal vein wall between two retention beads or to some other structure in the region to prevent kinking. The catheter should be checked for patency at this stage. Experience from liver transplantation experiments has shown

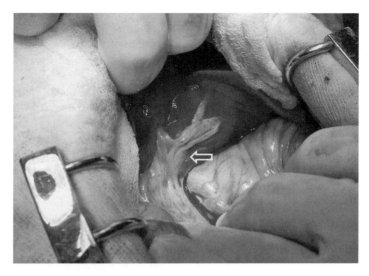

FIGURE 9.46 View of the hilum of the liver in the region of the branching of the portal vein (arrow).

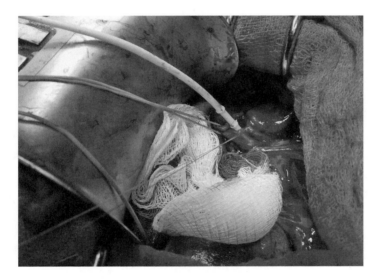

FIGURE 9.47 Direct catheterization of the portal vein through a purse-string suture.

that more than 15 min of occlusion of the portal vein leads to irreversible portal hypertension. The catheter may be exteriorized through the abdominal wall caudal to the ribs. If a vascular access port is used, it is placed on the lateral surface of the ribs. Experience from many laboratories does not give a consensus on the best type of catheter or technique to use for catheterization of this vessel. Most would consider 6 weeks of patency to be exceptional. Postoperative problems include thrombosis and erosion of the portal vein because of the low velocity in a thin-walled vessel.

The left branch of the portal vein may sometimes be located within the visceral surface of the left lateral liver lobe by palpation of a groove that corresponds to the entry of the branch into the liver parenchyma (Figure 9.46) (Drougas et al., 1996; Svendsen and Rasmussen, 1998). The vein may be catheterized in a retrograde manner by passing a trocar into the vessel and then inserting the catheter. The tip of the catheter should be passed into the main part of the vein where it can be palpated to determine that it is in the correct location. A catheter inserted in this manner must be sutured in place to the liver, and care should be taken to prevent kinking.

The portal vein can also be cannulated retrogradely from the splenic vein (Figure 9.48) or pancreatic vein (Figure 9.49) (Drougas et al., 1996; Kaiser et al., 2005). These approaches offer the advantage of ease of exposure, although it is more difficult to determine proper placement of the catheter tip with the splenic vein approach. This must be confirmed by either direct visualization or radiographic techniques. It is also possible for the catheter to advance into the wrong vein or kink or puncture the portal vein during placement. More rigid material than silicone may be required to advance the catheter, but this may cause postoperative erosion of the vessel wall. The pancreatic vein approach is relatively atraumatic and close to the hilus of the liver, so that catheter tip placement can be accurately determined (Kaiser et al., 2005).

In this method, the spleen is retracted caudally out of the abdomen, and the splenic vein is dissected free from the splenic artery close to the hilum of the organ (Drougas et al., 1996). This

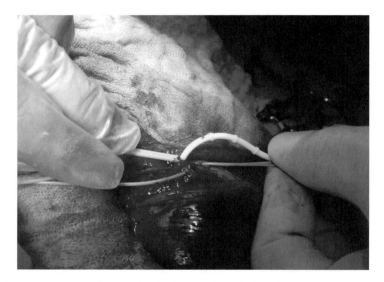

FIGURE 9.48 Catheterization of the portal vein through the splenic vein.

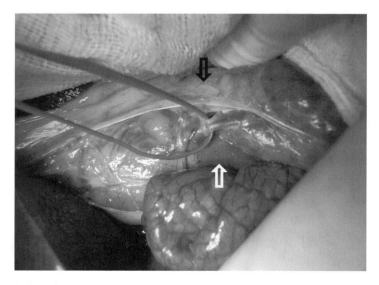

FIGURE 9.49 Isolation of a pancreatic vein entering the portal vein (white arrow). The pancreas is identified by the black arrow.

is the middle of the three major veins draining the spleen. The catheter must be passed slowly and guided with a finger on its tip to ensure that it follows the correct pathway into the portal vein. The catheter is fixed in place and exteriorized in the same manner as other abdominal catheters. The distal portion of the pancreatic vein can be isolated near the portal vein, which it enters as a side branch. It is cannulated in the same manner (Kaiser et al., 2005)

Other Blood Vessels

The cephalic vein may be used for chronic cannulation (Chapter 1, Figure 1.29) by locating the vein as it crosses the neck superficially from the point of the shoulder to the thoracic inlet. With the pig in dorsal recumbency, digital pressure is applied in the thoracic inlet, and the dilated vessel becomes apparent. It has the advantage of being more superficial in its location than the jugular veins; however, it has a much smaller diameter.

The external mammary vein is located along the lateral aspect of the mammary glands on the abdomen (Chapter 1, Figure 1.30). This vein may be located by putting digital pressure at either side of the sternum with the pig in dorsal recumbency. This vein is best utilized for short-term catheterization procedures because of its superficial location in an area easily traumatized by the pig. It is relatively small in immature pigs.

The medial saphenous artery (Figure 9.44; see also Chapter 2, Figure 2.18) is located over the medial aspect of the stifle (knee or femoral or tibial joint). Its pulse can be located superficially in all ages of animals. The artery is best utilized for short-term catheterization because of its location. Smaller catheters can be advanced into the femoral artery from this location. The vein is usually a plexus and is unreliable for cannulation.

Internal blood vessels may be cannulated by following the surgical approach for exposure of the organ or structure of interest. For instance, the left hemiazygous vein can be cannulated and the cannula threaded to the coronary sinus to measure venous coronary blood flow by following the applicable surgical instructions for the left total pneumonectomy described previously. Using these principles of catheter placement, reasonable success rates can be expected.

Postoperative Considerations

For survival procedures, meticulous aseptic techniques are obligatory not only intraoperatively, but also postoperatively. Every aspect of the use of chronic catheters must include attention to aseptic techniques. The outside of the catheter should be prepped with iodine solution, and personnel should wear gloves when injecting or withdrawing samples. Therapeutic levels of antibiotics at the time of surgery for device implantation have been shown to be useful, but chronic administration of antibiotics is not a reliable replacement for aseptic techniques. Infected implants will have to be surgically removed to resolve a chronic infection (Swindle et al., 1998, 2005). Analgesics help control the urge of the animal to rub the incision site and should be administered preemptively. When s.c. vascular access ports are implanted, the use of lidocaine or prilocaine (or both) topical adhesive patches provide topical anesthesia over the injection site for up to 12 h and should be used to prevent needle sensitivity when multiple injections are required over a short period of time.

Vascular Anastomosis

Anastomosis of blood vessels (Figure 9.50 and Figure 9.51) is a routine procedure required for experimental procedures, such as organ transplantation or implantation of vascular grafts. It may also be required clinically for trauma. The basic techniques of suturing are the same as for other species. Two characteristics of the porcine vascular system are important considerations. These are the tendency to vasospasm and the pig's rapid clotting time, which necessitates frequent administration of heparin for some procedures. The i.v. dosage of heparin is 100–300 units/kg as

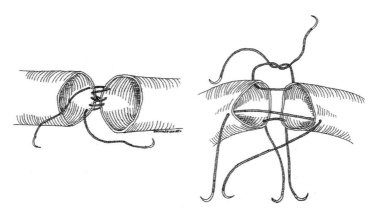

FIGURE 9.50 Anastomosis of the aorta using triangular and continuous suture patterns.

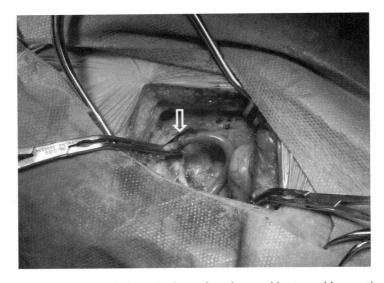

FIGURE 9.51 End-to-end anastomosis (arrow) of a graft to the carotid artery with a continuous pattern.

a priming dose with maintenance doses of 100–200 units/kg given approximately every 45 min (Gaymes et al., 1995; Smith et al., 1989; Swindle, 1983). Porcine graft implants have been shown to have a smooth fibrin surface and be relatively resistant to experimental infection; these characteristics may make them useful for some preclinical studies. Endothelialization of implanted biomaterials usually occurs. The pig is a definitive model for development of neointimal hyperplasia at the site of graft anastomosis, which occurs within a few months following surgery (Johnson et al., 2001; Kelly et al., 2002; Mehran et al., 1991; Rashid et al., 2003; Ricci et al., 1991a, 1991b; Rotmans et al., 2003).

The surgical approach to the blood vessels will be dictated by the procedure being performed. For instance, the abdominal aorta can be approached from either a retroperitoneal flank incision or a midline incision. If the procedure being performed is a simple anastomosis or implantation of a short graft segment, then the retroperitoneal approach should be considered because of the better exposure without the intestinal mass having to be retracted. On the other hand, if the aortic anastomosis is to be performed in conjunction with another procedure on the vena cava, then the midline incision may be more appropriate. Other vessels, such as the femoral or neck vessels, may be approached from the standard incisions described under vascular cannulation.

Isolation of the vessel and ligation of branches in the proximity of the anastomotic site should be performed gently to avoid vasospasm. The blood vessels to be anastomosed are cross-clamped with atraumatic vascular forceps, such as bulldog clamps for small vessels and Satinsky or DeBakey clamps for larger vessels. Cross-clamping resulting in total occlusion of blood flow is problematic in some regions, notably the aorta. When cross-clamping the aorta or other major vessels without substantial collateral circulation, heparin should always be administered. The total cross-clamp time of the prerenal descending aorta that is tolerated without ischemic damage to the spinal cord is approximately 15 min. Early ischemic preconditioning of 20 min followed by ischemia 80 min later has been demonstrated to provide some protection to spinal cord damage in a model of thoracic aortic occlusion (Toumpoulis et al., 2004). Likewise, mild hypothermia (32°C) has been shown to protect against up to 50 min of thoracic aortic occlusion (Strauch et al., 2004). Hypothermia with vena cava to left atrium bypass has also shown to be effective in prevention of spinal cord damage (Doty et al., 2002). Infrarenal cross-clamping results in the same syndromes of decreased cardiac index and increased arterial pressure that occur in humans (Alric et al., 2003).

The number of branches to the psoas musculature that are ligated during isolation of the aorta should be limited to the minimal number required for the procedure. Ligation of substantial numbers of these branches, i.e., four to six continuous pairs in most regions, can also result in spinal cord ischemia. Lymphatic vessels in the region of the aorta should be either circumvented or ligated to avoid leakage of chyle. Consequently, it is preferable that vascular surgery is performed using tangential clamps that only partially occlude the aorta. Bypass procedures can also be used as for some types of organ transplantation. Peripheral vessels are less of a problem when cross-clamped, but heparinization should be used if the goal of the procedure is to provide a patent vessel (Swindle, 1983; Qayumi et al., 1993).

Synthetic nonabsorbable 5/0–6/0 cardiovascular suture is indicated for most vascular anastomoses in swine. Larger vessels, such as the aorta, are sutured in a continuous pattern, and smaller vessels are sutured using simple interrupted sutures. For large vessels, the wall of the aorta most distal from the surgeon is the starting point. A double-armed cardiovascular suture is passed from inside the lumen to outside, and a knot is tied at the middle of the suture length to ensure that the knot is outside the lumen. Suture bites of approximately 2–3 mm are necessary to avoid tearing the vessel. The strands are tied in a continuous pattern to a position opposite the first knot one at a time toward the surgeon. The distal clamp may be partially released at this point to allow the vessel to fill and to remove air bubbles. The knot is tied, and the distal clamp is released slowly to check for leaks. This is followed by gradual release of the proximal clamp one notch at a time. If substantial leakage occurs, then the leaks can be repaired with simple interrupted sutures. If leakage is minor, then the anastomotic incision may be packed with gauze for 3–5 min. This is usually sufficient for clotting to occur at the needle puncture sites. Longitudinal incisions in blood vessels, such as the aorta, may also be utilized. They may be closed in a similar fashion or, if extra security is required, a continuous mattress suture with buffering tags at the knots may be used. This suture pattern is oversewn with simple continuous or continuous Lembert sutures.

When smaller vessels are repaired with simple interrupted patterns, the basic procedure is the same. The wall of the vessel distal from the surgeon is sutured first, and the sides are sutured alternatively until the portion of the wall most proximal to the surgeon is closed last. A triangular pattern may also be used for appropriately sized vessels with the first sutures placed distal to the surgeon as for the other patterns. Vascular picks are helpful in positioning the walls of the smaller vessels for proper alignment during suturing.

Veins may be sutured in the same manner as arteries; however, they are much more friable and easily torn with sutures. Closure of the surgical incision is routine for the area in which the vessel is located.

Femoral arterial ligation, excision, or both have been utilized as a model of arteriogenesis (Hoefer et al., 2006). Collateral arterial growth simulates the same phenomena in humans. Rodent and rabbit models are typically hyperresponders compared to the pig with some treatments.

Postoperative anticoagulant and antimicrobial therapy may be required for some procedures, such as the implantation of synthetic grafts. Oral coumarin and aspirin, 25 mg/kg once daily, are readily administered to swine in their food. Injectable and oral anticoagulants may also be administered. Individual sensitivity to these agents, including protracted bleeding, GI bleeding, and anaphylaxis, may be encountered. These supportive agents are discussed in Chapter 2. Antibiotics are given intraoperatively for graft implantation and postoperatively if contamination is suspected (Rogers et al., 1988).

ARTERIOVENOUS AND VENOVENOUS FISTULAS AND VASCULAR SHUNTS

Arteriovenous fistulas (Figure 9.52) and shunts are usually created in swine to produce a model of volume overload heart failure (Randsbaek et al., 1996; Wittnich et al., 1991) that leads to cardiac dilatation and subsequent eccentric cardiac hypertrophy (Carroll et al., 1995; Gardner and Johnson, 1988). They have been used to create a dilated vascular space for enhanced vascular access as for human dialysis patients (Johnson et al., 2001; Kelly et al., 2002; Rotmans et al., 2003).

The technique involves performing a side-to-side anastomosis between an artery and a vein or the suturing of a vascular prosthesis in an end-to-side vascular window technique between an artery and a vein to produce a left-to-right shunt. The more peripheral the location (femoral vessels), the longer the time for production of volume overload. Fistulation between the aorta and pulmonary trunk will have significant immediate effects. This is in contrast to a period of months for clinical effects if peripheral vasculature is used. A fistulation between the carotid artery and the internal jugular vein would be intermediate in time for development of clinical effects. The size of the shunt required differs with the age and breed of the pig and location of the shunt. Generally, the fistulation needs to be 2.5 times the outside diameter of the blood vessels in length for peripheral vessels. If a fistula of this size were used in an aorta-pulmonary shunt of a neonatal pig, it would die acutely. Miniature pigs are less susceptible to the effects of arteriovenous fistulas and shunts, at least in the acute and short-term phases. Because there are relatively few references in the literature to creation of this model in swine, no consensus on the best surgical technique or breed and age of pig has been reached.

A model of cyanotic heart disease can be produced by creating a fistula between the pulmonary artery and the left atrial appendage (Zhang et al., 1998). In a 12-kg swine a fistula of 4 × 6 mm created by partial occlusion of the pulmonary artery with vascular clamps and suturing to a similar incision in the atrial appendage results in the development of cyanotic heart disease over 4–6 weeks. It may be enhanced by placement of a nonrestrictive pulmonary arterial band distal to the fistula.

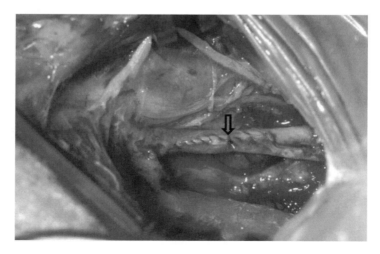

FIGURE 9.52 Femoral arteriovenous fistula (arrow).

A portocaval shunt may be created by side-to-side or end-to-side anastomosis of the portal vein and the posthepatic caudal vena cava. This model has been used to study the effects of the portocaval shunt on the metabolism of lipids and lipoproteins. Attempts to produce a model of portal hypertension with gastric ulcers and esophageal varices have been made in swine. This involves creation of an end-to-side anastomosis of the vena cava to the portal vein and gradual constriction of the portal vein with devices such as an ameroid constrictor. Collateral circulation in the region helps lower the portal pressure in swine. Irreversible portal hypertension has also been reported as a complication in hepatic transplantation with prolonged portal vein occlusion, and this should be avoided during portal vein surgery (Carew et al., 1976; Dupont et al., 1985; Gadacz, 1988; Jensen et al., 1983; Kahn et al., 1994; Nestruck et al., 1977).

An arteriovenous malformation model has been developed in swine by using a transorbital puncture in the cavernous sinus to create an arteriovenous communication between the rostral rete and the cavernous sinus. The model is possible because of the presence of a rete mirabile in the cavernous sinuses of the skull base (Chaloupka et al., 1994).

The surgical approaches to the vessels will be the routine approaches described for isolation of the vessels in the other sections, i.e., vascular cannulation for femorals or caudal celiotomy for the iliacs. The techniques for suturing the vessels are described in the section on vascular anastomosis.

ATRIOTOMY AND VENTRICULOTOMY

The atria on either side can be approached through the fourth or fifth intercostal space or a median sternotomy using the standard thoracotomy incisions described earlier. Indications would include cannulation procedures and surgical approaches to the foramen ovale, atrioventricular valves, and high membranous ventricular septal defects. Cannulation and other procedures should be performed in the atrial appendage if possible (Figure 9.53). However, this approach would not be useful for the valvular rings. Cardiopulmonary bypass (Chapter 2) would be required for most procedures except simple cannulations. The atria are extremely friable in swine and should be handled gently with appropriate instruments (Ehler et al., 1990; Hall et al., 1986; Horneffer et al., 1986; Smerup et al., 2004; Swindle et al., 1986).

The appropriate portion of the atrium is incised with a scalpel or punctured with a scalpel and the incision extended with scissors. Gentle handling of the tissues using cardiovascular instruments is essential to prevent tearing of the atrial incision. Care should be taken to avoid traumatizing the conduction system especially in the region of the sinoatrial (SA) node, atrioventricular (AV) node, and bundle of His in the right atrium.

After the procedure is performed, closure of the incision should be undertaken with great care. Synthetic monofilament nonabsorbable cardiovascular suture material 5/0–6/0 is usually indicated. A purse-string suture may be sufficient for the implantation of a catheter into the atrial appendage.

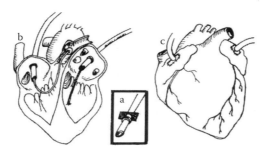

FIGURE 9.53 Atrial cannulation. A. Tip of silastic catheter showing placement of silastic ridge and sheeting. B. Cutaway view of heart showing a balloon tipped catheter in the main pulmonary artery and a biopsy catheter in the left ventricle. C. External view of the heart with left and right artial catheters sutured in place. (Reprinted from Smith et al., 1989, *J. Invest. Surg.* 2(2): 187–194. With permission.)

However, such simple suturing techniques for the atria will probably be insufficient, especially in immature animals. Continuous suture patterns can be used if care is taken with their placement and the tension on the suture line. The use of continuous horizontal mattress suture patterns with buttress pledgets at both ends of the suture line offer more security. This pattern may be oversewn with a simple continuous patten for control of leaks. Before tying the suture, the usual precautions for closure of cardiac incisions on bypass should be taken. This would include such procedures as the removal of air from the atrium and filling it with blood. If leakage occurs from the atrium, it may be repaired by either packing it with gauze sponges or the judicious placement of simple interrupted sutures. A small amount of leakage can be tolerated in a heparinized animal and controlled postoperatively with chest tube drainage. The use of protamine to counteract heparin is not recommended as a routine in swine; however, it can be administered slowly with monitoring of blood pressure if indicated.

Intracardiac surgery should be limited to atrial approaches if at all possible, because of the potential complications with ventricular incisions. The surgeon must take care to avoid compromising the coronary circulation and the conduction system. There is also the potential of developing a surgical scar causing arrhythmias. Consequently, most procedures are limited to small puncture wounds or windows with internal instrumentation except for outflow tract approaches and aneurysm repair. Examples would include cutting tendinous chordae or dilation of valves. When incising the ventricle without cardiopulmonary bypass, a purse-string suture should be preplaced around the entry site. Following the removal of the instrument, the purse-string suture is tightened.

Epicardial implantation of devices is easily performed if the same precautions concerning the blood supply and conduction system are taken. The ventricle is easily catheterized from peripheral vessels with or without the use of fluoroscopy, this being the preferred method of placing internal catheters. Cardiac catheterization is discussed in Chapter 12.

Closure of the incision and postoperative care techniques are the routine ones described for thoracotomy.

VALVULAR SURGERY

The AV valves, the pulmonary valve, and the aortic valve are approached for surgical replacement during cardiopulmonary bypass. The AV valves are usually approached using the appropriate atriotomy incision after a lateral thoracotomy at the fourth to fifth intercostal space on the appropriate side. A median sternotomy approach can also be used, as in humans, particularly for the right atrium. The mitral valvular approach is problematic regardless of the incision site selected and may require slight rightward rotation for visualization. The pulmonary and aortic valves are approached by longitudinal or transverse incisions over the site of the valve from a median sternotomy or, alternatively, a left lateral thoracotomy may be used for the pulmonary artery (Gallegos et al., 2005; Grehan et al., 2000; Gross et al., 1997; Hasenkam et al., 1988; Hazekamp et al., 1993; Litzke and Berg, 1977; Lomholt et al., 2002; Nguyen et al., 2004; Shimokawa et al., 1996; Smerup et al., 2004; Smith et al., 1994; Swindle et al., 1986). Bioprosthetic valves of 15- to 23-mm diameter have been percutaneously placed in the aorta using an expandable stent with porcine valves obtained at slaughterhouses in 64- to 76-kg pigs (Lutter et al., 2002).

The selected valve is sutured in place using the manufacturer's instructions (Figure 9.54). Most of the valves used will require sizing of the orifice and preplacement of a specified number of sutures using synthetic nonabsorbable suture material. The sutures are passed through the AV valvular tissue into the valve sleeve and then tied in turn. Experimentally, this procedure is usually performed to test new valves using a mitral valve implantation site. The porcine bioprosthesis valves prepared from glutaraldehyde fixed aortic valves collected at slaughterhouses are the preferred valvular implant if there is a choice. These valves offer the advantages of being of porcine origin and having minimal problems with thrombosis and emboli, thus eliminating the need for anticoagulant therapy. Sizing of the orifice for selecting a valve can be performed using two-dimensional

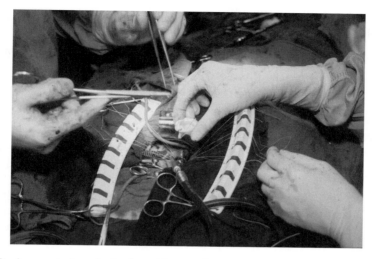

FIGURE 9.54 Replacement of a mitral valve with a porcine bioprosthesis.

echocardiography or may be performed intraoperatively. As a guideline 60-kg farm pigs have been determined to require 29-mm mitral valves and have a similar mitral valvular leaflet and tendinous chordae anatomy (Smerup et al., 2004). If mechanical valves of synthetic material are selected, lifetime anticoagulant therapy will be required.

Cutting of the valves to produce valvular regurgitation and creation of volume overload models of heart failure and eccentric ventricular hypertrophy can be performed from peripheral vessels without the use of thoracotomy or cardiopulmonary bypass. Chordal cutting (Figure 9.55) has been proposed as a treatment for ischemic mitral regurgitation causing distortion of the basal leaflet (Messas et al., 2001). Using fluoroscopic guidance, an instrument, such as urologic grasping forceps, is advanced into the ventricle, tendinous chordae are grasped and then torn. Cardiac catheterization or echocardiography can be utilized to judge the degree of regurgitation.

Closures of the atriotomy or blood vessel (or both) and the thoracotomy are routine. Emerging technology provides the opportunity to study minimally invasive intracardiac procedures such as

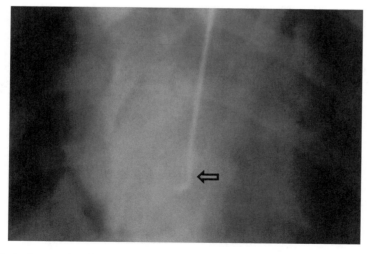

FIGURE 9.55 Urologic grasping forceps (arrow) being used to cut tendinous chordae using fluoroscopic guidance.

robotics (Chitwood et al., 2001) or three-dimensional echocardiography guidance (Suematsu et al., 2004) in porcine models. Postoperative care should include antimicrobial therapy as well as the usual analgesic and cardiothoracic precautions.

Aortic and Pulmonary Artery Banding, Ligation of the Ductus Arteriosus, and Chronic Instrumentation

The aorta and pulmonary artery are best approached through a left lateral thoracotomy in the third intercostal space. The pulmonary artery can also be approached throughout the fourth intercostal space in most animals. Both vessels can also be approached through a median sternotomy that does not bisect the manubrium. The ductus arteriosus also can be approached through the same lateral incision.

Indications for these surgical approaches to the aorta and pulmonary artery include cannulation for bypass procedures, implantation of devices or grafts, and constriction banding to produce pressure overload of the ventricles (Carroll et al., 1995; Dougherty, 1981; Gardner and Johnson, 1988; Harvey and Jones, 1982; Kaplan et al., 1995; Rabkin et al., 2004; Swindle et al., 1986). The ductus arteriosus can be ligated through the same approach if it is a patent ductus arteriosus (PDA). Banding of the great vessels produces a model of concentric ventricular hypertrophy as compared to the models of eccentric hypertrophy produced by AV fistulas as described previously. Banding of the aorta produces more severe postoperative consequences than banding of the pulmonary artery. The left pulmonary artery has been ligated and later reanastomosed to the pulmonary arterial trunk as a model to study pulmonary thromboendartectomy as a treatment for vasculopathy (Fadel et al., 2004). Normal function was shown to return after 5 weeks of reperfusion. Hypertrophic cardiomyopathy occurs spontaneously in both farm and miniature breeds (Lin et al., 2002; Swindle, 1992). The condition is characterized by increases in heart weight: body weight and increased thickness of the left-ventricular free wall and interventricular septum with myocardial fiber disarray, intramural arteriosclerosis and interstitial fibrosis (Figure 9.56). Attempts to produce a genetic model of this condition have been frustrating because many of the animals die prior to sexual maturity.

The surgical approach is routine, and the pericardium is incised, care being taken to avoid damage to the phrenic nerve. The most difficult part of the surgery is dissection and isolation of the blood vessels, especially in immature animals. Most models require that the dissection be proximal to the ductus arteriosus close to the base of the heart. The tissue is dissected bluntly using either right-angle forceps or Metzenbaum scissors. In older animals, there may be a fat pad present in this location. In younger animals, the thymus gland may also extend to this region. The most common problems during the dissection are tearing of the right atrium, tearing the ligamentum arteriosus, or tearing of the great vessels. The pulmonary artery is more easily dissected than the

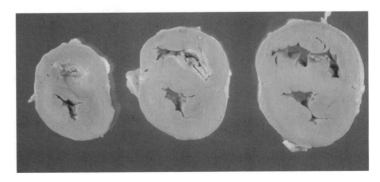

FIGURE 9.56 Hypertrophic cardiomyopathy.

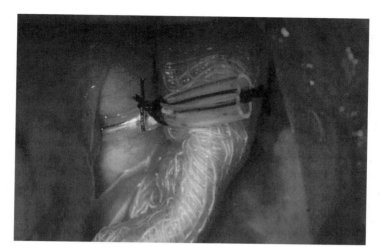

FIGURE 9.57 Pulmonary arterial banding technique.

aorta from the lateral incision; however, for complex instrumentation, the surgeon may prefer the sternotomy approach.

If the ductus arteriosus is to be ligated, the dissection is similar to that done to isolate the pulmonary artery. The vagus nerve crosses the region and should be retracted dorsally without damaging the structure. Atropine should be administered before this procedure. The ductus can be doubly ligated using nonabsorbable suture material. If a rupture occurs during this process, the aorta or pulmonary artery (or both) may have to be repaired by tangential clamping and suture closure of the tear. The method of reopening a closed ductus and using it as a model of PDA is discussed in Chapter 12.

Various methods have been utilized to band these blood vessels to produce a pressure gradient (Figure 9.57 and Figure 9.58). The method and type of banding material will be dictated by the research application. Generally, the bands are placed with a pressure gradient in mature animals, or they are placed loosely around the vessel in immature animals, allowing gradual constriction as

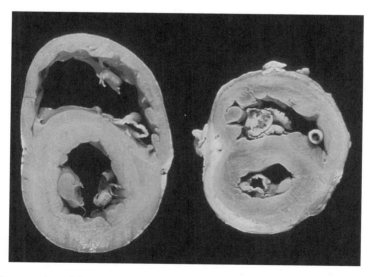

FIGURE 9.58 Cross section of the hearts of a Hanford control (left) and pulmonary arterial banded pig (right) after 4 months.

the animal grows. When bandings that result in an acute pressure gradient are made, it should ensure that the constriction produces a gradient of less than 20 torr. This varies with the age, weight, and breed of the animal but may be used as a general guideline. Bradycardia will be readily detectable with a tight banding procedure. Making too tight a constriction acutely can result in heart failure. Procedures using angioplasty balloon implantation between the band and the blood vessel to produce a gradual constriction by periodic inflation of the balloon have been used in the dog and could possibly be applicable in this species (Keech et al., 1997). A telemetry device has been developed (FloWatch®, EndoArt SA, Lausanne, Switzerland) which allows adjustable pulmonary arterial banding. The pressure gradient can be increased or decreased over time, and the device has proven to be functional for at least 6 months (Corno et al., 2003).

Erosion of the blood vessel and resultant fatal hemorrhage occurs to some degree with virtually all banding techniques. Erosion tends to be less than in some species because of the presence of a true vaso vasorum in the aorta. However, the incidence may be minimized by the design of the band. The same principles of constriction banding are true for both the aorta and the pulmonary artery. The band should be wide and without sharp edges. Constricting the vessel with either suture material or umbilical tape tends to have a high incidence of erosions. Polytetrafluoroethylene (PTFE) or teflon bands used clinically have fewer problems. Placing a piece of nonabsorbable suture material inside silicone tubing also has a low incidence of erosion and is the preferred technique. In this technique, the ends of the suture material can be tied after passing it through a piece of tubing that is long enough to encircle the blood vessel with some overlap. The ends of the tubing are then clamped together at a location to produce the appropriate amount of constriction. Enough overlap of the ends of the tubing to suture around it twice is needed to provide security against slippage. With this technique, only curved pieces of silicone tubing are in contact with the blood vessel, and neither the cut ends of the tubing or the knots in the suture material are in contact with the vessel walls.

A band that can be ruptured with balloon angioplasty techniques to reverse the stenosis can be developed by use of absorbable suture material within the silicone tubing. Inside a silicone constriction band, 3/0 polydiaxonone will lose its tensile strength within 2 months. The period of time it takes a band to lose enough tensile strength to be ruptured with balloon expansion can be varied with the type and size of absorbable suture material used. For instance, 3/0 polyglactin will lose its tensile strength in approximately one half the time as polydiaxonone. If these bands are not ruptured mechanically, they will eventually rupture from the pressure of the blood vessel. These same principles can be used to develop a model of coarctation of the aorta or peripheral vascular constriction in addition to the pulmonic and aortic stenosis models described here.

Closure of the incision is routine for thoracotomies as described previously. In addition to the usual analgesic and antimicrobial administration postoperatively, treatment for congestive heart failure may have to be administered. Generally, in neonates, bands that do not immediately cause constriction (loose banding) will require 2–3 months before significant constriction occurs. Banding in adults with a pressure gradient usually produces significant cardiac hypertrophy in the same period of time. Respiratory distress is usually the first clinical symptom detected. Monitoring with echocardiography should detect changes before the development of clinical symptoms. Furosemide should be the initial agent used in cases of congestive heart failure.

MYOCARDIAL INFARCTION AND ASSOCIATED ARRHYTHMIAS

Swine have been extensively used as animal models of myocardial infarction for the reasons discussed in the preceding text. These models have included acute and gradual onset occlusion of all the various coronary arteries and the study of arrhythmias associated with infarction (Bloor et al., 1986, 1992; Gardner and Johnson, 1988; Lee, 1986; Pak et al., 2003; Roberts et al., 1987; Stanley, 2000; Terp et al., 1999; Verdouw and Hartog, 1986; Verdouw et al., 1998; Watanabe et al., 1998; White et al., 1986).

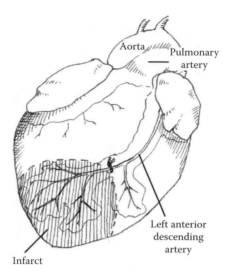

Aorta

Pulmonary artery

Left anterior descending artery

Infarct

FIGURE 9.59 Schematic of the occlusion of the left anterior descending coronary artery.

The surgical approach depends upon the vessel being instrumented. The left anterior descending (LAD or anterior interventricular) artery is best approached through a median sternotomy. The left circumflex (LCX) is best seen using a left lateral thoracotomy in the fourth intercostal space after lifting the left auricle. The proximal region of the LAD can also be seen through this approach. The right coronary artery (RCA) and its posterior interventricular branch are best seen from a right thoracotomy in the fourth intercostal space. The proximal portion of the RCA is also observed using a median sternotomy. All coronary vessels can be observed using a median sternotomy, if the heart is gently lifted from the pericardial cradle. However, prolonged lifting of the heart to see its dorsal aspect leads to compromise of the systemic circulation secondary to compression of the major blood vessels.

Occlusive techniques may either be intravascular or extravascular. Extravascular techniques include the use of snares, clips, and suture ligations for acute occlusion (Figure 9.59–Figure 9.61). Gradual occlusion with chronic models can be performed by encircling the vessel with an ameroid constrictor or inflatable cuffs. Intravascular techniques would include occlusion with angioplasty balloon catheters, injection of embolic substances or coils (Pak et al., 2003), such as 20- to 80-µm microspheres (Borrego et al., 1996; Terp et al., 1999) or sponge-type materials (Reffelmann et al., 2004), to block the vessel, or gradual occlusion by creating an atherosclerotic plaque. Atherogenic occlusion can be created after initiating endothelial damage with an inflated angioplasty balloon in conjunction with feeding an atherosclerotic diet. Global ischemia is produced by administering cardioplegic agents during cardiopulmonary bypass. The midsternal approach may be used for coronary artery bypass procedures between the internal thoracic artery and the LAD or by means of grafts between the aorta and LAD. Additional information on the intravascular procedures may be found in Chapter 12.

Because of the paucity of collateral circulation, swine develop a high incidence of ventricular fibrillation following acute occlusion. This is especially true of the LAD, which has less collateral circulation than other vessels, such as the LCX. The incidence of arrhythmias can be decreased in several ways. Using the gradual occlusion methods in miniature swine allows the collateral circulation to develop, as it does in humans.

In acute infarctions, the incidence of fatal arrhythmias can be decreased by limiting the time of occlusion, limiting the region of occlusion, or administering antiarrhythmics (Bloor et al., 1986; Horneffer et al., 1986; Swindle, 1994; Verdouw and Hartog, 1986; White et al., 1986). Generally,

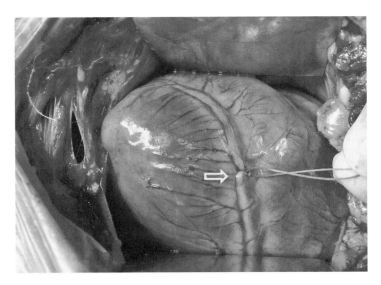

FIGURE 9.60 Ligation (arrow) of the left anterior descending (LAD) coronary artery using a midsternotomy approach.

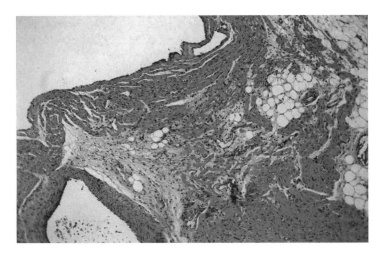

FIGURE 9.61 Histology of an infarct following 30 min of complete occlusion.

the incidence of arrhythmias increases substantially after 15 min and approaches 100% after 30 min. The survival rate for acute occlusion of the LAD can be increased by performing the occlusion distal to the main lateral branch at approximately two thirds of the length of the artery. Ligation of the posterior vessels of the RCA creates a high incidence of heart block and other damage to the conduction system in contrast to ligation of the LAD. Partial occlusion of blood flow also increases the survival rate. Use of antiarrhythmics, such as bretylium or amioidarone as a slow infusion, substantially decreases the risk of fatal arrhythmias. Pharmacological agents and anesthetic recommendations are discussed in Chapter 2. Miniature swine appear to be more resistant to the development of arrhythmias than farm animals. Arrhythmias in farm animals may vary in incidence among herds, possibly because of heritable factors. However, there is published data indicating that there is no difference in mortality rate between Yucatans and farm pigs in one laboratory (De Leon et al., 2003).

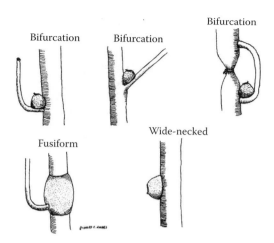

FIGURE 9.62 Examples of surgically created bifurcation, fusiform, and wide-necked aneurysms.

The predominant surgical problem associated with instrumenting the coronary vessels is the development of vasoconstriction. The incidence of vasospasm can be decreased by careful surgical technique and the infusion of lidocaine i.v. following a bolus injection. Care should be taken not to damage the atria during manipulation of vessels such as the LCX (Rogers et al., 1988; Swindle et al., 1986).

Following manipulation of the coronary artery, the thoracotomy incision is closed in a routine manner. Animals should be monitored postoperatively with electrocardiograms, as well as the usual procedures recommended for cardiac surgery. However, experience indicates that minimal handling and manipulation of the animals for the first three postsurgical days reduces the mortality that can occur in the first week up to 30%. Keeping the animals in a warm quiet location and using gentle handling and injection techniques are essential.

Vascular Aneurysms

Models of aortic aneurysm have been created in swine by making windows of various sizes in the aorta and suturing in graft materials such as bovine pericardium. These can be variable in their effectiveness in producing aneurysmal sacs. A variety of aneurysms have been created using the neck vessels as a model of intracranial aneurysms. True aneurysms, as they occur in humans, have not been reported in swine (Chaloupka et al., 1994; Dawson et al., 1995; Dion et al., 2003; Guglielmi et al., 1991; Marinov et al., 1997; Massoud et al., 1994, 1995; Maynar et al., 2003; Milner et al., 2004; Turjman et al., 1994; Uflacker and Brothers, 2006).

The classical work of Massoud et al. (1994, 1995) and Turjman et al. (1994) provides a detailed comparison of the various types of aneurysms (Figure 9.62) and their surgical creation in porcine models and will be summarized here. Using a combination of procedures on unilateral external jugular veins, carotid arteries, and ascending cervical arteries, three types of bifurcation aneurysms, two types of terminal aneurysms, wide-necked aneurysms, and fusiform aneurysms were created. The surgical approach is the same as that described for access to the cervical vessels. Blood vessels were treated with heparinized saline to prevent coagulation and papaverine to prevent vasospasm.

Bifurcation Aneurysms

One type was created by harvesting a 5-cm segment of ascending cervical artery and a segment of the external jugular vein. One end of the external jugular vein was ligated to form a venous pouch. End-to-side anastomosis of the arterial graft was performed on a segment of the carotid artery. At the caudad anastomosis of the ascending cervical artery, the venous pouch was included in the anastomosis at the V-shaped notch created between the vessels. The cephalad portion of the arterial graft was looped around the venous pouch and anastomosed to the carotid artery. Blood flow to the carotid artery was restricted between the two arterial anastomoses with an incomplete ligature to increase blood flow through the bypass loop.

A variation of the technique involved ligation of the ascending cervical artery at the caudal end and anastomosis as described previously. This created a bifurcation aneurysm with flow continued in both the carotid and ascending cervical artery. A third type was created by suturing a venous pouch at the bifurcation of two cranial branches of the ascending cervical artery. This resulted in a smaller aneurysm in a smaller blood vessel.

Terminal Aneurysms

As stated, a segment of the external jugular vein is isolated to be used as an aneurysmal sac. An additional 5-cm segment is isolated to be sewn to the carotid artery as a bypass loop. The venous pouch is sewn in the caudad notch of the bypass loop. When distended with blood, the aneurysm compresses the carotid artery, obviating the need for an incomplete ligature.

Another type is formed by the production of a carotid-bijugular fistula with an aneurysmal sac at the T junction. For this procedure, the external jugular vein is harvested for the aneurysm as before. The carotid artery on the same side has a 5-cm segment harvested, and two opposing elliptical arteriotomy sites are incised halfway along the segment. The carotid graft is sutured in an end-to-side manner to the carotid artery stump, and the aneurysmal pouch of the external jugular vein is sutured to the opposite arteriotomy. The ends of the carotid artery graft are then sutured end-to-side to the external jugular vein and the internal jugular vein. This will result in a rapid flow aneurysm with an arteriovenous fistula.

Fusiform Aneurysms

Fusiform aneurysms are produced by end-to-end anastomosis of the isolated external jugular vein segment to the carotid artery. A side branch may be added by anastomosing a segment of the anterior cervical artery in an end-to-side fashion with the external jugular vein segment on one end and ligating the other. The external jugular vein graft will dilate circumferentially, and the side branch will fill with blood as well if it is added.

Wide-Necked Aneurysms

For this model, the external jugular vein segment is anastomosed in an end-to-side fashion to the common carotid artery and the opposite end ligated. The model has had variations performed by suturing the venous pouch obliquely 45° through the carotid artery to give a more acute angle and improve flow to prevent spontaneous thrombosis and minimize the Venturi effect (Dawson et al., 1995; Guglielmi et al., 1991).

Similar types of aneurysms can be produced in the aorta using bovine pericardium, various biomaterials, or venous grafts sutured over oval windows in the distal aorta (Figure 9.63 and Figure 9.64). Infrarenal patches with peritoneum measuring 6–12 cm in length and 2–3 cm in width have been shown to grow and potentially rupture. Generally, shorter patches rupture less than longer patches and most ruptures occur within 3 weeks (Maynar et al., 2003; Uflacker and Brothers, 2006). All the various aneurysms are prone to spontaneous thrombosis but may be used for acute and chronic evaluation of various endovascular devices to occlude them. Use of antiplatelet therapy is useful in maintaining patency as discussed in Chapter 2.

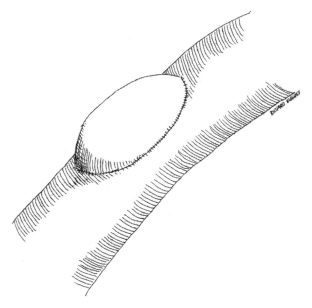

FIGURE 9.63 Schematic of an aortic aneurysm.

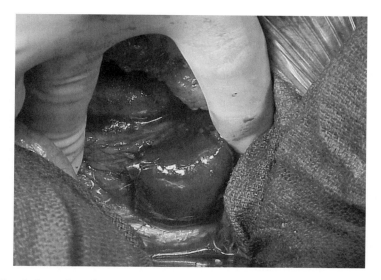

FIGURE 9.64 Surgical creation of an aortic aneurysm. (Courtesy of Renan Uflacker, Department of Radiology, Medical University of South Carolina.)

COARCTATION OF THE AORTA

Coarctation of the aorta may be created by surgically decreasing the size of the lumen of the aortic arch or descending aorta (Fossum et al., 2003; Lock et al., 1982; Morrow et al., 1994). Following a left thoracotomy in the fourth intercostal space, vascular clamps are applied to partially occlude the lumen proximally and distally to the ligamentum arteriosus. An elliptical excision of a portion of the aorta equal in length to one half of the circumference of the aorta is performed. Continuous cardiovascular sutures are placed to close the edges of the ellipse (Figure 9.65). After the clamps are removed, a defect that reduces the diameter of the aorta approximately 50% should be formed.

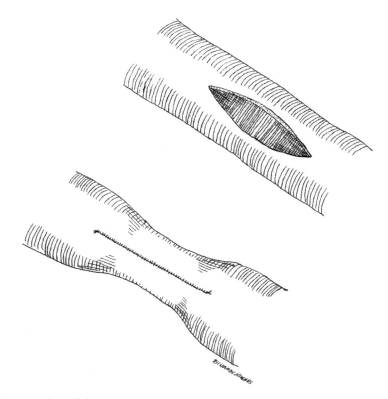

FIGURE 9.65 Coarctation of the aorta.

Large-sized absorbable sutures, such as 1 surgical gut or polydiaxonone ligatures, are placed around the narrowing of the wedge. The sutures are tied loosely, so that additional constriction of blood flow does not occur. The model may be used for angioplasty or stent placement.

A technique of implanting an inflatable occluder over a polytetrafluethylene soft tissue patch on the aorta has been developed to provide a model which can be gradually occluded in an awake animal. It offers the advantage of being reversible if clinical signs of heart failure occur. It was used to produce renal hypertension but has applications in other studies requiring coarctation (Fossum et al., 2003).

CARDIOMYOPLASTY

Cardiomyoplasty procedures are utilized as interim cardiac assist procedures for heart failure. The procedure involves isolating and wrapping the latissimus dorsi muscle around the heart and stimulating it to contract like cardiac muscle (Figure 9.66) (Borrego et al., 1996; Hansen et al., 1998; Kratz et al., 1994).

In swine, the latissimus dorsi muscle is large and thick and receives its primary blood and nerve supply from the thoracodorsal artery and nerve that enter the muscle close to its insertion at the second rib. The origin of the muscle is broad and extends caudally to the last ribs. Because of the size of the muscle and the thoracic wall in swine, the procedure would be difficult to perform except in smaller animals. A long oblique incision over the fifth intercostal space is made, and the skin is either undermined or an additional transverse incision is made to expose the origin of the muscle, which is transected. The muscle body is isolated to the area of insertion at approximately the 10th–11th rib while preserving the neurovascular pedicle. After isolating the muscle, the third, fourth, and fifth ribs (or such of these as required) are resected to allow space for the muscle to

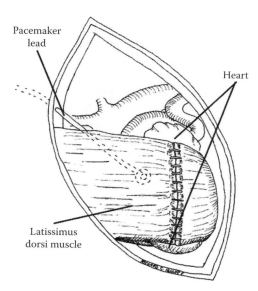

Pacemaker
lead

Heart

Latissimus
dorsi muscle

FIGURE 9.66 The cardiomyoplasty procedure.

be inserted into the thoracic cavity. The pericardium is incised in a U-shaped opening in such a manner as to allow the muscle to be wrapped around the heart. An epicardial sensor electrode is placed over the ventricle and muscular myostimulators are attached to the insertion of the muscle. The muscle is sutured with mattress sutures in such a way as to form a pocket around the ventricular region of the heart while preserving the blood and nerve supply to the muscle (Figure 9.66). It can also be anchored to the retracted pericardium to prevent slippage during the healing phase.

Either before or after performing the procedure the skeletal muscle must be trained to develop a predominance of type I muscle fibers, which are more resistant to fatigue. This is accomplished by resting the muscle for several weeks and then progressively stimulating it over several weeks to accomplish the task. Performing the procedure in a two-stage progression would involve isolating the muscle first and stimulating it before implanting it into the thorax.

This procedure impairs the mobility of swine and requires combination analgesic therapy with opioids and nonsteroidal anti-inflammatory drugs to control the pain. The thoracic incision is closed in the usual manner.

EPICARDIAL PACEMAKER AND DEVICE IMPLANTATION

Epicardial pacemaker implantation may be performed to test pacemaker devices and leads (Brownlee et al., 1997; Gillette et al., 1991; Hughes and Bowman, 1986; Schumann et al., 1994; Smith et al., 1997; Tong et al., 1995, 1996) or used to create a model of dilated cardiomyopathy and congestive heart failure from rapid epicardial pacing (240 beats per minute) (Caparas et al., 2000; Eble and Spinale, 1995; Hendrick et al., 1990; LeGrice et al., 1995; Spinale, 1995; Spinale et al., 1990; Yarbrough and Spinale, 2003). The model of dilated cardiomyopathy results in congestive heart failure developing over several weeks and requires intensive postoperative care with diuretics for medical management. Endocardial pacemaker lead implantation and electrophysiology are discussed in Chapter 12. Other devices that may be required for implantation on the epicardium include sonomicrometry crystals for measurement of cardiac dimensions and flow transducers on the coronary arteries.

The surgical approach to the heart may be either through a left lateral thoracotomy in the fourth to fifth intercostal space or via a substernal or median sternotomy. The approach is dictated by the desired placement of the electrode or device. The left lateral thoracotomy allows access to the left

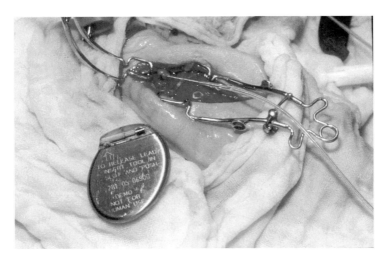

FIGURE 9.67 Pacemaker with epicardial lead for a fetal pig.

coronary artery and its branches, as well as both the left and right ventricles. The median sternotomy allows access to different regions of the same structures and improved access to the epicardium. A substernal approach through the ventral midline of the abdomen and the ventral attachment of the diaphragm and pericardium allows access to the apex of the heart only. The relatively noninvasive substernal approach allows more rapid recovery without many of the complications associated with a thoracotomy.

Two basic types of pacemaker electrodes with some variations are used. They are generally either screw-in leads or sutured leads (Figure 9.67). The manufacturer's recommendations should be followed. Regardless of which lead is used, the coronary artery and its branches should be avoided during implantation. Because of the characteristics of the coronary circulation discussed earlier, damage of these vessels could result in an infarct. Pacemaker leads are implanted subcutaneously using the same principles of surgery that apply to chronic catheterization. In general, this means that the lead is tunneled through the subcutaneous tissue from the thorax to the subcutaneous site where the pulse generator is to be implanted. Pacemaker pockets can be made in the subcutaneous tissues of the side of the chest or preferably the neck or flank if the lead is long enough. The subcutaneous pockets need to be dissected carefully to avoid having seepage of blood from small vessels, which will consistently lead to hematomas and seromas. The subcutaneous pocket needs to be large enough so that the device to be implanted is easily placed and does not cause tension leading to necrosis and dehiscence. This is especially a problem on the chest wall. The implantation of pacemakers with endocardial pacemaker leads in the jugular furrow of the neck is discussed in Chapter 12. The skin incision should never be directly over or ventral to the implanted device. Implanted devices tend to gravitate ventrally in animals, and the incision is best made either cranial or caudal to the device to be implanted. The pacemaker pocket needs to be closed with subcutaneous and subcuticular sutures, ensuring that the dead space is closed adequately. Skin sutures are placed as required.

Implantation of sonomicrometry crystals and flow transducers follows the principles of surgery discussed previously for ventriculotomy and coronary vessel procedures in myocardial infarction models. The model of epicardial pacing to produce congestive heart failure requires intensive postoperative observation and care especially for pulmonary edema. The use of furosemide as a diuretic is usually indicated. If high pacemaker rates (240 beats per minute [bpm]) are used, the pacing rate may have to be reduced or the pacemaker turned off in 14–21 d (Caparas et al., 2000; Hendrick et al., 1990; LeGrice et al., 1995; Spinale et al., 1990; Spinale, 1995).

Heart and Heart-Lung Transplantation

The pig has been utilized for all of the various forms of heart (Calne et al., 1976, 1978; Hall et al., 1986; Martin et al., 1999; Qayumi et al., 1991; Saito and Waters, 1994; Swindle et al., 1986; White and Lunney, 1979), heart-lung (Baumgartner et al., 1988; Hansen et al., 1987; Harjula and Baldwin, 1987; Qayumi et al., 1990, 1993; Saito and Waters, 1994), and lung (see preceding text) transplantation. However, swine are susceptible to apnea following total cardiopulmonary denervation and are usually reserved for acute and chronic heart and single-lung transplantation and acute heart-double lung transplantation. The growth of the pig makes it useful for the growing heart model as described previously (Brutel de la Riviere et al., 1983; Haworth and Hislop, 1981; Pae et al., 1981). A growing interest in the porcine model has developed because of the progress with xenotransplantation. It is likely that the pig will be the donor animal of choice for this procedure for multiple organs including the heart (Swindle, 1996).

The donor and recipient are operated on using a complete median sternotomy with a pericardial cradle for all these procedures. Bretylium or amiodarone are useful as a preventative for cardiac arrhythmias in both the donor and the recipient (see Chapter 2).

Heart Transplant

Donor

The donor is prepared by dissection of the cranial and caudal vena cava. The pericardium between the aorta and pulmonary artery is dissected completely. The donor is heparinized (300 IU/kg), and cardiectomy is initiated. The cranial vena cava is ligated and divided caudal to the azygous vein. The caudal vena cava is ligated, and the aorta is cross-clamped. The animal is exsanguinated, and the blood may be used for priming the bypass pump. Chilled cardioplegia solution (4°C) is infused into the aortic root, and the caudal vena cava is opened to allow drainage of the cardioplegia solution. The aorta and pulmonary arteries are transected distal to their first branches. The posterior wall of the left atrium is opened between the pulmonary veins and immersed in chilled preservation solution awaiting implantation.

Recipient

The recipient is prepared in a similar manner except that the animal is placed on cardiopulmonary bypass. Venous bypass cannulae are passed through the right atrial appendage and snared in the cranial and caudal vena cavae. The arterial line is placed in the aorta or femoral artery. Bypass parameters may vary among experiments; however, cooling to 28–30°C and flow rates of 50–80 ml/kg have been recommended.

The recipient cardiectomy is performed following cross-clamping of the aorta with an incision that follows the atrioventricular groove. The incision should preserve the coronary sinus. The pulmonary artery and aorta are transected at the level of the commissures of the valves.

Implantation of the donor heart is performed with a series of continuous sutures with 5/0–6/0 nonabsorbable cardiovascular suture. The atria are anastomosed first. Starting the anastomosis with either the left or right atrium have been described (Baumgartner et al., 1988; Saito and Waters, 1994). The heart must be rotated caudoventrally if the right atrium is anastomosed first, in order to accomplish anastomosis of the left atrium. The pulmonary artery and aorta are anastomosed next. Air is removed from the aorta before removing the cross-clamp.

The cardiac rhythm is restored with internal defibrillation if it does not return spontaneously during rewarming and weaning from bypass. Isoproterenol infusion to effect is used postoperatively to provide a regular heart rate and blood pressure as the catecholamine-induced heart rate recovers. Protamine may be used judiciously at a slow infusion rate of 1 mg/100 U heparin if clotting is a problem. A double chest tube with a Y connection should be used postoperatively.

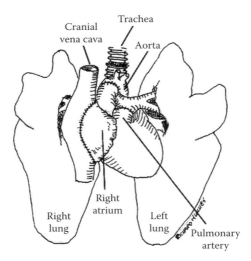

FIGURE 9.68 Heart and lung transplantation.

HEART-LUNG TRANSPLANT

The donor and recipient are prepared in a similar manner as for heart transplantation, except that the trachea is divided cranial to the bifurcation and the recipient is left with the right atrium with a portion of the interatrial septum. The phrenic nerves are preserved on pediciles during the dissection. The pulmonary artery and veins remain intact with the transplantation block. With this technique, the anastomosis of the right atrium, trachea, and aorta are required for implantation into the recipient. The right lung is passed dorsally to the vena cava and phrenic nerve (Figure 9.68). The donor vena cava is ligated.

Single-lung transplant (described earlier) provides an experimental model for evaluation of pulmonary transplant that is better than isolated double-lung transplant because of the physiological problems associated with respirator apnea postoperatively in the pig. Consequently, double-lung transplant is not described.

MISCELLANEOUS THORACIC PROCEDURES

THORACIC DUCT CANNULATION

Cannulation of the thoracic duct is performed to collect chyle for experimental studies (Figure 9.69 and Figures 6.12 through 6.16). The most frequent complication associated with collection of chyle is failure of the cannulation due to clotting shortly after the procedure. The reentry cannulation method described here may provide a longer collection period (Mendenhall et al., 1996). Lymphatic ultra-sonography has been performed to study the lymphatic system in the Sinclair malignant melanoma model and compared to the use of vital blue dyes and radiopharmaceuticals (Goldberg et al., 2004).

The thoracic duct courses dorsal to the aorta and ventral to the hemiazygous vein from the base of the heart caudally to the cisterna-chyli, which it drains. The duct is dorsolateral to the aorta in the left side of the thorax until approximately the fifth rib, then it is more accessible from the right thorax. Cannulation is usually performed in the right seventh to eighth intercostal space. Variations in ductal anatomy may occur, such as branching ducts, which make the procedure more difficult.

Cannulation of the duct is performed in the same manner as cannulation of blood vessels described earlier. However, the duct is easily damaged and difficult to locate in fat animals and animals that have been fasted for a prolonged period of time. Feeding of liquids containing a high proportion of fatty substances before anesthesia may help identify the duct.

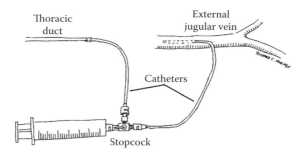

FIGURE 9.69 Cannulation of the thoracic duct with reentry into the external jugular vein.

The catheter needs to be small bore and composed of silicone or polyethylene. Coating with silicone or the use of heparin-impregnated catheters may be helpful to prevent catheter failure due to clotting. After cannulation, the catheter is passed through an intercostal space cranial to the cannulation site. It is tunneled subcutaneously in a cranial direction along the dorsum of the rib line. It is exteriorized several intercostal spaces cranial to the exit from the thorax. Chyle may be collected in this location, or the cannula can be placed into a reentry circuit to drain into the right external jugular vein. If it is drained back into the jugular vein, then a three-way valve is placed into the system at the exit site. The cannula is then passed subcutaneously to an incision into the right jugular furrow for cannulation into the jugular vein as described previously for vascular cannulation. The incisions are closed in a routine manner. The cannula tract is kept open until collection of chyle is desired, and then the three-way valve is closed on the cranial side. Meticulous aseptic handling of the exteriorized catheter is indicated. In a closed system, the catheter should be heparinized if continuous flow into a collection site is not provided.

Postoperative care is routine.

Esophageal Surgery

Esophageal surgery is usually performed in the thorax or the neck. The techniques are described in this section, because, experimentally, it is likely that the thoracic approach will be the one most likely used (see Chapter 4).

The esophagus courses from the pharynx dorsal to the larynx. It begins to course to the left dorsolateral aspect of the trachea at approximately the fourth cervical vertebra. In the thorax, it passes dorsal to the tracheal bifurcation and to the right of the aortic arch. It enters the esophageal hiatus of the diaphragm and joins the stomach shortly after entering the abdominal cavity.

The esophagus can be surgically approached in the neck through a ventral midline incision with lateral retraction of the trachea. In the cranial thorax, it is best approached using a median sternotomy. It may also be approached using a lateral thoracotomy in the cranial thorax; however, access and dissection are more difficult. In the caudal abdomen, it is approached through either a right or left lateral thoracotomy from the fourth to the ninth intercostal spaces. The esophageal sphincter can be approached using a midline celiotomy incision with caudal retraction of the stomach and cranial retraction of the liver. At any location, care should be taken to avoid injury to the recurrent laryngeal nerves and vagal trunks, which are located in the proximity of the esophagus. Striated and smooth muscle are included in the tunica muscularis of swine.

The esophagus may be fistulated in the neck, have a pharyngostomy tube placed into the cervical region, have an esophagotomy, or be anastomosed with or without a graft. The main problem associated with surgery of the esophagus is the retarded healing process because of the constant tension and peristalsis of the structure and the lack of a strong serosal layer to maintain sutures. The esophagus is usually closed in two layers. The inner layer is placed in the tunical mucosa and submucosa with continuous sutures using synthetic absorbable sutures. The outer muscular layers and adventitial layers are closed with simple interrupted or horizontal mattress sutures. For some chronic procedures, such as graft implantation, synthetic nonabsorbable sutures should be utilized. The surgical incisions are closed in the routine manner described for the region.

REFERENCES

Ackermann, M.R., 2001, Respiratory tract, in *Biology of the Domestic Pig,* Pond, W.G. and Mersmann, H.J., Eds., Ithaca, NY: Cornell University Press, pp. 502–532.

Alric, P., Ryckwaert, F., Branchereau, P., Marty-Ane, C., Mary, H., and Colson, P., 2003, A porcine model of systemic and renal haemodynamic responses to infrarenal aortic cross-clamping, *Eur. J. Vasc. Endovasc. Surg.*, 25(1): 72–78.

Bailie, M.B., Wixson, S.K., and Landi, M.S., 1986, Vascular access port implantation for serial blood sampling in conscious swine, *Lab. Anim. Sci.*, 36(4): 431–433.

Baumgartner, W.A., Kirkman, R.J., Pennington, L.R., Pritchard, T.J., Sarr, M.G., and Williams, G.M., 1988, Organ transplantation, in Swindle, M.M. and Adams, R.J., Eds., *Experimental Surgery and Physiology: Induced Animal Models of Human Disease*, Baltimore, MD: Williams and Wilkins, pp. 284–299.

Betjes, M.G.H. and van Agteren, M., 2004, Prevention of dialysis catheter-related sepsis with a citrate–taurolidine-containing lock solution, *Nephrol. Dial. Transplant.*, 19(6): 1546–1551.

Bloor, C.M., White, F.C., and Lammers, R.J., 1986, Cardiac ischemia and coronary blood flow in swine, in Stanton, H.C. and Mersmann, H.J., Eds., *Swine in Cardiovascular Research*, Vol. 2, Boca Raton, FL: CRC Press, pp. 87–119.

Bloor, C.M., White, F.C., and Roth, D.M., 1992, The pig as a model of myocardial ischemia and gradual coronary occlusion, in Swindle, M.M., Ed., *Swine as Models in Biomedical Research*, Ames, IA: Iowa State University Press, pp. 163–175.

Bobbie, D.L. and Swindle, M.M., 1986, Pulse monitoring, intramuscular, and intravascular injection sites in swine, in Tumbleson, M.E., Ed., *Swine in Biomedical Research*, New York: Plenum Press, pp. 273–277.

Borrego, J.M., Ordonez, A., Hernandez, A., and Perez, J., 1996, Neovascularization of the ischemic myocardium by cardiomyoplasty, in Tumbleson, M.E. and Schook, L.B., Eds., *Advances in Swine in Biomedical Research*, Vol. 2, New York: Plenum Press, pp. 653–661.

Brownlee, R.R., Swindle, M.M., Bertolet, R., and Neff, P., 1997, Toward optimizing a preshaped catheter and system parameters to achieve single lead DDD pacing, *PACE*, 20(SPT 1): 1354–1358.

Brutel de la Riviere, A., Quaegebeur, J.M., Hennis, P.J., Brutel de la Riviere, G., and Van Herpen, G., 1983, Growth of an aorta-coronary anastomosis: an experimental study in pigs, *J. Thorac. Cardiovasc. Surg.*, 86(3): 393–399.

Calne, R.Y., English, T.A., Dunn, D.C., McMaster, P., Wilkins, D.C., and Herbertson, B.M., 1976, Orthotopic heart transplantation in the pig: the pattern of rejection, *Transplant. Proc.*, 8(1): 27–30.

Calne, R.Y., Rolles, K., White, D.J., Smith, D.P., and Herbetson, B.M., 1978, Prolonged survival of pig orthotopic heart grafts treated with cyclosporin A, *Lancet*, 1(8075): 1183–1185.

Caparas, S.N, Clair, M.J., Krombach, R.S., Hendrick, J.W., Houck, W.V., Kribbs, S.B., Mukherjee, R., Tempel, G.E., and Spinale, F.G., 2000, Brain blood flow patterns after the development of congestive heart failure: effects of treadmill exercise, *Crit. Care Med.*, 28(1): 209–214.

Carew, T.E., Saik, R.P., Johansen, K.H., Dennis, C.A., and Steinberg, D., 1976, Low density and high density lipoprotein turnover following portocaval shunt in swine, *J. Lipid Res.*, 17(5): 441–450.

Carroll, S.M., Nimmo, L.E., Knoepfler, P.S., White, F.C., and Bloor, C.M., 1995, Gene expression in a swine model of right ventricular hypertrophy, *J. Mol. Cell. Cardiol.*, 27(7): 1427–1441.

Chaloupka, J.C., Vinuela, F., Robert, J., and Duckwiller, J., 1994, An *in vivo* arteriovenous malformation model in swine: preliminary feasibility and natural history study, *Am. J. Neuroradiol.*, 15(5): 945–950.

Chitwood, W.R., Jr., Wiley, N.L., Chapman, W.H.H., Felger, J.E., Bailey, B.M., Ballint, T., Mendleson, K.G., Kim, V.B., Young, J.A., and Albrecht, R.A., 2001, Robotic surgical training in an academic institution, *Ann. Surg.*, 234(4): 475–486.

Corin, W.J., Swindle, M.M., Spann, J.F., Jr., Frankis, M., Biederman, W.W.R., Smith, A., Taylor, A., and Carabello, B.A., 1988, The mechanism of decreased stroke volume in children and swine with ventricular septal defect and failure to thrive, *J. Clin. Invest.*, 82(2): 544–551.

Corno, A.F., Sekarski, N., Gernath, M.A., Payot, M., Tozzi, P., and von Segesser, L.K., 2003, Pulmonary artery banding: long-term telemetric adjustment, *Eur. J. Cardio. Thorac. Surg.*, 23(3): 317–322.

Dawson, R.C., Krisht, A.F., Barrow, D.L., Joseph, G.J., Shengelaia, G.G., and Bonner, B., 1995, Treatment of experimental aneurysms using collagen-coated microcoils, *Neurosurgery*, 36(1): 133–140.

De Leon, H., Duktig, K., Mulkey, S.P., Li, J., Shaw, L., Swenson, R.B., Chronos, N.A.F., and Robinson, K.A., 2003, Mortality rates of interventional and surgical procedures performed in domestic juvenile farm pigs and Yucatan mini-pigs, *Contemp. Top. Lab. Anim. Sci.*, 42(3): 29–33.

Dion, Y.M., deWailly, G.W., Thaveau, F., and Gourdon, J., 2003, Totally laparoscopic juxtarenal aortic anastomosis, *Surg. Laparosc. Endosc. Percutaneous Tech.*, 13(2): 111–114.

Doty, J.R., Walinsky, P.L., Salazar, J.D., Brawn, J., Haggerty, M., Redmond, J.M., Baumgartner, W.A., and Gott, V.L., 2002, Left atrial-inferior vena cava bypass achieves retroperfusion of the porcine spinal cord: morphologic and preliminary physiologic studies, *J. Surg. Res.*, 108(1): 157–164.

Dougherty, R.W., 1981, *Experimental Surgery in Farm Animals*, Ames, IA: Iowa State University Press.

Drougas, J.G., Barnard, S.E., Wright, J.K., Sika, M., Lopez, R.R., Stokes, K.A., Williams, P.E., and Pinson, C.W., 1996, A model for the extended studies of hepatic hemodynamics and metabolism in swine, *Lab. Anim. Sci.*, 46(6): 648–655.

Dupont, J., Lumb, W.V., Nelson, A.W., Seegmiller, J.P., Hotchkiss, D., and Chase, H.P., 1985, Portocaval shunt as a treatment for hypercholesterolemia: metabolic and morphological effects in a swine model, *Atherosclerosis*, 58(1–3): 205–222.

Eble, D.M. and Spinale, F.G., 1995, Contractile and cytoskeletal content, structure, and mRNA levels with tachycardia-induced cardiomyopathy, *Am. J. Physiol.*, 268(6 Pt. 2): H2426–39.

Ehler, W.J., Cissik, J.H., Smith, V.C., and Hubbard, G.B., 1990, Evaluation of Gore-Tex graft material in the repair of right ventricular outflow tract defect, *J. Invest. Surg.*, 3(2): 119–127.

Fadel, E., Michel, R.P., Eddahibi, S., Bernatchez, R., Mazmanian, G.M., Baudet, B., Dartevelle, P., and Herve, P., 2004, Regression of postobstructive vasculopathy after revascularization of chronically obstructed pulmonary artery, *J. Thorac. Cardiovasc. Surg.*, 127(4): 1009–1017.

Fossum, T.W., Baltzer, W.I., Miller, M.W., Aguirre, M., Whitlock, D., Solter, P., Makarski, L.A., McDonald, M.M., An, M.Y., and Humphrey, J.D., 2003, A novel coarctation model for studying hypertension in the pig, *J. Invest. Surg.*, 16(1): 35–44.

Gadacz, T.R., 1988, Portal hypertension, in Swindle, M.M. and Adams, R.J., Eds., *Experimental Surgery and Physiology: Induced Animal Models of Human Disease*, Baltimore, MD: Williams and Wilkins, pp. 250–253.

Gal, D. and Isner, J.M., 1992, Atherosclerotic Yucatan microswine as a model for novel cardiovascular interventions and imaging, in Swindle, M.M., Ed., *Swine as Models in Biomedical Research*, Ames, IA: Iowa State University Press, pp. 118–140.

Gallegos, R.P., Nockel, P.J., Rivard, A.L., and Bianco, R.W., 2005, The current state of *in-vivo* pre-clinical animal models for heart valve evaluation, *J. Heart Valve Dis.*, 14(3): 423–32.

Gardner, T.J. and Johnson D.L., 1988, Cardiovascular system, in Swindle, M.M. and Adams, R.J., Eds., *Experimental Surgery and Physiology: Induced Animal Models of Human Disease*, Baltimore, MD: Williams and Wilkins, pp. 74–124.

Gaymes, C.H., Swindle, M.M., Gillette, P.C., Harold, M.E., and Schumann, R.E., 1995, Percutaneous serial catheterization in swine: a practical approach, *J. Invest. Surg.*, 8(2): 123–128.

Gillette, P.C., Swindle, M.M., Thompson, R.P., and Case, C.L., 1991, Transvenous cryoablation of the bundle of His, *PACE*, 14(4 Pt. 1): 504–510.

Goldberg, B.B., Merton, D.A., Liu, J.B., Thakur, M., Murphy, G.F., Needleman, L., Tornes, A., and Forsberg, F., 2004, Sentinel lymph nodes in a swine model with melanoma: contrast enhanced lymphatic ultrasound, *Radiology*, 230(3): 727–734.

Gootman, P.M., 2001, Cardiovascular system, in Pond, W.G. and Mersmann, H.J., Eds., *Biology of the Domestic Pig*, Ithaca, NY: Cornell University Press, pp. 533–559.

Greenberg, S., McGowan, C., and Glenn, T.M., 1981, Pulmonary vascular smooth muscle function in porcine splanchnic arterial occlusion shock, *Am. J. Physiol.*, 241(1): H33–34.

Grehan, J.F., Hilbert, S.I., Ferrans, V.J., Droel, J.S., Salerno, C.T., and Bianco, R.W., 2000, Development and evaluation of a swine model to assess the preclinical safety of mechanical heart valves, *J. Heart Valve Dis.*, 9(5): 710–719.

Gross, D.R., Dewanjee, M.K., Zhai, P., Lanzo, S., and Wu, S.M., 1997, Successful prosthetic mitral valve implantation in pigs, *ASAIO J.*, 435(5): M382–386.

Guglielmi, G., Vinuela, F., Dion, J., and Duckwiler, G., 1991, Electrothrombosis of saccular aneurysms via endovascular approach, Part 2: Preliminary clinical experience, *J. Neourosurg.*, 75(1): 8–14.

Hall, T.S., Borkon, M., Baumgartner, W.A., Scott Stuart, R., Swindle, M.M., Galloway, E., and Reitz, B.A., 1986, Use of swine in heart transplantation research, in Tumbleson, M.E., Ed., *Swine in Biomedical Research*, Vol. 1, New York: Plenum Press, pp. 373–376.

Hand, M.S., Phillips, R.W., Miller, C.W., Mason, R.A., and Lumb, W.V., 1981, A method for quantitation of hepatic, pancreatic and intestinal function in conscious Yucatan miniature swine, *Lab. Anim. Sci.*, 31(6): 728–731.

Hansen, S.B., Nielsen, S.L., Christensen, T.D., Gravergaard, A.E., Baandrup, U., Bille, S., and Harjula, A., and Baldwin, J.C., 1987, Lung transplantation in the pig with successful preservation using prostaglandin E-1, *Appl. Cardiol.*, 2: 397.

Hansen, S.B., Nielsen, S.L., Christensen, T.D., Gravergaard, A.E., Baandrup, U., Bille, S., and Hasenkam, J.M., 1998, Latissimus dorsi cardiomyoplasty: a chronic experimental porcine model, feasibility study of cardiomyoplasty in Danish landrace pigs and Göttingen minipigs, *Lab. Anim. Sci.*, 48(5): 483–489.

Harjula, A. and Baldwin, J.C., 1987, Lung transplantation in the pig with successful preservation using prostaglandin E-1, *J. Appl. Cardiol.*, 2(5): 397–402.

Harvey, R.C. and Jones, E.F., 1982, A technique for bioinstrumentation of the thorax of miniature swine, *Lab. Anim. Sci.*, 32(1): 94–96.

Hasenkam, J.M., Østergaard, J.H., and Pedersen, E.M., 1988, A model for acute haemodynamic studies in the ascending aorta in pigs, *Cardiovasc. Res.*, 227: 464–471.

Haworth, S.G. and Hislop, A.A., 1981, Adaptation of the pulmonary circulation to extrauterine life in the pig and its relevance to the human infant, *Cardiovasc. Res.*, 15(2): 108–119.

Hazenkamp, M.G, Goffin, Y.A., and Huysmans, H.A., 1993, The value of the stentless biovalve prosthesis: an experimental study, *Eur. J. Cardiothorac. Surg.*, 710: 514–519.

Hendrick, D.A., Smith, A.C., Kratz, J.M., Crawford, F.A., and Spinale, F.G., 1990, The pig as a model of tachycardia and dilated cardiomyopathy, *Lab. Anim. Sci.*, 40(5): 495–501.

Hillinger, S., Hoerstrup, S.P., Zollinger, A., Weder, W., Schmid, R.A., and Stamberger, U., 2000, A new model for the assessment of lung allograft ischemia/reperfusion injury, *J. Invest. Surg.*, 13(1): 59–65.

Hoefer, I.E., van Royen, N., and Jost, M.M., 2006, Experimental models of arteriogenesis: differences and implications, *Lab Anim.*, 35(2): 36–44.

Horneffer, P.J., Gott, V.J., and Gardner, T.J., 1986, Swine as a cardiac surgical model, in Tumbleson, M.E., Ed., *Swine in Biomedical Research*, Vol. 1, New York: Plenum Press, pp. 321–326.

Hughes, H.C., 1986, Swine in cardiovascular research, *Lab. Anim. Sci.*, 36(4): 348–350.

Hughes, H.C. and Bowman, T.A., 1986, Intracardiac electrophysiology of swine for design and testing of cardiac pacemakers, in Tumbleson, M.E., Ed., *Swine in Biomedical Research*, Vol. 1, New York: Plenum Press, pp. 327–331.

Jangra, D., Powell, T., Kalloger, S.E., Guerra, H.L., Clifton, J., Coxson, H.O., Finley, R.J., and Mayo, J.R., 2005, CT-directed microcoil localization of small peripheral lung nodules: a feasibility study in pigs, *J. Invest. Surg.*, 18(5): 265–272.

Jensen, D.M., Machicado, G.A., Tapia, J.I., Kauffman, G., Franco, P., and Beilin, D., 1983, A reproducible canine model of esophageal varices, *Gastroenterology*, 84(3): 573–579.

Johnson, M.S., McLennan, G., Lalka, S.G., Whitfield, R.M., and Dreesen, R.G., 2001, The porcine hemodialysis access model, *J. Vasc. Interv. Radiol.*, 12(8): 969–977.

Jurewitsch, B. and Jeejeebhoy, K.N., 2005, Taurolidine lock: the key to recurrent catheter-related bloodstream infections, *Clin. Nutr.*, 24(3): 462–465.

Kahn, D., Hickman, R., Pienaar, H., and Terblanche, J., 1994, Liver transplantation in the pig, in Cramer, D.V., Podesta, L., and Makowka, L., Eds., *Handbook of Animal Models in Transplantation Research*, Boca Raton, FL: CRC Press, pp. 75–86.

Kaiser, G.M., Fruhauf, N.R., and Broelsch, C.E., 2005, New surgical technique for portal venous port system in swine, *Eur. Surg. Res.*, 37(5): 298–301.

Kaplan, D.K., Atsumi, N., D'Ambra, M.N., and Vlahakes, G.J., 1995, Distal circulatory support for thoracic aortic operations' effects on intracranial pressure, *Ann. Thorac. Surg.*, 59(2): 448–452.

Keech, G.B., Koide, M., Carabello, B., Smith, A.C., Defreyte, G., and Swindle, M., 1997, An adult canine model of progressive left ventricular pressure overload, *J. Invest. Surg.*, 10(5): 295–304.

Kelly, B.S., Heffelfinger, S.C., Whiting, J.F., Miller, M.A., Reaves, A., Armstrong, J., Narayana, A., and Roy-Chaudhury, P., 2002, Aggressive venous neointimal hyperplasia in a pig model of arteriovenous graft, *Kidney Int.*, 62(7): 2272–2280.

Koldehoff, M. and Zakrzewski, J.L., 2004, Taurolidine is effective in the treatment of central venous catheter related bloodstream infections in cancer patients, *Int. J. Antimicrob. Agents*, 24(5): 491–495.

Kratz, J.M., Johnson, W.S., Mukherjee, R., Hu, J., Crawford, F.A., and Spinale, F.G., 1994, The relation between latissimus dorsi skeletal muscle structure and contractile function after cardiomyoplasty, *J. Thorac. Cardiovasc. Surg.*, 107 (3): 868–878.

Lee, K.T., 1986, Swine as animal models in cardiovascular research, in Tumbleson, M.E., Ed., *Swine in Biomedical Research*, Vol. 3, New York: Plenum Press, pp. 1481–1496.

LeGrice, I.J., Takayama, Y., Holmes, J.W., and Covell, J.W., 1995, Impaired subendocardial function in tachycardia-induced cardiac failure, *Am. J. Physiol.*, 268(5 Pt. 2): H1788–1794.

Lin, J.H., Huang, S.Y., Lee, W.C., Liu, S.K., and Chu, R.M., 2002, Echocardiographic features of pigs with spontaneous hypertrophic cardiomyopathy, *Comp. Med.*, 52(3): 238–242.

Litzke, L.F. and Berg, R., 1977, Quantitative-morphological studies of the heart of mini-lewe miniature swine. 2: Atrioventricular and semilunar valves, *Arch. Exp.Veterinarmed.*, 31(4): 547–556.

Lock, J.E., Niemi, T., Burke, B.A., Einzig, S., and Castaneda-Zuniga, W., 1982, Transcutaneous angioplasty of experimental aortic coarctation, *Circulation*, 6(6): 1280–1286.

Lomholt, M., Nielsen, S.L., Hansen, S.B., Andersen, N.T., and Hasenkam, J.M., 2002, Differential tension between secondary and primary mitral chordae in an acute *in vivo* porcine model, *J. Heart Valve Dis.*, 113: 337–345.

Lutter, G., Kuklinski, D., Berg, B., von Samson, P., Martin, J., Handlke, M., Uhrmeister, P., and Beyersdorf, F., 2002, Percutaneous aortic valve replacement: an experimental study. I. Studies on implantation, *J. Thorac. Cardiovasc. Surg.*, 123(4): 768–776.

Marinov, G.R., Marois, Y., Paris, E., Roby, P., Formichi, M., Douville, Y., and Guidoin, R., 1997, Can the infusion of elastase in the abdominal aorta of the Yucatan miniature swine consistently produce experimental aneurysms?, *J. Invest. Surg.*, 10(2): 129–150.

Martin, J., Sarai, K., Yoshitake, M., Takahashi, N., Haberstroh, J., Lutter, G., Geiger, A., and Beyersdorf, F., 1999, Orthotopic transplantation of pig hearts harvested from non-heart-beating donors, *Transpl. Proc.*, 31(1): 153–154.

Massoud, T.F., Ji, C., Guglielmi, G., Vinuela, F., and Robert, J., 1994, Experimental models of bifurcation and terminal aneurysms: construction techniques in swine, *Am. J. Neuroradiol.*, 15(5): 938–944.

Massoud, T.F., Turjman, F., Ji, C., Vinuela, F., Guglielmi, G., Gobin, Y.P., and Duckwiller, G.R., 1995, Endovascular treatment of fusiform aneurysms with stents and coils: technical feasibility in a swine model, *Am. J. Neuroradiol.*, 16(10): 1953–1963.

Maynar, M., Qian, Z., Hernandez, J., Sun, F., DeMiguel, C., Crisostomo, V., Uson, J., Pineda, L.F., Espinoza, C.G., and Castaneda, W.R., 2003, An animal model of abdominal aortic aneurysm created with peritoneal patch: technique and initial results, *Cardiovasc. Interv. Radiol.*, 26(2): 168–176.

McKenzie, J.E., 1996, Swine as a model in cardiovascular research, in Tumbleson, M.E. and Schook, L.B., Eds., *Advances in Swine in Biomedical Research*, Vol. 1, New York: Plenum Press, pp. 7–18.

Mehran, R.J., Ricci, M.A., Graham, A.M., Carter, K., and Smyes, J.F., 1991, Porcine model for vascular graft studies, *J. Invest. Surg.*, 4(1): 37–44.

Mendenhall, H.V., Horvath, C., Piechowiak, M., Johnson, L., and Bayer, K., 1996, An external thoracic duct venous shunt to allow for long-term collection of lymph and blood in the conscious pig, in Tumbleson, M.E. and Schook, L.E., Eds., *Advances in Swine in Biomedical Research*, Vol. 3, New York: Plenum Press, pp. 621–627.

Messas, E., Guerrero, J.L., Handschumacher, M.D., Conrad, C., Chow, C.M., Sullivan, S., Yoganathan, A.P., and Levine, R.A., 2001, Chordal cutting: a new therapeutic approach for ischemic mitral regurgitation, *Circulation*, 104(16): 1958–1963.

Milner, R., Verhagen, H.J., Prinssen, M., and Blankensteijn, J.D., 2004, Noninvasive intrasac pressure measurement and the influence of type 2 and type 3 endoleaks in an animal model of abdominal aortic aneurysm, *Vascular*, 12(2): 99–105.

Mitchell, S.E., Anderson, J.H., Swindle, M.M., Strandberg, J.D., and Kan, J., 1994, Atrial septostomy: stationary angioplasty balloon technique, experimental work and preliminary clinical applications, *Pediatr. Cardiol.*, 15(1): 1–7.

Morrow, W.R., Smith, V.C., Ehler, W.J., Van Dellen, A.F., and Mullins, C.E., 1994, Balloon angioplasty with stent implantation in experimental coarctation of the aorta, *Circulation*, 89(6): 2677–2683.

Murphy, J.G., Schwartz, R.S., Edwards, W.D., Camrud, A.R., Vliestra, R.E., and Holmes, D.R., Jr., 1992, Percutaneous polymeric stents in porcine coronary arteries: initial experience with polyethylene terephthalate stents, *Circulation*, 86(5): 1596–1604.

Nestruck, A.C., Lussier-Cacan, S., Bergseth, M., Bidallier, M., Davignon, J., and Marcel, Y.L., 1977, The effect of portocaval shunt on plasma lipids and lipoproteins in swine, *Biochim. Biophys. Acta*, 488(1): 43–54.

Nguyen, K., Stauch, J.T., Srivastava, S., Lauten, A., Haldenwang, P., Zhang, N., Vlahakis, S., and Adams, D.H., 2004, Orthotopic mitral valve replacement with autologous pulmonary valve in a porcine model, *J. Thorac. Cardiovasc. Surg.*, 127(5): 1527–1529.

Nicolau, D.P., Feng, Y.J., Wu, A.H.B., Bernstein, S.P., and Nightingale, C.H., 1996, Swine model of continuous arteriovenous hemofiltration, *Lab. Anim. Sci.*, 46(3): 355–357.

Pae, W.E., Jr., Myers, J.L., Waldhausen, J.A., Prophet, G.A., and Pierce, W.S., 1981, Subclavian flap angioplasty: experimental study in growing piglets, *J. Thorac. Cardiovasc. Surg.*, 82(6): 922–927.

Pak, H.N., Qayyumi, J.M., Kim, D.T., Hamabe, A., Miyauchi, Y., Lill, M.C., Frantzen, M., Takizawa, K., Chen, L.S., Fishbein, M.C., Sharifi, B.G., Chen, P.S., and Makkar, R., 2003, Mesenchymal stem cell injection induces cardiac nerve sprouting and increased tenascin expression in a swine model of myocardial infarction, *J. Cardiovasc. Electrophysiol.*, 14(7): 841–848.

Purohit, D.M., Swindle, M.M., Smith, C.D., Othersen, H.B., Jr., and Kazanovicz, J.M., 1993, Hanford miniature swine model for extracoporeal membrane oxygenation (ECMO), *J. Invest. Surg.*, 6(6): 503–508.

Qayumi, A.K., Jamieson, W.R., Godin, D.M., Lam, S., Ko, K.M., Germann, E., and VandenBroek, J., 1990, Response to allopurinol pretreatment in a swine model of heart-lung transplantation, *J. Invest. Surg.*, 3(4): 331–340.

Qayumi, A.K., Jamieson, W.R., Rosado, L.J., Lyster, D.M., Schulzer, M., McConville, B., Gillespie, K.D., and Hudson, M.P., 1991, Comparison of functional and metabolic assessments in preservation techniques for heart transplantation, *J. Invest. Surg.*, 4(1): 93–102.

Qayumi, A.K., Godin, D.V., Jamieson, W.R., Ko, K.M., and Poostizadeh, A., 1993, Correlation of red cell antioxidant status and heart-lung function in swine pretreated with allopurinol (a model of heart-lung transplantation), *Transplantation*, 56(1): 37–43.

Rabkin, D.G., Cabreriza, S.E., Curtis, L.J., Mazer, S.P., Kanter, J.P., Weinberg, A.D., Hordof, A.J., and Spotnitz, H.M., 2004, Load dependence of cardiac output in biventricular pacing: right ventricular pressure overload in pigs, *J. Thorac. Cardiovasc. Surg.*, 127(6): 1713–1722.

Randsbaek, F., Riordan, C.J., Storey, J.H., Montgomery, W.D., Santamore, W.P., and Austin, E.H., III, 1996, Animal model of the univentricular heart and single ventricular physiology, *J. Invest. Surg.*, 9(4): 375–384.

Rashid, S.T., Salacinski, H.J., Hamilton, G., and Seifalian, A.M., 2003, The use of animal models in the discipline of cardiovascular tissue engineering: a review, *Biomaterials*, 23: 1627–1637.

Reffelmann, T., Sensebat, O., Birnbaum, Y., Stroemer, E., Hanrath, P., Uretsky, B.F., and Schwarz, E.R., 2004, A novel minimal-invasive model of chronic myocardial infarction in swine, *Coronary Artery Dis.*, 15(1): 7–12.

Rhee, P., Talon, E., Eifert, S., Anderson, D., Stanton, K., Koustova, E., Ling, G., Burris, D., Kaufmann, C., Mongan, P., Rich, N.M., Taylor, M., and Sun, L., 2000, Induced hypothermia during emergency department thoracotomy: an animal model, *J. Trauma Injury Infect. Crit. Care*, 48(3): 439–450.

Ricci, M.A., Mehran, R.J., Petsikas, D., Mohamed, F., Guidoin, R., Marois, Y., Christou, N.V., Graham, A., and Symes, J.F., 1991a, Species differences in the infectability of vascular grafts, *Invest. Surg.*, 4(1): 45–52.

Ricci, M.A., Mehran, R., Christou, N.V., Mohamed, F., Graham, A.M., and Smyes, J.F., 1991b, Species differences in the clearance of Staphylococcus aureus bacteremia, *J. Invest. Surg.*, 4(1): 53–58.

Roberts, S.L., Gilbert, M., and Tinker, J.H., 1987, Isoflurane has a greater margin of safety than halothane in swine with and without major surgery or critical coronary stenosis, *Anesth. Analg.*, 66(6): 485–491.

Rogers, G.P., Cromeens., D.M., Minor, S.T., and Swindle, M.M., 1988, Bretylium and diltiazem in porcine cardiac procedures, *J. Invest. Surg.*, 1(4): 321–326.

Rotmans, J.I., Velema, E., Verhagen, H.J.M., Blankensteijn, J.D., Kastelein, J.J.P., DeKleijn, D.P.V., Yo, M., Pasterkamp, G., and Stroes, E.S.G., 2003, Rapid arteriovenous graft failure due to intimal hyperplasia: a porcine bilateral, carotid arteriovenous graft model, *J. Surg. Res.*, 113(2): 161–171.

Rysavy, J.A., Lund, G.E., Lock, J.E., Bass, J.L., Einzig, S.S., and Amplatz, K., 1986, A method for nonsurgical creation of patent ductus arteriosus and its applications in piglets, in Tumbleson, M.E., Ed., *Swine in Biomedical Research*, Vol. 1, New York: Plenum Press, pp. 351–361.

Saito, R. and Waters, P.F., 1994, Heart, lung, and heart-lung transplantation in the dog and the pig, in Cramer, D.V., Podesta, L.G., and Makowks, L., Eds., *Handbook of Animal Models in Transplantation Research*, Boca Raton, FL: CRC Press, pp. 161–172.

Salminen, U.S., Maasilta, P.K., Taskinen, E.I., Alho, H.S., Ikonen, T.S., and Harjula, A.L.J., 2000, Prevention of small airway obliteration in a swine heterotopic lung allograft model, *J. Heart Lung Transpl.*, 19(2): 193–206.

Schumann, R.E., Swindle, M.M., Knick, B.J., Case, C.L., and Gillette, P.C., 1994, High dose narcotic anesthesia using sufentanil in swine for cardiac catheterization and electrophysiologic studies, *J. Invest. Surg.*, 7(3): 243–248.

Shimokawa, S., Matsumoto, H., Ogata, S., Komokata, T., Nishida, S., Ushijima, T., Saigenji, H., Moriyama, Y., and Taira, A., 1996, A new experimental model for simultaneous evaluation of aortic and pulmonary allograft performance in a composite graft, *J. Invest. Surg.*, 9(5): 487–493.

Smerup, M., Pedersen, T.F., Nyboe, C., Funder, J.A., Christensen, T.D., Nielsen, S.L., Hjortdal, V., and Hasenkam, J.M., 2004, A long-term porcine model for evaluation of prosthetic heart valves, *Heart Surg. Forum*, 7(4): E259–264.

Smith, A.C., Spinale, F.G., Carabello, B.A., and Swindle, M.M., 1989, Technical aspects of cardiac catheterization of swine, *J. Invest. Surg.*, 2(2): 187–194.

Smith, A.C., Spinale, F.G., and Swindle, M.M., 1990, Cardiac function and morphology of Hanford miniature swine and Yucatan miniature and micro swine, *Lab. Anim. Sci.*, 40(1): 47–50.

Smith, A.C., Dungan, L.J., and Swindle, M.M., 1994, Induced Heart Defects; Special Considerations, NRC (National Research Council), Institute of Laboratory Animal Resources, Committee on Dogs, Dogs: Laboratory Animal Management, Washington, D.C.: National Academy Press, pp. 76–130.

Smith, A.C., Knick, B., Swindle, M.M., and Gillette, P.C., 1997, A technique for conducting non-invasive cardiac electrophysiology studies in swine, *J. Invest. Surg.*, 10(1–2): 25–30.

Sparrow, M.P., 1996, Bronchial function in the porcine lung: from the fetus to the adult, in Tumbleson, M.E. and Schook, L.B., Eds., *Advances in Swine in Biomedical Research*, Vol. 1, New York: Plenum Press, pp. 33–44.

Spinale, F.G., 1995, Pacing tachycardia-induced congestive heart failure, *Heart Failure*, 11: 219–232.

Spinale, F.G., Hendrick, D.A., Crawford, F.A., Smith, A.C., Hamada, Y., and Carabello, B.A., 1990, Chronic supraventricular tachycardia causes ventricular dysfunction and subendocardial injury in swine, *Am. J. Physiol.*, 259(1 Pt. 2) (*Heart Circ. Physiol.* 28): H218–H229.

Stanley, W.C., 2000, *In vivo* models of myocardial metabolism during ischemia: application to drug discovery and evaluation, *J. Pharmacol. Toxicol. Methods*, 43: 133–140.

Stanton, H.C. and Mersmann, H.J., Eds., 1986, *Swine in Cardiovascular Research*, Vol. 1 and 2, Boca Raton, FL: CRC Press.

Strauch, J.T., Lauten, A., Spielvogel, D., Rinke, S., Zhang, N., Weisz, D., Bodian, C.A., and Griepp, R.B., 2004, Mild hypothermia protects the spinal cord from ischemic injury in a chronic porcine model, *Eur. J. Cardio. Thorac. Surg.*, 25(5): 708–715.

Suematsu, Y., Marx, G.R., Stoll, J.A., DuPont, P.E., Cleveland, R.O., Howe, R.D., Triedman, J.K., Mihaljevic, T., Mora, B.N., Savord, B.J., Salgo, I.S., and del Nido, P.J., 2004, Three dimensional echocardiography-guided beating-heart surgery without cardiopulmonary bypass: a feasibility study, *J. Thorac. Cardiovasc. Surg.*, 128(4): 579–587.

Svendsen, P. and Rasmussen, C., 1998, Anaesthesia of minipigs and basic surgical techniques, *Scand. J. Lab. Anim. Sci.*, 25(Suppl. 1): 31.

Swindle, M.M., 1983, *Basic Surgical Exercises Using Swine*, Philadelphia, PA: Praeger Press.

Swindle, M.M., 1986, Swine as models in thoracic surgery, in Powers, D.L., Ed., *Proc. 2nd Annu. Meet. Acad. Surg. Res.*, Clemson, SC: Clemson University Press, pp. 106–108.

Swindle, M.M., 1992, *Swine as Models in Biomedical Research*, Ames, IA: Iowa State University Press.

Swindle, M.M., 1994, Anesthetic and Perioperative Techniques in Swine: An Update, Charles River Technical Bulletin 12(1): 1–4.

Swindle, M.M., 1996, Considerations of specific pathogen free (SPF) swine in xenotransplantation, *J. Invest. Surg.*, 9(3): 267–271.

Swindle, M.M. and Adams, R.J., 1988, *Experimental Surgery and Physiology: Induced Animal Models of Human Disease*, Baltimore, MD: Williams and Wilkins.

Swindle, M.M. and Bobbie, D.L., 1987, Comparative Anatomy of the Pig, Charles River Technical Bulletin 4(1): 1–4.

Swindle, M.M., Horneffer, P.J., Gardner, T.J., Gott, V.L., Hall, T.S., Stuart, R.S., Baumgartner, W.A., Borkon, A.M., Galloway, E., and Reitz, B.A., 1986, Anatomic and anesthetic considerations in experimental cardiopulmonary surgery in swine, *Lab. Anim. Sci.*, 36(4): 357–361.

Swindle, M.M., Smith, A.C., and Hepburn, B.J.S., 1988, Swine as models in experimental surgery, *J. Invest. Surg.*, 1(1): 65–79.

Swindle, M.M., Wiest, D.B., Smith, A.C., Garner, S.S., Case, C.C., Thompson, R.P., Fyfe, D.A., and Gillette, P.C., 1996, Fetal surgical protocols in Yucatan miniature swine, *Lab. Anim. Sci.*, 46(1): 90–95.

Swindle, M.M., Smith, A.C., and Goodrich, J.A., 1998, Chronic cannulation and fistulation procedures in swine: a review and recommendations, *J. Invest. Surg.*, 11(1): 7–20.

Swindle, M.M., Nolan, T., Jacobson, A., Wolf, P., Dalton, M.J., and Smith, A.C., 2005, Vascular access port (VAP) usage in large animal species, *Contemp. Top. Lab. Anim. Sci.*, 44(3): 7–17.

Terp, K., Koudahl, V., Velen, M., Kim, W.Y., Andersen, H.R., Baandrup, U., and Hasenkam, J.M., 1999, Functional remodeling and left ventricular dysfunction after repeated ischaemic episodes, *Scand. Cardiovasc. J.*, 33(5): 265–273.

Tong, S.W., Ingenito, S., Anderson, J.E., Gootman, N., Sica, A.L., and Gootman, P.M., 1995, Development of a swine animal model for the study of sudden infant death syndrome, *Lab. Anim. Sci.*, 45(4): 398–403.

Tong, S., Ingenito, S., Frasier, I.D., Gootman, N., and Gootman, P.M., 1996, Differential effects of left and right cardiac sympathetic denervation on ventricular fibrillation threshold in developing swine, in Tumbleson, M.E. and Schook, L.B., Eds., *Advances in Swine in Biomedical Research*, Vol. 1, New York: Plenum Press, pp. 131–140.

Toumpoulis, I.K., Papakostas, J.C., Matsagas, M.I., Malamou-Mitsi, V.D., Pappa, L.S., Drossos, G.E., Derose, J.J., and Anagnostopoulos, C.E., 2004, Superiority of early relative to late ischemic preconditioning in spinal cord protection after descending thoracic aortic occlusion, *J. Thorac. Cardiovasc. Surg.*, 128(5): 724–730.

Turjman, F., Massoud, T.F., Ji, C., Guglielmi, G., Vinuela, F., and Robert, J., 1994, Combined stent implantation and endosaccular coil placement for treatment of experimental wide-necked aneurysms: a feasibility study in swine, *Am. J. Neuroradiol.*, 15(6): 1087–1090.

Uflacker, R. and Brothers, T., 2006, Filling of the aneurismal sac with DEAC-glucosamine in an animal model of abdominal aortic aneurysm following stent-graft repair, *J. Cardiovasc. Surg.*, 47(4): 425–436.

Unger, E.F., 2001, Experimental evaluation of coronary collateral development, *Cardiovasc. Res.*, 49: 497–506.

Verdouw, P.D. and Hartog, J.M., 1986, Provocation and suppression of ventricular arrhythmias in domestic swine, in Stanton, H.C. and Mersmann, H.J., Eds., *Swine in Cardiovascular Research*, Vol. 2, Boca Raton, FL: CRC Press, pp. 121–156.

Verdouw, P.D., van den Doel, M.A., de Zeeuw, S., and Duncker, D.J., 1998, Animal models in the study of myocardial ischaemia and ischaemic syndromes, *Cardiovasc. Res.*, 39(1): 121–135.

Wallace, M.J., Aharar, K., and Wright, K.C., 2003, Validation of US guided percutaneous venous access and manual compression for studies in swine, *J. Vasc. Interv. Radiol.*, 14: 481–483.

Watanabe, E., Smith, D.M., Delcarpio, J.B., Sun, J., Smart, F.W., Van Meter, C.H., and Claycomb, W.C., 1998, Cardiomyocyte transplantation in a porcine myocardial infarction model, *Cell Transplant.*, 7(3): 239–246.

White, D. and Lunney, J., 1979, Transplantation in pigs, *Transplant. Proc.*, 11(1): 1170–1173.

White, F.C., Roth, D.M., and Bloor, C.M., 1986, The pig as a model for myocardial ischemia and exercise, *Lab. Anim. Sci.*, 36(4): 351–356.

White, C.J., Ramee, S.R., Banks, A.K., Wiktor, D., and Price, H.L., 1992, The Yucatan miniature swine: an atherogenic model to assess the early potency rates of an endovascular stent, in Swindle, M.M., Ed., *Swine as Models in Biomedical Research*, Ames, IA: Iowa State University Press, pp. 156–162.

Wittnich, C., Belanger, M.P., Oh, B.S., and Salerno, T.A., 1991, Surgical model of volume overload-induced ventricular myocardial hypertrophy to study a clinical problem in humans, *J. Invest. Surg.*, 4(3): 333–338.

Yarbrough, W.M. and Spinale, F.G., 2003, Large animal models of congestive heart failure: a critical step in translating basic observations into clinical applications, *J. Nucl. Cardiol.*, 10(1): 77–86.

Zhang, J., Jamieson, W.R.E., Sadeghi, H., Gillespie, K., Marier, J.R., Mickleson, H., and McGibbon, R., 1998, Strategies of myocardial protection for operation in a chronic model of cyanotic heart disease, *Ann. Thorac. Surg.*, 66(5): 1507–1513.

10 Head and Neck Surgery/ Central Nervous System

GENERAL PRINCIPLES OF SURGERY AND SURGICAL ANATOMY

The use of swine in dental and neurologic research has been relatively uncommon, probably because of the anatomy of the head, neck, and oral cavity (Figure 10.1–Figure 10.10). The skull in Figure 10.3–Figure 10.10 is from a sexually mature boar. Its use in oral and maxillofacial surgery has recently increased (Bermejo et al., 1993; Curtis et al., 2001; Donovan et al., 1993; Drisco et al., 1996; North, 1988; Ouhayoun et al., 1992; Sims et al., 1997).

The dental formula for deciduous teeth in swine is 2(I 3/3, C 1/1, P 4/4) = 32. Permanent teeth have a dental formula of 2(I 3/3, C 1/1, P 4/4, M 3/3) = 44. Swine are born with the last incisors and canine teeth. The remainder of the incisors erupt between 2 weeks and 2 months of age. The premolars erupt between 4 d and 5 months. The molars are the first permanent teeth to erupt and appear between 4 months and 20 months of age. The incisors change between 8 and 20 months, the canines between 9 and 10 months, and the premolars between 12 and 15 months. The tooth eruption sequence of adult permanent teeth is P1/M1/I3/C/M2/I1/P3/P4/P2/I2/M3. In the boar, the canine teeth become the tusks and require trimming two to four times a year in the adult. Growth of the tusks is delayed in females and castrated males. The newborn's canines are called needle teeth and are usually trimmed shortly after birth to prevent damage to the sow during nursing. The dental formulas are identical among farm and miniature breeds, and eruption dates are similar. A full set of permanent teeth is usually present around 18 months of age. The size of the teeth is similar to human, and the tooth eruption and exfoliation of the primary teeth can be followed in a normal time sequence (Hargreaves and Mitchell, 1969; Sisson and St. Clair, 1975a, 1975b; Weaver et al., 1962).

There is a substantial difference in the conformation of the head and neck among different breeds; the breeds are illustrated in Chapter 1. The snout of the Yucatan, Göttingen, Sinclair, and most other miniature pigs is considerably shorter than that of domestic farm breeds and the Hanford miniature pig. The heads of miniature breeds tend to be more rounded than that of the farm breeds and the Hanford; the latter has a head and snout shape similar to wild pigs. Selection of a breed for oral and maxillofacial surgery should include a consideration of the differences in head and neck conformation.

The bones of the cranium and the mandible are massive. The temporomandibular joint has been compared to those of other species and humans in a detailed anatomic study (Bermejo et al., 1993). The authors concluded that the pig was an appropriate animal model to study temporomandibular joint abnormalities because it was most similar to humans. The pig has a reciprocally fitting meniscotemporal joint and a condylomeniscal joint of the condylar type. The size of the articular structures, the shape of the meniscus, and the omnivorous chewing characteristics of swine provided additional justification for the use of this model over that of rodents, rabbits, carnivores, and herbivores that were examined. Maxillofacial bone-healing studies have been performed in swine (North, 1988). Swine have also been found to have fluxes of autonomic tone in the nasal airway, identical to humans (Campbell and Kern, 1981).

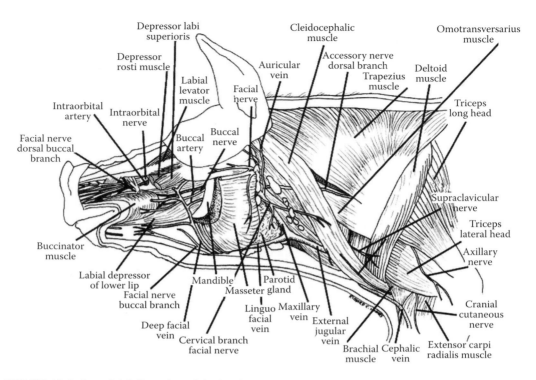

FIGURE 10.1 Superficial dissection of the head and neck.

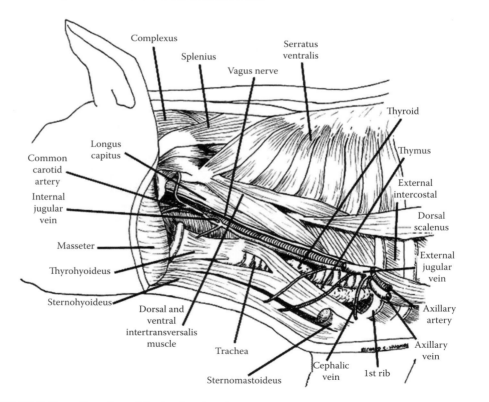

FIGURE 10.2 Deep dissection of the head and neck.

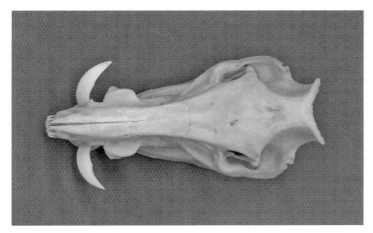

FIGURE 10.3 Dorsal view of the skull. (Courtesy of Mark Rodenberg and Joe Roberts, Elite Barber Shop.)

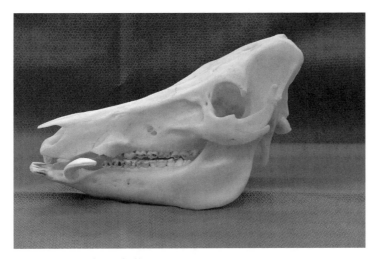

FIGURE 10.4 Left lateral view of the skull.

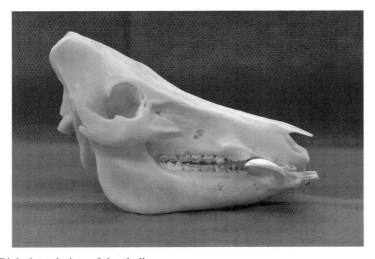

FIGURE 10.5 Right lateral view of the skull.

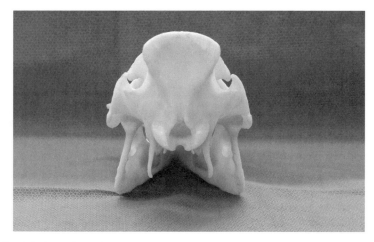

FIGURE 10.6 Caudal view of the skull.

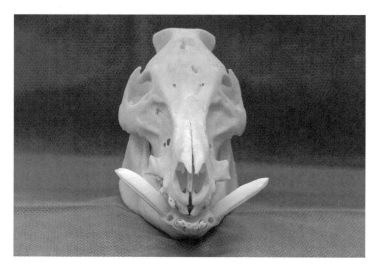

FIGURE 10.7 Frontal view of the skull.

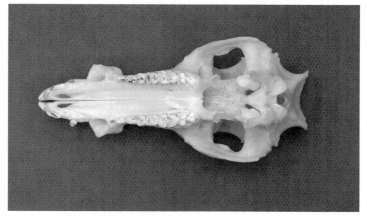

FIGURE 10.8 Ventral view of the maxilla and skull with the mandible removed.

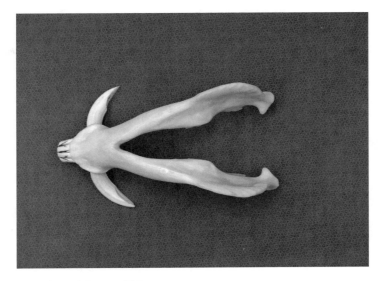

FIGURE 10.9 Ventral view of the mandible.

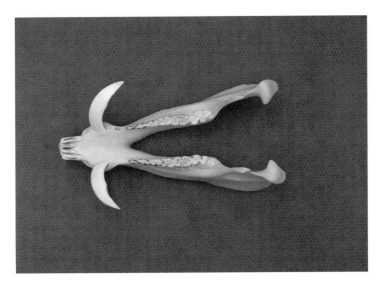

FIGURE 10.10 Dorsal view of the mandible.

The salivary glands of the pig are the parotid, the mandibular, and the sublingual. The parotid gland enters the oral cavity opposite the upper fourth or fifth cheek tooth and may have accessory glands along the duct. The mandibular gland enters near the frenulum. The sublingual glands are located in bilateral chains and have multiple openings into the floor of the mouth. A series of minor buccal glands are located opposite the upper and lower cheek teeth. In the pig, the parotid gland is serous, the sublingual gland is mucoid, and the mandibular and buccal glands are mixed in secretions.

Tonsils analogous to the palatine tonsils are embedded in the soft palate rather than in the lateral wall of the oropharynx as in other species. There is a pharyngeal diverticulum dorsal to the larynx in the caudal aspect of the nasopharynx; this structure may be damaged during the passing of gastric or endotracheal tubes. The thymus (Figure 10.11) extends from the thorax to the level of the larynx in the pig. The thyroid gland (Figure 10.12) has paired lobules that are fused on the ventral surface of the trachea near the thoracic inlet. The single pair of parathyroid glands are

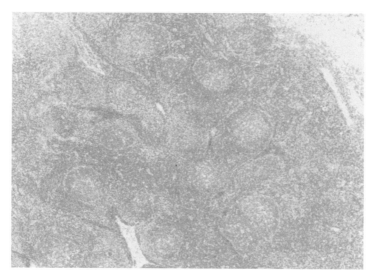

FIGURE 10.11 Histologic section of the thymus. H&E, ×40.

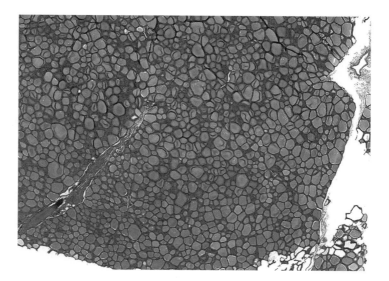

FIGURE 10.12 Histologic section of the thyroid. H&E, ×40.

minute and are associated with the cranial end of the thymus (Sack, 1982; Schantz et al., 1996; Sisson and St. Clair, 1975a, 1975b; Swindle and Bobbie, 1987). The dissection of the glands of the neck is illustrated in Figure 1.44.

The ophthalmic system of the pig has been previously reviewed and compared with other species of laboratory animals (Adams, 1988), and the pertinent comparisons are summarized here. The pig has an open field of vision with a pupil and retina similar to human. The seven extraocular muscles are attached to the orbital wall in deep fossae. A nictitating membrane, Bowman's membrane, and Descemet's membrane are present. A tapetum is absent. There may be either one or two puncta for lacrimal drainage. There is a deep gland of the third eyelid, Harder's gland. Pigs usually have brown or blue irises with a small amount of heterochromacity. The retina (Figure 10.13 and Figure 10.14) is completely vascularized (holangiotic). Spontaneous conditions found in the eyes of various miniature pigs are outlined in Table 10.1–Table 10.3.

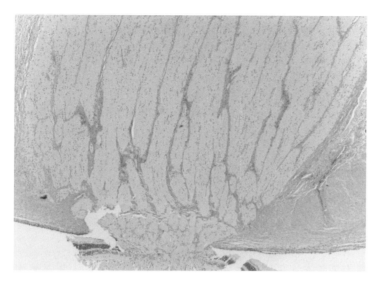

FIGURE 10.13 Histologic section of the optic nerve and retina. H&E, ×40.

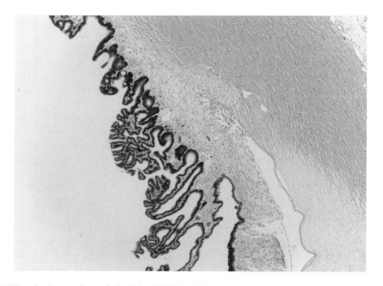

FIGURE 10.14 Histologic section of the iris. H&E, ×40.

The diameter of the adult eye is approximately 24 mm with an ocular power of 78 diopters, a binocular field of vision of 12°, and peripheral vision of 310° (Curtis et al., 2001). Specific eye measurements have been made in the Göttingen minipigs (Nielsen and Lind, 2005). In the adult pigs they measured, the following values were obtained: mean refractive error (+1.3 diopters), mean corneal power (44.1 diopters), and mean axial length (<19 mm). Additional comparisons of intraocular pressure measurements in 23 male Göttingen minipigs are illustrated in Figure 10.15.

In sexually mature 100-kg domestic swine, the physical properties of the lens have been measured as part of studies to develop artificial lenses and vitreous humor (Rapp et al., 2006; Ravi et al., 2005; Reilly et al., in press; Swindle et al., 2006a, 2006b). Their measurements were: refractive index 1.405, specific gravity 1.09, transmission 0.95, elastic modulus 1.2 kPa, and relaxation time constants 50–500 msec. Specific comparisons of the anterior lens capsule indicated that porcine lenses are thicker (50–66 µm) with a smaller accommodative amplitude than humans (Reilly et al.,

TABLE 10.1
Ophthalmologic Findings in 6- to 8-Week-Old Göttingen Minipigs

Observations	Males (N = 18)		Females (N = 18)		Both Sexes (N = 36)	
	n	%	n	%	n	%
Gross Findings						
Blepharitis	15	83.3	15	83.3	30	83.3
Conjunctivitis	8	44.4	8	44.4	16	44.4
Palpebral papilloma	—	—	1	5.6	1	2.8
Slight brown coloration of the sclera	—	—	1	5.6	1	2.8
Cornea						
Pinpoint opacities	1	5.6	—	—	1	2.8
Opalescence of the stroma	—	—	—	—	—	—
Iris						
Blue color	2	11.1	4	22.2	6	16.7
Blue/brown color	2	11.1	2	11.1	4	11.1
Brown color	14	77.8	12	66.7	26	72.2
Pupillary membrane remnants	6	33.3	6	33.3	12	33.3
Lens						
Suture line abnormality	1	5.6	—	—	1	2.8
Focal nuclear opacity	2	11.1	1	5.6	3	8.3
Posterior cortical pinpoint opacities	4	22.2	3	16.7	7	19.4
Posterior capsular opacities	—	—	3	16.7	3	8.3
Posterior capsular cataract	—	—	—	—	—	—
Vitreous						
Refringent points	2	11.1	—	—	2	5.6
Hyaloid artery remnants	14	77.8	16	88.9	30	83.3
Fundus						
Tigroid fundus	12	66.7	14	77.8	26	72.2
Retinal vascular abnormality	—	—	—	—	—	—
Retinal hemorrhage	—	—	—	—	—	—
Retinal degeneration	—	—	—	—	—	—
Optic disc abnormality	—	—	—	—	—	—

Note: N = number of animals examined, n = number with finding, % = percentage with finding.

Source: Reprinted from Loget, O. and Saint-Marcary, G., *Scand. J. Lab. Anim. Sci.*, Suppl. 1, pp. 173–179, 1998. With permission.

TABLE 10.2
Ophthalmologic Findings in 2- to 10-Month-Old Göttingen Minipigs

Observations	Males (N = 70)		Females (N = 92)		Both sexes (N = 162)	
	n	%	n	%	n	%
Gross Findings						
Blepharitis	3	4.3	2	2.2	5	3.1
Conjunctivitis	12	17.1	2	2.2	14	8.6
Palpebral papilloma	—	—	—	—	—	—
Slight brown coloration of the sclera	—	—	1	1.1	1	0.6
Cornea						
Pinpoint opacities	1	1.1	2	2.2	3	1.8
Opalescence of the stroma	1	1.4	—	—	1	0.5
Iris						
Blue color	5	7.1	9	9.7	14	8.6
Blue/brown color	8	4.7	21	22.8	29	15.9
Brown color	57	81.4	62	67.4	119	73.4
Pupillary membrane remnants	9	12.8	12	13.0	21	13.0
Lens						
Suture line abnormality	1	1.4	1	1.1	2	1.2
Focal nuclear opacity	2	2.8	6	6.5	8	4.9
Posterior cortical pinpoint opacities	8	11.4	11	11.9	19	11.7
Posterior capsular opacities	8	11.4	4	4.3	12	7.4
Posterior capsular cataract	—	—	—	—	—	—
Vitreous						
Refringent points	4	5.7	4	4.3	8	4.9
Hyaloid artery remnants	48	68.5	66	71.7	114	70.4
Fundus						
Tigroid fundus	50	71.4	64	69.5	107	70.4
Retinal vascular abnormality	—	—	—	—	—	—
Retinal hemorrhage	1	1.4	—	—	1	0.6
Retinal degeneration	—	—	1	1.1	1	0.6
Optic disc abnormality	1	1.4	1	1.1	2	1.2

Note: N = number of animals examined, n = number with finding, % = percentage with finding.

Source: Reprinted from Loget, O. and Saint-Marcary, G., *Scand. J. Lab. Anim. Sci.*, Suppl. 1, pp. 173–179, 1998. With permission.

TABLE 10.3
Ophthalmologic Findings in 7- to 12-Month-Old Yucatan Micropigs

Observations	Males (N = 112)		Females (N = 112)		Both Sexes (N = 224)	
	n	%	n	%	n	%
Gross Findings						
Blepharitis	—	—	—	—	—	—
Conjunctivitis	2	1.8	—	—	2	0.9
Palpebral papilloma	—	—	—	—	—	—
Cornea						
Corneal pigmentation	4	3.6	4	3.6	8	3.6
Pinpoint opacities	—	—	—	—	—	—
Opalescence of the stroma	—	—	—	—	—	—
Iris						
Brown color	112	100.0	112	100.0	224	100.0
Pupillary membrane remnants	70	62.5	78	69.6	148	66.1
Lens						
Suture line abnormality	—	—	8	7.1	8	3.6
Focal nuclear opacity	4	3.6	14	12.5	18	8.0
Nuclear cataract	2	1.8	8	7.1	10	4.5
Posterior cortical pinpoint opacities	26	23.2	20	17.9	46	20.5
Corticonuclear opacities	2	1.8	—	—	2	0.9
Posterior capsular pinpoint opacities	18	16.1	14	12.5	32	14.3
Posterior capsular cataract	6	5.4	2	1.8	8	3.6
Vitreous						
Refringent points	4	3.6	14	12.5	18	8.0
Hyaloid artery remnants	90	80.4	94	83.9	184	82.1
Fundus						
Tigroid fundus	58	51.8	54	48.2	112	50.0
Retinal vascular abnormality	—	—	2	1.8	2	0.9
Retinal hemorrhage	4	3.6	2	1.8	6	2.7
Retinal degeneration	2	1.8	4	3.6	6	2.7
Optic disc abnormality	—	—	4	3.6	4	1.8

Note: N = number of animals examined, n = number with finding, % = percentage with finding.

Source: Reprinted from Loget, O. and Saint-Marcary, G., 1998, *Scand. J. Lab. Anim. Sci.*, Suppl. 1, 173–179.
With permission.

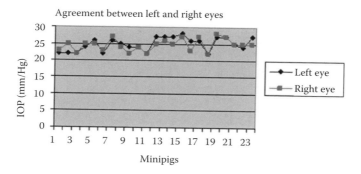

FIGURE 10.15 Intraocular pressure (IOP) agreement in measurements in 24 Göttingen minipigs. (Courtesy of Ellegaard Göttingen Minipigs.)

in press). In a recent study concerning the use of *ex vivo* eyes for laser safety testing (Fyffe et al., 2005) using 4- to 6-month-old Yucatan and Yorkshire pigs, differences from other published values were noted. They reported that a true Bowman's membrane is absent and the globe diameters were 30 mm, corneal thickness 1063 μm, and corneal epithelial thickness 47 μm, as compared to human values of 24 mm, 770 μm, and 35 μm, respectively. They reported an ED_{50} of 6.7 J cm^2 with infrared lasers. Differences between the minipigs and the farm pigs are likely because of the differences in body size. The ratio of body weight (BW) to eye weight is 2733:1. The extent of their color vision is uncertain, but they can distinguish wide wavelength differences.

Ultrastructural and other detailed studies of the retina have been performed (Chandler et al., 1999; Garca et al., 2005; Hendrickson and Hicks, 2002; Jackson et al., 2003; Jacobs et al., 2002; Ruiz-Ederra et al., 2004). Pigs have a high density of both rods and cones with a photoreceptor density (200,000 cells/mm) similar to humans. They lack a tapetum cellulosum and foveolar specialization. Overall, the porcine retina compares favorably with the human, as do the viscoelastic properties of the vitreous humor, and porcine eyes have been used to test development of artificial vitreous humor (Swindle et al., in press).

Pigs have highly developed auditory and olfactory systems (Curtis et al., 2001). Their hearing frequency range is 40 Hz–40 kHz, and they are able to localize sound very well. They are sensitive to sudden loud noises and may stampede if startled. They are capable of vocalizing distress at up to 5000 Hz and will vocalize loudly during feeding and cage cleaning, consequently, personnel should be provided with ear protection.

Stereotaxic atlases of the pig brain (Figure 10.16) have been published (Salinas-Zeballos et al., 1986; Felix et al., 1999). A method of making direct comparison between MRI digital images and histologic sections using a common coordinate has been published on the pig brain (Sørensen et al., 2000). The Göttingen minipigs were used in a study to define a stereotaxic coordinate system to clarify studies of radiotracer uptake with PET scanning. The study also defined the mean volumes of the main structures in the brain (Watanabe et al., 2001). The brain of a domestic pig weighs approximately 35 g at birth and 120 g in an adult (approximately 0.35% of BW). The spinal cord weighs approximately 30–40 g which is approximately 0.14% BW (Curtis et al., 2001). Normal intracranial pressure is usually <10 mmHg, brain blood flow is approximately 1 ml min^{-1}g^{-1}, and cerebral perfusion pressure is similar to the mean arterial pressure, which varies depending upon the anesthetic protocol (Cameron et al., 1992).

Comparisons in morphology and function of the porcine central nervous system (CNS) have been made (Felix et al., 1999; Larsen et al., 2004; Lind, 2005). Briefly, the similarities to humans are as follows: gyrencephalic morphology, distinct caudate and putamen structures in the striatal portion, cytoarchitectonic similarities in the cortex and hippocampus, and some dopanergic nuclei functions. In general, the patterns of distribution of gray and white matter, cerebral blood flow parameters, the size, and brain growth during development are similar.

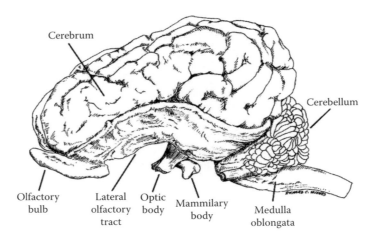

Cerebrum

Cerebellum

Olfactory   Lateral   Optic   Mammilary   Medulla
  bulb   olfactory   body   body   oblongata
                 tract

FIGURE 10.16 Lateral view of the brain.

A detailed description of the blood supply to the spinal cord and brain has also been published (Stodkilde-Jorgensen et al., 1986). The common carotid arteries leave the brachiocephalic trunk at the level of T1. The internal carotid artery provides most of the circulation to the brain. Vertebral arteries branch off the subclavian arteries at the level of C6–C7 and supply the vertebrae, muscle, and spinal cord at each level. The cranial portion of the vertebral artery provides some blood supply to the medulla as well. In studies that interrupted the blood supply of the branches of the vertebral artery at C1–C2, C4–C5, and C7–T1, the latter produced the least hemodynamic and systemic changes. Venous plexi from the brain and plexus enter the internal jugular vein at the level of C1–C2. The internal vertebral plexus enters the vertebral veins and drains into the azygous system at the level of C6. Venous drainage from the thoracic vertebrae enters the azygous veins cranial to the heart.

Principles of performing surgery on the head and neck of swine are the same as for other species. The principal problems involve the thickness of the cranium and the massive nature of the bones of the mandible and maxilla. Following intracranial procedures, cerebral edema and swelling must be controlled, usually by the use of diuretics such as 50% dextrose or furosemide. Laryngeal and tracheal procedures are discussed in Chapter 9.

The DVD attached to this book contains images of the head, neck, and brain.

DENTAL PROCEDURES AND TUSK TRIMMING

The principles of performing oral and dental surgery are the same as for other species, except that exposure is limited for the premolars and molars because of the narrowness of the oral cavity opening. Retractors are necessary to keep the mouth open for procedures on these teeth.

The tusks of the pig need to be trimmed periodically in adult animals, especially in boars, for personnel safety (Eubanks and Gilbo, 2005). To perform this procedure, pigs should have general anesthesia or chemical restraint. They may be trimmed in restraint slings with sedation (Figure 10.17 and Figure 10.18). The roots of the canine teeth are deep and difficult to extract; consequently, the tusks are usually trimmed at the gum line using either Gigli wire or saws. In the adult male, this procedure needs to be performed every 3–6 months. Tusks are slower growing in castrated males and females, and may not need to be trimmed. Veterinary advice should be sought to make this determination.

Dental extractions can be performed on the other teeth using standard methods of root elevation followed by extraction (Figure 10.19). Mucoperiosteal flaps may be reflected from the gingiva in the cranial aspects of the oral cavity, using standard techniques of incision and retraction of the

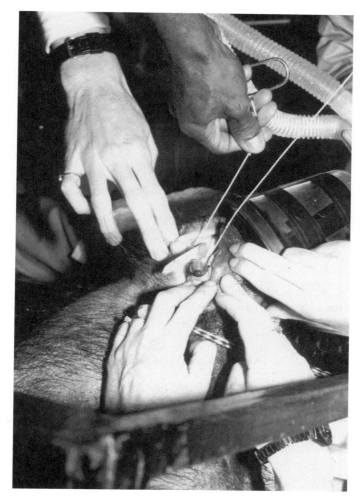

FIGURE 10.17 Cutting the tusks of a sedated boar with Gigli wire.

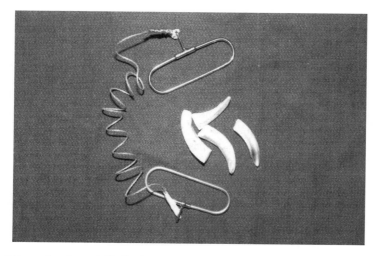

FIGURE 10.18 Trimmed tusks and Gigli wire.

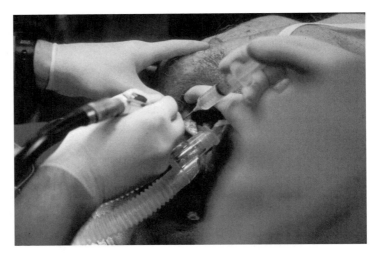

FIGURE 10.19 Elevation of the gum for dental extraction.

gingiva. Use of local anesthetics containing epinephrine as an adjunct to general anesthesia should aid hemostasis by the induction of local vasoconstriction. Oral incisions should be closed with absorbable sutures.

MAXILLOFACIAL AND CRANIOTOMY PROCEDURES

Swine have been used as models for both soft tissue and bone healing, including studies of grafting and implantation of biomaterials. Tissue engineering for bone augmentation and distraction osteogenesis has become an important area of research in maxillofacial surgery (Bradley, 1982; Donovan et al., 1993; Jensen, 2006; Kalkwarf et al., 1983; Ouhayoun et al., 1992; Robinson and Sarnat, 1955; Rosenquist and Rosenquist, 1982; Roth et al., 1984; Sims et al., 1997; Terheyden et al., 1999). Most of the studies have been performed on the mandible, maxilla, and temporomandibular joint. Surgical approaches will be described here.

The body of the mandible can be approached with the pig in dorsal recumbency. An incision made along the ventral aspect of the mandible will provide a relatively bloodless approach to the bone. Dorsal retraction of the skin and platysma muscle will expose the surface of the mandible. The facial vessels at the caudal end of the mandible should be avoided. The masseter muscle may be elevated with the periosteum to expose the lateral surface of the bone and inferior border of the mandible.

The temporomandibular joint may be approached using a lateral incision made dorsal to ventral from an area caudal to the ear and external auditory meatus to the ramus of the mandible following its caudal edge. This area may be readily palpated prior to making the incision. After incising the skin and platysma muscle, the dissection becomes difficult. Branches of the facial nerve and facial, temporal, and auricular arteries and veins should be retracted if possible. The parotid salivary gland should be retracted ventrally. The bodies of the parotidoauricularis muscle will have to be transected. The temporomandibular joint can then be accessed from a caudal direction under the zygomatic arch. If greater exposure is required, the zygomatic arch will have to be transected, taking care not to damage the blood vessels underlying it.

The dorsolateral aspects of the skull can be approached using a midline incision along the crest with the pig in sternal recumbency. The nuchal crest of the pig is quite prominent and is the thickest part of the bone. The superficial muscles along the midline are incised and retracted with the skin. This is followed by incision and retraction of the periosteum laterally from the midline. Using this approach the cranium, frontal sinus, parietal bone, and frontal bone may be approached.

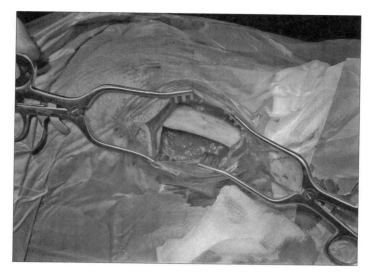

FIGURE 10.20 Exposure of the lateral and inferior border of the mandible. (Courtesy of T. Jensen, Aalborg Hospital, Aarhus University Hospital and Institute of Odontology, Faculty of Health Sciences, University of Copenhagen, Denmark.)

Swine have been developed as a model for endoscopic skull base surgery in the posterior fossa because of the similarities in anatomy with the human (Jarrahy et al., 1999). A curvilinear incision is made caudal to the auricle, and the soft tissue separated from the temporal bone. A burr hole is made down to the level of the intact dura. The endoscope can then be manipulated to visualize the cerebellum, midbrain, and cranial nerves V, VII, VIII, IX, X, and XI as well as the major blood vessels in the region. It is likely that this technique can be extrapolated to other areas of the brain.

The nasal bone, cranial aspects of the frontal sinus, and sinus cavity can be approached using a midline incision along the snout with the pig in sternal recumbency. The nasolabial muscles are incised with the skin and retracted subperiosteally, and then retracted laterally. The nasal bone can be fractured along its suture lines for exposure of the nasal cavity.

The use of Göttingen minipigs as an experimental model for augmentation of the maxillary sinus floor as a treatment for alveolar atrophy (Figure 10.20–Figure 10.24) (T. Jensen, personal communication) has been described by Terheyden and coworkers (Terheyden et al., 1999). This model is presently used to evaluate a mixture of autogenous bone graft and bone substitutes as graft material (Jensen, 2006). The maxillary sinus is exposed through an extraoral incision below the lower lid. A trap door is made with burrs in the lateral sinus wall and the Schneiderian membrane is elevated. The cavity created between the mucosa and the floor of the maxillary sinus can be packed with a grafting material around the inserted dental implant. The muscles, fascia, and skin are closed in a routine fashion.

These incisions may be closed routinely by repair of the bone with wires, screws, or dental acrylic if defects are created. Bone wax may be used to control bleeding. The muscles, fascia, and skin are closed in a routine fashion.

OCULAR SURGERY

The eyes of the pig are deeply embedded in the sockets, especially in anesthetized animals, and exposure requires the use of ocular retractors. Swine have rarely been used in ophthalmic research despite some of their anatomic similarities to humans, but they have been used for corneal procedures (Adams, 1988). The surgical procedures and approaches are the same as for other species. Enucleation of the eye will be described in this section.

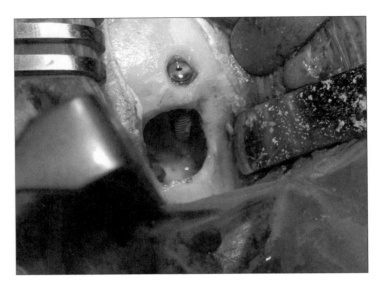

FIGURE 10.21 Insertion of the dental implant into the surgically created cavity. (Courtesy of T. Jensen, Aalborg Hospital, Aarhus University Hospital and Institute of Odontology, Faculty of Health Sciences, University of Copenhagen, Denmark.)

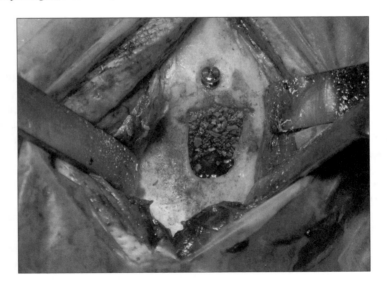

FIGURE 10.22 The entire sinus floor around the implant is packed with grafting material. (Courtesy of T. Jensen, Aalborg Hospital, Aarhus University Hospital and Institute of Odontology, Faculty of Health Sciences, University of Copenhagen, Denmark.)

Allis tissue forceps are used to clamp the margins of the eyelids together. The eyelids are incised in a circumferential fashion beyond their margins, and blunt dissection is initiated at the edge of the orbicularis oculi and into the conjunctiva. After the conjunctiva is dissected to the attachments of the ocular muscles, they are transected. After transection of the muscles, the globe is bluntly dissected free of its attachments except for the ocular nerve, artery, and vein. The globe may be drained using needle aspiration at this point to increase exposure. Right-angle forceps are passed behind the globe, and those structures are clamped. The globe is excised on the proximal side of the forceps, and the vessels and nerve are ligated together, followed by removal of the

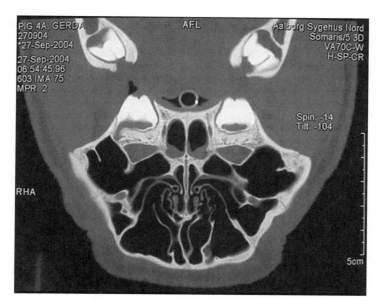

FIGURE 10.23 Preoperative CT scan of the maxillary sinuses. (Courtesy of T. Jensen, Aalborg Hospital, Aarhus University Hospital and Institute of Odontology, Faculty of Health Sciences, University of Copenhagen, Denmark.)

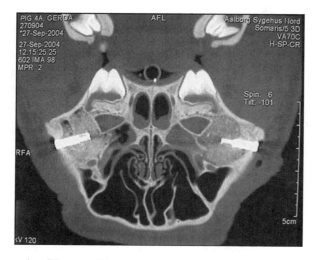

FIGURE 10.24 Postoperative CT scan of the maxillary sinuses with the grafting material packed around the dental implant. (Courtesy of T. Jensen, Aalborg Hospital, Aarhus University Hospital and Institute of Odontology, Faculty of Health Sciences, University of Copenhagen, Denmark.)

forceps. A biocompatible prosthesis may be inserted or the margins of the incision closed. Care should be taken prior to closure to ensure that all glandular structures have been excised and hemostasis is complete. The conjunctiva and skin are closed in a routine fashion.

Pigs have also been developed as models for retinal transplant (Del Priore et al., 2004; Ghosh et al., 2004; Warfvinge et al., 2005), retinal detachment (Jackson et al., 2003; Jacobs et al., 2002), visual prosthesis development (Sachs et al., 2005), and studies involving vitreous replacement (Rapp et al., 2006; Ravi et al., 2005; Swindle et al., 2006a, 2006b; Quiroz-Mercado et al., 2004). A rhodopsin transgenic pig (Petters et al., 1997; Warfvinge et al., 2005) with a retinitis pigmentosa-like disease has been developed. The mutation Pro347Leu reduces rod photoreceptors significantly by 4 months of age. Cones degenerate more slowly, following sexual maturity. In the cases of these models, the surgical procedures are the same as those performed in humans. In many cases, the procedure to be performed is the goal of the study. For procedures in which the vitreous is removed, it has to be replaced simultaneously with the test substance to prevent retinal detachment.

PHARYNGOSTOMY TUBES

A pharyngostomy tube may be surgically implanted when there is a necessity to chronically administer food or medication without mastication. However, it is relatively easy to pass a stomach tube with a mouth gag while the pig is immobilized in a restraint sling. This method of nonsurgical intervention is recommended over the surgical procedure.

The pharynx and proximal esophagus is approached using a ventral midline incision over the larynx. Blunt dissection is continued through the midline, and the esophagus is identified on the dorsum of the trachea by deviating laterally with the dissection when the sternohyoideus muscle is reached. After passing around the esophagus with elastic vessel loops, it is elevated, and a stab incision is made into the lumen. The proximal one half to two thirds of the muscle layers of the esophagus are striated muscle, which converts to smooth muscle in its distal length. A premeasured length of soft nasogastric tubing is passed into the stomach. The proper positioning can be determined when stomach gases are noted to be passing through the tube. The tubing is sutured in place with a purse-string suture. The tubing is tunneled subcutaneously to exit the skin behind the ear. A purse-string suture is placed in the exit site of the skin. The subcutaneous, muscle, and skin layers are closed routinely. The tubing may be taped to the ear for security.

THYROIDECTOMY

The approach to the thyroid gland (see Chapter 1, Figure 1.44) is made with the pig in dorsal recumbency. A ventral midline incision is made, cranial to the manubrium sterni in the last one third to one half of the neck (Swindle, 1983). The incision is continued between fascial planes of the sternohyoideus muscle until the thyroid is identified on the ventral surface of the trachea as a dark colored bilobular structure. The cranial and caudal thyroid artery and vein enter the gland from the dorsal surface and usually cannot be identified in advance. They are bisected and ligated during blunt dissection of the gland from the trachea. The fascial planes of the muscle, the subcutaneous tissues, and the skin are closed in a routine fashion.

PARATHYROIDECTOMY

The single pair of parathyroid glands (see Chapter 1, Figure 1.44) (parathyroid gland III) are difficult to identify (Sack, 1982; Swindle and Bobbie, 1987). They are located on the cranioventral surface of the thymus gland caudolateral to the larynx. A line drawn between the angles of the mandible will provide the surgeon with an approximate location. Because the thymus changes in size with age, the exact location of the dorsal end is variable. These grayish structures are minute (1–4 mm) but usually can be felt to be a definitive structure by rolling them between the thumb and forefinger.

They may either be approached using a ventral midline incision with lateral subcutaneous dissection or a ventral paramedian incision over the sternohyoideus and sternomastoideus muscles. Once the structures are identified, they are removed by blunt dissection. Histopathology is recommended to ensure that they have been removed. Alternatively, the cranial pole of the thymus may be removed if the structures cannot be identified. Hemorrhage is minimal, and vessels usually do not require ligation. The muscle fascia, subcutaneous, and skin layers are closed routinely.

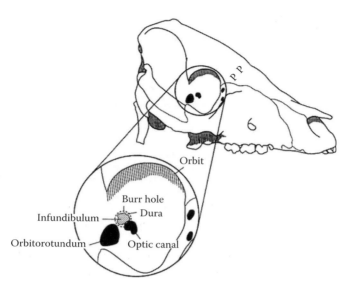

FIGURE 10.25 Hypophysectomy through the transorbital approach. (Reprinted from Drisko et al., *J. Invest. Surg.* 9(4): 305–311, 1996. With permission.)

HYPOPHYSECTOMY

The pituitary gland has been surgically removed in both fetal and adult animals (Drisko et al., 1996; Kraeling et al., 1986). The transsphenoidal and parapharyngeal approaches are difficult in swine because of the limitations in exposure through the open mouth and the extensive dissections involved from the ventral midline. The transfrontal, supraorbital approach has been used in the fetus and in gilts; however, the dissection in adult animals is much more difficult. The transorbital approach offers a minimally invasive technique in adult animals (Figure 10.25).

The first step is to perform a right-eye enucleation, including removal of the periosteum, as described previously. A 5-mm burr hole is drilled caudodorsal and parallel to the optic canal. The site is located dorsomedial to the foramen orbitorotundum. The drill is advanced carefully to the level of the dura overlying the juncture between the infundibulum and the infundibular stalk. Care should be taken to avoid the foramen orbitorotundum and the underlying internal carotid artery. If the hole requires enlargement, care should be taken to avoid damage to the underlying blood vessels and the optic chiasm. The dura is pulled away from the pituitary, and a small hole is made with a dura twist hook. Use of suction and microdissection will allow the surgeon to visualize the pituitary. It can be removed, transected, or cannulated at this point. When closing the incision, the burr hole is filled with bone wax to prevent leakage of cerebrospinal fluid. The socket can be filled with prosthetic material, such as dental acrylic, prior to closing the incision as described earlier for enucleation (Drisko et al., 1996).

The supraorbital frontal approach uses the surgical approach to the cranium described previously. A section of the frontal and parietal bone is removed, and care must be taken to avoid damage to the frontal artery and vein. The exposure and craniotomy is performed to expose the left and one half of the right cerebral hemispheres. The dura mater is incised taking care to avoid damaging the brain. A brain retractor is used to elevate the cerebral hemisphere and expose the region of the hypothalamus. The hypothalamus may be catheterized, transected, or removed as described earlier. The bone fragments are replaced, and the muscular, subcutaneous, and skin layers are closed in a routine manner. The authors recommend placement of a drain tube in the dorsum of the cranium for 48 h postoperatively and 50 mg of cortisone pre- and postoperatively. Mineral mix was added to the ration of hypophysectomized gilts as a permanent dietary supplement (Kraeling et al., 1986).

Administration of 100 ml of 10% saline i.v. intraoperatively may help reduce brain size. Also, an increase in mortality was noted when nitrous oxide was used in the anesthetic protocol (Kraeling et al., 1986). Postoperatively, analgesics are required, and the pig should be monitored closely to maintain homeostasis.

SPINAL CORD ISCHEMIA AND HEMORRHAGE

Spinal cord ischemia can be a complication of aortic surgery (see Chapter 9) or vascular damage. Spinal cord damage usually becomes clinically relevant after 20 min of cross-clamp time in the suprarenal aorta but may be extended in the postrenal aorta. Cross-clamping of the thoracic aorta distal to the branching of the left subclavian aorta for 30 min will consistently produce ischemic damage (Qayumi et al., 1997). Studies of healing of dural substitutes have also been performed following laminectomy (Chapter 11), excision of the dura, and implantation of substitutes such as biomaterials or allografts (Haq et al., 2004). An angiogram of the distal aorta and its branches is illustrated in Figure 10.26.

The model can be surgically produced by performing a left lateral thoracotomy (see Chapter 9) or a left-flank celiotomy (see Chapter 4 and Chapter 7) to approach the aorta. The aorta may either be clamped with vascular clamps or encircled with an umbilical tape snare. Alternatively, selected dorsal branches of the aorta may be ligated. Experience from aortic anastomosis (see Chapter 9) demonstrates that this must be more than two contiguous pairs of arteries.

Clamping of the prerenal aorta will produce hypertension that must be controlled with blood volume reduction or infusions of Na nitroprusside. Cross-clamping of the aorta will also produce hypoperfusion of all of the distal organs with the potential of dysfunction. Animals may become paraplegic.

If this model is performed as a survival procedure, intensive care of the animal postoperatively is imperative. Housing the animal in deep wood shavings or on padding is necessary. Nutritional support may have to be administered.

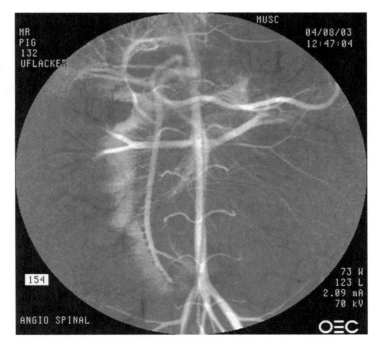

FIGURE 10.26 Angiogram of the distal aorta, renal, spinal and iliac arteries. (Courtesy of Renan Uflacker, Department of Radiology, Medical University of South Carolina.)

Similar types of clinical syndromes occur with spinal cord hemorrhage (Ganz and Zwetnow, 1990) associated with decompression injury models at a simulated dive depth of 200 ft of seawater with decompression after 43 min at 60 ft of seawater per second (Broome et al., 1997; Dick et al., 1997). Approximately two thirds of the swine will develop clinical neurologic syndromes related to petechia and ecchymoses in the spinal cord. Approximately 20% of the affected swine will die. Additional injuries due to dysbarism may occur and require treatment. This model avoids having to perform surgical procedures.

Experimental allergic encephalomyelitis (EAE) has been induced in minipigs at the National Institute of Health (NIH) by injection of spinal cord homogenate in Freund's adjuvant with or without pertussis toxin. Animals develop a transient monophasic illness with paresis, which can be graded clinically. The model is proposed as a preclinical animal to study treatments of multiple sclerosis (Singer et al., 2000).

STROKE MODELS

Pigs are emerging as a stroke model, mainly induced by ligation or occlusion of the middle cerebral artery (Olsen et al., 2003; Sakoh et al., 2000). In the author's experience, swine are protected against embolic cerebrovascular disease caused by such procedures as chronic catheterization, probably because of the anatomy of the rete mirabile. When swine experience embolic disease, it is characterized as transient blindness, which reverses within a few days.

However, a short-term acute model of inducing cerebral ischemia by injection of 0.5 ml of autologous clot into the ascending pharyngeal artery, causing occlusion of the internal carotid artery and rete mirabile, has been developed (Culp et al., 2004). Bilateral snare occlusion of the internal carotid arteries reduces cerebral blood flow, which is rapidly compensated by the basilar artery (Wang et al., 2005). Consequently, the chronic models will probably have to be produced by direct occlusion of the target artery in the brain. The artery of interest can be approached either via direct craniotomy or a transorbital approach. An acute model of intracranial hemorrhage and hematoma has been produced by direct infusion of blood into the frontal white matter (Wagner et al., 2000). For surgical occlusion models, the artery of interest is identified by angiography, and the area is approached surgically using the surgical techniques identified earlier. See the earlier sections on craniotomy and hypophysectomy for the surgical approaches.

In a chronic model of stroke, postoperative care will require intensive effort to prevent discomfort to the animal. If it has reduced mobility, it is recommended that the animal be housed either with soft padding on the floor and sides of the cage or, preferably, in deep wood shavings to prevent decubitus and scraping injury. Animals may require parenteral nutrition either i.v. or p.o. Unless analgesics are contraindicated by the protocol, they should be utilized. In direct surgical ligation models, cerebral edema may have to be controlled.

CEREBROSPINAL FLUID (CSF) COLLECTION AND
EPIDURAL INJECTION

Retrieval of CSF from the spinal cord and epidural administration of pharmacological agents may be necessary for some experimental procedures. Epidural administration of analgesics, such as morphine, may be desirable for preemptive analgesia for surgical procedures caudal to the thorax. The epidural cavity or space is the site of injection of substances such as analgesics. The subarachnoid cavity is the site of interest for obtaining CSF.

The vertebral bone structure in the pig is massive compared to other large animal species used in research. In addition, the intervertebral spaces are narrow and the dorsal processes of the vertebra tend to interfere with access to the vertebral spaces because of their size and caudal orientation. The pig does not normally have the ability to flex the spine as much as other species, giving them a more stiff posture. The vertebral formula is C7, T14–T15, L6–L7, S4, Cy20–Cy23. The sacral vertebrae are partially fused. The spinal cord terminates with the conus medullaris at S2–S3 and follows down the remaining vertebra with the cauda equina and the filum terminale. This is unlike the human in which the conus medullaris is located at L1–L2. The epidural space tends to contain fatty deposits. The cross section of the vertebral canal from outside to inside is as follows: dorsal longitudinal ligament, epidural cavity, dura mater, subdural cavity, arachnoid membrane, subarachnoid cavity, pia mater, and spinal cord.

Epidural Injection

Swine must be anesthetized for these procedures (Boogerd and Peters, 1986; Punto, 1980). Complete aseptic technique should be utilized when invading the spinal canal. This includes shaving, surgical skin preparation, and wearing sterile gloves. Most porcine spinal canals can be accessed using 20–22 g, 1.5–3.0 in. (3.8–7.6 cm) spinal needles (Figure 10.27).

Epidural administration of analgesics for preemptive analgesia is the most common procedure for which this technique is used. However, administration of test substances or radiopaque solutions may require this technique. Epidural administration is usually performed in the lumbar region because the regional analgesia is only effective for procedures caudal to the thorax. It is necessary to flex the spine to separate the intervertebral spaces. This is performed either by hanging the pig's rear legs off the end of a table while it is in sternal recumbency or by bending the rear legs forward under the abdomen in the same position.

An imaginary line is drawn between the most cranial aspects of the bilateral tuber coxae (wings of ileum), which are readily palpable. The intervertebral space cranial to this line will be L5–L6 or L6–L7. The needle is placed between the palpable dorsal spinous processes and advanced slowly through the intervertebral space until a popping sensation is felt and there is a lack of resistance. If the vertebral body is hit, the needle will not advance, and it should be withdrawn to try again. After entry into the site, the stylet is removed from the needle to ensure that blood or other fluid does not appear in the needle hub. The syringe is then attached, and the injection is given. There should not be any resistance to the injection if it is in the epidural space. Catheters can be passed into the epidural space by the same technique. Larger catheters may require a partial dorsal laminectomy to place them in this position.

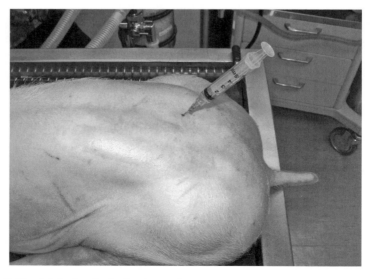

FIGURE 10.27 Epidural injection in the lumbar region.

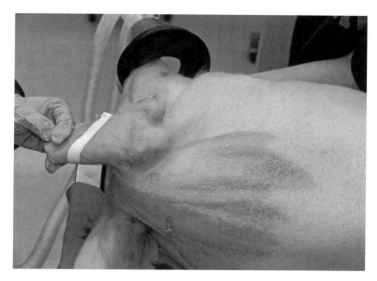

FIGURE 10.28 Spinal tap of the cisterna magna.

CSF COLLECTION

The area is prepped as per the directions above. CSF can be obtained from the lumbar region by use of the same technique and landmarks as described earlier. A greater volume can be obtained from the cisterna magna accessed through the foramen magnum (Figure 10.28). If this area is used, the pig's head is leaned off the end of a table to flex the neck. Alternatively, the pig may be placed in lateral recumbency and the neck flexed by an assistant. The caudal end of the occipital bone and the nuchal tubercles are palpated. The needle is passed slightly caudal to this area at an angle (approximately 60°) toward the oral cavity to enter the foramen magnum cranial to the body of the axis.

For CSF collection, the subarachnoid cavity is the site of interest. The spinal needle is passed into the epidural space as described earlier. Then a slight resistance is felt as the arachnoid membrane is penetrated. The stylet is removed from the needle and clear CSF fluid will drip from the needle if the location is correct. Passing the needle too deep will penetrate the spinal cord, and a reflex jerk will be observed. If blood comes from the needle, then either the venous plexus or a small artery has been hit. These problems should not occur if the needle is passed on the midline in the fashion described earlier. CSF catheters can be implanted chronically into the brain, using a burr hole in the cranium over the site of the central system in the brain (Figure 10.29). CSF catheters must be skillfully implanted to prevent infection and migration out of the burr hole.

An exact calculation is not available but, generally, administration of <5 ml of solution or collection of 5–10 ml of CSF twice a week is not harmful to 25- to 50-kg swine.

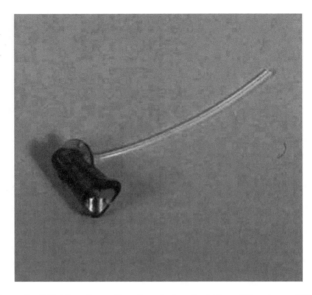

FIGURE 10.29 Cerebrospinal fluid catheter for chronic implantation. (Courtesy of Da Vinci Biomedical.)

REFERENCES

Adams, R.J., 1988, Opthalmic system, in Swindle, M.M. and Adams, R.J., Eds., *Experimental Surgery and Physiology: Induced Animal Models of Human Disease*, Baltimore, MD: Williams and Wilkins, pp. 125–153.

Bermejo, A., Gonzalez, O., and Gonzalez, J.M., 1993, The pig as an animal model for experimentation on the temporomandibular articular complex, *Oral Surg. Oral Med. Oral Pathol.*, 75(1): 18–23.

Boogerd, W. and Peters, A.C.B., 1986, A simple method for obtaining cerebrospinal fluid from a pig model of herpes encephalitis, *Lab. Anim. Sci.*, 36(4): 386–388.

Bradley, P.F., 1982, A two-stage procedure for reimplantation of autogenous freeze-treated mandibular bone, *J. Oral Maxillofac. Surg.*, 40(5): 278–284.

Broome, J.R., Dick, E.J., Jr., and Dutka, A.J., 1997, Neurological decompression illness in swine, *Avia. Space Environ. Med.*, 67: 207–213.

Cameron, D.E., Tam, V.K.H., Cheng, W., and Braxton, M., 1992, Studies in the physiology of cardiopulmonary bypass using a swine model, in Swindle, M.M., Ed., *Swine as Models in Biomedical Research*, Ames, IA: Iowa State University Press, pp. 185–196.

Campbell, W.M. and Kern, E.B., 1981, The nasal cycle in swine, *Rhinology*, 19(3): 127–148.

Chandler, M.J., Smith, P.J., Samuelson, D.A., and MacKay, E.O., 1999, Photoreceptor density of the domestic pig retina, *Vet. Opthalmol.*, 2: 179–184.

Culp, W.C, Porter, T.R., Lowery, J., Xie, F., Roberson, P.K., and Marky, L., 2004, Intracranial clot lysis with intravenous microbubbles and transcranial ultrasound in swine, *Stroke*, 35(10): 2407–2411.

Curtis, S.E., Edwards, S.A., and Gonyou, H.W., 2001, Ethology and psychology, in Pond, W.G. and Mersmann, H.J., Eds., *Biology of the Domestic Pig*, Ithaca, NY: Cornell University Press, pp. 41–78.

Del Priore, L.V., Tezel, T.H., and Kaplan, H.J., 2004, Survival of allogeneic porcine retinal pigment epithelial sheets after subretinal transplantation, *Invest. Opthalmol.*, 45(3): 985–992.

Dick, E.J., Jr., Broome, J.R., and Hayward, I.J., 1997, Acute neurologic decompression illness in pigs: lesions of the spinal cord and brain, *Lab. Anim. Sci.*, 47(1): 50–56.

Donovan, M.G., Dickerson, N.C., Hellstein, J.W., and Hanson, L.J., 1993, Autologous calvarial and iliac onlay bone grafts in miniature swine, *J. Oral Maxillofac. Surg.*, 51(8): 898–903.

Drisko, J.E., Faidley, T.D., Hora, D.F., Jr., Niebauer, G.W., Feeney, W.P., Friscino, B.H., and Hickey, G.J., 1996, Transorbital approach to the porcine pituitary, *J. Invest. Surg.*, 9(4): 305–311.

Eubanks, D.L. and Gilbo, K., 2005, Trimming tusks in the Yucatan minipigs, *Lab Anim.*, 34(9): 35–38.

Felix, B., Leger, M.E., Albe-Fessard, D., Marcilloux, J.C., Rampin, O., and Laplace, J.P., 1999, Stereotaxic atlas of the pig brain, *Brain Res. Bull.,* 49: 1–137.

Fyffe, J.G., Neal, T.A., Butler, W.P., and Johnson, T.E., 2005, The *ex vivo* pig eye as a replacement model for laser safety training, *Comp. Med.,* 55(6): 503–509.

Ganz, J.C. and Zwetnow, N.N., 1990, A quantitative study of some factors affecting the outcome of experimental epidural bleeding in swine, *Acta Neurochir. (Wien),* 102(3–4): 164–172.

Garca, M., Ruiz-Ederra, J., Hernandez-Barbachano, H., and Vecino, E., 2005, Topography of pig retinal ganglion cells, *J. Comp. Neurol.,* 486(4): 361–372.

Ghosh, F., Wong, F., Johansson, K., Bruun, A., and Petters, R.M., 2004, Transplantation of full-thickness retina in the rhodopsin transgenic pig, *Retina,* 24(1): 98–109.

Haq, I., Cruz-Almeida, Y., Siqueira, E.B., Norenberg, M., Green, B.A., and Levi, A.D., 2004, Postoperative fibrosis after surgical treatment of the porcine spinal cord: a comparison of dural substitutes, *J. Neurosurg. Spine,* 2: 50–54.

Hargreaves, J.A. and Mitchell, B., 1969, Features of the dentition of the pig for experimental work, *J. Dent. Res.,* 48(21): 1103.

Hendrickson, A. and Hicks, D., 2002, Distribution and density of medium and short wavelength selective cones in the domestic pig retina, *Exp. Eye Res.,* 74(4): 435–444.

Jackson, T.L., Hillenkamp, J., Williamson, T.H., Clarke, K.W., Almubarak, A.I., and Marshall, J., 2003, An experimental model of rhematogenous retinal detachment: surgical results and glial cell response, *IOVS,* 44(9): 4026–4034.

Jacobs, G.H., Calderone, J.B., Sakai, T., Lewis, G.P., and Fisher, S.K., 2002, An animal model for studying cone function in retinal detachment, *Doc. Opthalmol.,* 104(1): 119–132.

Jarrahy, R., Shahinain, H.K., Young, J., and Berci, G., 1999, Endoscopic skull base surgery II: a new animal model for surgery of the posterior fossa, *J. Invest. Surg.,* 12(3): 335–339.

Jensen, T., 2006, Personal communication, Ph.D. thesis (in progress), Aalborg Hospital, Aarhus University Hospital and Institute of Odontology, Faculty of Health Sciences, University of Copenhagen, Denmark.

Kalkwarf, K.L., Krejci, R.F., Edison, A.R., and Reinhardt, R.A., 1983, Subjacent heat production during tissue excision with electrosurgery, *J. Oral Maxillofac. Surg.,* 41(10): 653–657.

Kraeling, R.R., Barb, C.R., and Rampacek, G.B., 1986, Hypophysectomy and hypophysial stalk transection in the pig: technique and application to studies of ovarian follicular development, in Tumbleson, M.E., Ed., *Swine in Biomedical Research,* Vol. 1, New York: Plenum Press, pp. 425–436.

Larsen, M., Bjarkam, C.R., Østergaard, K., West, M.J., and Sørensen, J.C., 2004, The anatomy of the porcine subthalmic nucleus evaluated with immunohistochemistry and design based stereology, *Anat. Embryol.,* 208(3): 239–247.

Lind, N.M., 2005, Brain Dopamine Function in Pigs: Behavioral Aspects, Ph.D. thesis, Faculty of Health Sciences, University of Copenhagen, Denmark.

Nielsen, L.S. and Lind, N.M., 2005, Measurements of three ocular parameters in the Göttingen minipigs, *Scand. J. Lab. Anim. Sci.,* 32(1): 9–16.

North, A.F., 1988, Oral and maxillofacial surgery, in Swindle, M.M. and Adams, R.J., Eds., *Experimental Surgery and Physiology: Induced Animal Models of Human Disease,* Baltimore, MD: Williams and Wilkins, pp. 173–203.

Olsen, A.K., Watanabe, H., Bjarkam, C., Rodell, A., Zeidler, D., Blankholm, A.D., Cumming, P., and Gyldensted, C., 2003, A porcine model for long-term stroke studies, *Proc. Scand-LAS Annu. Symp.,* p. 56.

Ouhayoun, J.P., Shabana, A.H.M., Issahakian, S., Patat, J.L., Guillemin, G., Sawaf, M.H., and Forest, N., 1992, Histological evaluation of natural coral skeleton as a grafting material in miniature swine mandible, *J. Mater. Sci., Mater. Med.,* 3(3): 222–228.

Petters, R.M., Alexander, C.A., Wells, K.D., 1997, Genetically engineered large animal model for studying cone photoreceptor survival and degeneration in retinitis pigmentosa, *Nat. Biotechnol.,* 15(10): 965–970.

Punto, L., 1980, Lumbar leptomenigeal and radicular reactions after the subarachnial injection of water-soluble contrast media, meglumine iocarmate and metrizamide: an experimental study in the pig, *Acta Vet. Scand.,* 73(Suppl.): 1–52.

Qayumi, A.K., Nanusz, M.T., Lyster, D.M., and Gillespie, K.D., 1997, Animal model for investigation of spinal cord injury caused by aortic cross-clamping, *J. Invest. Surg.,* 10(1): 47–52.

Quiroz-Mercado, H., Suarez-Tata, L., Magdalenic, R., Murillo-Lopez, S., Garcia-Aguirre, G., Guerrero-Naranjo, J., and Rodriguez-Reyes, A.A., 2004, Perfluorocarbon perfused vitrectomy: animal studies, *Am. J. Opthalmol.*, 137(2): 287–293.

Rapp, B., Reilly, M.A., Hamilton, P.D., and Ravi, N., 2006, A comparison of the viscoelastic properties of porcine crystallins and OH terminal PANAM dendrimers, *Polym. Prepr.*, 47(1): 85–86.

Ravi, N., Aliyar, H.A., and Hamilton, P.D., 2005, Hydrogel nanocomposite as a synthetic inta-ocular lens capable of accommodation, *Macromol. Symp.*, 227: 191–201.

Robinson, I.B. and Sarnat, B.G., 1955, Growth pattern of the pig mandible, *Am. J. Anat.*, 96(41): 37–64.

Reilly, M.A., Hamilton, P.D., and Ravi, N., in press, Dynamic multi-arm radial lens stretcher: a machine analog of the ciliary body, *Invest. Ophthalmol. Vis. Sci.*

Rosenquist, J.B. and Rosenquist, K., 1982, Effects of bone grafting on maxillary bone healing in the growing pig, *J. Oral Maxillofac. Surg.*, 40(9): 566–569.

Roth, T.E., Goldberg, J.S., and Behrents, R.G., 1984, Synovial fluid pressure determinations in the temporo-mandibular joint, *Oral Surg. Oral Med. Oral Pathol.*, 57(5): 583–588.

Ruiz-Ederra, J., Garcia, M., Hicks, D., and Vecino, E., 2004, Comparative study of the three neurofilament subunits within pig and human retinal ganglion cells, *Mol. Vision*, 10(1): 83–92.

Sachs, H.G., Gekeler, F., Schwahn, H., Jakob, W., Kohler, M., Schulmeyer, F., Marienhagen, J., Brunner, U., and Framme, C., 2005, Implantation of stimulation electrodes in the subretinal space to demonstrate cortical responses in Yucatan minipig in the course of visual prosthesis development, *Eur. J. Opthalmol.*, 15(4): 492–499.

Sack, W.O., 1982, *Essentials of Pig Anatomy and Harowitz/Kramer Atlas of Musculoskeletal Anatomy of the Pig*, Ithaca, NY: Veterinary Textbooks.

Sakoh, M., Røhl, L., Gyldensted, C., Gjedde, A., and Østergaard, L., 2000, Cerebral blood flow and blood volume measured by magnetic resonance imaging bolus tracking after acute stroke in pigs: comparison with (^{15}O) H_2O positron emission tomography, *Stroke*, 31(8): 1958–1964.

Salinas-Zeballos, M.E., Zeballos, G.A., and Gootman, P.M., 1986, A stereotaxic atlas of the developing swine (Sus scrofa) forebrain, in Tumbleson, M.E., Ed., *Swine in Biomedical Research*, Vol. 2, New York: Plenum Press, pp. 887–906.

Schantz, L.D., Laber-Laird, K., Bingel, S., and Swindle, M., 1996, Pigs: applied anatomy of the gastrointestinal tract, in Jensen, S.L., Gregersen, H., Moody, F., and Shokouh-Amiri, M.H., Eds., *Essentials of Experimental Surgery: Gastroenterology*, New York: Harwood Academic Publishers, pp. 2611–2619.

Sims, C.D., Butler, P.E.M., Casanova, R., Randolph, M.A., and Yaremchuk, M.J., 1997, Prolonged general anesthesia for experimental craniofacial surgery in fetal swine, *J. Invest. Surg.*, 10(1–2): 53–57.

Singer, B.A., Tresser, N.J., Frank, J.A., McFarland, H.F., and Biddison, W.E., 2000, Induction of experimental allergic encephalomyelitis in the NIH minipig, *J. Neuroimmunol.*, 105(1): 7–19.

Sisson, S. and St. Clair, S.E., 1975a, Appendages, in Getty, R., Ed., *Sisson and Grossman's The Anatomy of the Domestic Animals*, 5th ed., Philadelphia, PA: WB Saunders, pp. 1222–1230.

Sisson, S. and St. Clair, S.E., 1975b, Porcine digestive system, in Getty, R., Ed., *The Anatomy of the Domestic Animals*, 5th ed., Philadelphia, PA: WB Saunders, pp. 1268–1282.

Sørensen, J.C., Bjarkam, C.R., Danielsen, E.H., Simonsen, C.Z., and Geneser, F.A., 2000, Oriented sectioning of irregular tissue blocks in relation to computerized scanning modalities: results from the domestic pig brain, *J. Neurosci. Methods*, 104(1): 93–98.

Stodkilde-Jorgensen, H., Frokiaer, J., Kirkeby, H.J., Madsen, F., and Boye, N., 1986, Preparation of a cerebral perfusion model in the pig: anatomic considerations, in Tumbleson, M.E., Ed., *Swine in Biomedical Research*, Vol. 1, New York: Plenum Press, pp. 719–725.

Swindle, K.E., Hamilton, P.D., and Ravi, N., 2006a, Advancements in the development of artificial vitreous humor utilizing polyacrylamide copolymers with disulfide crosslinkers, *Polym. Prepr.*, 47(1): 59–60.

Swindle, K.E., Hamilton, P.D., and Ravi, N., 2006b, Comparison of viscoelastic properties of porcine vitreous to copolymeric hydrogels evaluated as potential vitreous substitutes, *Assoc. Res. Vision Opthalmol.*, 1455/B919.

Swindle, K.E., Hamilton, P.D., and Ravi, N., in press, In situ formation of hydrogels as vitreous substitutes: viscoelastic comparison to porcine vitreous, *J. Biomed. Mater. Res.* In press.

Swindle, M.M., 1983, *Basic Surgical Exercises Using Swine*, Philadelphia, PA: Prager Publishers.

Swindle, M.M. and Bobbie, D.L., 1987, Comparative Anatomy of the Pig, Charles River Technical Bulletin 4(1): 1–4.

Terheyden, H., Jepsen, S., Möller, B., Tucker, M.M., and Rueger, D.C., 1999, Sinus floor augmentation with simultaneous placement of dental implants using a combination of deproteinized bone xenografts and recombinant human osteogenic protein-1, A histometric study in miniature pigs, *Clin. Oral Implants Res.*, 10: 510–521.

Wagner, K.R., Hua, Y., de Courten-Myers, G.M., Broderick, J.P., Nishimura, R.N., Lu, S.Y., and Dwyer, B.E., 2000, Tin-mesoporphyrin, a potent heme oxygenase inhibitor, for treatment of intracerebral hemorrhage: *in vivo* and *in vitro* studies, *Cell. Mol. Biol.*, 46(3): 597–608.

Wang, Y., Hosler, G., Zhang, T., and Okada, Y., 2005, Effects of temporary bilateral ligation of the internal carotid arteries on the low and high-frequency somatic evoked potentials in the swine, *Clin. Neurophysiol.*, 116(10): 2420–2428.

Warfvinge, K., Kiligaard, J.F., Lavik, E.B., Scherfig, E., Langer, R., Klassen, H.J., and Young, M.J., 2005, Retinal progenitor cell xenografts to the pig retina, *Arch. Opthalmol.*, 123(10): 1385–1393.

Watanabe, H., Andersen, F., Simonsen, C.Z., Evans, S.M., Gjedde, A., Cumming, P., and DaNeX Study Group, 2001, MR-based statistical atlas of the Göttingen minipigs brain, *Neuroimage*, 14: 1089–1096.

Weaver, M.E., Sorenson, F.M., and Jump, E.B., 1962, The miniature pig as an experimental animal in dental research, *Arch. Oral Biol.*, 7(1): 17–24.

11 Musculoskeletal System and Orthopedic Procedures

GENERAL PRINCIPLES OF SURGERY AND SURGICAL ANATOMY

The bones and musculature of the pig are massive (Figure 1.34 and Figure 1.35), which is consistent with the use of pork as a primary food source for humans. The cortex of the bones also tends to be thick compared to other animals, which provides the strength necessary to support an animal that tends to be heavy and have a small stature. Diseases of the joints occur frequently, probably because of the rapid weight gain on an immature skeleton in young animals (Sack, 1982). Swine have seldom been used as models for musculoskeletal or orthopedic experiments because of the conformation of the muscles and skeletal axis. However, the proportion and distribution of muscles and bones that support and provide locomotion for the body are similar between farm and miniature pigs, and they have been proposed as a model of growth of the system because of their rapid weight gain (Bobilya et al., 1991; Davies and Henning, 1986). They have also been used as models of bone healing and epiphyseal plate growth (Ahn et al., 1997; Alitalo, 1979; Allan et al., 1990; Peltonen et al., 1984), and of congenital hip dislocation (Salter, 1968) and experimentally produced scoliosis (MacEwen, 1973). Recently there has been an increased interest in the model for the evaluation of grafting techniques (Costa et al., 2003; Doll et al., 2001; Donovan et al., 1993; Ouhayoun et al., 1992; Schliephake and Langner, 1997), bone implants (Buser et al., 1991; Illi and Feldman, 1998), lumbar fusion (Li et al., 2004; Zou et al., 2004), osteonecrosis (Swiontkowski et al., 1993), osteochondral defects (Gotterbarm et al., 2006; Peretti et al., 2006; Vasura et al., 2006), and osteoporosis (Boyce et al., 1995). The temporomandibular joint (Chapter 10, Figure 10.8 and Figure 10.10) of swine has also been determined to be more similar to humans than many other species in a comparative macroscopic study (Bermejo et al., 1993).

There are conflicting data on the ability of cartilaginous lesions induced by 6- to 7-mm biopsy punches in the trochlear groove of the knee to heal in immature pigs. A study in Yorkshire pigs (Peretti et al., 2006) indicates that they do not spontaneously heal, whereas a study in Landrace pigs (Vasara et al., 2006) indicates that good spontaneous repair does occur. There may be a difference in this characteristic between breeds of farm pigs, and performing the studies in more mature Göttingen miniature pigs indicated that incomplete repair occurred (Gotterbarm et al., 2006). Also the study in Yorkshire pigs only lasted 8 weeks and that in Landrace pigs lasted longer. Unless the study involves examination of a pediatric model, it seems that more mature miniature pigs would provide a better chronic model, especially because these studies require months to years for complete evaluation.

Mammals have a predominance of Type II B muscle fibers (Figure 11.1) with a lesser extent of Type IIA, IIC, and IIX fibers. Locomotion characteristics of swine, as well as most other quadrupeds, are also dissimilar from those of humans (Adams, 1988; MacEwen, 1973; Salter, 1968). An extensive dissection atlas of the musculoskeletal system of the domestic pig has been published (Sack, 1982). Laboratory dissection manuals for the fetal pig are available (Chiasson et al., 1997; Donnelly and Wistreich, 1996), and a complete description of the anatomy and physiology of the musculoskeletal system in the domestic pig has been published (Novakofski and McCusker, 2001).

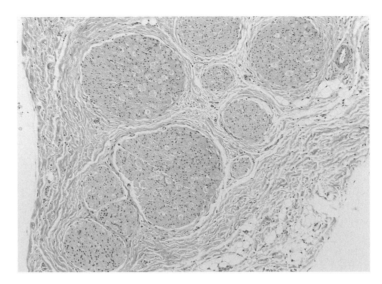

FIGURE 11.1 Histologic section of skeletal muscle and peripheral nerve. H&E, ×100.

There are differences in the closure of the epiphyses of the long bones among breeds of swine. The miniature pig breeds tend to have an earlier closure than domestic farm breeds, which typically have epiphyseal closure between 3 and 4 years of age (Sisson, 1975). Dates of epiphyseal closure for some of the breeds of miniature pigs are the following: Hanford, 2–4 years; Yucatan, 2–3 years; Yucatan micropig and Göttingen minipig, 1.5–2 years. Details of the vertebral formula for swine are in Chapter 1 and Chapter 10.

Muscles may be transected, dissected between muscular fibers, or preferably divided in the fascial plane between muscle bellies. The fascial sheath surrounding the muscle provides the predominant strength for holding sutures and must be included when suturing surgical incisions. Sutures may pass all the way through a muscle body, and the sheath on both sides of the muscle or the muscular sheath can be sutured by itself (Swindle, 1983).

AMPUTATION OF A DIGIT AND HOOF TRIMMING

The principal digits of the pig are numbers III and IV. Vestigial digits, numbers II and V, form the dewclaws, which are positioned caudal to the principal digits. All terminate in hooves that may periodically have to be trimmed, using hoof nippers on swine that are not housed on concrete floors or rough material that allows constant wear of the hoof (Figure 11.2). The dewclaws are non-weight-bearing, and their amputation does not result in any consequential debility to the pig. If the principal digits become injured or infected, they may require amputation. The pig will retain its locomotive ability as long as one of the pair is retained intact.

The digit is amputated in the joint between either the metacarpal bone and the proximal phalanx or between the proximal and middle phalanx, depending upon the extent of the lesion. A horizontal incision is made across the dorsal aspect of the digit distal to the joint in which the amputation is to be performed. Two vertical incisions are made, up the sides of the digit extending to the ventral surface of the joint in which the amputation is being performed. The dorsal flap is then bluntly dissected to the surface of the joint. The branches of the digital veins on the dorsal surface are ligated and the tendons severed at their insertions on the bones. A flap is then dissected on the palmar surface of the digit, and the vessels and tendons are similarly transected. The skin on the palmar surface is transected horizontally cranial to the joint. The joint is then disarticulated and amputated. The tendons and muscles are trimmed and tacked down across the ventral surface of

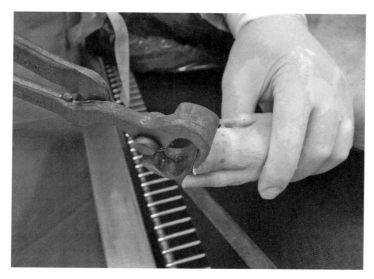

FIGURE 11.2 Trimming a hoof with hoof nippers.

the joint with stay sutures. The ventral aspect of the dorsal flap is sutured with simple interrupted sutures to the skin on the palmar surface of the joint. This will leave a skin flap that covers the joint from the dorsal to the palmar aspect of the joint.

The foot is bandaged leaving the intact digit uncovered. The animal should be housed in clean dry bedding, and the bandage changed daily for the first few days following surgery.

TENDON AND LIGAMENT REPAIR

The major tendons that are substantial in size and accessible through superficial surgical dissection are the common calcaneus and the popliteus. The digital extensor and flexor tendons are also readily accessible on the distal portion of the metacarpal and metatarsal bones, and on the cranial and palmar surfaces of the digits if small to midsized tendons are preferred. The patellar ligaments are the main superficial ligaments. These tendons and ligaments may be used in wound-healing studies and may also require clinical repair owing to trauma, especially of the digital extensor and flexor ligaments.

Methodology for suturing the ligaments is the same as for other species and has been described in the pig (Swindle, 1983). The common calcaneal tendon includes the tendons of the superficial flexor and the larger oval gastrocnemius tendon. It is approached with a caudal vertical incision along the distal end of the tibia ending at the tuber calcis. The popliteal tendon is approached using a similar incision along the caudal aspect of the humerus ending at the olecranon. The digital tendons can be palpated on the distal aspect of the legs and direct incisions made over them. The patellar ligaments can be approached using a vertical incision along the cranial aspect of the stifle joint, with the ventral patellar ligament being the most accessible.

After transecting the ligament or tendon, the edge is grasped with forceps and repaired using the Bunnell-Mayer technique (Figure 11.3). Starting well back from the edge of the incised tendon, a transection suture is placed through the tendon from side to side, using a double-armed suture with nonabsorbable material. The ends of the suture are left equidistant from the tendon. In an alternating pattern, the needles reenter the tendon at a 45° angle aimed distally. Sutures are continued distally in this crossing pattern until the outer edges of the severed tendon are exited. The same suture pattern is then placed in the distal end of the severed tendon. The ends of the sutures are tied along the lateral and medial edges of the tendon at the incised edge. The subcutaneous tissues

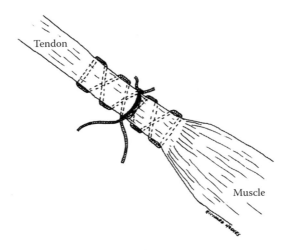

FIGURE 11.3 Suturing technique for repair of a tendon.

and skin are closed in a routine fashion. Postoperatively, the limb may require immobilization in a plaster cast or require some other form of support for a short time.

TAIL AMPUTATION

Swine routinely traumatize the tails of less dominant animals when housed in groups. This may require corrective surgery. The tail is amputated between the bodies of the coccygeal vertebrae in the joint. It is best to amputate the entire length of the tail to prevent further trauma.

A V-shaped flap is made with the long ends of the flap on the dorsal and ventral aspects of the tail. The blood vessels along the ventral and lateral surfaces of the tail are identified and ligated. The tail is disarticulated in the joint, and the flap is sutured using a simple interrupted pattern.

HERNIA REPAIR

Both umbilical and inguinal hernias occur spontaneously in swine. Inguinal hernias and retained testicles are more common on the left side (St-Jean and Anderson, 1999). Both conditions have a genetic predisposition.

For inguinal hernias, the pig is placed in dorsal recumbency. A skin incision is made directly over the inguinal canal, which can be readily palpated on a line drawn between the mid to cranial aspect of the cranial surface of the thigh and the midline. After the skin incision is made, the edges of the femoral ring are bluntly dissected away from the herniated tissues, which typically include omentum and fat without the intestines. The spermatic cord should not be damaged in this process. After the herniated tissue is free from attachments, it is bluntly replaced into the abdominal cavity. It may have to be held in place with a blunt instrument, or the pig's hindquarters directed upward, to move the herniated tissues and viscera away from the surgical site. The muscles surrounding the inguinal ring are sutured together with simple interrupted sutures using 2/0 or 3/0 nonabsorbable synthetic suture material. The inguinal canal should not be sutured so tightly as to constrict the blood flow to the blood vessels in the spermatic cord. The skin and subcutaneous tissues are closed in a routine manner.

An inguinal hernia may be created experimentally in small swine by making an incision over the inguinal ring and incising the muscles on the cranial edge of the ring (Garcia-Ruiz et al., 1998). This relaxation of the ring should lead to herniation postsurgically and can be tested at the time of surgery by applying pressure to the abdomen to cause the viscera to herniate.

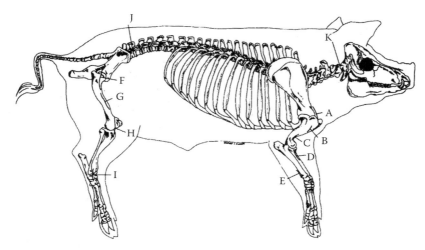

FIGURE 11.4 Surgical approaches to the bones and joints. A — shoulder joint, B — proximal humerus, C — distal humerus, D — proximal radius, E — ulna, F — hip joint, G — femur, H — stifle (knee) joint, I — tarsocrural (hock) joint, J — subarachnoid space injection site, K — cisterna magna injection site.

Umbilical hernias are usually closed around herniated omentum and fat, and are rarely clinically relevant. The umbilical hernia may be closed after making a skin incision directly over the herniation and by either replacing or excising the eviscerated material. The umbilicus is closed with nonabsorbable sutures as described previously.

SURGICAL APPROACHES TO BONES AND JOINTS

The surgical approaches (Figure 11.4 and Figure 11.5) to bones and joints of the pig can be determined by the surgeons using their knowledge of other species, and by anatomic inspection

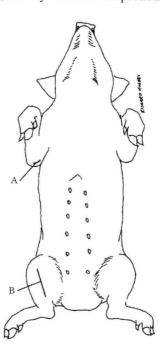

FIGURE 11.5 Surgical approaches to the bones and joints. A — medial aspect of the elbow, B — medial approach to the tibia.

and palpation of the animal prior to surgery. Surgical approaches to the major bones and joints that avoid major muscle dissection and vascular ligation are described here. Variations of these procedures may be dictated by the experimental protocol.

FORELEG

The shoulder joint is approached in the craniolateral aspect after flexion. The greater tubercle of the humerus is prominent, and the caudal part is readily palpated. The incision is made between the cranial and caudal portions of the tubercle alongside the infraspinatus tendon. The infraspinatus tendon may have to be transected at its attachment in order to be retracted caudally. The infraspinatus nerve should be avoided.

The humerus is not readily approached surgically because of the massiveness of the musculature. Surgical approaches from the lateral aspect will probably involve transecting musculature. The proximal shaft can be approached between the brachiocephalic muscle and the distal portion of the deltoideus. The distal portion of the shaft can be approached between the brachiocephalic and biceps brachii muscles cranially, and the lateral head of the triceps caudally. The radial nerve and deep branches of the brachial vessels should be avoided. The medial aspect is even more difficult to approach because of the close attachment of the leg to the trunk at that level. The distal shaft can be approached between the biceps brachii and the medial head of the triceps. The brachial artery and vein, and the ulnar nerve should be avoided.

The elbow joint is approached from a medial aspect between the medial epicondyle of the humerus and the tuber olecrani of the ulna. The tensor fasciae antebrachii muscle will have to be partially transected, and the medial head of the triceps reflected. Laterally, the approach can be made by reflecting the lateral head of the triceps proximally and incising the anconeus muscle.

The radius can be approached from a lateral incision between the common digital extensor and the ulnaris lateralis. The distal shaft of the radius can be approached medially between the extensor carpi radialis and the pronater teres with caudal reflection of the digital flexors. The radial artery and vein, and the median nerve should be avoided. The ulna is more accessible from the caudal aspect between the deep digital flexor and the ulnaris lateralis. The bones and joints of the distal limb can be readily palpated even in large swine and are easily approached from the cranial aspect.

HIND LIMB

The approach to the femoral head and neck and acetabulum is difficult even in small pigs. The trochanter major can be palpated with difficulty below a line drawn from the tuber coxae and the tuber ischiadicum. A curved incision starting above this area and following the line of the femur is made to expose the juncture of the gluteus medius, the gluteus superficialis, and the tensor fasciae latae. Dissection through this juncture of fascia and tendinous attachments with retraction of the vastus lateralis and biceps femoris caudally will expose the greater trochanter and cranial aspect of the hip joint. Depending upon the experimental procedure, full exposure of the femoral head and neck and the joint will require cutting the tendinous attachments of these muscles and further deep dissection.

The femoral shaft can be exposed by an incision following the lateral aspect of the bone and dissecting between the fascia of the tensor fascia latae and the biceps femoris.

The stifle (knee) joint is approached from a craniolateral incision after flexion. The incision is made lateral to the patella and the patellar ligament through the infrapatellar fat pad. The patella can be displaced laterally if required. The tibia is subcutaneous on the medial aspect and can be surgically approached at any level with minimal difficulty. The medial saphenous artery, vein, and nerve should be avoided.

The tarsocrural joint (hock) can be approached in either the lateral or medial aspect of the cranial border of the calcaneus. The malleolus of the fibula and the tuber olecrani can be palpated as landmarks, and the incision line should be between them. On the lateral aspect, the saphenous vein should be avoided. On the medial aspect, the collateral ligaments and tendons are more prominent. The digits may be approached as described for the foreleg and the amputation previously described.

VERTEBRAL COLUMN

The bones of the vertebral column of the pig are massive compared to many other species, and the intervertebral spaces are relatively narrow. With the pig in sternal recumbency, the vertebra can be approached from a dorsal midline incision as in other species (Haq et al., 2005; Li et al., 2002, 2004; Zou et al., 2004). In general, this involves stripping of the paravertebral muscles and retracting them laterally. A paramedian abdominal incision with a retroperitoneal approach has also been used (Zou et al., 2004). A laminectomy can then be performed to expose the spinal cord. Detailed studies of spinal cord fusion have been performed (Christensen, 2004). The Göttingen minipig was used for chronic studies because of its well-defined vertebral pedicles, which make screw-type techniques feasible, and because of its early growth plate closure at <2 years. Using posterior-lateral techniques, fusion can be achieved in 3 months with this model.

Injections into the subarachnoid space can be made between the last two lumbar vertebrae (see Chapter 10 for a complete description of the techniques). The lateral wings of L5 are at the level of the tuber coxae. More cranial positions are difficult because of the conformation of the spinous processes of the vertebrae and the difficulty in flexing the vertebral column. The pig is positioned with the hindquarters hanging over the end of a table to flex the vertebrae. A spinal tap needle is slowly inserted until either cerebrospinal fluid drips from the needle or the position is confirmed radiographically (Boogerd and Peters, 1986; Punto, 1980). The cisterna magna can be accessed by flexing the pig's head off the table or over a sandbag. The space is narrow, and the needle should be directed cranioventrally until access is confirmed by dripping of cerebrospinal fluid.

A ventral midline approach can be made to the cervical and lumbar vertebrae. For the cervical vertebrae, the trachea and esophagus must be directed laterally and care taken not to damage the vagal sheath. The lumbar vertebrae can be approached from a ventral midline incision (Alitalo, 1979). The viscera must be retracted and packed off with laparotomy sponges within the abdomen. The aorta, vena cava, and branching vessels must be retracted laterally to expose the vertebrae underlying the ventral longitudinal ligament. Care should be taken to not damage the lymphatics in the region or to ligate them if they are transected.

All of the musculoskeletal procedures should include the use of postoperative analgesics as part of the protocol. Use of phenylbutazone or other NSAIDs in combination with buprenorphine has been found to be superior to the use of either agent alone for procedures involving major muscular manipulations. Although NSAIDs have been found to delay cartilage and bone healing, it is unlikely that this would be significant with short-term use as preemptive or postoperative administration of a few days. Use of infusion pumps or catheters with local anesthetics is also effective.

BONE MARROW ASPIRATION

Bone marrow aspiration to collect samples may be performed with standard bone marrow aspiration needles. The medial aspect of the proximal tibia, approximately at the level of the tibial crest, is a suitable site for obtaining bone marrow samples in all ages of swine (Figure 11.6 and Figure 11.7). Bone marrow may also be aspirated from the dorsal aspect of the tuber coxae (Figure 11.8) and from the midsternum (Figure 11.9). Sternal samples are best obtained from neonatal and juvenile animals. After aseptic preparation of the skin, the bone marrow aspiration needle with a stylet is inserted through the skin and muscle to the bone. It is then rotated back and forth while exerting forward pressure. A popping sensation will be felt when the needle penetrates the cortex. The stylet is removed, and the sample is collected with a syringe containing saline or preservative. The needle

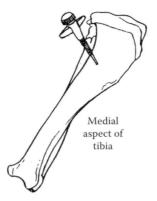

FIGURE 11.6 Bone marrow aspiration site in the medial aspect of the tibia.

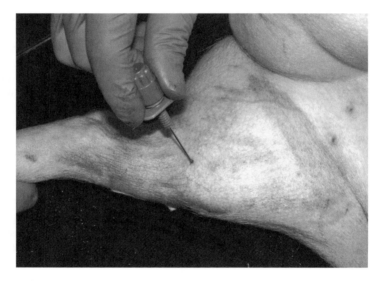

FIGURE 11.7 Aseptic approach to the medial tibial site for bone marrow aspiration or injection.

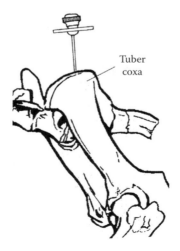

FIGURE 11.8 Bone marrow aspiration site in the tuber coxa (iliac crest).

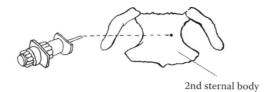

2nd sternal body

FIGURE 11.9 Bone marrow aspiration site in the second sternal body.

is removed when the sample is obtained. The same technique can be used to inject substances into the bone marrow. Bone marrow injections are absorbed in a similar manner to i.v. injections (Laber-Laird and Swindle, 1996).

REFERENCES

Adams, R.J., 1988, Musculoskeletal system, in Swindle, M.M. and Adams, R.J., Eds., *Experimental Surgery and Physiology: Induced Animal Models of Human Disease*, Baltimore, MD: Williams and Wilkins, pp. 10–41.

Ahn, D.K., Sims, C.D., Randolph, M.A., O'Connor, D., Butler, P.E., Amarante, M.T., and Yaremchuk, M.J., 1997, Craniofacial skeletal fixation using biodegradable plates and cyanoacrylate glue, *Plast. Reconstruct. Surg.*, 99(6): 1508–1515.

Alitalo, I., 1979, Ventral interbody implantation for fusion of the lumbar spine using polytetrafluoroethylene-carbonfiber and porous high density polyethylene: an experimental study in growing pigs, *Acta Vet. Scand.*, 71(Suppl.): 1–58.

Allan, D.G., Russell, G.G., Moreau, M.J., Raso, V.J., and Budney, D., 1990, Vertebral end plate failure in porcine and bovine models of spinal fracture instrumentation, *J. Orthop. Res.*, 8(1): 154–156.

Bermejo, A., Gonzalez, O., and Gonzalez, J.M., 1993, The pig as an animal model for experimentation on the temporomandibular articular complex, *Oral Surg. Oral Med. Oral Pathol.*, 75(1): 18–23.

Bobilya, D.J., Maurizi, M.G., Veum, T.L., and Allen, W.C., 1991, A bone biopsy procedure for neonatal pigs, *Lab Anim.*, 25(3): 222–225.

Boogerd, W. and Peters, A.C.B., 1986, A simple method for obtaining cerebrospinal fluid from a pig model of herpes encephalitis, *Lab. Anim. Sci.*, 36(4): 386–388.

Boyce, R.W., Ebert, D.C., Youngs, T.A., Paddock, C.L., Mosekilde, L., Stevens, M.L., and Gundersen, H.J.G., 1995, Unbiased estimation of vertebral trabecular connectivity in calcium restricted ovariectomized minipigs, *Bone*, 16(6): 637–642.

Buser, D., Schenk, R.K., Steinemann, S., Fiorellini, J.P., Fox, C.H., and Stich, H., 1991, Influence of surface characteristics on bone integration of titanium implants: a histomorphometric study in miniature pigs, *J. Biomed. Mater. Res.*, 25(7): 889–902.

Chiasson, R.B., Odlaug, T.O., and Radke, W.J., 1997, *Laboratory Anatomy of the Fetal Pig*, 11th ed., Dubuque, IA: Wm. C. Brown.

Christensen, G.B., 2004, Lumbar spinal fusion: outcome in relation to surgical methods, choice of implant and postoperative rehabilitation, *Acta Orthoped. Scand. Suppl.*, 313(75): 2–43.

Costa, C., Brokaw, J.L., Wang, Y., and Fodor, W.L., 2003, Delayed rejection of porcine cartilage is averted by transgenic expression of alpha 1,2-gucosyltransferase, *FASEB J.*, 17(1): 109–111.

Davies, A.S. and Henning, M., 1986, Use of swine as a model of musculoskeletal growth in animals, in Tumbleson, M.E., Ed., *Swine in Biomedical Research*, Vol. 2, New York: Plenum Press, pp. 839–848.

Doll, B., Sfeir, C., Winn, S., Huard, J., and Hollinger, J., 2001, Critical aspects of tissue-engineered therapy for bone regeneration, *Crit. Rev. Eukaryot. Gene Expr.*, 11(1–3): 173–198.

Donnelly, P.J. and Wistreich, G.A., 1996, *Laboratory Manual for Anatomy and Physiology: With Fetal Pig Dissections*, 2nd ed., Menlo Park, CA: Benjamin Cummings.

Donovan, M.G., Dickerson, N.C., Hellstein, J.W., and Hanson, L.J., 1993, Autologous calvarial and iliac onlay bone grafts in miniature swine, *J. Oral Maxillofac. Surg.*, 51(8): 898–903.

Garcia-Ruiz, A., Naitoh, T., and Gagner, M., 1998, A porcine model for laparoscopic ventral hernia repair, *Surg. Laparoscopy Endoscop.*, 8(1): 35–39.

Gotterbarm, T., Richter, W., Jung, M., Vilei, S.B., Mainil-Varlet, P., Yamashita, T., and Breusch, S.J., 2006, An *in vivo* study of a growth-factor enhanced, cell free, two-layered collagen-tricalcium phosphate in deep osteochondreal defects, *Biomaterials*, 27(18): 3387–3395.

Haq, I., Cruz-Almeida, Y., Siqueira, E.B., Norenberg, M., Green, B.A., and Levi, A.D., 2005, Postoperative fibrosis after surgical treatment of the porcine spinal cord: a comparison of dural substitutes, *J. Neurosurg. Spine*, 2(1): 50–54.

Illi, O.E. and Feldmann, C.P., 1998, Stimulation of fracture healing by local application of humeral factors integrated in biodegradable implants, *Eur. J. Pediatr. Surg.*, 8(4): 251–255.

Laber-Laird, K.E. and Swindle, M.M., 1996, Techniques for serial bone marrow aspirations in growing Yucatan minipigs, *Contemp. Top. Lab. Anim. Sci.*, 35(4): 73.

Li, H., Zou, X., Laursen, M., Egund, N., Lind, M., and Bunger, C., 2002, The influence of intervertebral disc tissue on anterior spinal interbody fusion: an experimental study on pigs, *Eur. Spine J.*, 11(5): 476–481.

Li, H., Zou, X., Xue, Q., Egund, N., Lind, M., and Bünger, C., 2004, Anterior lumbar interbody fusion with carbon fiber cage loaded with bioceramics and platelet-rich plasma: an experimental study in pigs, *Eur. Spine J.*, 13(4): 354–358.

MacEwen, G.D., 1973, Experimental scoliosis, *Clin. Orthop.*, 93: 69–74.

Novakofski, J.E. and McCusker, R.H., 2001, Skeletal and muscular systems, in Pond, W.G. and Mersmann, H.J., Eds., Ithaca, NY: Cornell University Press, pp. 454–501.

Ouhayoun, J.P., Shabana, A.H.M., Issahakian, S., Patat, J.L., Guillemin, G., Sawaf, M.H., and Forest, N., 1992, Histological evaluation of natural coral skeleton as a grafting material in miniature swine mandible, *J. Mater. Sci.: Mater. Med.*, 3(3): 222–228.

Peltonen, J., Alitalo, I., Karaharju, E., Helio, H., 1984, Distraction of the growth plate: experiments in pigs and sheep, *Acta Orthop. Scand.*, 55(3): 359–362.

Peretti, G.M., Xu, J.W., Bonassar, L.J., Kirchhoff, C.H., Yaremchuk, M.J., and Randolph, M.A., 2006, Review of injectable cartilage engineering using firbirn gel in mice and swine models, *Tissue Eng.*, 12(5): 1151–1168.

Punto, L., 1980, Lumbar leptomenigeal and radicular reactions after the subarachnial injection of water-soluble contrast media, meglumine iocarmate and metrizamide: an experimental study in the pig, *Acta Vet. Scand.*, 73(Suppl.): 1–52.

Sack, W.O., 1982, *Essentials of Pig Anatomy and Harowitz/Kramer Atlas of Musculoskeletal Anatomy of the Pig*, Ithaca, NY: Veterinary Textbooks.

Salter, R.B., 1968, Etiology, pathogenesis and possible prevention of congenital dislocation of the hip, *Can. Med. Assoc. J.*, 98(20): 933–945.

Schliephake, H. and Langner, M., 1997, Reconstruction of the mandible by prefabricated autogenous bone grafts: an experimental study in minipigs, *Int. J. Oral Maxillofac. Surg.*, 26(4): 244–252.

Sisson, S., 1975, Appendages, in Getty, R., Ed., *Sisson and Grossman's The Anatomy of the Domestic Animals*, 5th ed., Philadelphia, PA: WB Saunders, pp. 1222–1230.

St-Jean, G. and Anderson, D.E., 1999, Anesthesia and surgical procedures in swine, in Straw, B.E., D'Allaire, S., Mengeling, W.L., and Taylor, D.J., Eds., *Diseases of Swine*, 8th ed., Ames, IA: Iowa State University Press, pp. 1133–1154.

Swindle, M.M., 1983, *Basic Surgical Exercises Using Swine*, New York: Praeger Publishers.

Swiontkowski, M.F., Tepic, S., Rahn, B.A., Cordey, J., and Perren, S.M., 1993, The effect of fracture on femoral head blood flow: osteonecrosis and revascularization studied in miniature swine, *Acta Orthop. Scand.*, 64(2): 196–202.

Vasara, A.I., Hyttinen, M.M., Pulliainen, O., Lammi, M.J., Jurvelin, J.S., Peterson, L., Lindahl, A., Helminen, H.J., and Kiviranta, I., 2006, Immature porcine knee cartilage lesions show good healing with or without autologous chondrocyte transplantation, *Osteoarthritis Cartilage*, in press.

Zou, X., Li, H., Bünger, M., Egund, N., Lind, M., and Bünger, C., 2004, Bone ingrowth characteristics of porous tantalum and carbon fiber interbody devices: an experimental study in pigs, *Spine J.*, 4: 99–105.

12 Cardiovascular Catheterization, Electrophysiology, and Imaging Laboratory Procedures

INTRODUCTION

Swine have been used extensively in procedures involving the use of cardiovascular catheterization laboratories, fluoroscopic imaging, and interventional radiology techniques (Gaymes et al., 1995; Smith et al., 1989; Swindle et al., 1992, 1994). The anatomy and surgical procedures involving the cardiovascular system have been discussed in Chapter 9. The relationship of the vessels entering and exiting the heart is illustrated here (Figure 12.1). Recommended anesthetics for cardiovascular protocols and methods of prevention of cardiac arrhythmias are discussed in Chapter 2. The purpose of this chapter is to provide practical guidance to the use of swine in catheterization and fluoroscopy laboratories. Atherosclerosis is also discussed in this chapter because of the close relationship of angioplasty techniques to the study of that technique.

PERIPHERAL VASCULAR ACCESS FOR CARDIOVASCULAR CATHETERS

Access to the femoral and neck vessels (see Chapter 9, Figure 9.33–Figure 9.45) via surgical cutdown procedures has been discussed in detail in Chapter 9. The technique of catheterization of these vessels using percutaneous techniques (Seldinger technique) (Figure 12.2–Figure 12.8) for cardiovascular research has been published (Gaymes et al., 1995; Goldman and Shuros, 2000; Smith et al., 1989). Advantages of percutaneous techniques include minimal damage to the catheterized vessels, a shorter healing time than surgical procedures, and an increased likelihood that serial catheterizations can be performed in the same animal. The technique of locating and accessing blood vessels for percutaneous catheterization is discussed here. The technique can be guided with fluoroscopy or sonography (Goldman and Shuros, 2000).

The femoral vessels are located with the pig in dorsal recumbency, and the legs restrained caudolaterally. If the legs are stretched too tightly, it will be more difficult to determine the location of the vessels than if the hip joint remains slightly flexed. The medial saphenous artery may be routinely palpated as it crosses the medial aspect of the stifle (knee) joint. The arterial pulse may be palpated until it enters the deep muscles of the leg to join the femoral artery between the cranial sartorius and caudal gracilis muscles in the femoral canal (see Chapter 9, Figure 9.44). The femoral canal is palpated and the vessels are located lateral to the edge of the sartorius muscle. The femoral

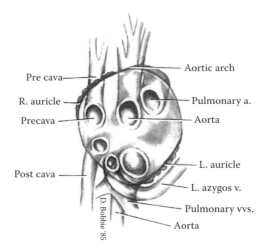

FIGURE 12.1 Relationship of the blood vessels entering and exiting the heart cap. (Reprinted from Swindle et al., *Lab. Anim. Sci.,* 36(4): 357–361, 1986. With permission.)

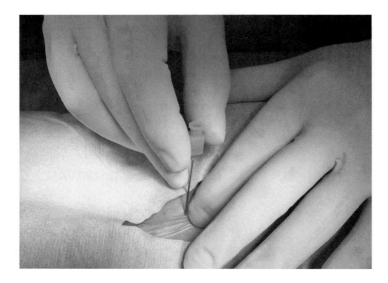

FIGURE 12.2 Seldinger technique: An introducer needle is guided into the femoral artery.

pulse is difficult to palpate, even in smaller animals, and the anatomic guide to location is usually more reliable.

A saline filled 19-gauge (ga) 1.5-in. percutaneous needle is inserted through the caudal edge of the sartorius muscle approximately one third to one half the distance from the entrance of the median saphenous artery into the femoral canal and the hip joint (Figure 12.2). The needle should enter the skin at a 45° angle in a craniolateral direction. The needle is advanced slowly until blood appears in the needle or the passage through the vessel is felt by a popping sensation. The tip of the needle is manipulated until a free flow of blood is obtained. Venous and arterial blood may be distinguished by pressure and color. The vein is usually encountered first, is caudal, and slightly overlaps the artery. The nerve is cranial to the artery. If the vessel cannot be catheterized percutaneously after three tries with the needle, a surgical cutdown should be performed because of the high probability of vasospasm.

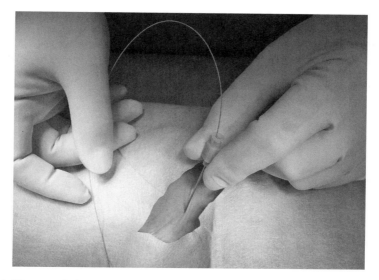

FIGURE 12.3 Seldinger technique: After arterial blood is noticed dripping from the needle, a guidewire is passed through the needle into the artery with the soft bent tip first.

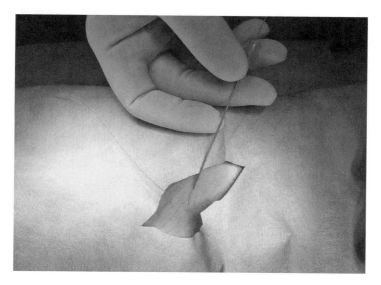

FIGURE 12.4 Seldinger technique: After the guidewire is passed into the artery, the needle is withdrawn.

When the vessel is accessed, as indicated by bleeding, a 0.021 guidewire is inserted into the needle with the soft tip first (Figure 12.3). It is advanced cranially to the site of interest using fluoroscopy for guidance. A skin nick is made at the site of needle entry, and the needle is removed (Figure 12.4), leaving the wire in place. A dilator inside a 5- to 7-French (Fr) sheath with a side arm is passed over the guidewire (Figure 12.5). It is advanced into the vessel using a gentle back-and-forth rotational movement. The dilator and sheath should be wetted and filled with saline prior to their introduction (Figure 12.6). After full advancement and demonstration of blood reflux, the dilator and guidewire are removed (Figure 12.7), and the sheath is flushed with heparinized saline (Figure 12.8). Two sheaths may be placed in the same vessel by passing a second guidewire into the first sheath, removing the sheath, and passing two smaller dilators and sheaths over the individual

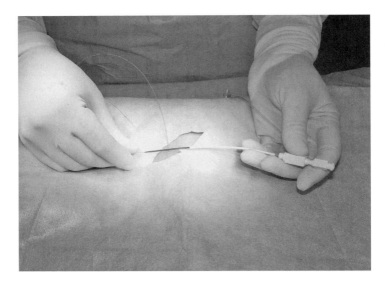

FIGURE 12.5 Seldinger technique: The dilator and sheath are passed over the guidewire into the artery. A small skin incision will facilitate passage of the device through the skin.

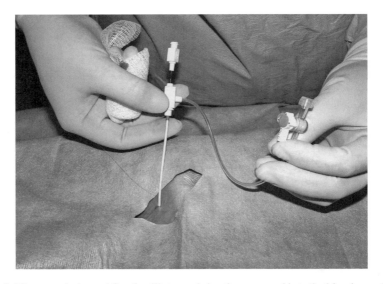

FIGURE 12.6 Seldinger technique: After the dilator and sheath are passed into the blood vessel, the guidewire is withdrawn.

wires. It is also possible to catheterize both the artery and vein on the same side. The medial saphenous artery, but not the vein, can be catheterized with a smaller needle and guidewire and can accommodate up to a 5-Fr catheter in 25- to 30-kg swine. It is possible to insert a small guidewire and cannulate the central cardiovascular system from this vessel. However, digital pressure will have to be applied at the juncture of the saphenous artery and the femoral artery to facilitate passage of the angle of the juncture between the vessels by directing the tip of the catheter more deeply.

It is possible to pass up to 11-Fr sheaths in 15-kg swine. However, use of the smallest possible size is advisable, because larger catheters are more likely to cause permanent damage to the vessels. For most procedures, 5- to 9-Fr sheaths suffice. When the sheath and catheters are removed, digital

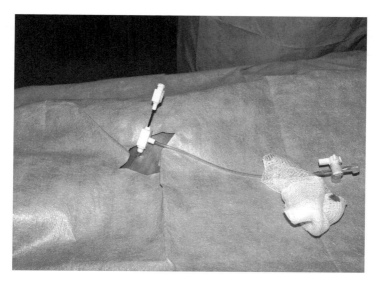

FIGURE 12.7 Seldinger technique: After the dilator and sheath are passed fully into the artery, the dilator is withdrawn.

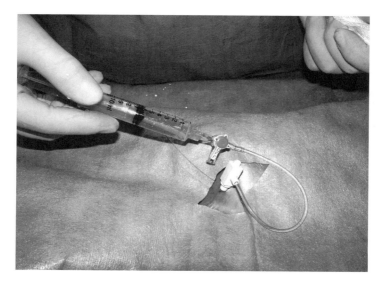

FIGURE 12.8 Seldinger technique: The sheath is now filled with heparinized saline and is ready for catheter passage into the circulatory system.

pressure should be applied for approximately 5 min to prevent the formation of a hematoma. If the animal has been systemically heparinized, the activated clotting time (ACT) should be allowed to return to baseline before removal of the sheath. The skin can usually be repaired with a single suture.

The external jugular vein, internal jugular vein, and carotid artery can be catheterized using a similar technique (see Chapter 9, Figure 9.33–Figure 9.36). Larger sheath sizes can be used, especially in the external jugular vein. The pig is placed in dorsal recumbency, and the forelegs are restrained caudally. The anatomic locations for percutaneous needle insertion can be identified. A triangle is identified with the cranial surface of the first rib as the base, the apex represented by the jugular furrow. At the middle of this triangle along the lateral aspect of the jugular furrow, the needle is inserted through the juncture of the sternohyoideus and sternomastoideus muscles. This location is approximately one quarter of the distance between the manubrium sterni and the ramus of the mandible. The carotid arterial pulse and the wings of the cervical vertebrae can usually be palpated, even in large swine, along the lateral aspect of the trachea. The internal jugular vein, carotid artery, and vagus nerve are located in a sheath on the floor of the cervical vertebrae. Depending upon whether the catheterization direction is cranial or caudal, the needle is still inserted at an angle in the appropriate direction.

Other vessels (Chapter 1, Figure 1.21–Figure 1.33), such as the auricular and cranial abdominal vessels, can be cannulated to gain access into the central circulation in large swine, depending upon the indications for catheterization. These techniques, as well as the chronic catheterization techniques previously described, can be modified for a pig of any size.

ANESTHETICS AND ADJUNCT DRUGS

General anesthetic and analgesic techniques have been described in detail in Chapter 2 with additional dosages in Chapter 9; however, some specific recommendations for cardiac catheterization procedures can be made. As a general rule, isoflurane should be the default agent unless it is contraindicated by the protocol. When procedures involve the heart and great vessels, caution should be taken to avoid anesthetic agents that are proarrhythmic or cardiodepressant. Agents that have been associated with adverse cardiac events in these procedures include halothane, xylazine, tiletamine-zolazepam, and propofol.

When performing intracardiac procedures or catheterization of the coronary arteries, prophylactic treatment for prevention of arrhythmias and vasospasm should be utilized (Table 12.1). A complete listing of cardiac emergency drugs and procedures is in Chapter 2.

Swine are very prone to development of ventricular fibrillation when the myocardium is irritated or coronary blood flow is restricted. Bretylium (class III) and amiodarone (class I and class III) are antiarrhythmics, and either of these should be administered i.v. prior to cardiac manipulation until the procedure is completed. Amiodarone has individual variation and the mean arterial pressure should be monitored and the i.v. rate titrated to prevent significant hypotension. Diltiazem (class IV) is an antiarrhythmic and Ca channel blocker, useful as prophylaxis prior to performing intra-

TABLE 12.1
Adjunct Agents for Interventional Procedures

Drug	Dosage	Indication
Amiodarone	10–12 mg/kg i.v. as a bolus followed by 0.5–3.5 mg/kg/h infusion	Antiarrhythmic, class I and class III
Aspirin	10 mg/kg p.o., sid	Platelet inhibition
Bretylium	5 mg/kg i.v. slowly q 30 min	Antiarrhythmic, class III
Clopidogrel	75 mg/d (25–50 kg pig) p.o., sid	Platelet aggregation inhibition
Dalteparin	50–75 µg/kg s.c., sid or bid	Antithrombotic
Diltiazem	2–4 mg/kg p.o., tid	Antiarrhythmic, class IV, Ca^+ channel blocker
Heparin	150–300 IU/kg, i.v. q 1–2 h	Anticoagulant, increase ACT
Hirudin	1 mg/kg i.v. followed by 1 mg/kg s.c., sid	Thrombin inhibition
Indomethacin	50 mg rectal suppository the day prior to the procedure	Antiprostaglandin effect
Lidocaine	2–4 mg/kg i.v. bolus followed by 50 µg/kg/min i.v. infusion	Vessel antispasmotic, antiectopic
Nitroglycerine	200 µg diluted into 2 ml saline i.v. slow infusion to effect	Vessel dilation
Reviparin	200–300 IU /kg s.c., sid	Anticoagulant

coronary procedures. It is generally administered orally the day before the surgery. Lidocaine infusions are antiectopic and help prevent vasospasm when the blood vessels are invaded by catheters. Nitroglycerin may be administered slowly as an i.v. infusion at the aortic root to provide short-term vasodilation for catheterization of the coronaries.

Anticoagulation is indicated during some procedures and in the postoperative period when some intravascular devices or grafts are implanted. Aspirin is relatively safe but may be insufficient for some protocols. If the pig shows signs of gastric upset, aspirin with Maalox® or separate administration of antacids may be used to counter the condition. Heparin is generally administered intraoperatively for short-term anticoagulation by increasing the ACT. It is generally not necessary to administer protamine to reverse it because it has a short-term effect of approximately 45 min in swine. Low molecular weight heparin injections or oral preparations (reviparin, clopridogrel, hirudin, dalteparin) may be administered long term for the acute phase of healing of implanted devices or grafts. Pigs show a wide individual variation in their sensitivity to these agents. If a pig is sensitive to the injectable preparations, bleeding from the injection site is a frequent occurrence. Changes in the feces indicative of intraintestinal bleeding should be monitored for oral preparations. The exact dosages of these agents in swine have not been determined. If a problem with hemorrhage occurs, administration of the agent should be halted or the dosage reduced. In our laboratories, the most common agents administered for these effects are aspirin in combination with clopidogrel and reviparin.

Indomethacin suppositories help prevent the prostaglandin-stimulating effects of some procedures and help alleviate pulmonary platelet clotting, which can result in pulmonary hypertension. There can be severe toxic effects with this agent if it is administered orally or as an injection. Inserting a rectal suppository the night before a procedure has been demonstrated to be safe and effective.

HEMODYNAMICS

Hemodynamic measurements may be taken employing the cardiovascular catheterization techniques described in the preceding text, using fluoroscopic guidance to see the catheter placement, and noting the morphology of the pressure waves (Figure 12.9). Standard-sized catheters used for measurements in humans, such as Swan-Ganz catheters in the 5- to 7-Fr range of sizes, work for most laboratory swine. The length of the catheter to be used should be determined in advance. As a general rule, pediatric lengths work best in swine. Echocardiography can also be used as a noninvasive technique for obtaining some measurements. Chronic cardiovascular catheterization, as described in Chapter 9, may be performed if it is desirable to take hemodynamic measurements without sedation. Peripheral cuff measurements from the tail or the medial saphenous artery can also be used for limited measurements of systemic pressure. Physiological and monitoring equipment used for other species is appropriate for swine.

Pulse oximetry is a useful technique for monitoring swine for oxygenation (Chapter 2, Figure 2.14–Figure 2.17). Human finger cuffs may be used on the dewclaws, tail, ear, or tongue. If the soft tissues are chosen, the cuff will periodically have to be repositioned because of vascular compression. Arterial blood gases may be measured using the same techniques that are applicable to humans and other species.

Hemodynamic values are affected by age, weight, breed, measurement technique, body temperature, ventilation, anesthetic administration, and pathological conditions. Consequently, comparison to normal values in the literature should be made with caution. In cases of measurements taken under anesthesia, it is not always possible to reproduce the exact anesthetic level from the description in the literature. If possible, each animal should be used as its own control and experimental measurements compared to the baseline. As a general rule, sexually mature miniature swine have hemodynamics that closely resemble those of adult humans.

The animals should be matched for age, body weight (BW), and breed, if possible. Hemodynamic values should be indexed to body surface area (BSA). Formulas are based on dissection and

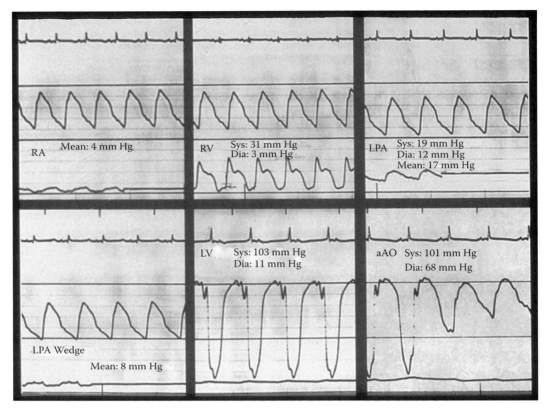

FIGURE 12.9 Pressure wave recording. RA — right atrium, RV — right ventricle, LPA — left pulmonary artery, LPA wedge — left pulmonary artery wedge, LV — left ventricle, AO — aorta.

measurement of the skin of farm pigs. One formula, BSA = 0.097 × BW in $kg^{0.633}$ (Brody and Kibler, 1944), should be used with caution because the conformation of farm pigs has changed substantially since the time of that publication. The formulas were recalculated more recently to reflect those differences. Kelley et al. (1973) provided two formulas: BSA (cm^2) = 734 $(BW_{kg})^{0.656}$ and BSA (cm^2) = 3996 + 110(BW_{kg}). The first is a geometric formula and correlates better with other formulas than the second linear formula. Wachtel et al. (1972) used a different formula to calculate BSA in miniature swine, which were determined to be different from farm pigs. That formula is as follows: BSA (m^2) = 0.121 $BW_{kg}^{0.575}$. Another formula based upon metabolism has been described in Göttingen minipigs (Bollen et al., 2000), BSA (m^2) = (70 × $BW^{0.75}$)/1000. The author has used the formulas in comparison to farm pigs of various sizes and the final results are reasonably close to each other regardless of the formula used. Another formula was determined for BSA in neonatal swine less than 2 kg (DeRoth and Bisaillon, 1979). That formula is as follows: BSA (cm^2) = 337.2 + 0.553 BW (g). The formulas that are most applicable to current research are probably the Kelley formula: BSA (cm^2) = 734 $BW_{kg}^{0.656}$ or BSA (m^2) = 0.0734 BW_{kg} for farm pigs and the Wachtel formula BSA (m^2) = 0.121 $BW_{kg}^{0.575}$ for miniature breeds. The neonatal and Göttingen formulas may be more applicable for some studies.

All anesthetic protocols have some effects on hemodynamics; however, they can be minimized as discussed in Chapter 2. A complete review of the effects of hemorrhagic shock on the hemodynamics of domestic farm swine as well as hemodynamic methods has been published (Hannon, 1992; McKirnan et al., 1986). In addition, there have been published the effects of age on hemodynamics in domestic farm swine under pentobarbital anesthesia (Buckley et al., 1979) and comparison to different breeds of swine, dogs, and humans (Benharkate et al., 1993; Konrad et al.,

TABLE 12.2
Cardiac Morphometrics for Three Groups of Miniature Swine

	Hanford	Minipig	Micropig
Heart weight (g)			
Total	117 ± 4[b,c]	61 ± 2	53 ± 2
Right-ventricular (RV) free wall	23 ± 1[b,c]	13 ± 1	11 ± 1
Left-ventricular (LV) free wall	39 ± 1[b,c]	23 ± 1	19 ± 1[a]
Wall thickness (cm)			
Right ventricular	4.1 ± 0.1	4.4 ± 0.2	4.5 ± 0.2
Left ventricular	10.4 ± 0.3	11.2 ± 0.3	10.2 ± 0.3
Heart weight/body weight	4.6 ± 0.1[b,c]	5.7 ± 0.1	5.5 ± 0.1
LV weight/body weight	1.5 ± 0.1[b,c]	2.2 ± 0.1	2.0 ± 0.1
RV weight/body weight	0.9 ± 0.1[b,c]	1.2 ± 0.1	1.2 ± 0.1

Note: All values are reported as mean ± standard error of the mean.

[a] Significant *(p <.05)* difference between minipig vs. micropig.
[b] Significant *(p <.05)* difference between minipig vs. Hanford.
[c] Significant *(p <.05)* difference between micropig vs. Hanford.

Source: Reprinted from Smith et al., *Lab. Anim. Sci.,* 40(1), 47–50, 1994. With permission.

2000; McKenzie, 1996; Vogl et al., 1997). In general, blood pressure increases and heart rate decreases with age. Some examples of hemodynamic values and cardiac sizes from the literature are listed in Table 12.2–Table 12.5. Hemodynamics associated with particular systems are also discussed in Chapter 5 and Chapter 9, and in the appendix.

Comparisons were made among 4-month-old Hanford miniature swine, Yucatan miniature swine, and Yucatan microswine under a surgical plane of isoflurane anesthesia (Smith et al., 1990). Table 12.5 compares hemodynamic values and Table 12.2 compares cardiac morphometrics from this study. Table 12.3 contains measurements that were made in 20- to 22-week-old Yucatan micropigs under isoflurane anesthesia (Corin et al., 1988). Table 12.4 contains measurements that were made in domestic farm swine, 10–15 kg, without anesthesia. They previously had chronic atrial lines implanted (Smith et al., 1989). Serial hemodynamic values from unanesthetized farm pigs can be found in Table 5.3.

ANGIOPLASTY BALLOON TECHNIQUES, INTRAVASCULAR DEVICE IMPLANTATIONS, AND RESTENOSIS

Swine have been used for testing angioplasty balloon techniques, implantation of intravascular devices, and interventional radiology procedures (Amin et al., 1999; Anfinsen et al., 1999; Derdeyn et al., 1997; Dondelinger et al., 1998; Gal and Isner, 1992; Gepstein et al., 1999; Grifka et al., 1993; Jumrussirikul et al., 1998; Lock et al., 1982, 1985; Lund et al., 1984; Magee et al., 1998; Massoud et al., 1997; Mitchell et al., 1994; Morrow et al., 1994; Mukherjee et al., 2003; Murphy et al., 1992; Pawelec-Wojtalik et al., 2005; Randsbaek et al., 1996; Rashkind et al., 1987; Rogers et al., 1988; Schalla et al., 2005; Schwartzman et al., 2001; Sideris et al., 2002; Solomon et al., 1999; Swindle et al., 1992; Uflacker and Brothers, 2006; White et al., 1992; Windhagen-Mahnert et al., 1998; Wood et al., 2005) (Figure 12.10). The techniques of using these devices involve the procedures described previously for vascular access, as well as the procedures for surgical approaches to peripheral vessels and cannulations described in Chapter 9. Models of aneurysm for endovascular device closure are also discussed in the same chapter. The anatomic depictions of the

TABLE 12.3
Yucatan Swine Hemodynamic Data

QP/QS	Controls (mean ± SEM)
Age (weeks)	21 ± 1
Wt (kg)	21 ± 2
HR (beats per minute)	116 ± 13
LVMI (g/kg)	2.4 ± 0.4
EDVI (ml/kg)	1.9 ± 0.5
ESVI (ml/kg)	0.8 ± 0.3
EF (%)	0.58 ± 0.08
IP (mmHg)	81 ± 8
PAP (mmHg)	21 ± 10
PCW (mmHg)	4 ± 4
V_2 (ml m^{1}kg^{-1})	2.6 ± 0.3
FSVI (ml/kg)	1.1 ± 0.26
CI (l min^{-1}kg^{-1})	0.12 ± 0.03
SVRI (dyn sec/cm^5 kg)	152 ± 71
PVRI (dyn sec/cm^5 kg)	37 ± 17
EDS (dyn/cm^2)	9 ± 5
ESS (dyn/cm^2)	111 ± 28
$Emax$	2.2 ± 0.7
$Emax_c$	84 ± 27
V_{cf50} (circ/sec)	1.04 ± 0.14
V_{cf100} (circ/sec)	0.68 ± 0.14

Note: QP/QS = ratio of pulmonary to systemic blood flow, Wt =
body weight, HR = heart rate, LVMI = left-ventricular muscle mass
index, EDVI = end-diastolic volume index, ESVI = end-systolic
volume index, EF = ejection fraction, IP = incisural pressure, PAP
= mean pulmonary artery pressure, PCW = pulmonary capillary
wedge pressure, V_2 = oxygen consumption, FSVI = forward stroke
volume index, CI = systemic cardiac index, SVRI = systemic vascular resistance index, PVRI = pulmonary vascular resistance index,
EDS = end-diastolic stress, ESS = end-systolic stress, $Emax$ = maximum systolic elastance, $Emax_c$ = Emax corrected for end-diastolic
volume, V_{cf50} and V_{cf100} = mean velocity of circumferential fiber
shortening at a common end-systolic stress of 50 and 100 kdyn/cm^2.

Source: Reprinted from Corin et al., *J. Clin. Invest.*, 82: 544–551,
1988. With permission.

vessels in a subsequent section of this chapter, Angiography, and the additional images in the DVD
attached to this book may be of use in designing protocols and approaches for these procedures.
Sizes of the heart and blood vessels may be estimated from these images. The manufacturer's
directions for use of these devices should be followed.

Angioplasty balloon techniques (Figure 12.11) have been utilized to reopen intracardiac and
intravascular shunts in neonates, to provide models of shunt patency for device closure, to produce
left-to-right shunts for volume overload cardiac hypertrophy, and to study the effects of angioplasty
on stenosed valvular structures and atherosclerotic lesions (Lock et al., 1985; Lund et al., 1984;
Mitchell et al., 1994; Rashkind et al., 1987; Sideris et al., 2002; Smith et al., 1997; Thomsen et
al., 1998). Transient decreases in systemic blood pressure will probably be noted with the inflation
of angioplasty balloons. The angioplasty balloon should be filled with contrast material to observe

TABLE 12.4
Weekly Catheterization Results of Chronic Atrial Line Implantation: Control of Animals

	Week 1
Left ventricle	
Ejection fraction (%)	59 ± 1
End-diastolic volume (cc)	54 ± 4
Peak systolic pressure (mmHg)	104 ± 4
End-diastolic pressure (mmHg)	2 ± 1
Right ventricle	
Ejection fraction (%)	53 ± 3
End-diastolic volume (cc)	56 ± 4
Peak systolic pressure (mmHg)	24 ± 1
End-diastolic pressure (mmHg)	2 ± 1

Note: Data presented as mean ± standard error of the mean. There was no significant difference in weekly values. ($p < .75$, $n = 4$).

Source: Reprinted from Smith et al., *J. Invest. Surg.,* 2 (2): 187–194, 1989. With permission.

TABLE 12.5
Hemodynamic Parameters for Three Groups of Miniature Swine

	Hanford	Minipig	Micropig
Heart rate (beats per minute [bpm])	105 ± 7	112 ± 3	106 ± 5
Left ventricle			
Systolic pressure (mmHg)	116 ± 4[b,c]	58 ± 2	59 ± 3
Diastolic pressure (mmHg)	4 ± 1	3 ± 1	6 ± 2
Right ventricle			
Peak pressure (mmHg)	30 ± 1[b]	24 ± 2	27 ± 2
Diastolic pressure (mmHg)	4 ± 1[b]	2 ± 1	5 ± 1[a]
Mean arterial pressure (mmHg)	89[b,c]	48 ± 3	53 ± 2
Mean pulmonary artery pressure (mmHg)	19 ± 1[b]	15 ± 1[a]	20 ± 2
Right atrial pressure (mmHg)	9 ± 1 [b,c]	3 ± 1[a]	6 ± 1
Pulmonary capillary wedge pressure (mmHg)	12 ± 1	12 ± 2	11 ± 1

Note: Measurements taken under isoflurane anesthesia. All values are reported as mean ± standard error of the mean.

[a] Significant *(p <.05)* difference between minipig vs. micropig.
[b] Significant *(p <.05)* difference between minipig vs. Hanford.
[c] Significant *(p <.05)* difference between micropig vs. Hanford.

Source: Reprinted from Smith et al., *Lab. Anim. Sci.,* 40(1): 47–50, 1994. With permission.

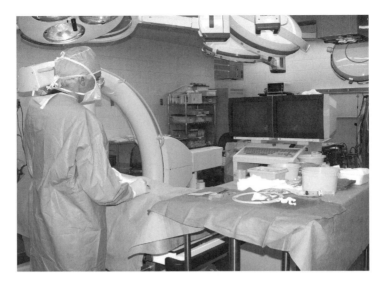

FIGURE 12.10 Catheterization laboratory using C-arm fluoroscopy.

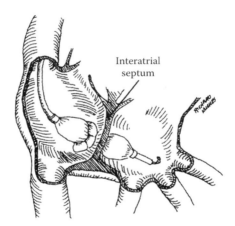

FIGURE 12.11 Method of using angioplasty balloon catheter inflation to create a shunt.

inflation better and to observe for leaks. Catheters filled with air may cause air embolism if the balloon ruptures.

Atrial septostomy has been performed in 18- to 27-kg domestic swine to produce a patent foramen ovale (Mitchell et al., 1994) (Figure 12.11). A transseptal catheter was advanced from the femoral vein to cross the closed fossa ovalis. After exchanging the catheter with an angioplasty balloon catheter, the balloon was inflated three times with 3–4 atm of pressure for 10–15 sec. No reclosures of the septum were noted with balloon sizes greater than 12 mm during long-term studies. Modifications of this technique have been used in larger pigs, 28–33 kg (Thompsen et al., 1998). Smaller pigs (10–13 kg) have also been used to produce this model for study of transcatheter patch occlusion (Sideris et al., 2002). Histologically, the septums healed with collagenous scar tissue and reendothelization (Mitchell et al., 1994; Sideris et al., 2002). Acute studies have been performed with larger angioplasty balloons (18 mm) in swine 20–40 kg, which produced similar-sized defects, measured postmortem or by fluoroscopy or magnetic resonance imaging (MRI) (Schalla et al., 2005).

Domestic swine weighing 5 kg were used to create a model of patent ductus arteriosus (PDA). A 0.035-in. guidewire was passed distal to the aortic arch from the right femoral artery. A 5-Fr

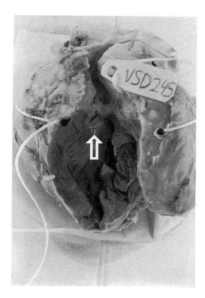

FIGURE 12.12 Subaortic ventricular septal defect (arrow). (Courtesy of R.P. Thompson, PhD, Medical University of South Carolina.)

curved catheter was advanced over the guidewire, and the guidewire was advanced across the PDA into the right ventricle. The catheter was exchanged for a 6-mm diameter angioplasty balloon. The balloon was inflated to 8–10 atm of pressure for 2–5 min. No reclosures of the PDA were noted in long-term studies (Lund et al., 1984). This method offers an alternative to keeping the PDA open with multiple injections and long-term infusions of prostaglandins (Starling et al., 1978).

A genetic model of subaortic ventricular septal defect (VSD) (Figure 12.12), which develops clinical syndromes similar to humans, exists in Yucatan minipigs (Amin et al., 1999; Corin et al., 1988; Fu et al., 2006; Swindle et al., 1990, 1992). This perimembranous defect has been used to test interventional closure devices. Swine have also been used as models to refine techniques of closure of ventricular defects using larger catheter devices (Figure 12.13 and Figure 12.14). A

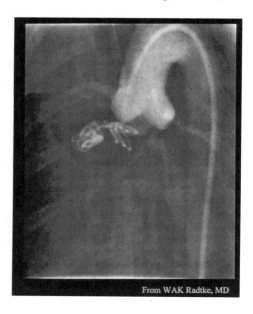

FIGURE 12.13 Fluoroscopic view of coil after placement into a VSD. (Courtesy of W.A.K. Radtke, MD, Nemours Cardiac Center, Wilmington, DE.)

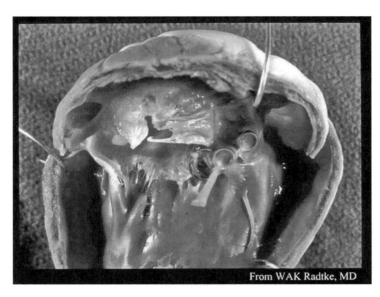

From WAK Radtke, MD

FIGURE 12.14 The VSD has been closed by a fibrous membrane which has formed over the coil. (Courtesy of W.A.K. Radtke, Nemours Cardiac Center, Wilmington, DE.)

hybrid procedure of performing a substernal incision, opening the pericardium, and inserting the device through the left-ventricular apex (Pawelec-Wojtalik et al., 2005) as well as a technique for passing the devices through the free wall of either ventricle (Amin et al., 1999) have been described.

A model of restenosis of the coronary artery following balloon angioplasty or stent implantation (Figure 12.15 and Figure 12.16) has been developed in swine (Murphy et al., 1992; Willette et al., 1996). The model may be produced by either overinflation with a balloon angioplasty catheter of 25–75% (20 sec, 10 atm of pressure) repeated three times. Neointimal formation occurs in approximately 50% of the miniature or domestic swine subjected to this procedure. The implantation of various stents reliably produces 100% neointimal formation. The stent needs to be oversized (>30%) in the coronary artery (Willette et al., 1996). The restenosis following the procedure may be noted in as short a period as 2 weeks but consistently occurs in 4–6 weeks with some stents.

In one of the investigations, it was noted that pigs developed postinfarction ventricular aneurysm similar to the clinical syndrome in humans. The infarctions and aneurysms occurred in all animals

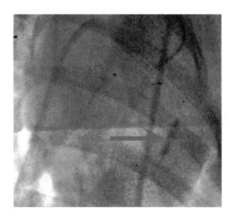

FIGURE 12.15 Fluoroscopic view of a stent (arrow) being placed in the circumflex coronary artery. (Courtesy of Michael Sturek, PhD, Indiana University.)

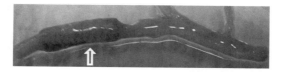

FIGURE 12.16 Necropsy specimen of a coronary artery with an implanted stent (arrow). (Courtesy of Michael Sturek, PhD, Indiana University.)

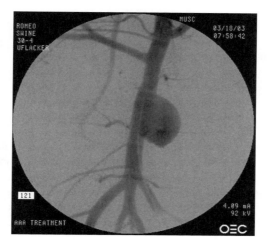

FIGURE 12.17 Fluoroscopic image of an artificially created aneurysm on the distal aorta (Chapter 9 for technique). (Courtesy of Renan Uflacker, MD, Department of Radiology, Medical University of South Carolina.)

that developed occlusion following implantation of the stent. This model provides distinct advantages to surgical implantation of graft material into windows created in the ventricular wall. It can be performed without a thoracotomy and provides a more similar pathogenesis to the human situation (Murphy et al., 1992).

Interventional catheter techniques are also utilized for embolotherapy (Derdeyn et al., 1997), closure of arteriovenous malformations (Massoud et al., 1997), and tracking techniques during intervention (Solomon et al., 1999; Wood et al., 2005). They have also been used for development of stent devices for closure of aneurysms (Figure 12.17 and Figure 12.18). Creation of these lesions is discussed in Chapter 9. Postoperative and intraoperative antithrombotic therapy may be necessary in the models of stent implantation.

As a general rule, vascular growth in a young domestic pig can be expected to increase in diameter 35–40% and length, 25–30% over a 6-month time period. Growth in miniature pigs is substantially less. Heart and vessel sizes are discussed in Chapter 9, and data are available in Table 9.1–Table 9.3. As a guideline for sizing of devices, sample measurements are provided in the following text and in the appendix:

> Göttingen miniature swine weighing 20–25 kg had the following diameter measurements *in vivo*: left anterior descending coronary artery, 1.4 mm ID (inside diameter) and 1.9 mm OD (outside diameter) (N. Grand, personal communication).
>
> Yucatan microswine weighing 14–33 kg had the following diameter measurements *in vivo*: iliac arteries, 5 mm; femoral arteries, 3.5 mm; popliteal arteries, 2.0 mm (Gal and Isner, 1992).
>
> Yucatan miniature swine weighing 10–20 kg had the following measurements *in vivo*: coronary arteries, 2.0–3.5 mm; iliac artery, 2.5–4.0 mm (White et al., 1992).
>
> Hanford miniature swine weighing 15 kg had coronary artery diameters of 2.0–2.5 mm (Rogers et al., 1988).

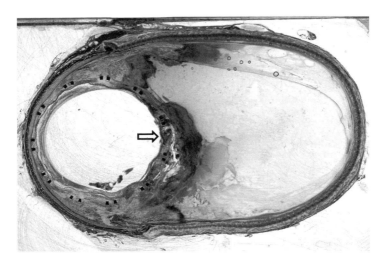

FIGURE 12.18 Histologic section of a stent (arrow) implanted into the lumen of the aortic aneurysm in Figure 12.17. (Courtesy of Renan Uflacker, MD, Department of Radiology, Medical University of South Carolina.)

Necropsy measurements of the diameters of various arteries and veins were collected by the author. *In vivo*, it can be expected that these vessel sizes can be expanded. The measurements recorded were the following:

Yucatan micropig (29 kg): aortic arch — 1.2 cm, abdominal aorta — 6 mm, external iliac artery — 2 mm, internal iliac artery — 1 mm, portal vein — 1.0 cm, postcava — 2 cm

Yucatan miniature pig (47.6 kg): carotid — 4 mm, external jugular — 6 mm, internal jugular — 4 mm, aortic arch — 1.1 cm, pulmonary trunk — 1.1 cm, renal artery — 4 mm, heart weight — 0.2 kg, heart length — 95 mm, heart circumference — 230 mm, LV chamber length — 48 mm, RV chamber length — 75 mm, coronary sinus — 10 mm, mitral valve diameter — 63 mm, tricuspid valve diameter — 65 mm

Yucatan miniature pig (109 kg): aortic arch — 1.1 cm, abdominal aorta — 6 mm, external iliac artery — 4 mm, internal iliac artery — 3 mm, renal artery — 2 mm

Hanford miniature pig (43.6 kg): aortic arch — 1.3 cm, abdominal aorta — 4 mm, external iliac artery — 3 mm, internal iliac artery — 2 mm, postcava — 4 mm

Landrace domestic pig (70 kg): aortic arch — 1. 2 cm, abdominal aorta post renal — 5 mm, external iliac artery — 4 mm, internal iliac artery — 3 mm, renal artery — 2 mm, carotid artery — 3.5 mm, coronary artery — 3.0 mm

Yorkshire domestic pig (25 kg): aortic arch — 2.1 cm, abdominal aorta pre renal — 11 mm, abdominal aorta post renal — 10 mm, external iliac — 6 mm, internal iliac — 3 mm, carotid artery — 5 mm, pulmonary artery — 2.1 cm, precava — 12 mm, postcava — 12 mm, portal vein — 16 mm, renal artery — 4 mm, vena cava — 11 mm

Yorkshire domestic pig (47.5 kg): aortic arch — 2.2 cm, abdominal aorta prerenal — 15 mm, abdominal aorta post renal — 8 mm, external iliac — 6 mm, internal iliac — 4 mm, renal artery — 5 mm, coronary — 3 mm

ATHEROSCLEROSIS

Models of atherosclerosis (Figure 12.19) can be produced by inflation of angioplasty balloons in the artery and denudation of the endothelium by pulling back on the inflated balloon in swine fed an atherogenic diet (Attie et al., 1992; Gal and Isner, 1992; Lee et al., 1986; Rogers et al., 1988;

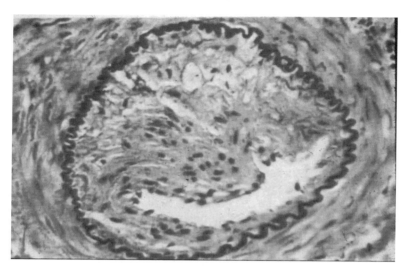

FIGURE 12.19 Coronary arterial atherosclerotic plaque. H&E, ×100.

White et al., 1992). The denudation procedure should be repeated two to three times. Fogarty embolectomy catheters (5–6 Fr) may be used for this technique after being inflated to 6–8 atm of pressure. Other angioplasty catheters can also be used. Animals must be fed an atherogenic diet of 0.5–4.0% cholesterol. The cholesterol is added as a supplement in lard, or atherogenic food oils, and fats are mixed in standard diets. Alternatively, diets may be commercially prepared by food manufacturers. No universal standard for the amount of cholesterol to be included in the diet has been developed, but it is likely that 2% cholesterol is adequate for most studies. The diet should be fed to the animals starting 2 weeks prior to the procedure. The diet has to be continued for up to 12 weeks following the procedure to have radiographically visible occlusal lesions. Swine fed atherogenic diets alone may not develop significant atherogenic lesions within a year. The arteries most utilized in these techniques are the coronaries and the iliacs. The iliacs are approached from catheters introduced into the carotid artery and the coronaries from the femoral artery. Anesthetic and ancillary drug administration for coronary artery catheterization is discussed in Chapter 2.

Gal and Isner (1992) concluded that the Yucatan micropig may be a more favorable model for the development of these lesions than other miniature swine and domestic swine after comparing their results with the literature. The model can then be tested for balloon angioplasty of the occlusal lesions, atherectomy techniques, stent implantation, and local and systemic drug therapies.

Goodrich et al. (2003) developed a Yucatan minipig model of menopause and atherosclerosis. Sexually mature Yucatan micropigs are ovariectomized and fed a 4% cholesterol diet free of plant phytoestrogens with 40% of the calories from fat for 6 months. This model results in generalized atherosclerotic plaques including significant lesions in the coronary arteries. Swine are hyperresponders in serum lipid levels and C-reactive protein levels may be measured.

Expandable stents can be placed in atherogenic and normal arteries to provide patency and for local drug delivery. The technique involves placing an expandable stent over an inflatable balloon and then inflating the balloon after the stent is in the proper location (Figure 12.15 and Figure 12.16). The balloon is then deflated and the catheter removed. Stents are most commonly employed to study percutaneous transluminal coronary angioplasty (PCTA) but have also been used for other vascular models such as surgically produced coarctation of the aorta or iliac artery stenosis (Gal and Isner, 1992; Grifka et al., 1993; Lock et al., 1982; Morrow et al., 1994; Murphy et al., 1992; White et al., 1992).

ELECTROPHYSIOLOGY AND ELECTROCARDIOGRAPHY (ECG) AND TELEMETRY

Swine have been used as models for study of cardiac electrophysiology and cardiac arrhythmias (Gillette et al., 1991; Huang et al., 2001; Hughes, 1986; Khan et al., 2001; Lin et al., 1999; Nahas et al., 2002; Schumann et al., 1993, 1994; Smith et al., 1997; Verdouw and Hartog, 1986). The position of the heart in the pig as well as other quadrupedal animals is different from the human, and the ECG monitoring is slightly different. In the Göttingen, minipig triangular leads (Nehb-Spöri leads) have been shown to be better than bipolar or unipolar leads for monitoring QRS patterns while being restrained in a sling (Nahas et al., 2002). The cubital and stifle joint areas are the preferred location for standard limb leads. The dorsolateral neck, sacrum, and xiphoid process are the preferred positions for triangular leads. The authors recommended these positions based on a detailed study of the minipig and the topographical relationship of the heart to the sternum. The heart projection is from the second to the fifth intercostal space, and the right ventricle forms a sharp angle to the sternum. Adhesive leads typically need to be taped in position as well although cleaning the skin with alcohol helps with their security. Various software programs used in humans can be utilized to process and analyze continuous ECG recordings and look for abnormalities. Illustrations of lead placement techniques and recordings are illustrated in Figure 12.20–Figure 12.23. Table 12.6–Table 12.8 contain selected ECG parameters for minipigs.

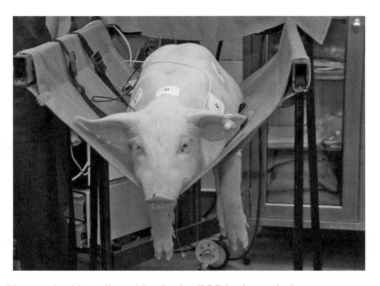

FIGURE 12.20 Pig restrained in a sling with adhesive ECG leads attached.

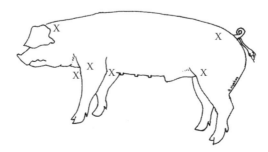

FIGURE 12.21 ECG lead placement is marked by an X on each location (limbs, sternum, manubrium, neck, sacrum). The limb leads are bilateral.

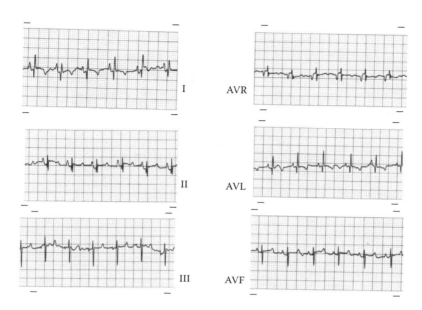

FIGURE 12.22 Surface ECG tracings of leads I, II, III, aV$_R$, aV$_L$, and aV$_F$ recorded at 25 mm/sec. The leads were placed in the cubital position over the elbow joint of the forelegs and the knee joint of the hind limbs while the pig was restrained in the sternal position in a sling. The 22-kg domestic pig was unsedated.

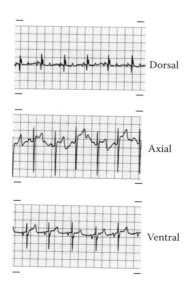

FIGURE 12.23 Triangular ECG tracings with the electrodes placed behind the ear, on the sacrum, and on the sternum. This is the same pig as in Figure 12.22.

TABLE 12.6
Selected ECG Parameters for Göttingen Miniature Swine

	Male (N = 24)			Female (N = 24)		
	Average	SD (+/–)	# of Measurements	Average	SD (+/–)	# of Measurements
Age (months)	4.0	0.3	24	3.8	0.3	24
Heart rate (bpm)	119	29	47	126	23	48
P (msec)	34	5	46	36	5	48
PR (msec)	78	11	47	75	8	48
QRS (msec)	36	6	47	39	4	48
QRT (msec)	240	22	47	235	17	48

Source: Courtesy of Ellegard Göttingen Minipigs ApS, Dalmose, Denmark.

TABLE 12.7
Selected ECG Results for Juvenile and Young Adult Hanford Miniature Swine

	Male				Female			
	N	Average	SD	Range	N	Average	SD	Range
HR (bpm)	24	115	17.7	84–144	24	118	18.4	84–144
RR (msec)	24	536	83.3	417–714	24	523	84.5	417–714
PR (msec)	24	106	15.6	80–140	24	115	15.3	80–140
QRS (msec)	24	35	5.1	30–40	24	35	5.1	30–40
QT (msec)	24	261	23.3	220–300	24	258	25.8	210–300
QTc (Fridericia's formula) (msec)	24	322	21.0	277–365	24	321	24.5	273–361

Note: Age: ~4–8 Months.

Source: Courtesy of Sinclair Research Center, Auxvasse, MO.

TABLE 12.8
Selected ECG Parameters for Juvenile Sinclair Miniature Swine

	Male			Female		
	Average	SD	Range	Average	SD	Range
RR (sec)	0.36	0.08	0.24–0.56	0.37	0.07	0.28–0.50
HR (bpm)	172	36	108–252	168	30	120–216
PR (mm)	4.16	0.46	3.39–5.52	4.10	0.57	3.20–5.61
QT (mm)	10.79	1.45	8.27–13.78	10.79	1.04	8.46–12.72
QT (sec)	0.22	0.03	0.17–0.28	0.22	0.02	0.17–0.25
QTc (Bazett's) (sec)	0.36	0.02	0.33–0.40	0.36	0.02	0.32–0.40

Note: N = 32, age = ~3–4 months.

Source: Courtesy of Sinclair Research Center, Auxvasse, MO.

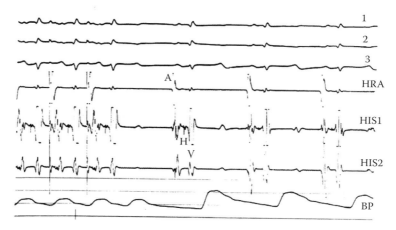

FIGURE 12.24 Surface and intracardiac electrocardial recordings. 1,2,3 — surface leads, HRA — high right atrium, HIS 1 and HIS 2 — distal and proximal bundle of His catheter recordings, BP — blood pressure, A — atrium, H — bundle of His spike, V — ventricle. (Reprinted from Gaymes et al., *J. Invest. Surg.*, 8(2): 123–128, 1995. With permission.)

The anatomy of the conduction system of the porcine heart has been compared to other species, including humans (Bharati et al., 1991; Truex and Smythe, 1965). The principal difference between the porcine conduction system and that of humans is the presence of large numbers of adrenergic and cholinergic nerve fibers in the atrioventricular (AV) node and bundle branches. Nerve cells are lacking in the fibers. The Purkinje fibers are large, well differentiated, and easily identifiable in the endocardium (Chapter 9, Figure 9.9 and Figure 9.10). Humans have some nerve fibers, no ganglia, and smaller Purkinje fibers. Swine may have more of a neuromyogenic rather than predominantly a myogenic component to the conduction system because of these differences.

The sinus rhythm rate and conduction system velocity rates vary depending upon the age and weight of the pig; in smaller pigs, they are more rapid (Huang et al., 2001; Lin et al., 1999). Cardiac maturity in minipigs is achieved at approximately 60 d of age (Lin et al., 1999). In general, heart rates are more rapid than for humans of equivalent maturity. Heart conduction system rates are also affected by the anesthetic protocol. Long QT segments, with the T wave sometimes becoming superimposed with the following P wave, may be observed in deep surgical anesthesia. Ketamine-midazolam or sufentanil infusions (see Chapter 2) may be used to shorten the QT interval if required (Schumann et al., 1993, 1994). Swine have been demonstrated to have similar enough conduction system parameters (Figure 12.24 and Figure 12.25) to be used for pacemaker testing (Brownlee et al., 1997; Hughes, 1986; Smith et al., 1997) and for study of ventricular arrhythmias (Verdouw and Hartog, 1986). Arrhythmias following myocardial infarction are discussed in Chapter 2 and Chapter 9. Right cardiac vagal denervation created by surgery in neonatal pigs leads to decreased QT and RR intervals 6 weeks following surgery and sudden pauses in sinus rhythm (Khan et al., 2001). The electrophysiological (EP) testing techniques of Gillette and Garson (1981) and Gillette and Griffin (1986) have been modified for use in swine (Smith et al., 1997). Noninvasive programmable stimulation (NIPS) that performs EP using a telemetry system has also been successfully used in Hanford miniature swine (Smith et al., 1997). Examples of intracardiac electrophysiological parameters in anesthetized domestic swine used for pacemaker testing are listed in Table 12.9–Table 12.11.

The NIPS program is summarized below as follows:

1. Verify programming parameters of the pacemaker. Surface electrocardiogram should be recorded simultaneously.

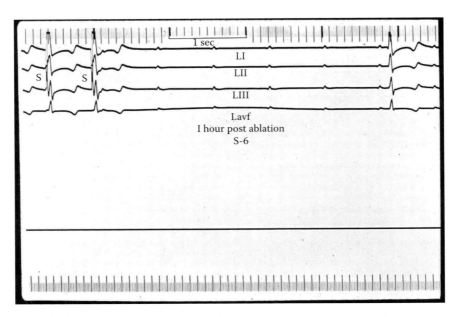

FIGURE 12.25 Surface leads demonstrating complete heart block following cryoablation of the bundle of His. The heart block is illustrated when the pacemaker has been turned off.

TABLE 12.9
Threshold Voltage (Volts) Requirements:
Domestic Swine 25–30 kg

Electrode Location	Mean Pulse Duration (msec)	Pig (range)
SA node	1.0	0.36–0.58
	0.5	0.58–0.96
Atrial appendage	1.0	0.26–0.60
	0.5	0.27–1.21
Right ventricle	1.0	0.15–0.35
	0.5	0.23–0.51
Left ventricle	1.0	0.17–0.43
	0.5	0.31–0.69

Source: Reprinted from Hughes, *Lab. Anim. Sci.*, 36(4): 348–350, 1986. With permission.

2. Retrieve diagnostic data collected by the NIPS.
3. Intracardiac electrogram is checked for proper lead placement.
4. The stimulation threshold is determined for atrial and ventricular leads by pacing at 50 msec shorter than the shortest sinus rhythm cycle.
5. AAI and VVI modes are used to perform pacing stimulation protocols for the atrium and ventricle separately.
6. Pacing procedures:
   a. Eight beats of burst pacing (300 msec) and determination of the rate at which 2:1 block occurs (decrease cycle by 10 msec each time).

TABLE 12.10
Threshold Current (mA) Requirements:
Domestic Swine 25–30 kg

Electrode Location	Mean Pulse Duration (msec)	Pig (range)
SA node	1.0	0.81–1.25
	0.5	1.54–2.70
Atrial appendage	1.0	0.37–1.55
	0.5	0.47–2.87
Right ventricle	1.0	0.24–0.74
	0.5	0.43–1.21
Left ventricle	1.0	0.38–0.80
	0.5	0.72–1.44

Source: Reprinted from Hughes, *Lab. Anim. Sci.,* 36(4): 348–350, 1986. With permission.

b. Deliver a single premature beat into the paced chamber (SPRA/V). Start at 400 msec for 8 beats and deliver a premature beat at 380 msec. Decrease the interval of premature beat delivery by 20 msec until 300 msec. The interval at which the premature beat was introduced is decreased by 10 msec until capture discontinues. The shortest interval without capture of either chamber is the atrial or ventricular effective refractory period (AERP or VERP).

c. Deliver 2 premature beats into the paced chamber (DPPRA/V) after 8 beats of 400 msec. The 2 premature beats are introduced at a cycle length 50 msec greater than AERP or VERP. The introduction of each premature beat is decreased by 10-msec intervals until it is no longer captured. The protocol is concluded when AERP or VERP is reached.

7. Reprogram the pacemaker to DDD mode for previous pacing parameters.

Table 12.11 contains values recorded from this technique in Hanford miniature swine (Smith et al., 1997). Other telemetry devices have been developed for swine. The telemetry units illustrated in Figure 12.26 may be used for blood pressure, temperature, and a variety of biopotential measurements. Devices may be customized for studies in swine.

The LifeShirt System® for data collection in animals is being modified for swine from an established human ambulatory monitoring technology (A. Derchak, personal communication) (Figure 12.27 and Figure 12.28). This noninvasive equipment is an alternative to implanted telemetry units and chronic catheterization for the continuous long-term collection of respiratory and cardiovascular data in unanesthetized animals. Respiratory data are collected with two respiratory inductance plethysmography bands, one circling the thoracic cavity and the other circling the abdomen. The respiratory signals provide breathing frequency and all timing aspects of the respiratory cycle (e.g., inspiratory time, expiratory time, total time, duty cycle, etc.). Potentially other parameters can be collected if there is calibration using a spirometer (tidal volume, minute ventilation, inspiratory flow, and expiratory flow). Electrocardiography (ECG) is captured with a single-lead arrangement, which can be applied in a species-specific manner, and activity and postural changes are continuously monitored with a triaxial accelerometer. Additional data streams, including SpO_2, skin temperature, and other measures, can be collected on a protocol-specific basis. Currently, all data are recorded to removable flash memory for subsequent analysis (Figure 12.28). However, addition of radio transmission of high-resolution waveforms to a computer for real-time evaluation is under development.

TABLE 12.11
Noninvasive Programmable Stimulation Values for Hanford Miniature Swine

	VTHRESH	VBURST	VERP	DPPRV		ATHRESH	ABURST	AVNERP	AERP	DPPRA	
				S2	S3					S2	S3
Mean	0.07	220.98	228.51	226.45	163.01	0.25	233.55	249.88	210.25	221.15	166.73
Standard deviation	0.07	29.01	20.54	19.54	27.22	0.20	35.09	27.91	30.51	34.53	33.77
Range, minimum	0.03	140.00	180.00	170.00	110.00	0.03	160.00	210.00	150.00	140.00	100.00
Range, maximum	0.45	290.00	320.00	330.00	260.00	1.00	370.00	340.00	320.00	310.00	270.00

Note: Refer to the description of electrophysiological testing in text for explanation of pacing protocols. VTHRESH = ventricular threshold, VBURST = ventricular burst pacing, VERP = ventricular effective refractory period, DPPRV = double premature beats into paced right ventricle, S2 = first premature beat, S3 = second premature beat, ATHRESH = atrial threshold, ABURST = atrial burst pacing, AVNERP = AV node effective refractory period, AERP = atrial effective refractory period, DPPRA = double premature beats into paced right atrium.

Source: Reprinted from Smith et al., *J. Invest. Surg.*, 10(1–2): 25–30, 1997. With permission.

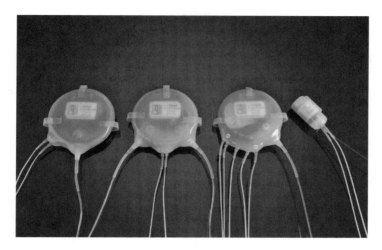

FIGURE 12.26 Data Sciences telemetry transmitters. The unit on the left measures blood pressure, temperature, and one biopotential channel. The second unit measures two pressure channels and one biopotential channel. The third unit measures one pressure channel and two biopotential channels. The unit on the right is for rats and provides a size comparison. These units are for pigs >2.5 kg. Biopotential channels can be used for ECG, EEG, or EMG. (Courtesy of Data Sciences International.)

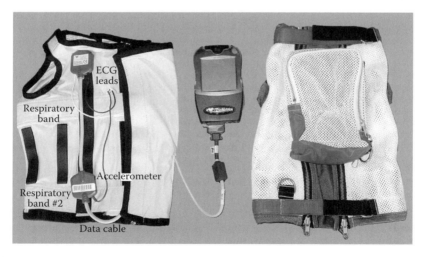

FIGURE 12.27 Complete LifeShirt System — the LifeShirt garment is on the left. The data recorder contains a removable flash memory card, the battery, and an interactive touch screen that can be used to mark study events (treatment, dosing, etc.), as well as to display waveforms for the evaluation of signal quality. The jacket on the back provides protection for the equipment and contain a pouch in which the data recorder is stored during recording periods. (Courtesy of A. Derchak, VivoMetrics, Inc.)

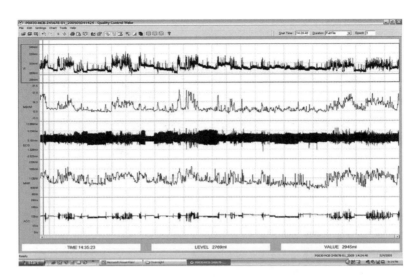

FIGURE 12.28 Example of LifeShirt data — 19 h and 25 min of data. VT — tidal volume, MBr/M — minute median breathing frequency, ECG — electrocardiogram, MHR — minute median heart rate. Activity and postural changes can be noted in the accelerometer trace (ACC). The multiple signals provide researchers with the ability to evaluate unrestrained data and make comparisons between periods of similar activity and/or body orientation. (Courtesy of A. Derchak, VivoMetrics, Inc.)

PACEMAKER IMPLANTATION AND ENDOCARDIAL PACEMAKER LEADS

The technique for epicardial pacemaker implantation is described in Chapter 9. In this section, the implantation of endocardial pacemaker leads and the implantation of the pulse generator in the neck is described.

Hanford miniature swine weighing >45 kg have similar intracardiac measurements to the human heart, and single-pass 11- to 13-cm pacemaker leads designed for adult humans can be inserted for testing (Figure 12.29 and Figure 12.30) (Brownlee et al., 1997). Smaller swine of the same breed have been used for pacemaker implantation after conduction system ablation (Gillette et al., 1991; Rabkin et al., 2004; Smith et al., 1997). Both single-pass leads and separate atrial and ventricular leads have been used for dual chamber pacing. The angle of entry into the heart is different in swine, as it is in other quadrupedal animals, and adjustments in the technique of passing a lead into the heart using fluoroscopic guidance must be made.

A left external jugular cutdown surgery is performed as described in Chapter 9. The pacemaker generator will be implanted in the pocket formed by this surgery (Figure 12.31 and Figure 12.32); consequently, dorsal dissection between the muscle planes along the path of the external jugular vein to accommodate the device will be required. Elastic vessel loops are applied to the external jugular vein, and a venotomy is made with iris scissors. The pacemaker leads are passed into the heart through the venotomy. The ventricular lead is implanted first if two leads are required. Either screw-in or tined lead tips will work in the ventricle; however, screw-in leads work best in the atrium.

When the ventricular lead tip is observed at the tricuspid valve, the insertion wire is retracted 1–5 cm so that the tip of the lead is floppy and can be manipulated through the valve. The internal guidewire can be slightly curved along the distal end to facilitate the manipulation. Depending upon the location of the lead tip, either a counterclockwise or a clockwise twist is performed on the lead while inserting it through the valve. The tendency of the lead will be to pass into the postcava, and multiple insertion attempts to correct the angle usually have to be made. Once the lead tip is in the ventricle, the tip will pass into the pulmonary outflow tract if it is passed between tendinous chordae.

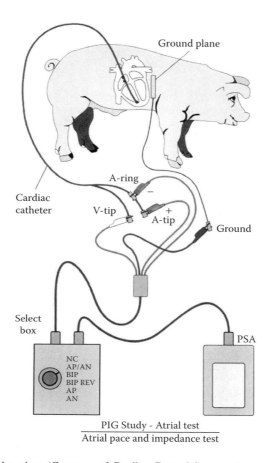

FIGURE 12.29 Atrial lead testing. (Courtesy of Cardiac Control Systems.)

The goal of the insertion is to implant it into the apex. This can be accomplished by inserting the internal guidewire fully into the pacemaker lead after it has been passed into the ventricle.

For single-pass leads (Figure 12.33) after the ventricular tip is secured, the electrodes are placed close to the entrance of the precava into the atrium. For atrial screw-in leads the implantation site should be the high right atrium. Care must be taken when inserting this lead to avoid overmanipulation that will dislodge the ventricular lead. The internal guidewire is retracted slightly to place the lead in the proper location using a counterclockwise twist. The tip is then screwed into the atrial wall.

After the electrode tips are implanted, they are tested to ensure that appropriate impedance and threshold values are obtained. The manufacturer's instructions for the electrodes should be followed, and similar electrophysiology values to humans can be expected with implantation of these devices in swine (Brownlee et al., 1997; Hughes, 1986; Smith et al., 1997). The phrenic nerve runs along the course of the pre- and postcava, and diaphragmatic stimulation may occur with improper positioning of the lead electrodes or too high a threshold value. The pacemaker leads are secured in place with nonabsorbable suture ligatures around the proximal and distal venotomy sites and around the suture sleeves on the leads. The pacemaker generator is attached, and excess lead material is coiled around the device. The device is implanted into the pocket, and its placement is checked to ensure that it is not stimulating the skeletal muscle in the region. The pocket is enclosed by suturing the muscles over the pacemaker generator. The closure between the sternohyoideus and the sternomastoideus muscles should completely cover the device. Leaving dead space in the pocket

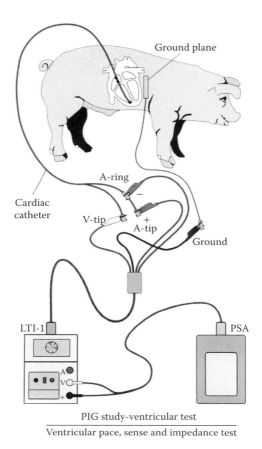

FIGURE 12.30 Ventricular lead testing. (Courtesy of Cardiac Control Systems.)

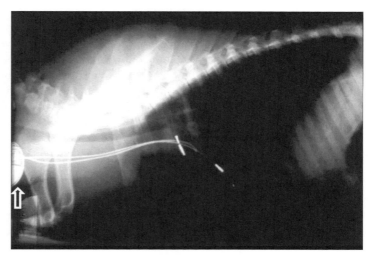

FIGURE 12.31 Lateral radiographs of placement of atrial and ventricular leads. The pacemaker generator has been implanted in the neck (arrow).

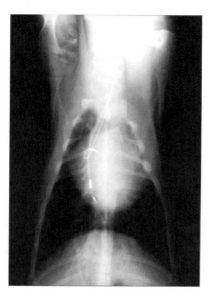

FIGURE 12.32 Ventrodorsal radiograph of placement of atrial and ventricular leads.

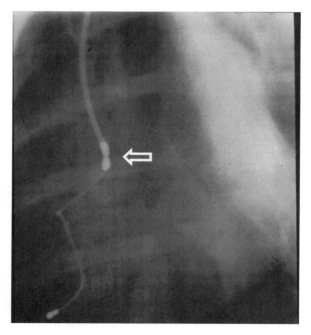

FIGURE 12.33 Single-pass pacemaker lead implantation. The atrial lead rolls in the atrium (arrow), and the ventricular lead is implanted in the apex. The indentation in the lead half way between them is the lead passing through the tricuspid valve.

will lead to seroma formation. The fascial layers are closed using synthetic absorbable sutures, and a subcuticular suture pattern is used to close the skin.

Pacemaker wand telemetry systems should be able to communicate with the device through the skin and muscle if it is held next to the skin. Some manipulation of the wand may be necessary to achieve the desired communication. The wand should be checked for its ability to communicate with the pacemaker generator prior to closing the muscle layers.

CONDUCTION SYSTEM ABLATION

Conduction system ablation is used to study electrophysiology of the heart, techniques for ablation of aberrant conduction system pathways, and the function of cardiac pacemakers. Heart block and regional ablation of the conduction system of the heart has been produced in animals by traumatic damage to the area of interest using surgical techniques. These have included cutting, thermal damage, tight sutures, and injection of formalin into the SA node, AV node, bundle of His, and bundle branches. Some of these techniques involve the use of a right atriotomy, and most have a high failure rate (Gardner and Johnson, 1988). Transvenous ablation of the conduction system has been developed using catheter delivery of cryothermia (Figure 12.25, Figure 12.34, and Figure 12.35), radiofrequency, direct current, microwave, ultrasonic, and laser trauma to the conduction system. These methods have been utilized in swine (Anfinsen et al., 1999; Fujino et al., 1991;

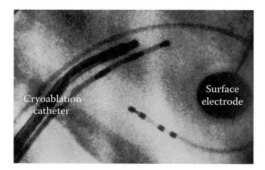

FIGURE 12.34 Cryoablation catheter at the bundle of His (large catheter). The other catheters are electrodes for recording the intracardiac electrogram (small catheters). The round object is a surface ECG lead.

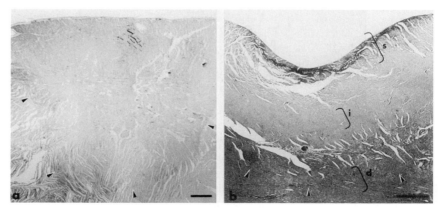

FIGURE 12.35 Histologic section comparing cryoablation (left) and radiofrequency (right) lesions in the heart. The cryoablation lesion is a homogeneous scar and the radiofrequency lesion is a cratered char-type lesion. (Courtesy of R.P. Thompson, PhD, Medical University of South Carolina.)

Fujino et al., 1993; Gepstein et al., 1999; Gillette et al., 1991; Jumrussirikul et al., 1998; Mukherjee et al., 2003; Ohkubo et al., 1998; Schwartzman et al., 2001; Smith et al., 1997; Windhagen-Mahnert et al., 1998).

The technique of transvenous ablation involves the positioning of intracardiac tripolar electrode catheters into the heart to record electrical signals of the heart. The area of interest is positioned between two of the electrodes. An ablation catheter is guided fluoroscopically until the tip of the catheter can be seen at the area of interest, and the energy to ablate the conduction system is delivered using the applicable generator. Recordings of the electrical signals of the heart will indicate when a lesion has been delivered. When producing heart block, it is necessary to provide ventricular pacing. Currently, the two most common types of energy delivery systems in use are radiofrequency and cryothermia. The catheters are usually introduced into the heart from the femoral vessels, as described earlier.

The catheter size, amount of energy delivered, length of delivery of energy, and necessity to repeat the procedure vary depending upon the type of ablation selected and the design characteristics of the catheter and equipment. From our experience, the following examples are given for cryoablation and radiofrequency ablation in 14- to 22-kg Hanford pigs. Cryoablation of the bundle of His: 11-Fr catheter, 60°C, 180 sec, three freeze-and-thaw cycles. Radiofrequency ablation of the bundle of His: 5-Fr catheter, 50-W energy output, 70–90°C, 30 sec, repeated once.

ANGIOGRAPHY

Angiography may be performed in swine in a similar fashion to other species. A complete anatomic study of the vascular system using angiography has been published as a guide for using farm pigs in training in interventional radiology (Dondelinger et al., 1998). The angiographic images included in this section are provided to give anatomic guidance of structures of major importance in research in swine (Figure 12.36–Figure 12.50). They were taken in 16-kg Yorkshire swine with iodine contrast solution (iohexol 350 mg/ml). An 8-Fr 110-cm Cordis catheter (inside dimension, 1.2 mm) with side holes was used. A Cordis automated injector was set at a volume of 14 ml, a delay of

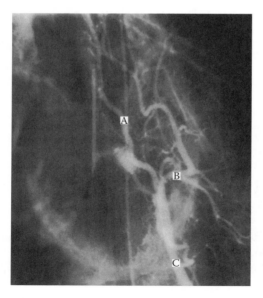

FIGURE 12.36 Ventrodorsal view of a cerebral angiogram with the catheter placed in the carotid artery. A — rostral cerebral artery, B — external carotid artery and branches, C — internal carotid artery.

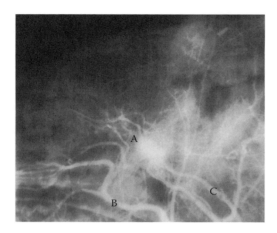

FIGURE 12.37 Lateral view of a cerebral angiogram with the catheter placed in the carotid artery. A — rostral cerebral artery, B — facial artery, C — internal carotid artery.

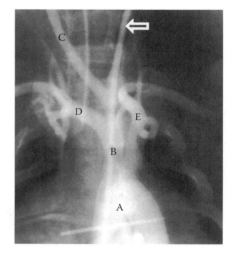

FIGURE 12.38 Ventrodorsal view of the arteries of the cranial thorax and neck with the catheter (arrow) placed at the aortic root. A — aorta, B — brachiocephalic trunk, C — right carotid artery, D — right subclavian artery, E — left subclavian artery.

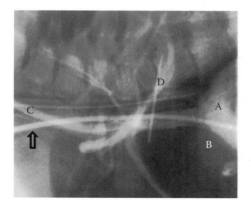

FIGURE 12.39 Lateral view of the arteries of the cranial thorax and neck with the catheter (arrow) placed at the aortic root from the left carotid artery. A — aorta, B — brachiocephalic trunk, C — right carotid artery, D — costocervical trunk, E — internal thoracic artery, F — left subclavian artery.

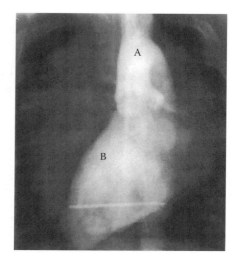

FIGURE 12.40 Ventrodorsal view of the left-ventricular chamber. A — aorta, B — left ventricle.

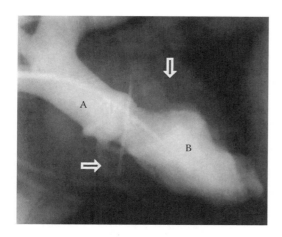

FIGURE 12.41 Lateral view of the left-ventricular chamber. The coronary arteries are apparent (arrows). A — aorta, B — left ventricle.

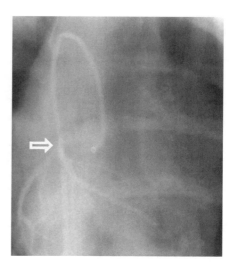

FIGURE 12.42 Left coronary (arrow) arteriogram, ventrodorsal view.

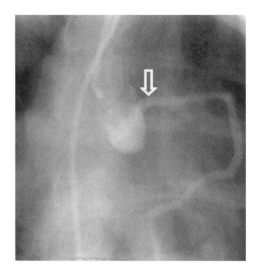

FIGURE 12.43 Right coronary (arrow) arteriogram, ventrodorsal view.

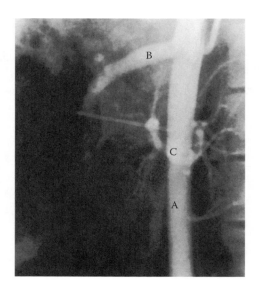

FIGURE 12.44 Ventrodorsal view of the root of the celiac and cranial mesenteric arteries. A — aorta, B — celiac artery, C — cranial mesenteric artery.

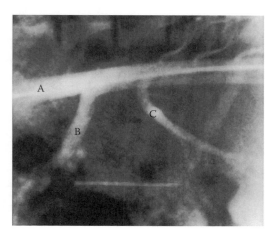

FIGURE 12.45 Lateral view of the root of the celiac and cranial mesenteric arteries. A — aorta, B — celiac artery, C — cranial mesenteric artery.

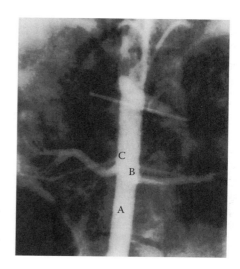

FIGURE 12.46 Ventrodorsal view of the renal arteries. A — aorta, B — right renal artery, C — left renal artery.

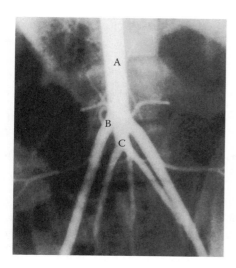

FIGURE 12.47 Ventrodorsal view of the iliac arteries. A — aorta, B — external iliac artery, C — internal iliac artery.

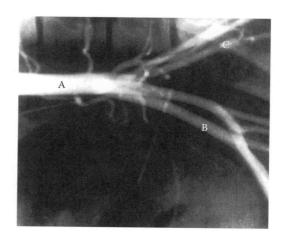

FIGURE 12.48 Lateral view of the iliac arteries. A — aorta, B — external iliac artery, C — internal iliac artery.

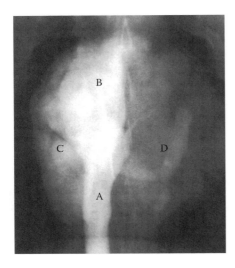

FIGURE 12.49 Ventrodorsal views of the right side of the heart. A — caudal vena cava, B — right atrium, C — right ventricle, D — reflux of contrast into the coronary sinus and left azygous (hemiazygous) vein.

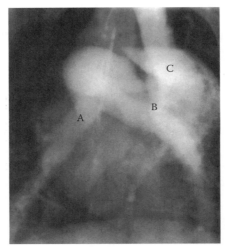

FIGURE 12.50 Ventrodorsal view of the pulmonary veins. A — right pulmonary artery, B — left pulmonary artery, C — left atrium.

0.15 sec, a pressure of 490 psi, and a rate of 14 ml/sec. The coronary arteriograms were taken using 7-Fr Judkins left and right coronary artery catheters with the same contrast material in a 43-kg Hanford pig. Instead of an automated injector, 10 ml of contrast solution was injected manually during cinefluorography. The size marker in the films is an 18-ga 1.5-in. hypodermic needle. Additional images can be seen in the DVD attached to this book.

ECHOCARDIOGRAPHY

Echocardiography can be challenging in swine because of the narrow intercostal spaces and wide ribs. Standard equipment used in humans can be utilized for porcine studies. Echocardiographic images of domestic, miniature, and fetal swine have been published (Konrad et al., 2000). The figures in this chapter (Figure 12.51–Figure 12.58) are examples of images of the heart in an 8-month-old female Hanford miniature pig weighing 36.5 kg. Comparisons of normal hearts with hypertrophic hearts are made in Table 12.12. Normal echocardiographic values for Göttingen minipigs are located in Table 12.13–Table 12.15. Additional images are on the companion DVD.

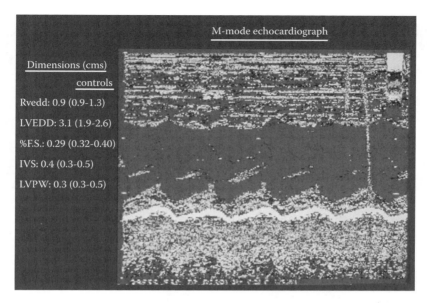

FIGURE 12.51 M mode echocardiogram. RVEDD — right-ventricular end diastolic dimension. LVEDD — left-ventricular end diastolic dimension, %FS — fractional shortening, IVS — interventricular septum, LVPW — left-ventricular posterior wall.

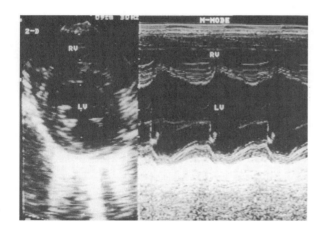

FIGURE 12.52 2D directed M mode electrocardiogram short axis view. LV — left ventricle, RV — right ventricle.

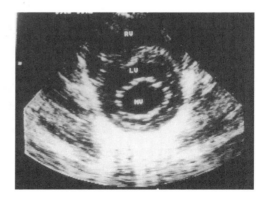

FIGURE 12.53 2D short axis view electrocardiogram. RV — right ventricle, LV — left ventricle, MV — mitral valve.

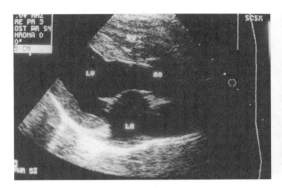

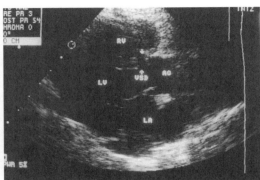

FIGURE 12.54 2D long axis view (parasternal) echocardiogram. LV — left ventricle, AO — aorta, LA — left atrium.

FIGURE 12.55 2D long axis view echocardiogram of a pig with a ventricular septal defect (VSD). RV — right ventricle, LV — left ventricle, AO — aorta, LA — left atrium.

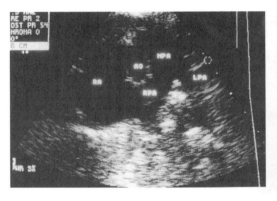

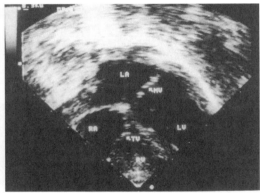

FIGURE 12.56 2D short axis view (great vessels). AO — aorta, MPA — main pulmonary artery, LPA — left pulmonary artery, RPA — right pulmonary artery, RA — right atrium.

FIGURE 12.57 2D apical four chamber view echocardiogram. LA — left atrium, MV — mitral valve, RA — right atrium, LV — left ventricle, RV — right ventricle, TV — tricuspid valve.

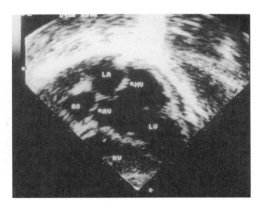

FIGURE 12.58 2D four chamber long axis view. LA — left atrium, AO — aorta, MV — mitral valve, AV — aortic valve, LV — left ventricle, RV — right ventricle.

TABLE 12.12
Demographic and Morphologic Characteristics of Pigs with Hypertrophic Cardiomyopathy (HCM) and of Clinically Normal Control Pigs

Parameters	Pigs with HCM	Control Pigs	P Value
No. of Pigs	8	25	NA
Age (months)	7.3 ± 1.3	7.2 ± 0.8	NS
Male (%)	75	44	NS
Body weight (kg)	114.0 ± 32.0	112.0 ± 16.0	NS
IVS (mm)			
End diastolic	16.2 ± 1.0	13.1 ± 7.5	< 0.01
End systolic	22.4 ± 1.6	17.1 ± 1.0	< 0.01
LV caudal free wall (mm)			
End diastolic	14.5 ± 2.5	13.1 ± 1.4	NS
End systolic	23.4 ± 1.6	20.2 ± 0.9	NS
LV cavity dimension (mm)			
End diastolic	44.0 ± 12.9	47.3 ± 6.3	NS
End systolic	26.0 ± 7.6	28.4 ± 6.1	NS
Fraction shortening (%)	36.7 ± 13.9	39.1 ± 10.8	NS
Left arterial dimension (mm)	29.0 ± 10.1	28.0 ± 4.3	NS
Aortic root dimension (mm)	27.3 ± 10.0	28.6 ± 3.8	NS

Note: Data are expressed as mean ± SEM. Echo measurements of Landrace pigs under anesthesia. LV = Left ventricular, IVS = intraventricular septum, NS = not significant, NA = not applicable.

Source: Reprinted from Lin JH, et al., *Comp Med* 52 (3): 238–242, 2002. With permission.

TABLE 12.13
Echocardiographic Values in Female Göttingen Minipigs

Parameter	Mean	SD	Minimum	Maximum
Body weight (kg)	13.15	3.25	8.1	21.9
Motor activity[a]	1.77	0.65	1	3
Heart rate (bpm)	115.10	20.65	84	216
Rhythm[b]	0.96	0.22	0	1
IVSD (cm)	0.59	0.13	0.41	1.01
IVSS (cm)	1.07	0.24	0.62	1.99
LVCWD (cm)	0.61	0.14	0.38	1.09
LVCWS (cm)	1.1	0.21	0.69	1.59
LVDD (cm)	2.96	0.33	2.02	4.08
LVDS (cm)	1.53	0.33	0.96	2.56
FS (%)	48.63	8.03	27.65	67.06
EF	0.86	0.07	0.62	0.96
PIVST (%)	0.81	0.30	0.194	1.43
PLVCWT (%)	0.84	0.34	0.18	1.67
EDV (ml)	35.30	12.63	13.05	73.36
ESV (ml)	6.96	4.32	1.84	23.67
SV (ml)	28.34	10.38	5.58	60.16
CO (ml/min)	3,254.78	1,265.57	624.96	6,256.64
CI (ml min^{-1}kg^{-1})	248.43	86.47	77.15	509

Note: N = 58, bpm = beats per minute, IVSD = diastolic diameter of interventricular septum, IVSS = systolic diameter of IVS, LVCWD = diastolic diameter of left-ventricular caudal wall, LVCWS = systolic diameter of LV caudal wall, LVDD = LV diastolic diameter, LVDS = LV systolic diameter, FS = fractional shortening, EF = ejection fraction, PIVST = percentage of thickening of IVS, PLVCWT = percentage of thickening of LV caudal wall, EDV = end diastolic volume, ESV = end systolic volume, SV = stroke volume, CO = cardiac output, and CI = cardiac index.

[a] 0 = Calm and cooperative animal, 3 = maximal excitation, no cooperation.
[b] Binary — 0 = no arrhythmia, 1 = arrhythmia present.

Source: Reprinted from Konrad D, et al., *Comp Med* 50(4): 405–409, 2000. With permission.

TABLE 12.14
Sonograhic Values for Aortic Parameters in Göttingen Minipigs

Parameter	Mean	SD	Minimum	Maximum
AD prox ARS (cm) (ADP)	0.75	0.09	0.61	1.18
AD dist ARS (cm) (ADDi)	0.75	0.09	0.61	1.11
ADD (cm)	0.82	0.12	0.62	1.21
ADS (cm)	0.88	0.13	0.69	1.29
ADD:ADS	0.93	0.03	0.85	0.98
Vmax (m/sec)	1.94	0.45	1.09	2.95
Aortic morphology	0.03	0.18	0.00	1.00
Systolic window [a]	1	0	1	1
Doppler color [b] variegation	0	0	0	0

Note: N = 58 female pigs, AD prox ARS = aortic diameter proximal to the right renal artery, AD dist. ARS = aortic diameter distal to the right renal artery, ADD = aortic diastolic diameter, ADSS = aortic systolic diameter, ADD:ADS = ratio of ADD to ADS, and Vmax = maximum flow speed.

[a] Systolic window — 1 = present, 0 = not present.
[b] Doppler color variegration — 0 = not present.

Source: Reprinted with permission from Konrad D, et al., *Comp Med* 50(4): 405–409, 2000. With permission.

TABLE 12.15
Effect of Body Weight on Echocardiographic Parameters

Parameter	Equation for Regression	Coefficient of Correlation
LVDD	1.739 + 0.093 W	0.69**
LVDS	0.821 + 0.054 W	0.53**
EDV	0.885 + 2.618 W	0.67**
ESV	−2.764 + 0.740 W	0.56**
SV	3.644 + 1.881 W	0.59**
CO	344.63 + 221.39 W	0.57**

Note: N = 58 female minipigs, W = body weight (kg), **$P < .001$, LVDD = LV diastolic diameter, LVDS = LV systolic diameter.

Source: Reprinted with permission from Konrad D, et al., *Comp Med* 50(4): 405–409, 2000. With permission.

REFERENCES

Amin, Z., Gu, X., Berry, J.M., Titus, J.L., Gidding, S.S., and Rocchini, A.P., 1999, Perventricular closure of ventricular septal defects without cardiopulmonary bypass, *Ann. Thorac. Surg.*, 68(1): 149–153.

Anfinsen, O.G., Aass, H., Kongsgaard, E., Foerster, A., Scott, H., and Amlie, J.P., 1999, Temperature controlled radiofrequency catheter ablation with a 10 mm tip electrode creates larger lesions without charring in the porcine heart, *J. Interv. Card. Electrophysiol.*, 3(4): 343–351.

Attie, A.D., Aiello, R.J., and Checovich, W.J., 1992, The spontaneously hypercholesterolemic pig as an animal model of human hypercholesterolemia, in Swindle, M.M., Ed., *Swine as Models in Biomedical Research*, Ames, IA: Iowa State University Press, pp. 141–155.

Benharkate, M., Zanini, V., Blanc, R., Boucheix, O., Coyez, F., Genevois, J.P., and Pairet, M., 1993, Hemodynamic parameters of anesthetized pigs: a comparative study of farm piglets and Gottingen and Yucatan miniature swine, *Lab. Anim. Sci.*, 43(1): 68–72.

Bharati, S., Levine, M., Shoei, K., Huang, S., Handler, B., Parr, G.V.S., Bauernfeind, R., and Lev, M., 1991, The conduction system of the swine heart, *Chest*, 100(1): 207–212.

Bollen, P.J.A., Hansen, A.K., and Rasmussen, H.J., 2000, *The Laboratory Swine*, Boca Raton, FL: CRC Press.

Brody, S. and Kibler, H.H., 1944, Table for Measuring the Body Surface Area of Swine, Missouri University Agricultural Experimental Station Research Bulletin 380.

Brownlee, R.R., Swindle, M.M., Bertolet, R., and Neff, P., 1997, Toward optimizing a preshaped catheter and system parameters to achieve single lead DDD pacing, *PACE*, 20(5, Pt. 1): 1354–1358.

Buckley, N.M., Gootman, P.M., Brazeau, P., Matanic, B.P., Frasier, I.D., and Gentles, E.L., 1979, Cardiovascular function in anesthetized miniature swine, *Lab. Anim. Sci.*, 29(2): 200–208.

Corin, W.J., Swindle, M.M., Spann, J.F., Jr., Frankis, M., Biederman, W.W.R., Smith, A., Taylor, A., and Carabello, B.A., 1988, The mechanism of decreased stroke volume in children and swine with ventricular septal defect and failure to thrive, *J. Clin. Invest.*, 82(2): 544–551.

Derchak, A., 2006, personal communication, VivoMetrics, Inc.

Derdeyn, C.P., Graves, V.B., Salamat, M.S., and Rappe, A., 1997, Collagen-coated acrylic microspheres for embolotherapy: *in vivo* and *in vitro* characteristics, *AJNR*, 18: 647–653.

DeRoth, L.A. and Bisaillon, A., 1979, Determination of body surface area in neonatal swine, *Lab. Anim. Sci.*, 29(2): 249–250.

Dondelinger, R.F., Ghysels, M.P., Brisbois, D., Donkers, E., Snaps, F.R., Saunders, J., and Deviere, J., 1998, Relevant radiological anatomy of the pig as a training model in interventional radiology, *Eur. Radiol.*, 8(7): 1254–1273.

Fu, Y.C., Bass, J., Amin, Z., Radtke, W., Cheatham, J.P., Hellenbrand, W.E., Balzer, D., Cao, Q.L., and Hijazi, Z.M., 2006, Transcatheter closure of perimembranous ventricular septal defects using the new Amplatzer membranous VSD occluder: results of the U.S. phase I trial, *J. Am. Coll. Cardiol.*, 47(2): 319–325.

Fujino, H., Thompson, R.P., Germroth, P.G., Swindle, M.M., Case, C.L., and Gillette, P.C., 1991, Histological comparison of cryothermia and radiofrequency catheter ablation in swine, *Circulation*, 84(4)II: 514.

Fujino, H., Thompson, R.P., Germroth, P.G., Harold, M.E., Swindle, M.M., and Gillette, P.C., 1993, Histological study of chronic catheter cryoablation of atrioventricular conduction in swine, *Am. Heart J.*, 125(6): 1632–1637.

Gal, D. and Isner, J.M., 1992, Atherosclerotic Yucatan microswine as a model for novel cardiovascular interventions and imaging, in Swindle, M.M., Ed., *Swine as Models in Biomedical Research*, Ames, IA: Iowa State University Press, pp. 118–140.

Gardner, T.J. and Johnson, D.L., 1988, Cardiovascular system, in Swindle, M.M. and Adams, R.J., Eds., *Experimental Surgery and Physiology: Induced Animal Models of Human Disease*, Baltimore, MD: Williams and Wilkins, pp. 74–124.

Gaymes, C.H., Swindle, M.M., Gillette, P.C., Harold, M.E., and Schumann, R.E., 1995, Percutaneous serial catheterization in swine: a practical approach, *J. Invest. Surg.*, 8(2): 123–128.

Gepstein, L., Hayam, G., Shpun, S., Cohen, D., and Ben-Haim, S.A., 1999, Atrial linear ablations in pigs, Chronic effects on atrial electrophysiology and pathology, *Circulation*, 100(4): 419–426.

Gillette, P.C. and Garson, A., Jr., Eds., 1981, *Pediatric Cardiac Dysrhythmias*, New York: Grune and Stratton.

Gillette, P.C. and Griffin, J.C., Eds., 1986, *Practical Cardiac Pacing*, Baltimore, MD: Williams and Wilkins.

Gillette, P.C., Swindle, M.M., Thompson, R.P., and Case, C.L., 1991, Transvenous cryoablation of the bundle of His, *PACE*, 14(4 Pt. 1): 504–510.

Goldman, J.A. and Shuros, A., 2000, Percutaneous femoral artery access in a swine model: a novel and reproducible fluoroscopic technique, *Lab Anim.*, 29(7): 48–50.

Goodrich, J.A., Clarkson, T.B., Cline, J.M., Jenkins, A.J., and Del Signore, M.J., 2003, Value of the micropig model of menopause in the assessment of benefits and risks of postmenopausal therapies for cardiovascular and reproductive tissues, *Fertil. Sterility*, 79(Suppl. 1): 779–788.

Grifka, R.G., Vick, G.W., III, O'Laughlin, M.P., Myers, T.J., Morrow, W.R., Nihill, M.R., Kearney, D.L., and Mullins, C.E., 1993, Balloon-expandable intravascular stents: aortic implantation and later furthur dilation in growing mini-pigs, *Am. Heart J.*, 126(4): 979–984.

Hannon, J.P., 1992, Hemorrhage and hemorrhagic shock in swine: a review, in Swindle, M.M., Ed., *Swine as Models in Biomedical Research*, Ames, IA: Iowa State University Press, pp. 197–245.

Huang, S.Y., Lin, J.H., Lin, E.C., Yang, P.C., and Tsou, H.L., 2001, Effects of birth season, breed, sex, and sire family on cardiac morphology determined in pigs (*Sus scrofa domestica*) by use of echocardiography, *Comp. Med.*, 51(6): 545–549.

Hughes, H.C., 1986, Swine in cardiovascular research, *Lab. Anim. Sci.*, 36(4): 348–350.

Jumrussirikul, P., Chen, J.T., Jenkins, M., Hui, R., Taylor, K., Wang, P.J., Hutchins, G.M., and Calkins, J., 1998, Prospective comparison of temperature guided microwave and radiofrequency catheter ablation in the swine heart, *Pacing Clin. Electrophysiol.*, 21(7): 1364–1374.

Kelley, K.W., Curtis, S.E., Marzan, G.T., Karara, H.M., and Anderson, C.R., 1973, Body surface area of female swine, *J. Anim. Sci.*, 36(5): 927–930.

Khan, M.S., Zhao, N., Sica, A.L., Gootman, N., and Gootman, P.M., 2001, Changes in R-R and Q-T intervals following cardiac vagotomy in neonatal swine, *Exp. Biol. Med.*, 226(1): 32–36.

Konrad, D., Weber, K., Corney, S., Allen, T.R., and Terrier, C., 2000, Echocardiography, color-coded Doppler imaging, and abdominal sonograpy, a non-invasive method for investigation of heart and aortic morphology and function in female Göttingen minipigs: method and reference values for M-mode, B-mode and flow parameters, *Comp. Med.*, 50(4): 405–409.

Lee, K.T., Kim, D.N., and Thomas, W.A., 1986, Atherosclerosis in swine, in Stanton, H.C. and Mersmann, H.J., Eds., *Swine in Cardiovascular Research*, Vol. 1, Boca Raton, FL: CRC Press, pp. 33–48.

Lin, J.H., Chu, R.M., Yang, P.C., Weng, C.N., Lin, P.H., Liu, S.K., and Mao, S.J.T., Influence of age on the electrocardiographic waves in Taiwanese Lan Yu miniature pigs, *Contemp. Top. Lab. Anim. Sci.*, 38(5): 36–41.

Lock, J.E., Niemi, T., Burke, B.A., Einzig, S., and Castaneda-Zuniga, W., 1982, Transcutaneous angioplasty of experimental aortic coarctation, *Circulation*, 66(6): 1280–1286.

Lock, J.E., Bass, J.L., Lund, G., Rysavy, J.A., and Lucas, R.V., Jr., 1985, Transcatheter closure of patent ductus arteriosus in piglets, *Am. J. Cardiol.*, 55(6): 826–829.

Lund, G., Rysavy, J., Cragg, A., Salomonowitz, E., Vlodaver, Z., Zuniga, W.C., and Amplatz, K., 1984, Long-term patency of the ductus arteriosus after balloon dilatation: an experimental study, *Circulation*, 69(4): 772–775.

Magee, A.G., Wax, D., Saiki, Y., Rebekya, I., and Benson, L.N., 1998, Experimental branch pulmonary artery stenosis angioplasty using a novel cutting balloon, *Can. J. Cardiol.*, 14(8): 1037–1041.

Massoud, T.F., Ji, C., Guglielmi, G., and Vinuela, F., 1997, Endovascular treatment of arteriovenous malformations with selective intranidal occlusion by detachable platinum electrodes: technical feasibility in a swine model, *AJNR*, 17: 1459–1466.

McKenzie, J.E., 1996, Swine as a model in cardiovascular research, in Tumbleson, M.E. and Schook, L.B., Eds., *Advances in Swine in Biomedical Research*, Vol. 1, New York: Plenum Press, pp. 7–18.

McKirnan, M.D., White, F.C., Guth, B.D., and Bloor, C.M., 1986, Exercise and hemodynamic studies in swine, in Stanton, H.C. and Mersmann, H.J., ed., *Swine in Cardiovascular Research*, Vol. 2, Boca Raton, FL: CRC Press, pp. 105–120.

Mitchell, S.E., Anderson, J.H., Swindle, M.M., Strandberg, J.D., and Kan, J., 1994, Atrial septostomy: stationary angioplasty balloon technique, experimental work and preliminary clinical applications, *Pediatr. Cardiol.*, 15(1): 1–7.

Morrow, W.R., Smith, V.C., Ehler, W.J., Van Dellen, A.F., and Mullins, C.E., 1994, Balloon angioplasty with stent implantation in experimental coarctation of the aorta, *Circulation*, 89(6): 2677–2683.

Mukherjee, R., Laohakunakorn, P., Welzig, M.C., Cowart, K.S., and Saul, J.P., 2003, Counter intuitive relations between *in vivo* RF lesion size, power, and tip temperature, *J. Interv. Card. Electrophysiol.*, 9(3): 309–315.

Murphy, J.G., Schwartz, R.S., Edwards, W.D., Camrud, A.R., Vliestra, R.E., and Holmes, D.R., Jr., 1992, Percutaneous polymeric stents in porcine coronary arteries: initial experience with polyethylene terephthalate stents, *Circulation*, 86(5): 1596–1604.

Nahas, K., Baneux, P., and Detweiler, D., 2002, Electrocardiographic monitoring in the Göttingen minipig, *Comp. Med.*, 52(3): 258–264.

Ohkubo, T., Okishige, K., Goseki, Y., Matsubara, T., Hiejima, K., and Ibukiyama, C., 1998, Experimental study of catheter ablation using ultrasound energy in canine and porcine hearts, *Jpn. Heart J.*, 39(3): 399–409.

Pawelec-Wojtalik, M., von Segesser, L.K., Liang, M., and Bukowska, D., 2005, Closure of left ventricle perforation with the use of muscular vsd occluder, *Eur. J. Cardiothorac. Surg.*, 27: 714–716.

Rabkin, D.G., Cabreriza, S.E., Curtis, L.J., Mazer, S.P., Kanter, J.P., Weinberg, A.D., Hordof, A.J., and Spotnitz, H.M., 2004, Load dependence of cardiac output in biventricular pacing: right ventricular pressure overload in pigs, *J. Thorac. Cardiovasc. Surg.*, 127(6): 1713–1722.

Randsbaek, F., Riordan, C.J., Storey, J.H., Montgomery, W.D., Santamore, W.P., and Austin, E.H., III, 1996, Animal model of the univentricular heart and single ventricular physiology, *J. Invest. Surg.*, 9(4): 375–384.

Rashkind, W.J., Mullins, C.E., Hellenbrand, W.E., and Tait, M.A., 1987, Nonsurgical closure of patent ductus arteriosus: clinical application of the Rashkind PDA occluder system, *Circulation*, 75(3): 583–592.

Rogers, G.P., Cromeens, D.M., Minor, S.T., and Swindle, M.M., 1988, Bretylium and diltiazem in porcine cardiac procedures, *J. Invest. Surg.*, 1(4): 321–326.

Schalla, S., Saeed, M., Higgins, C.B., Weber, O., Martin, A., and Moore, P., 2005, Balloon sizing and transcatheter closure of acute atrial septal defects guided by magnetic resonance fluoroscopy: assessment and validation in a large animal model, *J. Magn. Reson. Imaging*, 21(2): 204–211.

Schumann, R.E., Harold, M., Gillette, P.C., Swindle, M.M., and Gaymes, C.H., 1993, Prophylactic treatment of swine with bretylium for experimental cardiac catheterization, *Lab. Anim. Sci.*, 43(3): 244–246.

Schumann, R.E., Swindle, M.M., Knick, B.J., Case, C.L., and Gillette, P.C., 1994, High dose narcotic anesthesia using sufentanil in swine for cardiac catheterization and electrophysiologic studies, *J. Invest. Surg.*, 7(3): 243–248.

Schwartzman, D., Ren, J.F., Devine, W.A., and Callans, D.J., 2001, Cardiac swelling associated with linear radiofrequency ablation in the atrium, *J. Interv. Card. Electrophysiol.*, 5(2): 159–166.

Sideris, E.B., Sideris, C.E., Stamatelopoulos, S.F., and Moulopoulos, S.D., 2002, Transcatheter patch occlusion of experimental atrial septal defects, *Cathet. Cardiovasc. Interv.*, 57(3): 404–407.

Smith, A.C., Spinale, F.G., Carabello, B.A., and Swindle, M.M., 1989, Technical aspects of cardiac catheterization of swine, *J. Invest. Surg.*, 2(2): 187–194.

Smith, A.C., Spinale, F.G., and Swindle, M.M., 1990, Cardiac function and morphology of Hanford miniature swine and Yucatan miniature and micro swine, *Lab. Anim. Sci.*, 40(1): 47–50.

Smith, A.C., Zellner, J.L., Spinale, F.G., and Swindle, M.M., 1991, Sedative and cardiovascular effects of midazolam in swine, *Lab. Anim. Sci.*, 41(2): 157–161.

Smith, A.C., Knick, B., Swindle, M.M., and Gillette, P.C., 1997, A technique for conducting non-invasive cardiac electrophysiology studies in swine, *J. Invest. Surg.*, 10(1–2): 25–30.

Solomon, S.B., Magee, C., Acker, D.E., and Venbrux, A.C., 1999, TIPS placement in swine, guided by electromagnetic real-time needle tip localization displayed on previously acquired 3-D CT, *Cardiovasc. Interv. Radiol.*, 22(4): 411–414.

Starling, M.B., Neutze, J.M., Elliott, R.L., Taylor, I.M., and Elliott, R.B., 1978, The effects of some methyl prostaglandin derivatives on the ductus arteriosus of swine *in vivo*, *Prostaglandins Med.*, 1(4): 267–281.

Swindle, M.M., Thompson, R.P., Carabello, B.A., Smith, A.C., Hepburn, B.J.S., Bodison, W., Corin, W., Fazel, A., Biederman, W.W.R., Spinale, F.G., and Gillette, P.C., 1990, Heritable ventricular septal defect in Yucatan micropigs, *Lab. Anim. Sci.*, 40(2): 155–161.

Swindle, M.M., Thompson, R.P., Carabello, B.A., Smith, A.C., Green, C., and Gillette, P.C., 1992, Congenital cardiovascular disease, in Swindle, M.M., Ed., *Swine as Models in Biomedical Research*, Ames, IA: Iowa State University Press, pp. 176–184.

Swindle, M.M., Smith, A.C., Laber-Laird, K., and Dungan, L., 1994, Swine in biomedical research: management and models, *ILAR News*, 36(1): 1–5.

Thomsen, A.B., Schneider, M., Baandrup, U., Stenbøg, E.V., Hasenkam, J.M., Bagger, J.P., and Hausdorf, G., 1998, Animal experimental implantation of an atrial septal defect occluder system, *Heart*, 80: 606–611.

Truex, R.C. and Smythe, M.Q., 1965, Comparative morphology of the cardiac conduction tissue in animals, *Ann. NY Acad. Sci.*, 127: 19–23.

Uflacker, R. and Brothers, T., 2006, Filling of the aneurismal sac with DEAC-glucosamine in an animal model of abdominal aortic aneurysm following stent-graft repair, *J. Cardiovasc. Surg.*, 47(4): 425–436.

Verdouw, P.D. and Hartog, J.M., 1986, Provocation and suppression of ventricular arrhythmias in domestic swine, in Stanton, H.C. and Mersmann, H.J., Eds., *Swine in Cardiovascular Research*, Vol. 2, Boca Raton, FL: CRC Press, pp. 121–156.

Vogl, H.W., Colletti, A.E., and Zambraski, E.J., 1997, Nitric oxide inhibition causes an exaggerated pressor response in Yucatan miniature swine, *Lab. Anim. Sci.*, 47(2): 161–166.

Wachtel, T.L., McCahan, G.R., Jr., Watson, W.I., and Gorman, M., 1972, Determining the Surface Areas of Miniature Swine and Domestic Swine by Geometric Design, A Comparative Study, USAARL Report 73–5, Fort Rucker, AL.

White, C.J., Ramee, S.R., Banks, A.K., Wiktor, D., and Price, H.L., 1992, The Yucatan miniature swine: an atherogenic model to assess the early potency rates of an endovascular stent, in Swindle, M.M., Ed., *Swine as Models in Biomedical Research*, Ames, IA: Iowa State University Press, pp. 156–162.

Willette, R.N., Zhang, H., Louden, C., and Jackson, R.K., 1996, Comparing porcine models of restenosis, in Tumbleson, M.E. and Schook, L.B., Eds., *Advances in Swine in Biomedical Research*, Vol. 2, New York: Plenum Press, pp. 595–606.

Windhagen-Mahnert, B., Bokenkamp, R., Bertram, H., Peuster, M., Hausdorf, G., and Paul, T., 1998, Radio-frequency current application on immature porcine atrial myocardium: no evidence of areas of slow conduction after 12 month follow up, *J. Cardiovasc. Electrophysiol.*, 9(12): 1305–1309.

Wood, B.J., Zhang, H., Durrani, A., Glossop, N., Ranjan, S., Lindisch, D., Levy, E., Banovac, F., Borgert, J., Kruger, S., Kruecker, J., Viswanathan, A., and Cleary, K., 2005, Navigation with electromagnetic tracking for interventional radiology procedures: a feasibility study, *J. Vasc. Interv. Radiol.*, 16(4): 493–505.

13 Endoscopic, Laparoscopic, and Minimally Invasive Surgery

M. Michael Swindle and Robert H. Hawes

INTRODUCTION

With the advent of laparoscopic cholecystectomy, there has been an explosion in the development of laparoscopic tools to enhance not only cholecystectomy but also laparoscopic Nissen fundoplication, laparoscopic colon resection, and other techniques. The bulk of experimental work in developing these devices, as well as the enormous task of training surgeons to perform these new laparoscopic procedures, has utilized the swine model (Bailey et al., 1991; Freeman, 1994; Kopchok et al., 1993; Lyons and Sosa, 1992; Santos Garcia-Vaquero and Uson Gargallo, 2002; Soper and Hunter, 1992) (Figure 13.1). In parallel with laparoscopic interventions, therapeutic procedures using flexible endoscopes have also seen tremendous growth. Taking the lead from our laparoscopic colleagues, the bulk of experimental work for the development of devices has been done utilizing the swine model (Freys et al., 1995; Gutt et al., 2004; Ma and Fang, 1994; Noar, 1995; Pasricha et al., 1995; Rey and Romanczyk, 1995). The porcine model has also been a key player in endoscopic training. Given this tremendous activity over the last decade, it is important to provide an update in this chapter. The chapter will be broken down into sections on models for device and technique development and the models for teaching.

GENERAL CONSIDERATIONS

Methodologies of prepping and anesthetizing the animals for these procedures, as well as the anatomy, are discussed in the various system chapters and in Chapter 2. Fasting instructions and methods of bowel evacuation for gastrointestinal procedures are discussed in Chapter 4. Fasting for 48 h in a cage without contact bedding is essential for these procedures. It is not desirable to eliminate water unless it is of importance to a particular gastric procedure. Electrolyte or glucose and protein supplements, as described in Chapter 4, may be given as liquid diets during the 48-h fast without producing significant residue. This also provides the animals with a form of nutrition that will prevent them from being compromised physiologically for these procedures. Animals should be fully anesthetized and intubated when performing laparoscopic or endoscopic procedures (Chapter 2).

ANATOMIC CONSIDERATIONS FOR FLEXIBLE ENDOSCOPIC RESEARCH

Porcine models in the 20- to 34-kg weight range are acceptable as models for most endoscopic procedures in clinical practice (Freys et al., 1995; Ma and Fang, 1994; Noar, 1995; Pasricha et al., 1995; Rey and Romanczyk, 1995). The porcine model has both advantages and disadvantages as a model for these techniques (Figure 13.2–Figure 13.6). The porcine esophagus is on average 10 cm longer than the human, and the swine stomach has a tighter J-shaped curve. These two features

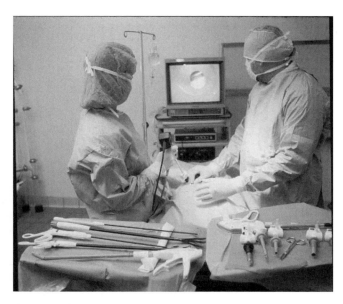

FIGURE 13.1 Operating room for laparoscopic surgery.

make it difficult to intubate the duodenum. The swine stomach has a muscular outpouching, the torus pyloricus, which is located adjacent to the pylorus (Freys et al., 1995; Rey and Romanczyk, 1995). This structure can serve as an excellent tool to teach the use of various endoscopic cutting devices where precision in movement is mandatory. The biliary papilla is located 1–2 cm distal to the pylorus, just behind the torus pyloricus and is separate from the pancreatic papilla. The orifice of the pancreatic duct is located 7–12 cm distal to the biliary papilla and is extremely difficult to find endoscopically but is readily identifiable in open surgery. The biliary sphincter serves as an excellent model for the study of the human sphincter of Oddi (see Chapter 5). Sphincter of Oddi dysfunction is a disorder in humans characterized by episodes of epigastric or right upper quadrant (RUQ) pain with or without abnormal liver tests during episodes of pain, or a dilated bile duct. Detection of this disorder is best accomplished with an endoscopic test called *sphincter of Oddi manometry*. Our understanding of the human condition has been greatly enhanced by studying the swine sphincter using sphincter manometry (Noar, 1995; Pasricha et al., 1995). The pig demonstrates basal sphincter pressures as well as phasic waves, in which the rate and amplitude can be recorded and studied, including pharmacological manipulation (Bak et al., 2000). The functions of the pancreas and pancreatic duct (see Chapter 6) are similar to those of humans, even though the gross anatomy is different (Mullen et al., 1992; Pasricha et al., 1995; Stump et al., 1988).

The conformation of the swine colon is very different from that of the human (Chapter 4). The colon forms a spiral, which does not exactly simulate the human colon when studying colonoscopy. There have been described techniques in which the swine colon is "unspiraled" in open surgery and tacked down so as to simulate the conformation of the human colon. In experiments that require colon cleansing, we have found that use of sodium phosphate (NaP) in a pill-based colon cleansing prep works very well in humans (Visicol®, InKine Pharmaceuticals, Inc., Blue Bell, PA). The pills are included in the feedings and are well tolerated by the pigs.

PERFORMING ENDOSCOPY

The basic technique of gastrointestinal endoscopy involves careful passage of the lubricated endoscope to the area of interest. Frequently, overtubes are passed over the endoscope once the scope is in the distal esophagus. The overtubes are designed with spiral coils in the wall to prevent kinking

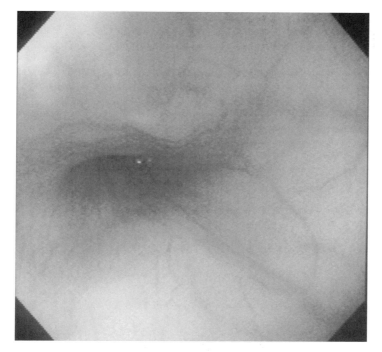

FIGURE 13.2 Endoscopic view of the esophagus.

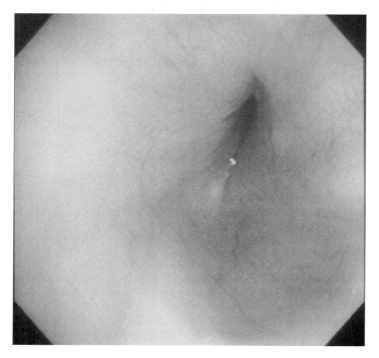

FIGURE 13.3 Endoscopic view of the lower esophageal sphincter.

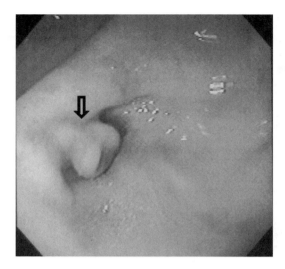

FIGURE 13.4 Endoscopic view of the gastric antrum and the torus pyloricus (arrow).

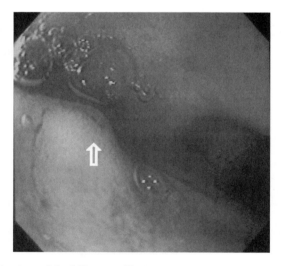

FIGURE 13.5 Endoscopic view of the biliary papilla (arrow).

and have a bite block fixed to the end, which fits securely in the pig's mouth. The overtubes are usually 45–54 French (15–18 mm diameter) and facilitate repeated intubation of the pig, which is often required when performing therapeutic procedures. The bite block protects the scope from the pig's teeth (which can easily tear the plastic covering of the scope shaft) and has a soft valve covering the end, which allows easy movement of the scope in and out but prevents air from escaping. Air insufflation is a routine and important part of endoscopic procedures. It is also essential in endoscopic procedures to avoid overinsufflation (>8 mmHg) of the gut lumen. This can produce a vagal response resulting in cardiac arrest. Insufflation should be performed slowly and judiciously as required for observation rather than continually administering air.

Intubation can be a particularly difficult aspect of performing endoscopy in the swine. The pharyngeal anatomy is different from the human, and care should be taken to avoid passing the device into the pharyngeal diverticulum when entering the esophagus. If this occurs and too much pressure is exerted, one can easily cause a pharyngeal perforation.

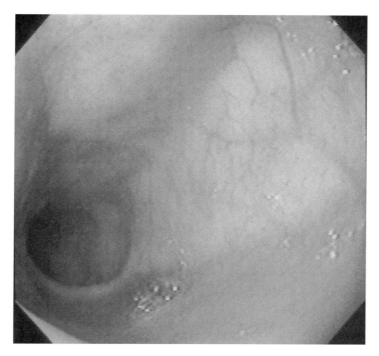

FIGURE 13.6 Endoscopic view of the duodenum.

Gut motility can be a problem, especially when working in the small bowel, and when needed, Glucagon® (Eli Lilly, Indianapolis, IN) can be administered i.v. to slow peristalsis. It is administered in 0.25- to 0.5-mg dosages by slow injection as required.

Once the proximal esophagus is entered, it is relatively easy to pass the scope into the stomach. There is inherent angulation between the distal esophagus and the stomach, and this must be carefully negotiated. Within the stomach, there is invariably some bile-stained fluid or residual food, which can be aspirated through the scope. The scope must be advanced quite far along the greater curvature of the stomach before one approaches the pylorus. Intubation of the pylorus can be difficult because of the extreme J shape of the stomach (Figure 13.3–Figure 13.5). Once past the pylorus, the opening of the bile duct can be identified in a location approximately 1 cm distal to the torus pyloricus. One needs a side viewing endoscope to locate the opening, and the instrument must have an elevator function to be successful in passing an endoscopic accessory into the bile duct. The pancreatic orifice is indistinct but can be located in most animals, with experience (Noar, 1995; Pasricha et al., 1995). The small intestine may be observed using the same methodologies as for other species. Air or saline tonometry can be used to estimate gastrointestinal mucosal carbon dioxide tension in swine (Salzman et al., 1994).

ENDOSCOPIC RETROGRADE CHOLANGIOPANCREATOGRAPHY (ERCP)

ERCP is a technique (Figure 13.7) for which the pig may have particular usage, even with the differences in anatomy noted in the preceding text (Gholson et al., 1990; Noar, 1995). The pig is the primary model for biliary sphincterotomy and biliary stenting. Nonhuman primates and cats have a common opening for the biliary and pancreatic duct; however, cats are too small for most equipment, and appropriately sized primates, such as the baboon (Siegel and Korsten, 1989), are expensive and difficult to obtain. The dog also has problems with availability, and size of the

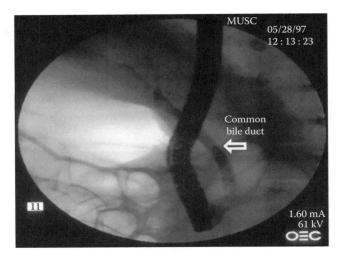

FIGURE 13.7 Retrograde cholangiogram of the common bile duct with retrograde flow into the intrahepatic biliary system.

structures can vary substantially among animals of the same weight because of breed differences. The pig has a unique ability to tolerate total biliary obstruction, which makes it a unique and ideal model for testing devices that relieve bile duct obstruction, such as stents (Sahai et al., 1998). The bile duct is ligated laparoscopically and dilates over the course of a couple of weeks. The ligation model, however, prevents endoscopic access to the bile duct and provides access only transhepatically. However, biliary stricture models have also been described in which a cautery probe (heater probe or bipolar probe) are passed into the bile duct via the biliary papilla, and then the mid bile duct wall is cauterized. This reproducibly creates a bile duct stricture within a few weeks (Rumalla et al., 2003). One can then go on to test new types of biliary stents or devices to dilate strictures. Implantation of gallstones into the biliary tree has also been described to create an opportunity to teach biliary sphincterotomy and stone extraction, which is a common procedure performed in humans (Griffith et al., 1989).

ENDOSCOPIC HEMOSTASIS (GASTROINTESTINAL BLEEDING)

Diagnosis and treatment of gastrointestinal (GI) bleeding is an important application of endoscopy in humans. Animal models are needed to help develop endoscopic techniques and therapeutic devices, as well as teach the techniques of endoscopic hemostasis. The two most common causes of GI bleeding are esophageal and gastric varices in patients with portal hypertension and bleeding from peptic ulcer disease. The dog has been found to be uniquely useful in the study of variceal bleeding because of its ability to produce portal hypertension and thus create esophageal and gastric varices (Jensen et al., 1983; Kulling et al., 1999). Swine, however, can be used to study ulcer bleeding and can develop portal hypertension (Chapter 5). A model has been described in which the short gastric artery is carefully exposed along a 2-cm segment on the side facing the stomach (Hu et al., 2005a, 2005b). The artery is then anchored to a small gastrostomy made at the posterior wall near the vessel. An inflatable plastic cuff is placed around the base of the artery to control flow. This model is capable of simulating arterial hemorrhage from a gastric ulcer. In the report, an endoscopic suturing device (Eagle Claw®, Olympus, Tokyo, Japan) was tested to determine its capability to oversew and stop ulcer bleeding (Hu et al., 2005a, 2005b). Recently, a model of delayed portal vein thrombosis has been created in swine following radiofrequency ablation procedures in the portal vein (Frich et al., 2006). The model has only been followed for less than a week but it has the potential of developing chronic hepatic disease and portal hypertension.

COLONOSCOPY

Entering the animal rectally for colonoscopy requires the same caution as for oral entry to avoid rupture of the colon. The colon may be observed in the same manner as for other species, with the exception of the spiral colon, which is located in the left upper quadrant of the abdomen (Chapter 4). Currently, there are a number of technologies being developed to perform screening colonoscopy in humans. These devices are self-propelling and automated. One such device was recently reported after preliminary testing in the pig colon (Pfeffer et al., 2006).

LARYNGOSCOPY AND BRONCHOSCOPY

Laryngoscopy and bronchoscopy can also be performed in swine. The anatomy is discussed in Chapter 9. Two precautions are necessary when using this technology. The epiglottis and larynx are very prone to spasm and edematous swelling with manipulation. The lateral ventricles of the larynx are also easily ruptured resulting in subcutaneous emphysema. The larynx should always be sprayed with topical anesthetics, and appropriate-sized devices should be used to prevent trauma. Swine are also very susceptible to vagal stimulation and bradycardia with manipulation of the airway. Animals should always be atropinized during the entire procedure (Chapter 2). Isoproterenol is useful to prevent bronchospasm.

TRAINING IN FLEXIBLE ENDOSCOPY

The porcine model has proved very beneficial in endoscopic and laparoscopic training. In some circumstances, it remains the best model. Training in endoscopic ultrasound (EUS) is a case in point. This technology involves attaching a miniaturized ultrasound probe on the end of a flexible endoscope (Figure 13.8). The endoscope serves as the "hands" of the endoscopist and allows one to place the transducer in various positions within the upper gastrointestinal track or rectum. The target organ is either the gut wall, structures (lymph nodes), or organs that lie adjacent to the gut (pancreas, bile duct, liver, etc.). With this technology, it is possible to place a needle down the biopsy channel of the endoscope, and then the needle can be advanced under real-time ultrasound guidance into a target outside the gut wall (lymph node, pancreatic mass, etc.) (Figure 13.9). Cells are then aspirated from the target and read by a cytopathologist. This technique has become very

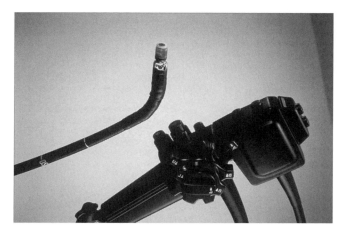

FIGURE 13.8 A picture showing the distal end of a radial scanning echoendoscope. This is a standard endoscope with oblique-forward viewing optics with an ultrasound transducer mounted on the distal tip. The ultrasound transducer is rotated 360° around the long axis of the scope producing a 360° image.

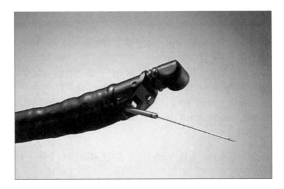

FIGURE 13.9 A picture showing a linear array echoendoscope. The transducer on this instrument is constructed of multiple piezoceramic elements aligned parallel to the shaft of the scope. When a needle is passed through the biopsy channel, it comes out in the plane of imaging allowing real-time, ultrasound-guided fine needle aspiration (FNA) cytology.

important in the practice of gastrointestinal endoscopy but requires considerable training. The learning curve can be shortened by doing preliminary work on the swine model (Bhutani et al., 1998; Bhutani et al., 2000). Although computer and inanimate models have been developed to aid EUS training (Burmester 2004, Sorbi 2003), they do not provide an adequate substitute for the live pig model.

Although some training requires anesthetized swine, animal conservation is important. As a result, over the last 5 years, there has been an explosion in the use of *ex vivo* swine tissue for endoscopic training. This model was first conceived by Martin Neumann in Erlangen, Germany (Neumann et al., 2000). It was first developed as a potential laparoscopic training model, but it quickly became apparent that its greatest utility would be for flexible endoscopic training. The concept involves harvesting the upper gastrointestinal tract (which can include the liver and biliary tree, as well as the respiratory tree with lungs and the colon) from a pig that has been slaughtered for meat. The specimen is cleaned and prepared followed by freezing. When needed, the specimen is thawed and tacked down with sutures within a plastic form that allows the anatomy to be displayed as if it were human (Figure 13.10). Various "pathologies" can be created, such as implantation of

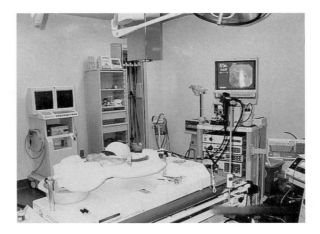

FIGURE 13.10 A picture taken from the Medical University of South Carolina (MUSC) Digestive Disease Center animal lab showing the Erlanger model where the upper gastrointestinal (GI) tract of the swine has been mounted in the plastic tray to simulate the human anatomy. An endoscopic system has been set up in preparation for a teaching session on therapeutic endoscopy.

a small piece of the splenic artery into the gastric wall to simulate a bleeding ulcer. The extralumenal end of the artery is hooked to a pump, which instills red-dye-colored fluid to simulate blood. An endoscope is passed into the stomach, and the pump is started. From the endoscopist's perspective, this looks just like arterial bleeding from an ulcer. Various therapeutic techniques can then be taught to stop the bleeding such as injection therapy, cautery with a heater or bipolar probe, or clips (Hochberger et al., 2004, 2005). One can create polyps, esophageal varices, and various pancreatobiliary pathologies to teach various therapeutic endoscopic procedures. The model serves as a very useful teaching tool and utilizes a readily available (and otherwise wasted) resource. The impact of these *ex vivo* training models is increasing (Neumann et al., 2001; Hochberger et al., 2001, 2002; Matthes et al., 2005). These same models can be used for preliminary testing of endoscopic devices as well.

LAPAROSCOPIC, CELIOSCOPIC, AND THORACOSCOPIC SURGERY

The minimally invasive surgical techniques that are rapidly developing will continue to replace many of the open surgical techniques now in clinical practice. The porcine model has proved to be invaluable in both training and development. The basic techniques involve insufflating a body cavity with CO_2, placing trocars, and using camera guidance to perform surgical techniques with specialized instruments through the trocars. Specialized suturing and instrument-handling techniques, different from those of open surgery, are required. The techniques may have fewer complications, such as adhesions, as compared to open techniques (Gutt et al., 2004).

When using swine for training, nonsurvival techniques are preferred, because they allow the surgeon the chance to perform multiple procedures and do not require close attention to aseptic techniques. Training courses should include the use of inanimate models or computer simulations prior to performing the techniques on live animals. Most procedures and instruments can be utilized in swine weighing 25–35 kg. Reviews of recommendations for training of surgeons have been published (Bailey et al., 1991; Freeman, 1994; Kopchok et al., 1993; Lyons and Sosa, 1992; Soper and Hunter, 1992; Srinivasan et al., 1999).

Swine are usually positioned in dorsal recumbency for these procedures, but the positioning may have to be varied for retroperitoneal and thoracic procedures. The positioning of the trocars and the insufflation needle depends upon the procedure being performed. Standard positions are described here as an example (Figure 13.11). A Veress needle is positioned at the umbilicus, and the abdomen is inflated to 12–14 mmHg with CO_2. As a minimum, a trocar is required for insertion of a camera, usually near the umbilicus, so that the procedure can be viewed on a TV screen, and a second trocar is required to insert and manipulate the surgical instruments. As many as four secondary trocars for instrumentation may be required, depending upon the procedure and types of instruments. Instrumentation trocars are positioned so that the area of surgical interest can be seen and manipulated with the least interference with surrounding structures.

Insufflation of the abdomen and thorax causes hemodynamic changes, and monitoring the intra-abdominal pressure is essential. Creating a pneumoperitoneum with CO_2 increases the arterial pCO_2 and reduces the pH. It has been demonstrated that using helium as the gas eliminates this respiratory acidosis (Leighton et al., 1993). Both the reverse Trendelenburg position and the increase in intra-abdominal pressure caused by insufflation reduce the venous blood flow from the lower limbs, which could predispose to venous thrombosis and pulmonary embolism (Jorgensen et al., 1994). The effects of insufflation during thoracoscopy are even more dramatic. Significant decreases in cardiac index, mean arterial pressure, stroke volume, and left-ventricular stroke work index were noted with pressures greater than 5 mmHg. In the same study, central venous pressure increased (Jones et al., 1993). In pigs, 25–35 kg, routinely used for these procedures, the mediastinum is thin and easily ruptured, and precautions should be taken both with the use of insufflation and the

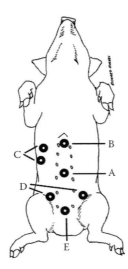

FIGURE 13.11 Drawing of a pig showing examples of laparoscopic trocar insertion points. A — Veress needle and camera trocar, B — large trocar site for upper abdominal procedures, C — small trocars in paramedian and lateral positions, D — small trocars for caudal abdominal procedures, E — large trocar for lower abdominal procedures.

placement of chest tubes (Chapter 9). The diaphragmatic communication between the peritoneal and pleural cavities in young swine is easily ruptured, and gas in either cavity is likely to penetrate the other cavity if the pressure is high enough (Freeman, 1994; Swindle et al., 1988). At the end of the procedure, the cavity is examined for hemostasis and proper tissue apposition. Following desufflation, the peritoneum, muscle, and skin layers penetrated by the trocars are closed with sutures or staples.

Freeman (1994) and Srinivasan (1999) have written succinct reviews of the most common techniques used for training in swine; these publications, in conjunction with the technical descriptions provided by others, will be used as examples of the types of technical variations that are used in performing various laparoscopic surgical techniques.

CHOLECYSTECTOMY

Three trocars, two 5-mm and one 10- or 12-mm, are inserted into the cranial abdomen. The gallbladder (Figure 13.12) is bluntly dissected to the cystic duct and ligated. The gallbladder is removed through the large trocar and may be emptied with suction prior to removal (Pasricha et al., 1995; Rodriguez et al., 1993; Soper et al., 1991, 1993; Srinivasan et al., 1999). The open technique is described in Chapter 5.

SMALL INTESTINAL ANASTOMOSIS

Four 10- or 12-mm trocars are inserted in the paramedian position over the area of interest. The standard techniques of identification of a segment, isolation, and anastomosis are described in Chapter 4 and are performed with laparoscopic instruments, sutures, and staples. The anastomosis must be checked for patency, and the mesenteric defect closed with this technique as well. The excised segment is removed through one of the trocars after closure. Laparoscopic techniques have been demonstrated to be as effective as open techniques when wound healing and complications were compared (Fleshman et al., 1993; Noel et al., 1994; Olson et al., 1995; Pietrafitta et al., 1992; Soper et al., 1993; Srinivasan et al., 1999).

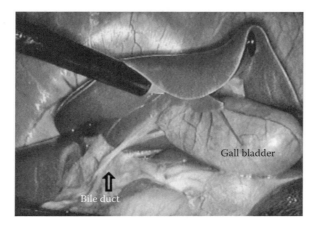

FIGURE 13.12 Laparoscopic view of the gallbladder and bile duct.

COLONIC ANASTOMOSIS

As for small intestinal anastomosis, four secondary 10- or 12-mm trocars are positioned in the paramedian position; however, they are in the caudal abdomen. A staple anastomosis is performed after mobilization of the segment to be excised. Both intracorporeal and extracorporeal techniques have been utilized. For the extracorporeal technique, the proximal segment is externalized through the right lower quadrant. The circular stapler may be placed through the anus if the anastomotic site is distal. Colonic anastomosis using these techniques has been demonstrated to be as effective as the open techniques described in Chapter 4 (Fleshman et al., 1993; Noel et al., 1994; Olson et al., 1995; Pietrafitta et al., 1992; Soper et al., 1993; Srinivasan et al., 1999).

VAGOTOMY AND HIATAL PROCEDURES

Four 5-mm or 10- to 12-mm trocars are used in the cranial abdomen. The vagus nerve can be identified along the margin of the esophagus, or selective vagotomy procedures at the level of the stomach can be performed (Figure 13.13). Hiatal hernias can be created and repaired as well as the performance of fundoplications. Procedures in this region require atropinization of the animal

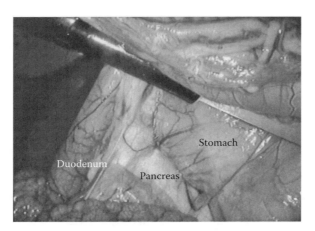

FIGURE 13.13 Laparoscopic view of the pancreas, duodenum, and stomach.

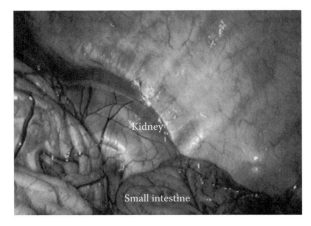

FIGURE 13.14 Laparoscopic view of the right kidney and small intestine.

to prevent vagal-induced bradycardia. Pneumothorax is also a potentially fatal complication associated with the dissection and must be monitored by the anesthetist and relieved with chest tubes, if necessary (Freeman, 1994; Josephs et al., 1992; Srinivasan et al., 1999).

Nephrectomy and Renal Ablation

Either a paramedian or a retroperitoneal approach may be made to the kidney with three 10- or 12-mm trocars (Figure 13.14). After dissection and ligation of the blood vessels, the kidney may be removed with a larger trocar or a specimen retrieval bag after morcellation (Chiu et al., 1992; Kerbl et al., 1993). Laparoscopic and percutaneous procedures of the kidney have also involved removal and ablation of tissue with radiofrequency (Bernardo and Gill, 2002; Desai et al., 2005; Gill et al., 2000; Hsu et al., 2000; Wagner et al., 2005). The open techniques are described in Chapter 7.

Inguinal Herniorrhaphy

Spontaneous inguinal hernias of swine or dissected inguinal rings (Figure 13.15) of male swine may be used as models. Two secondary 10- or 12-mm trocars are introduced in the caudal abdomen. For this procedure, the edges of the peritoneum around the inguinal ring are dissected free from

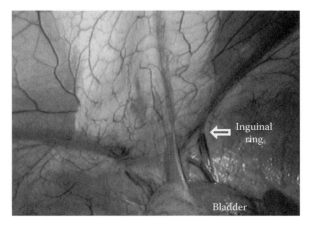

FIGURE 13.15 Laparoscopic view of the inguinal ring and urinary bladder.

the inguinal ring, and a prosthetic mesh is inserted and stapled in place. The insufflation pressure is reduced to facilitate proper alignment of the tissues prior to placing the last staples and closure of the peritoneum (Layman et al., 1993). The inguinal ring may also be repaired using a preperitoneal approach. From the midline, the trocars are inserted without penetration of the peritoneum. After insufflation, the operating trocars are inserted lateral to the midline below the umbilicus and cranial to the pubis (Freeman, 1994; Srinivasan et al., 1999). Inguinal hernias are discussed in Chapter 11.

Appendectomy

The pig does not have an appendix; however, one can be created as an acute model for training purposes from a loop of small intestine or uterine horn. For this procedure, two 10- or 12-mm trocars are introduced on either side of the midline. A loop of the structure has its blood supply ligated, and pretied loop ligatures are placed at the base of the loop (Freeman, 1994; Srinivasan et al., 1999).

Splenectomy

The spleen may be removed after placing four secondary 10- or 12-mm trocars in the cranial abdomen. The vascular supply is ligated or stapled and the organ reduced in size with a morcellation device prior to removal. The spleen can be removed through a 33-mm trocar site (Freeman, 1994; Srinivasan et al., 1999). Splenectomy is discussed in Chapter 6.

Adrenalectomy

With the pig in ventral recumbency, a unilateral adrenalectomy may be performed in the retroperitoneal space. Trocars are placed in the flank without penetrating the peritoneum, and the retroperitoneal space is insufflated. After ligation of the blood vessels and removal of the structure through 10- or 12-mm trocars, the retroperitoneal space is desufflated and closed in a routine fashion. Care should be taken to avoid penetration of the diaphragm from this position with a trocar (Brunt et al., 1993). Adrenalectomy is discussed in Chapter 7.

Urinary Bladder Procedures

Urinary procedures are discussed in Chapter 7. Laparoscopic urinary incontinence procedures have been described (Ou et al., 1993; Vancaillie, 1993). Two or three 10- or 12-mm trocars are placed in the right and left caudal quadrants of the abdomen. After tissue dissection to expose the urethra, a mesh or sutures are placed in the perivaginal tissue and anchored to Cooper's ligament.

Reproductive Procedures

The uterus of the pig is bicornuate with a small body (Chapter 8). The anatomy of the structure is dissimilar to human anatomy, and the goat is the preferred model for uterine body procedures and hysterectomy (Freeman, 1994). However, the porcine model may be used for ovarian and Fallopian tube procedures, such as ovariectomy and tubal ligation.

Thoracoscopy

Because of the precautions described in the preceding text and in Chapter 9, the procedure should not be performed with insufflation of the thoracic cavity. Rather, single lung ventilation can be performed after unilateral intubation of the right main-stem bronchus. Auscultation can be used to confirm the correct placement of the tube. Pneumothorax on the left side will be produced when the trocars are inserted and the lung collapses. Depending upon the procedure that is performed, the trocars can be inserted into the appropriate intercostal spaces with the pig in dorsal, ventral, or lateral recumbency (Freeman, 1994). Techniques for slowing the heart rate include using high-dose opioid infusion anesthetic techniques and beta blockers. The heart rate should be maintained >60 beats per minute (bpm) in swine. These techniques are discussed in Chapter 2.

LAPAROSCOPIC ULTRASONOGRAPHY

A semiflexible ultrasound transducer introduced through a laparoscopic port has been utilized to visualize abdominal structures. The transducer used both gray-scale and color Doppler techniques to observe normal structures, to aid dissection and also to diagnose abnormalities, such as gallstones. In one study, a 9.6-mm diameter catheter with a 5.0–7.5 mHz transducer was found to be applicable in both miniature swine and humans (Liu et al., 1995). Many modifications of imaging techniques, including CT, ultrasound, and MRI, have been utilized to aid in these types of procedures, and their use is demonstrated in the DVD attached to this book.

POSTOPERATIVE CARE FOR LAPAROSCOPIC AND ENDOSCOPIC PROCEDURES

If the surgeries are performed as survival procedures, appropriate postoperative care, including the use of postoperative analgesics, must be administered. Discomfort may be associated secondary to the introduction of CO_2 into the peritoneal cavity and gas in the intestines leading to ileus. Animals should also be monitored for respiratory acidosis and the potential of a tension pneumothorax.

NATURAL ORIFICE TRANSLUMINAL ENDOSCOPIC SURGERY (NOTES)

This is an emerging new surgical discipline, which is a hybrid between flexible endoscopy and laparoscopic surgery. This involves passing a flexible endoscope into the stomach, creating a hole in the gastric wall and entering the peritoneal cavity. An intervention is then performed followed by withdrawal of the endoscope back into the gastric lumen and closure of the gastrotomy. This may seem far-fetched, but basic work is now being done to test the hypothetical advantages of this new approach. The perceived advantages include a "perfect" cosmetic surgery, more rapid healing, avoidance of wound infections, and less pain. The first report of this procedure, from a group at Johns Hopkins, was on transgastric peritoneoscopy in a pig (Kalloo et al., 2004). This was followed by a report of the long-term survival of a pig that underwent a gastrojejunostomy performed with a flexible endoscope by the transgastric approach (Kantsevoy et al., 2005). Since these two early reports, there has been considerable activity in this area. Laparoscopic surgeons feel threatened that this new approach could eclipse laparoscopic interventions. Experts in flexible endoscopy now see this as a potential expansion of therapeutic options. Experiments are now under way looking at numerous transgastric procedures, including tubal ligation (Jagannath et al., 2005), splenectomy (Kantsevoy et al., 2006), cholecystectomy (Park et al., 2005), and appendectomy. In fact, though not yet reported in peer-reviewed form, the team of G.V. Rao (laparoscopic surgeon) and Nagy Reddy (expert endoscopist) from Hyderabad, India, have successfully performed transgastric appendectomy in a human. This promises to be an exciting new area of development, and the techniques and devices developed will largely be done using the porcine model. The porcine stomach is thicker and more robust than the human stomach but, interestingly, attempts to experimentally suture the stomach (for example, in gastric reduction experiments to produce weight loss) have shown that sutures easily migrate through the gastric wall under the slightest tension (Hu et al., 2005a, 2005b), which may be related to the immaturity of the animals used. For some of this work, the dog model may be preferred.

SURGICAL ROBOTICS

Surgical robotics is another evolving hybrid technology that embraces some of the aspects of laparoscopic and endoscopic procedures (Chitwood et al., 2001; Gourin and Terris, 2004; Kumar et al., 2005; Martinez and Wiegand, 2004; Oleynikov et al., 2005; Rentschler et al., 2004). The technology grew out of National Aeronautics and Space Administration (NASA) studies involving virtual reality. Semiactive and passive computer-controlled robots have been used as an extension of minimally invasive surgery and laparoscopic techniques. No truly active robot that performs a surgical procedure without a surgeon has been developed. In the case of robotic surgery as it is currently practiced, the techniques have proved to be helpful in increasing precision in micro tasks. Another form of robotic surgery involves the use of a remote console by the surgeon distant from the patient. In this procedure, referred to as *telerobotic* or *telepresence*, the surgeon can be thousands of miles distant from the patient and operate using a virtual three-dimensional procedure. In all these cases, intense training must be performed using both *in vitro* and *in vivo* models. The pig has proved to be an applicable model for training and development of these procedures. It is expected that this technology will continue to evolve and improve (Figure 13.16 and Figure 13.17).

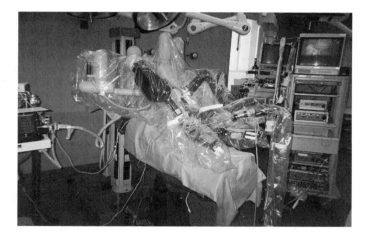

FIGURE 13.16 Advanced surgical training using the Da Vinci surgical robot. The pig is in the Trendelenberg position. (Courtesy of P. Rand Brown, DVM, Johns Hopkins University.)

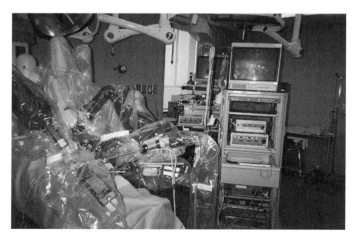

FIGURE 13.17 Surgical robot training using a porcine model. (Courtesy of P. Rand Brown, DVM, Johns Hopkins University.)

REFERENCES

Bailey, R.W., Imbembo, A.L., and Zucker, K.A., 1991, Establishment of a laparoscopic cholecystectomy training program, *Am. Surgeon*, 57(4): 231–236.

Bak, A., Perini, R.F., Muscara, M., Cotton, P.B., Hawes, R.H., and Wallace, J.L., 2000, An endoscopic animal model of sphincter of Oddi dysfunction, *Gastroenterology*, 120(5): AB2000.

Bernardo, N.O. and Gill, I.S., 2002, Laparoscopic partial nephrectomy: current status, *Arch. Esp. Urol.*, 55(7): 868–880.

Bhutani, M.S., Hoffman, B.J., and Hawes, R.H., 1998, A swine model for teaching endoscopic ultrasound (EUS) imaging and intervention under EUS guidance, *Endoscopy*, 30(7): 605–609.

Bhutani, M.S., Aveyard, M., and Stills, H.F., Jr., 2000, Improved model for teaching interventional EUS, *Gastrointest. Endosc.*, 52(3): 400–403.

Brunt, L.M., Molmenti, E.P., Kerbl, K., Soper, N.J., Stone, A.M., and Clayman, R.V., 1993, Retroperitoneal endoscopic adrenalectomy: an experimental study, *Surg. Laparosc. Endosc.*, 3(4): 300–306.

Burmester, E., Leineweber, T., Hacker, S., Tiede, U., Hutteroth, T.H., and Hohne, K.H., 2004, EUS meets Voxel-man: three-dimensional anatomic animation of linear-array endoscopic ultrasound images, *Endoscopy*, 36(8): 726–730.

Chitwood, W.R., Jr., Wiley, N.L., Chapman, W.H.H., Felger, J.E., Bailey, B.M., Ballint, T., Mendleson, K.G., Kim, V.B., Young, J.A., and Albrecht, R.A., 2001, Robotic surgical training in an academic institution, *Ann. Surg.*, 234(4): 475–486.

Chiu, A.W., Chen, M.T., Huang, W.J., Young, S.T., Cheng, C., Huang, S.W., Chu, C.L., and Chang, L.S., 1992, Laparoscopic nephrectomy in a porcine model, *Eur. Urol.*, 22(3): 250–254.

Desai, M.M., Desai, M.R., and Gill, I.S., 2005, Percutaneous endopyeloplasty: current clinical status, *BJU Int.*, 95(Suppl. 2): 106–109.

Fleshman, J.W., Brunt, L.M., Fry, R.D., Birnbaum, E.H., Simmang, C.L., Mazor, A., Soper, N., Freeman, L., and Kodner, I.J., 1993, Laparoscopic anterior resection of the rectum using a triple stapled intracorporeal anastomosis in the pig, *Surg. Laparosc. Endosc.*, 3(2): 119–126.

Freeman, L.J., 1994, Laparoscopic surgery courses, in Smith, A.C. and Swindle, M.M., Eds., *Research Animal Anesthesia, Analgesia and Surgery*, Greenbelt, MD: Scientists Center for Animal Welfare, pp. 15–24.

Freys, S.M., Heimbucher, J., and Fuchs, K.H., 1995, Teaching upper gastrointestinal endoscopy: the pig stomach, *Endoscopy*, 27(1): 73–76.

Frich, L., Hol, P.K., Roy, S., Mala, T., Edwin, B., Clausen, O.P.F., and Gladhaug, I.P., 2006, Experimental hepatic radiofrequency ablation using wet electrodes: electrode-to-vessel distance is a significant predictor for delayed portal vein thrombosis, *Eur. Radiol.*, in press.

Gholson, C.F., Provenza, J.M., Silver, R.C., and Bacon, B., 1990, Endoscopic retrograde cholangiography in the swine: a new model for endoscopic training and hepatobiliary research, *Gastrointest. Endosc.*, 36(6): 600–603.

Gill, I.S., Hsu, T.H.S., Fox, R.L., Matamoros, A., Miller, C.D., LeVeen, R.F., Grune, M.T., Sung, G.T., and Fidler, M.E., 2000, Laparoscopic and percutaneous radiofrequency ablation of the kidney: acute and chronic porcine study, *Urology*, 56(2): 197–200.

Gourin, C.G. and Terris, D.J., 2004, Surgical robotics in otolaryngology: expanding the technology envelope, *Curr. Opin. Otolaryngol. Head Neck Surg.*, 12(3): 204–208.

Griffith, S.L., Burney, B.T., Fry, F.J., and Franklin, T.D., Jr., 1989, A large animal model (swine) to study the diagnosis and treatment of cholelithiasis, *Invest. Radiol.*, 24(2): 110–114.

Gutt, C.N., Oniu, T., Schemmer, P., Mehrabi, A., and Buchler, M.W., 2004, Fewer adhesions induced by laparoscopic surgery?, *Surg. Endosc.*, 18: 898–906.

Hochberger, J., Maiss, J., Magdeburg, B., Cohen, J., and Hahn, E.G., 2001, Training simulators and education in gastrointestinal endoscopy: current status and perspectives in 2001, *Endoscopy*, 33(6): 541–549.

Hochberger, J., Maiss, J., and Hahn, E.G., 2002, The use of simulators for training in GI endoscopy, *Endoscopy*, 34(9): 727–729.

Hochberger, J., Euler, K., Naegel, A., Hahn, E.G., and Maiss, J., 2004, The compact Erlangen active simulator for interventional endoscopy: a prospective comparison in structured team-training courses on "endoscopic hemostasis" for doctors and nurses to the "Endo-Trainer" model, *Scand. J. Gastroenterol.*, 39(9): 895–902.

Hochberger, J., Matthes, K., Maiss, J., Koebnick, C., Hahn, E.C., and Cohen, J., 2005, Training with the compact EASIE biologic endoscopy simulator significantly improves hemostatic technical skill of gastroenterology fellows: a randomized controlled comparison with clinical endoscopy training alone, *Gastrointest. Endosc.*, 61(2): 204–215.

Hsu, T.H., Fidler, M.E., and Gill, I.S., 2000, Radiofrequency ablation of the kidney: acute and chronic histology in porcine model, *Urology*, 56: 872.

Hu, B., Chung, S.C., Sun, L.C., Kawashima, K., Yamamoto, T., Cotton, P.B., Gostout, C.J., Hawes, R.H., Kalloo, A.N., Kantsevoy, S.V., and Pasricha, P.J., 2005a, Eagle Claw II: a novel endosuture device that uses a curved needle for major arterial bleeding: a bench study, *Gastrointest. Endosc.*, 62(2): 266–270.

Hu, B., Chung, S.C., Sun, L.C., Kawashima, K., Yamamoto, T., Cotton, P.B., Gostout, C.J., Hawes, R.H., Kalloo, A.N., Kantsevoy, S.V., and Pasricha, P.J., 2005b, Transoral obesity surgery: endolumenal gastroplasty with an endoscopic suture device, *Endoscopy*, 37(5): 411–414.

Hu, B., Chung, S.C., Sun, L.C., Lau, J.Y., Kawashima, K., Yamamoto, T., Cotton, P.B., Gostout, C.J., Hawes, R.H., Kalloo, A.N., Kantsevoy, S.V., and Pasricha, P.J., 2005c, Developing an animal model of massive ulcer bleeding for assessing endoscopic hemostatic devices, *Endoscopy*, 37(9): 847–851.

Jagannath, S.B., Kantsevoy, S.V., Vaughn, C.A., Chung, S.S., Cotton, P.B., Gostout, C.J., Hawes, R.H., Pasricha, P.J., Scorpio, D.G., Magee, C.A., Pipitone, L.J., Kalloo, A.N., 2005, Peroral transgastric endoscopic ligation of fallopian tubes with long-term survival in a porcine model, *Gastrointest. Endosc.*, 61(3): 449–453.

Jensen, D.M., Machicado, G.A., Tapia, J.I., Kauffman, G., Franco, P., and Beilin, D., 1983, A reproducible canine model of esophageal varices, *Gastroenterology*, 84(3): 573–579.

Jones, D.R., Graeber, G.M., Tanguilig, G.G., Hobbs, G., and Murray, G.F., 1993, Effects of insufflation on hemodynamics during thoracoscopy, *Ann. Thorac. Surg.*, 55(6): 1379–1382.

Jorgensen, J.O., Gillies, R.B., Lalak, N.J., and Hunt, D.R., 1994, Lower limb venous hemodynamics during laparoscopy: an animal study, *Surg. Laparosc. Endosc.*, 4(1): 32–35.

Josephs, L.G., Arnold, J.H., and Sawyers, J.L., 1992, Laparoscopic highly selective vagotomy, *J. Laparoendosc. Surg.*, 2(3): 151–153.

Kalloo, N.N., Singh, V.K., Jagannath, S.B., Niiyama, H., Hill, S.L., Vaughn, C.A., Magee, C.A., and Kantsevoy, S.V., 2004, Flexible transgastric peritoneoscopy: a novel approach to diagnostic and therapeutic interventions in the peritoneal cavity, *Gastrointest. Endosc.*, 60(1): 114–117.

Kantsevoy, S.V., Jagannath, S.B., Niiyama, H., Chung, S.S., Cotton, P.B., Gostout, C.J., Hawes, R.H., Pasricha, P.J., Magee, C.A., Vaughn, C.A., Barlow, D., Shimonaka, H., and Kalloo, A.N., 2005, Endoscopic gastrojejunostomy with survival in a porcine model, *Gastrointest. Endosc.*, 62(2): 287–292.

Kantsevoy, S.V., Hu, B., Jagannath, S.B., Vaughn, C.A., Beitler, D.M., Chung, S.S., Cotton, P.B., Gostout, C.J., Hawes, R.H., Pasricha, P.J., Magee, C.A., Pipitone, L.J., Talamini, M.A., and Kalloo, A.N., 2006, Transgastric endoscopic splenectomy: is it possible?, *Surg. Endosc.*, 20(3): 522–525.

Kerbl, K., Figneshau, R.S., Clayman, R.V., Chadhoke, P.S., Kavoussi, L.R., Albala, D.M., and Stone, A.M., 1993, Retroperitoneal laparoscopic nephrectomy: laboratory and clinical experience, *J. Endourol.*, 7(1): 23–26.

Kopchok, G.E., Cavaye, D.M., Klein, S.R., Mueller, M.P., Lee, J.L., and White, R.A., 1993, Endoscopic surgery training: application of an in vitro trainer and *in vivo* swine model, *J. Invest. Surg.*, 6(4): 329–337.

Kulling, D., Vournakis, J.N., Woo, S., Demcheva, M.V., Tagge, D.U., Rios, G., Finkielstein, S., and Hawes, R.H., 1999, Endoscopic injection of bleeding esophageal varices with a poly-N-acetyl glocosamine gel formation in the canine portal hypertension model, *Gastrointest. Endosc.*, 49(6): 764–771.

Kumar, R., Hemal, A.K., and Menon, M., 2005, Robotic renal and adrenal surgery: present and future, *BJU Int.*, 96: 244–249.

Layman, T.S., Burns, R.P., Chandler, K.E., Russell, W.L., and Cook, R.G., 1993, Laparoscopic inguinal herniorrhaphy in a swine model, *Am. Surg.*, 59(1): 13–19.

Leighton, T.A., Liu, S.Y., and Bongard, F.S., 1993, Comparative cardiopulmonary effects of carbon dioxide versus helium pneumoperitoneum, *Surgery*, 113(5): 527–531.

Liu, J.B., Feld, R.I., Goldberg, B.B., Barbot, D.J., Nazarian, L.N., Merton, D.A., Rawool, N.M., Rosato, F.E., Winkel, C.A., and Gillum, D.R., 1995, Laparoscopic gray-scale and color Doppler U.S.: preliminary animal and clinical studies, *Radiology*, 194(3): 851–857.

Lyons, J.M. and Sosa, R.E., 1992, Laparoscopy: new applications of an established technique, *Urol. Nurs.*, 12(1): 2–8.

Ma, S. and Fang, R.H., 1994, Endoscopic mandibular angle surgery swine model, *Ann. Plast. Surg.*, 33(5): 473–475.

Martinez, B.D. and Wiegand, C.S., 2004, Robotics in vascular surgery, *Am. J. Surg.*, 188(Suppl.): 57S–62S.

Matthes, K., Cohen, J., Kochman, M.L., Cerulli, M.A., Vora, K.C., and Hochberger, J., 2005, Efficacy and costs of a one-day hands-on EASIE endoscopy simulator train-the-trainer workshop, *Gastrointest. Endosc.*, 62(6): 921–927.

Mullen, Y., Taura, Y., Nagsta, M., Miyazawa, K., and Stein, E., 1992, Swine as a model for pancreatic beta-cell transplantation, in Swindle, M.M., Ed., *Swine as Models in Biomedical Research*, Ames, IA: Iowa State University Press, pp. 16–34.

Noar, M.D., 1995, An established porcine model for animate training in diagnostic and therapeutic ERCP, *Endoscopy*, 27(1): 77–80.

Noel, P., Fagot, H., Fabre, J.M., Mann, C., Quenet, F., Guillon, F., Baumel, H., and Domergue, J., 1994, Resection anastomosis of the small intestine by celioscopy in swine: comparative experimental study between manual and mechanical anastomosis, *Ann. Chir.*, 48(10): 921–929.

Neumann, M., Mayer, G., Ell, C., Felzmann, T., Reingruber, B., Horbach, T., and Hohenberger, W., 2000, The Erlangen endo-trainer: life-like simulation for diagnostic and interventional endoscopic retrograde cholangiography, *Endoscopy*, 32(11): 906–910.

Neumann, M., Hochberger, J., Felzmann, T., Ell, C., and Hohenberger, W., 2001, Part 1. The Erlanger endo-trainer, *Endoscopy*, 33(10): 887–890.

Oleynikov, D., Rentschler, M.E., Dumpert, J., Platt, S.R., and Shane, S.M., 2005, *In vivo* robotic laparoscopy, *Surg. Innovation*, 12(2): 177–181.

Olson, K.H., Balcos, E.G., Lowe, M.C., and Bubrick, M.P., 1995, A comparative study of open, laparoscopic intracorporeal and laparoscopic assisted low anterior resection and anastomosis in pigs, *Am. Surg.*, 61(3): 197–201.

Ou, C.S., Presthus, J., and Beadle, E., 1993, Laparoscopic bladder neck suspension using hernia mesh and surgical staples, *J. Laparoendosc. Surg.*, 3(6): 563–566.

Park, P.O., Bergstrom, M., Ikeda, K., Fritscher-Raven, A., and Swain, P., 2005, Experimental studies of transgastric gallbladder surgery: cholecystectomy and cholecystogastric anastomosis (videos), *Gastrointest. Endosc.*, 61(4): 601–606.

Pasricha, P.J., Tietjen, T.G., and Kalloo, A.N., 1995, Biliary manometry in swine: a unique endoscopic model for teaching and research, *Endoscopy*, 27(1): 70–72.

Pfeffer, J., Grinshpon, R., Rex, D., Levin, B., Rosch, T., Arber, N., and Halpern, Z., 2006, The Aer-O-Scope: proof of the concept of a pneumatic, skill-independent, self-propelling, self-navigating colonoscope in a pig model, *Endoscopy*, 38(2): 144–148.

Pietrafitta, J.J., Schultz, L.S., Graber, J.N., and Hickok, D.F., 1992, An experimental technique of laparoscopic bowel resection and anastomosis, *Surg. Laparosc. Endosc.*, 2(3): 205–211.

Rentschler, M.E., Hadzialic, A., Dumpert, J., Platt, S.R., Farritor, S., and Oleynikov, D., 2004, *In vivo* robots for laparoscopic surgery, *Stud. Health Technol. Inf.*, 98: 316–322.

Rey, J.F. and Romanczyk, T., 1995, The development of experimental models in the teaching of endoscopy: an overview, *Endoscopy*, 27(1): 101–105.

Rodriguez, J., Kensing, K., Cardenas, C., and Stoltenberg, P., 1993, Laparoscopy-guided subhepatic cholecystostomy: a feasibility study in swine, *Gastrointest. Endosc.*, 39(2): 176–178.

Rumalla, A., Petersen, B.T., Baron, T.H., Burgart, L.J., Herman, L.J., Wiersema, M.J., and Gostout, C.J., 2003, Development of a swine model for benign stenosis of the bile duct by endoscopic ultrasound application of intraluminal thermal injury, *Gastrointest. Endosc.*, 57(1): 73–77.

Sahai, A.V., Hoffman, B.J., and Hawes, R.H., 1998, Endoscopic ultrasound-guided hepaticogastrostomy to palliate obstructive jaundice: preliminary results in pigs, *Gastrointest. Endosc.*, 47: AB37 (abstract).

Salzman, A.L., Strong, K.E., Wang, H.L., Wollert, P.S., Vandermeer, T.J., and Fink, M.P., 1994, Intraluminal balloonless air tonometry new method for determination of gastrointestinal mucosal carbon dioxide tension, *Crit. Care Med.*, 22(1): 126–134.

Santos Garcia-Vaquero, A. and Uson Gargallo, J., 2002, Training in laparoscopy: from the laboratory to the operating room, *Arch. Esp. Urol.*, 55(6): 643–657.

Siegel, J.H. and Korsten, M.A., 1989, ERCP in a nonhuman primate, *Gastrointest. Endosc.*, 35(6): 557–559.

Soper, N.J. and Hunter, J.G., 1992, Suturing and knot tying in laparoscopy, *Surg. Clin. N. Am.*, 72(5): 1139–1152.

Soper, N.J., Barteau, J.A., Clayman, R.V., and Becich, M.J., 1991, Safety and efficacy of laparoscopic cholecystectomy using monopolar electrocautery in the porcine model, *Surg. Laparosc. Endosc.*, 1(1): 17–22.

Soper, N.J., Brunt, L.M., Fleshman, J., Jr., Dunnegan, D.L., and Clayman, R.V., 1993, Laparoscopic small bowel resection and anastomosis, *Surg. Laparosc. Endosc.*, 3(1): 6–12.

Sorbi, D., Vazquez-Sequeiros, E., and Wiersema, M.J., 2003, A simple phantom for learning EUS-guided FNA, *Gastrointest. Endosc.*, 57(4): 580–583.

Srinivasan, A., Trus, T.T., Conrad, A.J., Scarbrough, T.J., and Swindle, M.M., 1999, Common laparoscopic procedures in swine: a review, *J. Invest. Surg.*, 12(1): 5–14.

Stump, K.C., Swindle, M.M., Saudek, C.D., and Strandberg, J.D., 1988, Pancreatectomized swine as a model of diabetes mellitus, *Lab. Anim. Sci.*, 38 (4): 439–443.

Swindle, M.M., Smith, A.C., and Hepburn, B.J.S., 1988, Swine as models in experimental surgery, *J. Invest. Surg.*, 1(1): 65–79.

Vancaillie, T.G., 1993, Laparoscopic bladder neck suspension, in Winfield, H.N., Ed., *Atlas of the Urologic Clinics of North American Urologic Laparoscopic Surgery*, Philadelphia, PA: WB Saunders, pp. 73–86.

Wagner, A.A., Solomon, S.B., and Su, L.M., 2005, Treatment of renal tumors with radiofrequency ablation, *J. Endourol.*, 19(6): 643–653.

14 Xenotransplantation and Transgenic Technologies

INTRODUCTION

Xenotransplantation procedures involving both whole organs and tissues will probably be developed to a level of clinical relevance within the next decade (Alisky, 2004; Dorling, 2002; Hoerbelt and Madsen, 2004; Ye et al., 1994). Transgenic technologies will continue to be involved in the development of organs that would be resistant to host rejection phenomena. Most likely, a combined strategy of transgenic manipulation and improvement of immunosuppressive agents and techniques will be required to achieve success. Xenografic tissue implants, such as islet cells for diabetic patients, are likely to be developed prior to whole-organ transplantation of such organs as the heart, liver, and kidneys. Swine are generally considered to be the most likely species to be utilized in clinical xenografic procedures. Primates are likely to be utilized only during initial experimental procedures because of supply, public health, and ethical considerations.

The technical aspects of the surgery involved in the xenotransplant procedures are the same as those described previously in the various system chapters in this textbook. Other considerations include ethical aspects, public health considerations, husbandry practices, and pre- and postsurgical monitoring procedures for both donors and recipients. Swine to nonhuman primate transplantations, especially baboons, are the most likely experimental procedures to be utilized during development of these procedures. For artificial organs and tissue or cellular implantations of porcine origin, other species may be used during some aspects of development if the xenografic devices provide a barrier to immunologic insult from the recipient.

The Institute of Medicine and the Food and Drug Administration held public hearings in 1995 and 1998 to discuss the various aspects of xenotransplantation and to develop draft guidelines, which have been updated since then (Institute of Medicine, 1996; Food and Drug Administration, 1999, 2002, 2003; Public Health Service, 1996). In addition, the World Health Organization (WHO), U.S. Department of Health and Human Services (USDHHS) through its Secretary's Advisory Committee on Xenotransplantation (SACX), and the Organization for Economic Cooperation and Development (OECD) held a series of hearings and also drafted documents on the procedures (OECD, 2001; WHO, 1998, 2001; USDHHS, 2004a, 2004b). The emphasis of these proceedings is on public health considerations.

ETHICAL CONSIDERATIONS

Millions of swine per year are consumed as food by the human population, and they are not an endangered species. These two considerations, combined with the physiological, immunologic, and zoonotic disease considerations, make swine the predominant choice as a donor animal for xenographic procedures. More of the general population would have ethical concerns with the use of primates. The entire captive population of some species of primates, such as baboons, could be consumed by clinical requests within a few years. The ethical considerations of xenographic transplant have been reviewed (Institute of Medicine, 1996; Prentice et al., 1994).

The number of human donors for whole organs has not kept up with the demand, and patients routinely die while on waiting lists for organ transplants. This problem could be greatly alleviated, if not eliminated, by a significant increase in the number of humans willing to donate organs. This solution has obvious advantages over the development of xenografic organ donations; however, it is unlikely to be successful because of the reluctance of surviving family members to donate organs, and the fact that many organs would not have the necessary physiological function at the time of donation. However, campaigns to increase the number of organ donors should be conducted to decrease the need for xenografts.

Tissue transplants involve an additional consideration. They are being developed for diseases, such as diabetes, because of the potential improvement in therapy that could be derived from not having to control the disease with insulin injections. The potential for curative therapy with these xenografic therapies is a significant consideration in their development. Some tissue xenografts have already been performed for Parkinson's disease (Brevig et al., 2000).

The risk-benefit ratio of these therapies must include a consideration of the potential for transmission of zoonotic diseases, which is minimal with swine compared to species such as nonhuman primates.

With all of these considerations, it is probable that the majority of the human population will accept the necessity of using swine as xenografic donors with minimal moral and ethical reservations.

IMMUNOLOGIC AND PHYSIOLOGICAL CONSIDERATIONS

The immunologic and physiological considerations associated with xenografic transplantation have been summarized in the Institute of Medicine study (1996) and in the scientific literature (Binns and Pabst, 1996; Brevig et al., 2000; Chang et al., 2002; Cramer and Makowka, 1994; Diamond et al., 2001; Dor et al., 2005; Gonzalez-Stawinski et al., 2001; Harrison et al., 2004; Kaufmann et al., 1995; Kuwaki et al., 2005; Laber et al., 2002; Lai et al., 2002; Lai and Prather, 2002; Lin and Platt, 1996; Loss et al., 2001; Matthews and Beran, 1996; Milland et al., 2005; Mirenda et al., 2005; Nagashima et al., 2003; Nash et al., 1999; Phelps et al., 2003; Pursel et al., 1996; Smith and Beattie, 1996; Schroeder et al., 2005; Tseng et al., 2005; USDHHS, 2004b; Yamada et al., 2005).

Phylogenetically distant species experience hyperacute rejection phenomena when donor endothelium is attacked by circulating antibodies. In pig-to-higher-primate grafts, these are associated with sugar (carbohydrate) antigens, such as Gal (1-3) on the donor tissue epithelium. These antigens are not present in humans and higher nonhuman primates. These xenoreactive antibodies attach to the endothelium of the discordant organ, and the complement system is activated. Within a few hours, the vascularized graft develops edema and hemorrhage followed by clotting, which decreases the blood supply to the transplanted organ. Techniques that reduce circulating antibodies, such as plasmapheresis or immunoabsorption, prolong the period of time that is required for the hyperacute rejection to occur.

Acute vascular rejection is a delayed response occurring days to weeks after the transplant. This delayed reaction is likely to be a sequela of hyperacute rejection caused by genetic upregulation of different genes in the endothelium of the graft. T-cell immune responses related to the major histocompatibility complex (MHC), as occurring in allografts, are likely to be the next phase of rejection to be overcome. These complex reactions may be successfully overcome with immunosuppressive drugs.

Chronic rejection occurs months to years following the transplant procedure and is the result of combined humeral and cellular responses. This phenomenon occurs in allografts, but no xenografic procedure has been successful for a long enough period of time to determine whether or not it will occur with xenografts.

Cellular grafts can be protected from the chronic rejection phenomenon by protection against circulating antibodies using encapsulation or protective filtration of the cells. Whole-organ transplantation offers more formidable obstacles. Research approaches to prevention of the various types of rejection include pharmaceutical development of immunosuppressive agents, modification of the source tissue, modification of the host immune system, and encapsulation and protection methodologies for the donor tissue or organ.

Donor modification includes transgenic modification, breeding inbred lines for MHC or SLA (swine leucocyte antigen) alleles, gene knockout, blocking of complementary fragments of ribonucleic acid (antisense RNA), human complement regulatory proteins (DAF, CD59), stem cell therapy, and antibody masking. All these technologies are being evolved to block the immune response of the host. Transgenic/knockout modification is currently the most advanced of the methods (Alisky, 2004; Chen et al., 2003; Dorling, 2002; Gonzalez-Stawinski et al., 2001; Hoerbelt and Madsen, 2004; Laber et al., 2002; Pinkert, 1994; Sachs, 1992; Ye et al., 1994).

The host response may be modified by bone marrow chimerism or microchimerism phenomena discovered in long-term transplant recipients and caused by gradual lymphocytic release from transplanted tissue. Bone marrow chimerism has not been tried between swine and humans. It would involve ablation of the host bone marrow and replacement with bone marrow from the donor animal. The procedure was unsuccessful in a single trial with baboon-to-human chimerism. This is the procedure that stimulated the Institute of Medicine study (1996).

Semipermeable barriers for encapsulation of tissues and cells are currently feasible but are unlikely to be developed for whole-organ transplantation without new technology.

STRATEGIES FOR DEVELOPMENT OF TRANSGENIC ANIMALS

Transgenic/knockout swine are being developed to eliminate barriers to xenotransplantation, develop new models in biomedical research, and improve agricultural animals. Prather has summarized the strategies currently being used, which are described in later text (Prather, 2005). Transgenic technologies involve manipulating the chromosome by adding a functional gene, adding an inhibitory gene, or disabling a gene. The National Swine Resource and Research Center at the University of Missouri provides supportive services for these technologies: (http://www.nsrrc.missouri.edu/).

Methodologies for producing transgenic pigs are pronuclear injection, oocyte transduction, sperm-mediated transfer, and nuclear transfer (Chang et al., 2002; Diamond et al., 2001; Dor et al., 2005; Gonzalez-Stawinski et al., 2001; Harrison et al., 2004; Kuwaki et al., 2005; Lai et al., 2002; Lai and Prather, 2002; Milland et al., 2005; Nagashima et al., 2003; Phelps et al., 2003; Schroeder et al., 2005; Yamada et al., 2005). Pronuclear transfer involves injecting a DNA construct into the pronucleus of a fertilized zygote at the 2- or 4-cell stage. Oocyte transduction involves integrating the construct with a replication-deficient retrovirus into an unfertilized oocyte. Sperm-mediated transfer involves mixing the construct with sperm and then fertilizing the oocyte. Nuclear transfer involves integrating the construct into fetal-cell-derived donor populations and replacing the nuclei of oocytes with the new nucleus, which clones the animal.

All these techniques have been utilized in swine, but there are problems with low percentages of integration, the site of integration, and offspring with unintended defects. Oocyte transduction was used to produce pigs that expressed the Green Fluorescent Protein (eGFP) marker (Cabot et al., 2001). Nuclear transfer is probably the most significant development because it provides increased specificity over the other techniques and was essential to the knockout technology for α-Gal-deficient pigs (Lai et al., 2002; Phelps et al., 2003). Cloning techniques for pigs are also under development (Du et al., 2005; Kragh et al., 2005). Techniques of embryo transfer and artificial insemination are discussed in Chapter 8.

REGULATORY GUIDELINES

Since the Institute of Medicine (1996) conference, the international community has developed guidelines and regulations concerning potential public health issues, recommendations for protocol approval, animal sources, clinical issues, and the need for a national or international registry and archive (Institute of Medicine, 1996; Food and Drug Administration, 1999, 2002, 2003; OECD, 2001; Public Health Service, 1996; WHO, 1998, 2001; USDHHS, 2004a, 2004b). Many countries have also developed their own specific guidelines and regulations concerning xenotransplantation. Summaries of the general recommendations of these guidelines and regulations are discussed in this section, with most of the discussion related to the documents from the U.S. and WHO.

The protocol issues include the composition of the xenotransplant team, the site, the protocol review, health surveillance plans, and the need for informed consent. The transplant team should include an infectious disease physician with knowledge of zoonoses, a veterinarian with expertise in zoonotic disease and animal husbandry, a transplant immunologist, a hospital epidemiologist or infection control specialist, and the director of the clinical microbiology laboratory at the transplantation site, in addition to the transplant surgical team. In the U.S., the transplantation site has to be accredited and associated with the Organ Procurement and Transplantation Network. The protocol has to be reviewed by the following institutions: Animal Care and Use Committee, the Biosafety Committee, and the Institutional Review Board for Human Research. All these committees must have expertise in zoonotic diseases and disease control. In addition, these protocols may be subject to regulation by the Food and Drug Administration. The protocol must include a plan for screening of the animal, organ, and the source herd. It must also include provisions for written informed consent and education of the recipient.

The major portion of many of these documents relate to the regulation of animal sources of xenotransplant tissues. Animals have to be bred and reared in captivity, herds have to be closed and serologically screened, and tissues and organs from slaughterhouses cannot be used. Biomedical research animal facilities should be accredited by the Association for the Assessment and Accreditation of Laboratory Animal Care (AAALAC) International to ensure compliance with all federal guidelines. The facility has to maintain and follow detailed standard operating facilities for quarantine and disease surveillance. Standard laboratory animal procedures for sanitation of facilities need to be followed, and the feed source and quality should be controlled to prevent the use of rendered products. Preclinical screening of the herd for potential zoonoses is required. Herd health maintenance programs include both prevention and treatment of potential zoonotic problems. The use of sentinel animals is suggested for monitoring serology, microbiology, and necropsy studies. Individual animals to be used as donors must also be screened. Biopsies of the actual xenograft are recommended.

The clinical issues deal with the safety of the recipient and the medical personnel and require lifetime monitoring and archiving. It also requires educating the recipient about informing close contacts. The archived information must be made available to a national archiving registry.

The World Health Organization (1998, 2001) prepared similar documents. However, they recommend the use of gnotobiotic animals that have been cesarean-derived and maintained in barrier facilities. Recognizing the impracticality of this source of animals, they provide for the use of animals from a similar health and husbandry situation as that described in the PHS document. They provide a criteria list for developing an exclusion list of infectious agents for xenograficorgan donation. Their criteria for the clinical arena is similar to the PHS document; however, it is not as detailed.

These guidelines are so rigorous as to preclude the conduction of xenotransplants in centers other than major medical ones with accredited laboratory animal programs. Very few commercial producers of swine could provide the required husbandry without substantial modification of their facilities and programs. Many of the existing guidelines and regulations are in draft form and most are continuously modified as the science of xenotransplantation develops.

PUBLIC HEALTH CONSIDERATIONS

Pig-to-human xenotransplantation carries little risk compared to other species, such as primates. A proposed set of practical considerations on herd maintenance and surveillance has been published (Swindle, 1996, 1998). Viruses with the highest potential for zoonotic infection in immunocompromised recipients or damage to tissue and cellular xenotransplants include swine influenza, human influenza, encephalomyocarditis virus, porcine rotavirus, porcine lymphotropic herpesvirus, porcine reovirus, parainfluenza virus, porcine adenovirus, porcine cytomegalovirus, porcine circovirus, porcine pneumovirus, hepatitis E, pseudorabies, and porcine retrovirus. The incidence of occurrence and potential of pathogenicity vary widely among these infectious agents. The primary agents of concern are the influenza viruses and retrovirus. There is also concern that some of these viruses, such as herpesvirus, may lead to the development of lymphoproliferative disorders.

Bacterial pathogens and commensals of concern include those of the following genera: *Salmonella*, *Pasteurella*, *Brucella*, *Erysipelothrix*, *Streptococcus*, *Campylobacter*, *Staphylococcus*, *Coxiella*, *Leptospira*, and *Mycobacterium*. The pathogenicity of these organisms varies widely depending upon the species and serotype.

Parasitic organisms should also be considered in the screening. *Balantidium coli* is the primary protozoal organism of concern. Nematodes can generally be controlled by anthelmintics; however, some, such as *Ascaris suum*, can also be associated with visceral larval migrans and damage of donor organs such as the liver.

The potential list of pathogens is much longer and includes organisms such as dermatomycoses, and immunocompromised patients may experience infection from organisms not previously associated with zoonotic disease. Summaries of the infectious risks associated with xenotransplantation and strategies for eliminating them have been published (Cooper et al., 1991; Fishman, 2000; Kalter and Heberling, 1995; Michaels, 2002; Michaels and Simmons, 1994; Swindle, 1996, 1998; Tucker et al., 2004; Ye et al., 1994). Specific pathogen-free (SPF) swine, as discussed in Chapter 1, could be used as a starter herd source for animals; however, they would not be considered to have the pathogen-free status necessary for xenotransplantation by current guidelines. There is a suggestion that a term such as *xenografic-defined flora animals* should be used, rather than SPF, to differentiate these two standards (Swindle, 1996).

MANAGEMENT AND HUSBANDRY STRATEGIES

Management and husbandry strategies are discussed in the FDA (1999, 2002) and PHS (1996) guidelines, and by Swindle (1996, 1998). AAALAC-accredited biomedical research facilities with ABSL 2 facilities are more likely to be capable of handling the quarantine and disease control standards required for xenotransplantation. The standard operating procedures for husbandry and the construction of the facilities should be adequate to meet these guidelines in such accredited research facilities. Their standards could be used as a guideline for the development of xenografic transplant facilities for housing donor herds of animals.

The use of a sentinel animal system for monitoring herds, similar to those used in rodent facilities for biomedical research, should be instituted. The use of multiple rooms with an all-in/all-out management system for batch procurement of tissues and organs is probably the most practical method to ensure compliance.

OTHER CONSIDERATIONS

Besides the immunologic and zoonotic problems to be overcome through research and management techniques, there are other issues to be considered. Swine may have congenital defects or genetic diseases, such as malignant hyperthermia; physiological function may be poor. There are also nonflexible regulations related to the shipment of swine and porcine tissues between states and countries that are in effect for agricultural and economic control purposes. Swine used for xenografts will either have to receive an exception to these regulations or be in compliance, depending upon the destination locale (Swindle, 1996).

It is likely that guidelines will continue to be revised as additional scientific meetings and public forums are held on the subject.

REFERENCES

Alisky, J.M., 2004, Xenografts are an achievable breakthrough, *Med. Hypotheses*, 63(1): 92–97.

Binns, R.M. and Pabst, R., 1996, The functional structure of the pig's immune system, resting and activated, in Tumbleson, M.E. and Schook, L.B., Eds., *Advances in Swine in Biomedical Research*, Vol. 1, New York: Plenum Press, pp. 253–266.

Brevig, T., Holgersson, J., and Widner, H., 2000, Xenotransplantation for CNS repair: immunological barriers and strategies to overcome them, *Trends Neurosci.*, 23(8): 337–344.

Cabot, R.A., Kuhholzer, B., Chan, A.W., Lai, L., Park, K.W., Chong, K.Y., Schatten, G., Murphy, C.N., Abeydeera, L.R., Day, B.N., and Prather, R.S., 2001, Transgenic pigs produced using *in vitro* matured oocytes infected with a retroviral vector, *Anim. Biotechnol.*, 12(2): 205–214.

Chang, K., Qian, J., Jiang, M.S., Liu, Y.H., Wu, M.C., Chen, C.D., Lai, C.K., Lo, J.L., Hsiao, C.T., Brown, L., Bolen, J., Jr., Huang, J.I., Ho, P.Y., Shih, P.Y., Yao, C.W., Lin, W.J., Chen, C.H., Wu, F.Y., Lin, Y.J., Xu, J., and Wang, K., 2002, Effective generation of transgenic pigs and mice by linker based sperm-mediated gene transfer, *BMC Biotechnol.*, 2: 5–18.

Chen, F.X., Tang, J., Li, N., Shen, B.H., Zhou, Y., Xie, J., and Chou, K.Y., 2003, Novel SLA class I alleles of Chinese pig strains and their significance in xenotransplantation, *Cell Res.*, 13(4): 285–294.

Cooper, D.K.C., Ye, Y., Rolf, L.L., Jr., and Zuhdi, N., 1991, The pig as a potential organ donor for man, in Cooper, D.C.K., Kemp, E., Reemtsma, K., and White, D.J.G., Eds., *Xenotransplantation: The Transplantation of Organs and Tissues Between Species*, Berlin: Springer-Verlag, pp. 481–500.

Cramer, D.V. and Makowka, L., 1994, The use of xenografts in experimental transplantation, in Cramer, D.V., Podesta, L.G., and Makowka, L., Eds., *Handbook of Animal Models in Transplantation Research*, Boca Raton, FL: CRC Press, pp. 299–310.

Diamond, L.E., Quinn, C.M., Martin, M.J., Lawson, J., Platt, J.L., and Logan, J.S., 2001, A human CD46 transgenic pig model system for the study of discordant xenotransplantation, *Transplantation*, 71(1): 132–142.

Dor, F.J.M.F., Kuwaki, K., Tseng, Y.L., Shimizu, A., Houser, S.L., Yamada, K., Hawley, R.J., Patience, C., Awwad, M., Fishman, J.A., Robson, S.C., Sachs, D.H., Schuurman, H.J., Cooper, D.K.C., 2005, Potential of aspirin to inhibit thrombotic microangiopathy in 1,3-galactosyltransferase gene-knockout pig hearts after transplantation in baboons, *Transpl. Proc.*, 37(1): 489–490.

Dorling, A., 2002, Clinical xenotransplantation: pigs might fly?, *Am. J. Transpl.*, 2: 695–700.

Du, Y., Kragh, P.M., Zhang, X., Purup, S., Yang, H., Bolund, L., and Vajta, G., 2005, High overall *in vitro* efficiency of porcine handmade cloning (HMC) combining partial zona digestion and oocyte trisection with sequential culture, *Cloning Stem Cells*, 7(3): 199–205.

Fishman, J.A., Xenotransplantation from swine: making a list, checking it twice, 2000, *Xenotransplantation*, 7(2): 93–95.

Food and Drug Administration (FDA), 1999, PHS Guideline on Infectious Disease Issues in Xenotransplantation, U.S. Dept. of Health and Human Services, Center for Biologics Evaluation and Research, http://www.fda.gov/cber/guidelines.htm.

Food and Drug Adminstration (FDA), 2002, Precautionary Measures to Reduce the Possible Risk of Transmission of Zoonoses by Blood and Blood Products from Xenotransplantation Product Recipients and Their Intimate Contacts, Draft guidance for Industry, U.S. Dept. of Health and Human Services, Center for Biologics Evaluation and Research, http://www.fda.gov/cber/guidelines.htm.

Food and Drug Administration (FDA), 2003, Source Animal, Product, Preclinical, and Clinical Issues Concerning the Use of Xenotransplantation Products in Humans, U.S. Dept. of Health and Human Services, Center for Biologics Evaluation and Research, http://www.fda.gov/cber/guidelines.htm.

Gonzalez-Stawinski, G.V., Lin, S.S., and Platt, J., 2001, Xenotransplantation, in Pond, W.G. and Mersmann, H.J., Eds., *The Biology of the Domestic Pig*, Ithaca, NY: Comstock Publishing, pp. 712–728.

Harrison, S., Boquest, A., Grupen, C., Faast, R., Guildolin, A., Giannakis, C., Crocker, L., McIlfatrick, S., Ashman, R., Wengle, J., Lyons, I., Tolstoshev, P., Cowan, P., Robins, A., O'Connell, P., D'Apice, A.J., and Nottie, M., 2004, An efficient method for producing alpha(1,3)-galactosyltransferase gene knock-out pigs, *Cloning Stem Cells*, 6(4): 327–331.

Hoerbelt, R. and Madsen, J.C., 2004, Feasibility of xeno-transplantation, *Surg. Clin. N. Am.*, 84(1): 289–307.

Institute of Medicine, 1996, *Xenotransplantation: Swine, Ethics and Public Policy*, Washington, D.C.: National Academy Press.

Kalter, S.S. and Heberling, R.L., 1995, Xenotransplantation and infectious diseases, *ILAR J.*, 5(37) 31–37.

Kaufmann, C.L., Gaines, B.A., and Ildstad, S.T., 1995, Xenotransplantation, *Annu. Rev. Immunol.*, 13(3): 339–367.

Kragh, P.M., Du, Y., Corydon, T.J., Purup, S., Bolund, L., and Vajta, G., 2005, Efficient *in vitro* production of porcine blastocysts by handmade cloning with a combined electrical and chemical activation, *Theriogenology*, 64(7): 1536–1545.

Kuwaki, K., Tseng, Y.L., Dor, F.J., Shimizu, A., Houser, S.L., Sanderson, T.M., Lancos, C.J., Prabharasuth, D.D., Cheng, J., Moran, K., Hisashi, Y., Mueller, N., Yamada, K., Greenstein, J.L., Hawley, R.J., Patience, C., Awwad, M., Fishman, J.A., Robson, S.C., Schuurman, H.J., Sachs, D.H., Cooper, D.K., 2005, Heart transplantation in baboons using alpha1,3–galactosyltransferase gene-knockout pigs as donors: initial experience, *Nat. Med.*, 11(1): 29–31.

Laber, K., Whary, M., Bingel, S.A., Goodrich, J.A., Smith, A.C., and Swindle, M.M., 2002, Biology and diseases of swine, in Fox, J.G., Anderson, L.C., Loew, F., and Quimby, F.W., Eds., *Laboratory Animal Medicine*, 2nd ed., New York: Academic Press, pp. 615–675.

Lai, L., Kolber-Simonds, D., Park, K.W., Cheong, H.T., Greenstein, J.L., Im, G.S., Samuel, M., Bonk, A., Rieke, A., Day, B.N., Murphy, C.N., Carter, D.B., Hawley, R.J., and Prather, R.S., 2002, Production of Alpha-1,3-Galactosyltransferase Knockout Pigs by Nuclear Transfer Cloning, *Science*, 295(5557), pp. 1089–1092.

Lai, L. and Prather, R.S., 2002, Progress in producing knockout models for xenotransplantation by nuclear transfer, *Annal. Med.*, 34(7–8): 501–506.

Lin, S.S. and Platt, J.L., 1996, Immunologic advances towards clinical xenotransplantation, in Tumbleson, M.E. and Schook, L.B., Eds., *Advances in Swine in Biomedical Research*, Vol. 1, New York: Plenum Press, pp. 147–162.

Loss, M., Schmidtko, J., Przemeck, M., Kunz, R., Arends, H., Jalali, A., Lorenz, R., Piepenbrock, S., Klempnauer, J., and Winkler, M., 2001, A primate model for discordant pig to primate kidney xenotransplantation without hyperacute graft rejection, *J. Invest. Surg.*, 14(1): 21–29.

Matthews, P.J. and Beran, G.W., 1996, Assessment of public health aspects of porcine xenotransplantation, in Tumbleson, M.E. and Schook, L.B., Eds., *Advances in Swine in Biomedical Research*, Vol. 1, New York: Plenum Press, pp. 163–170.

Michaels, M.G., 2002, Xenozoonoses: the risk of infection after xenotransplantation, in Fox, J.G., Anderson, L.C., Loew, F.M., and Quimby, F.W., *Laboratory Animal Medicine*, 2nd ed., New York: Academic Press, pp. 1107–1116.

Michaels, M.G. and Simmons, R.L., 1994, Xenotransplant-associated zoonoses: strategies for prevention, *Transplantation*, 57(1): 1–7.

Milland, J., Christiansen, D., and Sandrin, M.S., 2005, 1,3-galactosyltransferase knockout pigs are available for xenotransplantation: are glycosyltrnasferases still relevant?, *Immunol. Cell Biol.*, 83(6): 687–693.

Mirenda, V., Golshayan, D., Read, J., Berton, I., Warrens, A.N., Dorling, A., and Lechler, R.I., 2005, Achieving permanent survival of islet xenografts by independent manipulation of direct and indirect T-cell responses, *Diabetes*, 54(4): 1048–1055.

Nagashima, H., Fujimura, T., Takahagi, Y., Kurome, M., Wako, N., Ochial, T., Esaki, R., Kano, K., Saito, S., Okabe, M., and Murakami, H., 2003, Development of efficient strategies for the production of genetically modified pigs, *Theriogenology*, 59(1): 95–106.

Nash, K., Chang, Q., Watts, A., Treter, S., Oravec, G., Ferrara, V., Buhler, L., Basker, M., Gojo, S., Sachs, D.H., White-Scharf, M., Down, J.D., and Cooper, D.K.C., 1999, Peripheral blood progenitor cell mobilization and leukapheresis in pigs, *Lab. Anim. Sci.*, 49(5): 645–648.

National Swine Resource and Research Center, University of Missouri, (http://www.nsrrc.missouri.edu/).

Organisation for Economic Co-operation and Development (OECD)/World Health Organization (WHO), 2001, Consultation on Xenotransplantation Surveillance: Summary. Geneva, WHO, http://whqlibdoc.who.int/hq/2001/WHO_CDS_CSR_EPH_2001.1.pdf.

Phelps, C.J., Koike, C., Vaught, T.D., Boone, J., Wells, K.D., Chen, S.H., Ball, S., Specht, S.M., Polejaeva, I.A., Monahan, J.A., Jobst, P.M., Sharma, S.B., Lamborn, A.E., Garst, A.S., Moore, M., Demetris, A.J., Rudert, W.A., Bottino, R., Bertera, S., Trucco, M., Starzy, T.E., Dai, Y., and Ayares, D.L., 2003, Production of 1,3-galactosyltransferase-deficient pigs, *Science*, 299(5605), pp. 411–414.

Pinkert, C.A., 1994, *Transgenic Animal Technology*, New York: Academic Press.

Prather, R.S., 2005, Transgenic approaches to developing swine models, *Proceedings of the Swine in Biomedical Research Conference: Update on Animal Models Symposium*, 56th Annual AALAS Meeting, St. Louis, MO.

Prentice, E.D., Fox, I.J., Dixon, R.S., Antonson, D.L., and Lawson, T.A., 1994, History, donor considerations and ethics of xenotransplantation, in Smith, A.C. and Swindle, M.M., Eds., *Research Animal Anesthesia, Analgesia and Surgery*, Greenbelt, MD: Scientists Center for Animal Welfare, pp. 25–36.

Public Health Service, 1996, Draft Public Health Service Guideline on Infectious Disease Issues in Xenotransplantation, *Fed. Regist.*, 61(185): 49920–49932.

Pursel, V.G., Solomon, M.B., and Wall, R.J., 1996, Genetic engineering of swine, in Tumbleson, M.E. and Schook, L.B., Eds., *Advances in Swine in Biomedical Research*, Vol. 1, New York: Plenum Press, pp. 189–206.

Sachs, D.H., 1992, MHC-Homozygous miniature swine, in Swindle, M.M., Ed., *Swine as Models in Biomedical Research*, Ames, IA: Iowa State University Press, pp. 3–15.

Schroeder, C., Allan, J.S., Nguyen, B.N., Wu, G., Zhang, T., Azimzadeh, A.M., Madsen, J.C., Schuurman, H.J., Sachs, D.H., and Pierson, R.N., III, 2005, Hyperacute rejection is attenuated in GalT knockout swine lungs perfused *ex vivo* with human blood, *Transpl. Proc.*, 37(1): 512–513.

Smith, T.P.L. and Beattie, C.W., 1996, Identifying tumor initiator/suppressor and penetrance associated genes by gene mapping, in Tumbleson, M.E. and Schook, L.B., Eds., *Advances in Swine in Biomedical Research*, Vol. 1, New York: Plenum Press, pp. 239–249.

Swindle, M.M., 1996, Considerations of specific pathogen free swine (SPF) in xenotransplantation, *J. Invest. Surg.*, 9(3): 267–271.

Swindle, M.M., 1998, Defining appropriate health status and management programs for specific pathogen free (SPF) swine for xenotransplantation, *Ann. NY Acad. Sci.*, 62: 111–120.

Tseng, Y.L, Sachs, D.H., and Cooper, D.K.C., 2005, Porcine hematopoietic progenitor cell transplantation in nonhuman primates: a review of progress, *Transplantation*, 79(1): 1–9.

Tucker, A.W., Foweraker, J.E., Belcher, C.E., Moloo, B., Bell, J.A., Humar, A., Mazzulli, T., and Grant, D., 2004, Control of microbial contamination during surgical harvest of pig renal xenografts, *Xenotransplantation*, 11(1): 91–6.

U.S. Department of Health and Human Services (USDHHS), Secretary's Advisory Committee on Xenotransplantation (SACX), 2004a, Informed consent in clinical research, Draft, http://www4.od.nih.gov/oba/SACX/reports/IC_draft_030905.pdf.

U.S. Department of Health and Human Services (USDHHS), Secretary's Advisory Committee on Xenotransplantation (SACX), 2004b, Report on the state of the science in xenotransplantation, Draft, http://www4.od.nih.gov/oba/SACX/reports/Sci_draft_030905.pdf.

World Health Organization (WHO), 2001, WHO Guidance on Xenogeneic Infection/Disease Surveillance and Response: A Strategy for International Cooperation and Coordination. Geneva: World Health Organization (WHO), 1998, Xenotransplantation: Guidance on Infectious Disease Prevention and Management, Geneva, Switzerland: WHO. http://whqlibdoc.who.int/hq/1998/WHO_EMC_ZOO_98.1.pdf.

Yamada, K., Yazawa, K., Shimizu, A., Iwanaga, T., Hisashi, Y., Nuhn, M., O'Malley, P., Nobori, S., Vagefi, P.A., Patience, C., Fishman, J., Cooper, D.K.C., Hawley, R.J., Greenstein, J., Schuurman, H.J., Awwad, M., Sykes, M., and Sachs, D.H., 2005, Marked prolongation of porcine renal xenograft survival in baboons through the use of alpha 1,3-galactosyltransferase gene-knockout donors and the cotransplantation of vascularized thymic tissue, *Nat. Med.*, 11(1): 32–34.

Ye, Y., Niekrasz, S., Kosanke, R., Welsh, R., Jordan, H.E., Fox, J.C., Edwards, W.C., Maxwell, C., and Cooper, D.K.C., 1994, The pig as a potential organ donor for man, *Transplantation*, 57(6): 694–703.

15 Toxicology

Ove Svendsen

INTRODUCTION

The pig was domesticated from wild swine by the Chinese more than 7000 years ago. Within the last few centuries, the pig has increasingly been used in biomedical research. Today, more than 60,000 pigs are used in the EU every year for scientific procedures. The number of minipigs used for scientific purposes is relatively low. The minipig was introduced in Europe in the early 1970s for scientific purposes. In the mid-1980s the minipig was introduced in toxicology as an alternative to nonrodent species because of the many biochemical, anatomic, and physiological similarities with humans compared to other nonrodent species (Swindle and Smith, 1998). Their extensive use since then has highlighted details of the areas in which the minipig has become a particularly useful animal species for toxicological studies and toxicity testing.

DOMESTIC PIGS AND MINIPIGS

The use of the domestic pig (*Sus scrofa domestica*) in biomedical research is well established, particularly in surgical and physiological research. For years both pigs and minipigs have been used in pharmacology and toxicology to answer specific questions when the more conventional species were found unsuitable. The development of minipigs has resulted in strains of more manageable size than the domestic pig. Because of the aforementioned well-accepted physiological and other similarities to humans, the minipig has becoming increasingly attractive as an animal model in toxicology. There are several strains of minipigs (Göttingen, Yucatan, Sinclair, Hanford and others). This chapter is based on the experience of this author primarily with the Göttingen minipig.

There is an increasing interest in minipigs because they share many similarities with humans anatomically and physiologically; in particular, the skin and kidney are very similar to those of humans (Montiero-Riviere et al., 1996; Mortensen et al., 1998; Swindle, 1998). They are available as purpose-bred specific pathogen-free (SPF) high-quality animals and in addition, there is a growing amount of background data and increased regulatory acceptability. There are advantages over the traditional non-rodent species in relation to the ethical difficulties of using animals in biomedical research. The minipig has been shown to be sensitive to a wide variety of drugs and chemicals and exhibits specific responses to particular drug classes. It has been demonstrated that minipigs can be used for all routes of oral and parenteral administration. In many cases, they are preferable to dogs or primates for metabolic or pharmacological reasons. As an example, they have recently been developed as an alternative to other large animal species for vaginal irritancy testing (D'Cruz et al., 2005). Consequently, there are scientific, economic, and sociological reasons that make minipigs good animal models in toxicology and other scientific disciplines. The principal disadvantage is that in toxicity testing the minipig may require more test compound than the traditional smaller nonrodent species.

STRAINS OF MINIPIGS

There are several advantages to using the Göttingen strain of minipigs. This strain was developed by Göttingen University in the 1960s by cross-breeding of the Minnesota minipig, first with

Vietnamese potbellied pigs, and then with German Landrace to obtain pale skin. The Göttingen minipig is now a white nonpigmented and small-sized minipig with an adult body weight of 30–40 kg if kept on a restricted diet. They have been purpose-bred in Europe for years and are now also used in the U.S., making them readily available. They are of very high microbiological and parasitic quality. There is a full genetic background available, and background toxicology control data have accumulated in the scientific literature.

Other strains of minipigs are particularly available in the U.S., such as the Yucatan miniature and micropig, Sinclair, and Hanford, which may be used for the same purposes as the Göttingen minipig. The Yucatan micropig strain is of a similar size to the Göttingen minipig, whereas the Sinclair and Hanford minipig strains are considerably larger. A comparison of body weights of the various breeds of minipigs is included in Chapter 1. Farm breeds of pigs are generally too large to be useful in chronic toxicology studies because of their rapid growth and the need to use a greater quantity of test substances.

PHARMACOKINETICS AND METABOLISM

Pharmacokinetic studies are easily performed in the minipig with repeated blood sampling or sampling of other body fluids or tissues as demonstrated by Anzenbacherová et al. (2003) and Witkamp and Monschouwer (1998). The cytochrome P450 liver metabolic pattern has been studied in detail by Skaanild and Friis (1997, 1999, 2005) and compared to that of humans. This topic has recently been reviewed by Skaanild (2006). Most recently, the regulation of gender-dependent CYP2A expression in pigs has been described by Gillberg et al. (2006). In the past few years, by using primary hepatocyte cultures or hepatocyte microsomes, several subfamilies of cytochrome P450 have been characterized in the pig and minipig, such as CYP1A, CYP2A, CYP2B, CYP2C, CYP2E, and CYP3A. The porcine cytochrome P450 isoenzymes CYP1A, CYP2A, and CYP3A metabolize the same substrates as the human isoenzymes. However, with regard to metabolism the isoenzymes CYP2B, CYP2D, and CYP2E seem to be different from their human counterparts. In this respect, it is very important that CYP2D, in particular, be different from that of humans because this enzyme in humans is responsible for the existence of subgroups of fast or slow metabolizers, which is related to the level of CYP2D expression. In drug development, there is some concern if a new potential drug is primarily metabolized by this isoenzyme. The isoenzymes that are similarity to those of humans are identical in about 75% of their cDNA sequence. In early drug development, quantitative structure–activity relationship (QSAR) can be used to predict which CYPs may be expected to be involved, to help decide the most appropriate animal species for toxicity testing. In this respect, the minipig seems to be a good choice, in case CYP1A, CYP2A, or CYP3A are important in metabolism of the drug candidate. Actual testing by using porcine primary hepatocyte cultures or hepatocyte microsomes may confirm their usefulness.

In general, some comparisons can be made between pigs and humans in phase II enzyme biotransformation. Pigs have relatively high glucuronidation activity, low sulfation activity, and high acetylation activity. There are large differences between the plasma elimination of some drugs in pigs and humans, and these differences also exist between other species and humans. Consequently, one must be cautious when making direct comparisons between humans and animals without comparative data (Witkamp and Monshouwer, 1998).

REPEAT DOSE TOXICOLOGY

In addition to the traditional routes of dosing, porcine use in general toxicology testing employing the continuous intravenous infusion, dermal, or inhalation route has been described in detail in the literature and is discussed in Chapter 9. Background data on toxicological endpoints (ophthalmology, clinical pathology, ECG, organ weight, histopathology, and reproduction parameters) have been well established, allowing studies to be interpreted. Normal values are given in the various system chapters of this book as well as in the appendix. In the context of regulatory toxicity testing, histopathology and toxicopathological data of spontaneous or drug-induced origin have been published in the scientific literature (Svendsen et al., 1998; Dincer and Svendsen, 2006; Skydsgaard et al., 2006).

ROUTES OF DOSE ADMINISTRATION

The most common route of dosing is oral, either by gavage or dietary dosing in a medicated diet. Dosing by oral gavage in conscious minipigs may be stressful for the animals, but because of anatomic and physiological similarities with human skin the minipig is particularly useful for dermal studies. This route has been used for acute and repeat dose dermal toxicology studies, dermal absorption studies, phototoxicity studies, and photosensitization studies. Parenteral dosing can be applied by intramuscular, subcutaneous, intradermal, and intravenous injection. The latter can be applied either by bolus injection or as continuous intravenous infusion. The details of continuous intravenous infusion in the minipig have been described by Brinck (2000a), who has also described the surgical preparation for the application of continuous intravenous infusion (Brinck, 2000b). Other routes, such as nasal dosing or inhalation dosing (Koch et al., 2001), have also been successfully applied in minipigs. Techniques of dosing pigs are discussed in Chapter 1.

OBSERVATIONS AND SAMPLING TECHNIQUES

The observations required in toxicity testing, such as clinical signs, body weight, ophthalmoscopy, and electrocardiography (Nahas et al., 2002), are routine procedures in toxicity testing with the minipig. In addition, control hematologic and clinical chemistry data are available in the scientific literature and in the appendix (Ellegaard et al., 1995; Damm Jørgensen et al., 1998a). Parameters of immunotoxicity may be included (Hinton, 2000). Blood-sampling techniques have been described in detail in Chapter 1 and by Bollen et al. (2000) and Swindle (1998).

NECROPSY PROCEDURE

Pathology plays an important role in toxicology because it provides information about the differences in tissue and organ morphology that establish the presence or absence of lesions and whether there are dose–effect relationships in respect of such lesions. This information is critical in establishing toxic and other effects of a substance. In regulatory toxicity testing, samples of the tissues and organs listed in Table 15.1 have to be fixed for subsequent microscopic examination. When sampling specimens from tissues and organs for microscopic examination, it is crucial that the sampling procedure be highly standardized in order to avoid sampling bias.

When conducting postmortem procedures in minipigs, some major differences from other nonrodent species have to be taken into consideration. These include the gastrointestinal tract, thymus, thyroid, parathyroid, and brain. In minipigs, the cecum and colon are very large and, in addition, the colon is shaped spiral. Most of the thymus is located in the cervical region and the rest in the thoracic cavity. However, microscopic examination is usually performed on the thoracic portion, as in other species. The thyroid is located on the ventral part of the trachea cranial to the thoracic inlet. As another variation, the two lobes of the thyroid are merged into one organ. The parathyroids are not embedded or attached to the thyroids, but are located instead in the cranial part of the thymus in 90% of the cases. It is not unusual that the parathyroids are located in the most cranial part of the thymus caudal to the hyoid bone. It requires significant skill to be able to locate both glands routinely. The portion of the skull covering the brain of the minipig is rather thick owing to well-developed pneumatic sinuses and thick bones, rendering extraction of the brain (cerebrum, cerebellum, and medulla oblongata) complicated. After removal of skin, eyes, and

TABLE 15.1
Organs and Tissues for Histology

Abdominal organs	Endocrine/exocrine/glandular
Kidney	Adrenals
Liver (all lobes) and gallbladder	Epididymis
Spleen	Mammary gland
Ureters	Ovaries
Urinary bladder	Pancreas
Uterus (horns, cervix, oviduct)	Parathyroids
Vagina	Pituitary
Cardiovascular	Prostate
Aorta (thoracic)	Salivary glands
Bone marrow smear	Seminal vesicle
Heart (septum, left ventricle)	Testes
Vena cava	Thymus
Central nervous system	Thyroid
Cerebral cortex	Respiratory
Cerebellar cortex	Bronchiolar lymph nodes
Eyes with optic nerve	Larynx
Medulla	Lungs (bilateral cranial and caudal lobes)
Pons	Trachea
Spinal cord (cervical, thoracic, lumbar)	Skin/musculoskeletal/head
Gastrointestinal	Femur (medial condyle)
Cecum	Sciatic nerve
Colon	Mandibular lymph node
Duodenum	Skeletal muscle
Esophagus	Rib
Ileum	Skin
Jejunum	Sternum with bone marrow
Mesenteric lymph node	Tongue
Rectum	Tonsils
Stomach (glandular and nonglandular)	Also include any lesion observed grossly

muscle tissue from the skull, five cuts with an oscillating saw can be made. The first two cuts can be made from the foramen magnum dorsolaterally on the right and left side toward the temporal region. Another two cuts can then be made ventromedially in the right and left side, directed toward the entrance of the optic nerve in the eye cavity. Finally, a transverse cut can be made horizontally just in front of the olfactory bulbs. In this manner, the portion of the skull covering the brain is loosened and by use of a screwdriver, chisel, or similar instrument placed in the transverse cut, the complete skull bone can be removed without damaging the brain.

In the sampling sequence of the tissues and organs listed in Table 15.1, it is important to organize the sampling in such a manner that organs most likely to undergo the quickest postmortem changes are sampled first. This applies in particular to the tissues of the gastrointestinal tract and the eyes. The mucosa of the gastrointestinal tract undergoes rapid autolysis and retinal dislocation may occur in the eyes.

HISTOPATHOLOGY

The Göttingen minipig is a barrier-raised pig, free from any porcine bacterial, viral, or parasitic disease. Extensive studies of the histopathology of this breed have been performed. Histopathological findings of a spontaneous nature are few and, in general, focal and mild (Svendsen et al., 1998; Dincer and Svendsen, 2006). The most recent and most extensive collection of control data is reported by Skydsgaard et al. (2006). There are four significant spontaneous findings: (1) arteritis (scattered, focal, necrotic/fibrinoid), (2) tubular atrophy/hypoplasia in testis (focal), (3) serous atrophy (bone marrow fat cells, mainly femur/tibia), and (4) hemorrhagic syndrome. The etiology of all four features is unknown. Thrombocytopenia is extensive in the hemorrhagic syndrome and probably associated with an immune-complex-mediated condition and marked degenerative or regenerative megakaryocytic changes (Carrasco et al., 2003). Normal histology of the various organs and tissues are located in the system chapters of this book. Table 15.2 contains incidental microscopic findings in Göttingen minipigs used as controls in toxicological studies.

REPRODUCTIVE TOXICOLOGY

In testing for reproductive toxicity, in general, two animal species have to be used, a rodent and a nonrodent species. The two species routinely used are the rat and the rabbit, and in special cases the dog or nonhuman primate. The minipig may be an alternative species in teratogenicity and reproductive studies in which traditional species as mice, rats, or rabbits are not suitable. Nonhuman primates have supply and conservation considerations and the majority have single offspring. Minipigs can be purpose-bred to SPF standards, are relatively inexpensive, and have a number of similarities with humans. The reproductive characteristics of the Göttingen minipig have been described by Damm Jørgensen (1998a) together with a teratogenicity-testing protocol and historical control data. Additional information on reproductive and fetal techniques can be found in Chapter 8.

The testing protocol can be summarized as follows. Sexual maturity in minipigs is reached before the animals are 6 months of age. In general, minipig gilts are 5–10 months of age when included in studies. In teratogenicity studies, the treatment period extends from the start of implantation (day 11) to the closure of the hard palate (day 35), inclusive of gestation. Different routes of administration can be used. Although the oral route is the most commonly used, continuous intravenous infusion can also be applied (McAnulty, 2000). Pregnancy status can be ascertained by ultrasonography in week 4 or 5 of gestation. The sows are killed on day 110 to 112 of gestation. At term, the fetuses weigh 350–400 g, and it is possible to perform a full necropsy on them. In general, the protocol includes fetal examinations after removal from the uterus, alizarin staining of the skeleton, and free-hand sectioning of Bouins-fixed heads. For skeletal examination, radiographs may be added because the bones of the skull and bone densities are better visualized by them than with alizarin staining (Damm Jørgensen, 1998a). The historical data include skeletal diagnoses from 220 fetuses and spontaneous malformation data from more than 3700 newborn or stillborn fetuses. This protocol has shown that the Göttingen minipig is highly susceptible to the teratogenic effects of tretinoin with malformations resembling retinoic acid teratogenicity in humans (Damm Jørgensen, 1998b). Hematologic and clinical chemical control data of pregnant Göttingen minipigs have been reported by Damm Jørgensen et al. (1998a).

The Göttingen minipig has also proved useful as a model for studying effects on male fertility (Damm Jørgensen et al., 1998b). The reported data support the assumption that the male minipig may prove to be more susceptible to chemicals, with adverse effect on fertility, than the male rat. The minipig has closer similarities to humans with respect to fertility rate, percentage of morphologically similar sperm, percentage of sperm with progressive motility, and it has a spontaneous incidence of cryptorchidism.

JUVENILE STUDIES

So-called juvenile studies were introduced in the nonclinical testing program because it was realized that several drugs were administered in pediatric clinics to children without test data, justifying the safe use of the drugs in this particular age group. Standard nonclinical studies using adult animals, or safety information from adult humans, cannot always adequately predict these differences in safety profiles for all pediatric age groups, especially reactions on immature systems such as the

TABLE 15.2
Incidences of Microscopic Findings in 51 Male and 51 Female Göttingen Minipigs Used as Control Animals in 4-, 13-, and 26-Week General Toxicity Studies

Findings	Up to 4 weeks		13 weeks		26 weeks	
	M (39)	F (39)	M (7)	F (7)	M (5)	F (5)
Liver						
Inflammatory cell infiltration, focal	6	7	1	1	1	1
Haematopoiesis		2				
Single cell necrosis of hepatocytes		2				
Lungs						
Inflammatory cell infiltration, focal	2					
Granulomas		2				
Mineralization, focal	1	2	1		2	
Haemorrhage, alveolar	5	6	1	1		
Macrophages, alveolar	4	4	1	2	2	2
Pneumonia/bronchopneumonia, focal	1	1	1	1		
Arteritis						1
Pancreas						
No findings						
Skin						
Inflammation, focal	1	3				
Spleen						
Arteritis/fibrinoid necrosis		1				
Adrenals						
Haematopoiesis	2	2				
Lymphoid cell infiltration, focal	2	3				
Bone marrow (femur/tibia/sternum)						
Serous atrophy of fat cells	11	5			5	3
Brain						
Mineralization, focal	1	1			2	
Lymphoid cell infiltration, focal	1	1				
Gallbladder						
Oedema, subserosal		1				
Hypoplasia	1					
Cholecystitis		1		1		
Heart						
Lymphoid cell infiltration, focal		1				
Oedema, epicardial		1				
Haemorrhage, subendo./interstitial	1			1		1
Arteritis	1					
Kidneys						
Lymphoid/inflammatory cell infiltration, focal		1	1	1	1	
Basophilia/dilation, tubular		7		3		
Mineralization, focal	2	1				
Cysts		2				
Arteritis/periarteritis/fibrinoid necrosis		2				

Note: M = males, F = females; number of animals in parentheses.

Source: Reprinted from Svendsen, O., Skydsgaard, M., Aarup, V., and Klastrup, S., 1998, *Scand. J. Lab. Anim. Sci.* (Suppl. 1), 231–234. With permission.

developing brain, pulmonary system, kidneys, reproductive, and immune systems. This motivated the U.S. Food and Drug Administration and the European Medicines Agency to issue draft guidelines for nonclinical testing of human pharmaceuticals in juvenile animals for pediatric indications. Traditionally, rats and dogs have been the species of choice for such testing, but other species, such as the pig, may be more appropriate in some circumstances.

The appropriateness of the minipig in this type of testing has been evaluated by scientists at Scantox in Denmark and the results presented at various scientific conferences (Harling and Makin, personal communication, 2005). The optimal protocols for the conduct of juvenile studies includes cross-fostering, in order to handle all animals allocated to one mother as one study group and thus avoid a litter effect. Cross-fostering of juvenile minipigs for performance of juvenile toxicology studies is a realistic practical proposition, using estrus synchronization with mating in breeder facilities and subsequent housing in the testing laboratory. Properly controlled synchronization results in delivery of all minipigs within a few days, allowing for cross-fostering. Various standard techniques, such as oral or parenteral dosing, ophthalmoscopy, ECG, and repeated collection of blood samples for clinical pathology and toxicokinetics are practical and feasible. Implantation of vascular access ports was successful from day 7 and onward for daily intravenous dosing. Background clinical pathology data are important, because many of the standard parameters change rapidly with increasing age (Damm Jørgensen et al., 1998a). Techniques for synchronization and breeding are discussed in Chapter 8 and vascular access port implantation is discussed in Chapter 9.

REGULATORY ACCEPTANCE

The pig and minipig as a model in toxicity testing of pharmaceuticals and other chemicals has now been well accepted by Japan, EU, and the U.S. (Ikeda et al., 1998). The pig and minipig are specifically mentioned as a potential nonrodent species in the guidelines of Japan and Canada. The OECD 409 guideline lists pig and minipig as optional species. However, evidence should be provided that it is a suitable species, and there is still some regulatory resistance or unfamiliarity related to issues with background data and spontaneous and toxicological pathology.

CONCLUSIONS FOR TOXICOLOGICAL MODELS

The minipig is a useful nonrodent animal species in investigations of safety issues in drug development. However, selection of the most suitable nonrodent species is a complex issue. Many pharmaceutical industries still hold the dog as the first choice and move from the dog only when there is a specific justification. The minipig may be discounted merely on the basis of body weight because it requires larger quantities of test article. The quality of minipigs is generally high. However, housing barrier-raised breeds such as the Göttingen minipig in some laboratories requires isolation from other species and other breeds of pigs because this strain is raised under conditions that result in some immunologic naivety. There is still some regulatory resistance or unfamiliarity related to issues with background data and spontaneous and toxicological pathology; however, this is changing. The key area with maximum benefit for the pharmaceutical industry is that there is a significant justification for selecting the minipig when developing dermally applied drugs.

ACKNOWLEDGMENTS

The contributions of Robert J. Harling and Andrew Makin, Scantox A/S, DK-4623 Lille Skensved, Denmark, are highly appreciated.

REFERENCES

Anzenbacherová, E., Anzenbacher, P., Svoboda, Z., Ulrichová, J., Kvetina, J., Zoulová, J., Perlík, F., and Martínková, J., 2003, Minipig as a model for drug metabolism in man: comparison of *in vitro* and *in vivo* metabolism of propafenone, *Biomed. Pap.*, 147: 155–159.

Bollen, P.J.A., Hansen, A.K., Rasmussen, H.J., Eds., 2000, *The Laboratory Swine*, London: CRC Press.

Brinck, P., 2000a, Multidose infusion toxicity studies in the minipig, in Healing, G. and Smith, D., Eds., *Handbook of Pre-Clinical Continuous Intravenous Infusion*, London: Taylor and Francis, pp. 233–240.

Brinck, P., 2000b, Surgical preparation of the minipig, in Healing, G. and Smith, D., Eds., *Handbook of Pre-Clinical Continuous Intravenous Infusion*, London: Taylor and Francis, pp. 225–232.

Carrasco, L., Madsen, L.W., Salguero, F.J., Nunez, A., Sanchez-Cordon, P., and Bollen, P., 2003, Immune complex-associated thrombocytopenic purpura syndrome in sexually mature Göttingen minipigs, *J. Comp. Pathol.*, 128: 25–32.

Damm Jørgensen, K., 1998a, Minipig in reproduction toxicology, in Svendsen, O., Ed., The minipig in toxicology, *Scand. J. Lab. Anim. Sci.*, 25(Suppl. 1): 63–75.

Damm Jørgensen, K., 1998b, Teratogenic activity of tretionoin in the Göttingen minipig, in Svendsen, O., Ed., The minipig in toxicology, *Scand. J. Lab. Anim. Sci.*, 25(Suppl. 1): 235–243.

Damm Jørgensen, K., Ellegaard, L., Klastrup, S., and Svendsen, O., 1998a, Haematological and clinical chemical values in pregnant and juvenile Göttingen minipigs, in Svendsen, O., Ed., The minipig in toxicology, *Scand. J. Lab. Anim. Sci.*, 25(Suppl. 1): 181–190.

Damm Jørgensen, K., Kledal, T.S.A., Svendsen, O., and Skakkebæk, N.E., 1998b, The Göttingen minipig as a model for studying effects on male fertility, in Svendsen, O., Ed., The minipig in toxicology, *Scand. J. Lab. Anim. Sci.*, 25(Suppl. 1): 161–169.

D'Cruz, O.J., Erbeck, D., and Uckun, F.N., 2005, A study of the potential of the pig as a model for the vaginal irritancy of benzalkonium chloride in comparison to the nonirritant microbicide PHI-443 and the spermicide vanadocene dithiocarbamate, *Toxicol. Path.*, 33(4): 465–476.

Dincer, Z. and Svendsen, O., 2006, Pathology of Göttingen minipig: background and incidentally occurring changes, in Gad, S.C., Ed., *Animal Models in Toxicology*, 2nd ed., New York: Marcel Dekker.

Ellegaard, L., Dam Jørgensen, K., Klastrup, S., Kornerup Hansen, A., and Svendsen, O., 1995, Haematologic and clinical chemical values in 3 and 6 months old Göttingen minipigs, *Scand. J. Lab. Anim. Sci.*, 22: 239–248.

Gillberg, M., Skaanild, M.T., and Friis, C., 2006, Regulation of gender-dependent CYP2A expression in pigs: involvement of androgens and CAR, *Basic Clin. Pharmacol. Toxicol.*, in press.

Hinton, D.M., 2000, US FDA "Redbook II" immunotoxicity testing guidelines and research in immunotoxicity evaluations of food chemicals and new food proteins, *Toxicol. Pathol.*, 28: 467–478.

Ikeda, G.J., Friedman, L., and Hattan, D.G., 1998, The minipig as a model in regulatory toxicity testing, in Svendsen, O., Ed., The minipig in toxicology, *Scand. J. Lab. Anim. Sci.*, 25(Suppl. 1): 99–105.

Koch, W., Windt, H., Walles, M., Borlak, J., and Clausing, P., 2001, Inhalation studies with the Göttingen minipig, *Inhalation Toxicol.*, 13: 249–259.

McAnulty, P., 2000, Reproductive infusion toxicity studies in the minipig, in Healing, G. and Smith, D., Ed., *Handbook of Pre-Clinical Continuous Intravenous Infusion*, London: Taylor and Francis, pp. 241–250.

Montiero-Riviere, N.A. and Riviere, J., 1996. The pig as a model for cutaneous pharmacology and toxicology research, in Tumbleson, M.E. and Schook, L.B., Eds., *Advances in Swine in Biomedical Research*, Vol. 2, New York: Plenum Press, pp. 425–458.

Mortensen, J.T., Brinck, P., and Lichtenberg, J., 1998, The minipig in dermal toxicology, A literature review, In Svendsen, O., Ed., The minipig in toxicology, *Scand. J. Lab. Anim. Sci.*, 25(Suppl. 1): 77–83.

Nahas, K., Baneux, P., and Detweiler, D., 2002, Electrocardiographic monitoring in the Göttingen minipig, *Comp. Med.*, 52: 258–264.

Skaanild, M.T., 2006, Porcine cytochrome P450 and metabolism, *Curr. Pharm. Des.*, 12: 1421–1427.

Skaanild, M.T. and Friis, C., 1997, Characterization of the P450 system in Göttingen minipigs, *Pharmacol. Toxicol.*, 80(Suppl. 11): 28–33.

Skaanild, M.T. and Friis, C., 1999, Cytochrome P450 sex differences in minipigs and conventional pigs, *Pharmacol. Toxicol.*, 85: 174–180.

Skaanild, M.T. and Friis, C., 2005, Porcine CYP2A polymorphisms and activity, *Basic Clin. Pharmacol. Toxicol.*, 97: 115–121.

Skydsgaard, M., Harling, S.M., and Nielsen, G., 2006, Background pathology in Göttingen minipigs, *Exp. Toxicol. Pathol.*, in press.

Svendsen, O., Skydsgaard, M., Aarup, V., and Klastrup, S., 1998, Spontaneously occurring microscopic lesions in selected organs of the Göttingen minipig, in Svendsen, O., Ed., The minipig in toxicology, *Scand. J. Lab. Anim. Sci.*, 25(Suppl. 1): 230–234.

Swindle, M.M., 1998, *Surgery, Anaesthesia and Experimental Techniques in Swine*, Ames, IA: Iowa State University Press.

Swindle, M. and Smith, A.C., 1998, Comparative anatomy and physiology of the pig, in Svendsen, O., Ed., The minipig in toxicology, *Scand. J. Lab. Anim. Sci.*, 25(Suppl. 1): 10–21.

Witkamp, R.F. and Monshouwer, M., 1998, Pharmacokinetics *in vivo* and *in vitro* in swine, in Svendsen, O., Ed., The minipig in toxicology, *Scand. J. Lab. Anim. Sci.*, 25(Suppl. 1): 45–56.

16 Radiobiology

Swine were among the earliest large animal models used in radiobiology research (Brown and Johnson, 1970, 1971; Lefaix and Daburon, 1998), but largely became replaced by the dog, because of the difficulties in handling them in the laboratory in the 1950s and 1960s. There is a resurgence of the use of swine for particular types of radiobiology research, in part, owing to the improved technical procedures in handling and anesthesia that have been developed since then. Specifically, the areas in which swine are utilized are for studies involving total body irradiation, immune suppression, skin and muscular damage, pulmonary fibrosis, CNS paralysis, digestive system damage, tissue and bone marrow transplant, and vascular injury. This section provides an overview of the most significant areas of interest for using porcine models.

Some confusion may exist in comparing the older literature to the current publications, in that it was conventional in the U.S. for rad units (radiation dose) to be utilized rather than gray units. For practical purposes, 1 gray (Gy) = 100 rad or 1cGy = 1 rad. One Gy is the absorption of 1 J of radiation energy by 1 kg of matter (1 Gy = 1 J/kg = 1 $m^2 \cdot sec^{-2}$). Typically, a total-body dose of approximately 10–20 Gy is uniformly fatal to humans and swine. There is variation in swine owing to age and source of radiation, but typically dosages less than 7 Gy are not fatal. Short-term death is usually due to bone marrow suppression and long-term death is usually due to infection following dermal or organ pathology, and some long-term survivors develop neoplasia (Brown and Johnson, 1970, 1971). Whole-body irradiation with 6 Gy demonstrated that lymphocytic and neutrophilic suppression in conjunction with alterations in LDH, ALT, AST, amylase, and urea can be useful in prediction of radiation injury (Donnadieu-Claraz et al., 1999).

Bone marrow transplantation and suppression may be useful as part of transplantation and xenotransplantation protocols (Dor et al., 2004; Gollackner et al., 2003; Pennington et al., 1986). Total-body irradiation was used by Pennington (1986), who administered 900 rads (9 Gy) of irradiation for bone marrow transplant and Dor (2004) and Gollackner (2003), who administered 100 cGy for adjunct immunosuppression in organ transplantation. Thymic irradiation (700 cGy) was also used by the latter two authors for the same purpose.

Radiation fibrosis has been studied extensively in the pig (Douglas et al., 1985; Hopewell et al., 1994; Lefaix et al., 1996; Lefaix et al., 1993; Martin et al., 1993; Rezvani et al., 2000; Sabatier et al., 1992; van den Aardweg et al., 1990). Fibrosis of the skin, subcutaneous tissue, and muscle model is readily induced in swine with different sources of radiation usually applied focally in dosages ranging from 4 to 340 Gy. Epithelial, microvascular, vascular, and muscular changes have been demonstrated in addition to alterations in biochemical, collagen, myoglobin, and other morphological changes. This particular model seems to be one in which swine can replace other large animal species in development of treatments.

Pulmonary fibrosis can be induced in swine with 6–40 Gy (ED_{50} 21–26 Gy) either as homogeneous sequential dosages or, in some cases, single dosage to produce the syndrome that occurs in humans (Baumann et al., 2000; Kasper et al., 1993; Kasper et al., 1994; Takahashi et al., 1995). The model has been used for both treatment and diagnostic development. The syndrome is characterized by consolidation, thickening of bronchioalveolar tissues, thickened septum, edema, hemorrhage, and inflammation.

Radiation-induced nephropathy has also been studied in the pig (Robbins et al., 1989; Robbins et al., 1991a, 1991b, 1993; Zimmerman et al., 1995). Selective kidney damage, including arteritis, necrosis, scarring, and calcification, along with alterations in glomerular filtration rate, blood flow, and hematocrit can be induced with a wide range of localized dosages of radiation 3–100 Gy. The ED_{50} in mature pigs is approximately 11 and 8 Gy for immature pigs.

CNS paralysis following radiation injury has also been studied (van den Aardweg et al., 1994, 1995). In sexually mature farm pigs the ED_{50} dose was 27–28 Gy when delivered as a single dose to varying lengths of the cervical spinal cord. Paralysis occurred in 7–16 weeks postexposure. White matter necrosis leading to neuropathy was histologically detectable. The syndrome had a rapid onset of less than 48 h to paralysis, when the first clinical signs were noticed. Immature pigs less than 23 weeks old had spontaneous recovery.

Pigs have also been studied for the effects of radiation enteritis due to both ingestion and administration of radiation doses (Scanff et al., 1999). Increasingly, pigs are being utilized in the evaluation of radiation therapies and safety evaluation in a variety of organs and systems (Antoch et al., 2004; Baumann et al., 2000; Fajardo et al., 2002; Hom et al., 2005; Li et al., 2005; Radfar and Sirois, 2003; Stepinac et al., 2005). It is likely that the use of pigs in radiobiology-related research will increase in the future as the pig becomes recognized as a replacement for canine models in many of these areas.

REFERENCES

Antoch, G., Kaiser, G.M., Mueller, A.B., Metz, K.A., Zhang, H., Kuehl, H., Westermann, S., Broelsch, C.E., Mueller, S.P., Bockisch, A., and Debatin, J.F., 2004, Intraoperative radiation therapy in liver tissue in a pig model: monitoring with dual modality PET/CT, *Radiology*, 230(3): 753–760.

Baumann, M., Appold, S., Geyer, P., Knorr, A., Voigtmann, L., and Herrmann, T.H., 2000, Lack of effect of small high dose volumes on the dose response relationship for the development of fibrosis in distant parts of the ipsilateral lung in minipigs, *Int. J. Radiat. Biol.*, 76(4): 477–485.

Brown, D.G. and Johnson, D.F., 1970, Clinical and gross pathological findings in swine relative to late effects of mixed gamma-neutron and X-irradiation, *Radiat. Res.*, 44: 498–511.

Brown, D.G. and Johnson, D.F., 1971, Unilateral and bilateral exposure of swine to fission neutrons, *Health Phys.*, 21: 537–545.

Donnadieu-Claraz, M., Benderitter, M., Joubert, C., and Voisin, P., 1999, Biochemical indicators of whole body γ-radiation in the pig, *Int. J. Radiat. Biol.*, 75(2): 165–174.

Dor, F.J.M.F., Doucette, K.E., Mueller, N.J., Wilkinson, R.A., Bajwa, J.A., McMorrow, I.M., Tseng, Y.L., Kuwaki, K., Houser, S.L., Fishman, J.A., Cooper, D.K.C., and Huang, C.A., 2004, Posttransplant lymphoproliferative disease after allogeneic transplantation of the spleen in miniature swine, *Transplantation*, 78(2): 286–291.

Douglas, B.G., Grulkey, W.R., Chaplin, D.J., Lam, G., Skarsgard, L.D., and Denekamp, J., 1985, Pions and pig skin: preclinical evaluation of RBE for early and late damage, *Int. J. Radiat. Oncol. Biol. Phys.*, 12: 221–229.

Fajardo, L-G.L.F., Prionas, S.D., Kaluza, G.L., and Raizner, A.E., 2002, Acute vasculitis after endovascular brachytherapy, *Int. J. Radiat. Oncol. Biol. Phys.*, 53(3): 714–719.

Gollackner, B., Dor, F.J., Knosalla, C., Buhler, L., Duggan, M., Huang, C.A., Houser, S.L., Sachs, D.H., Kawai, T., Ko, D.S., and Cooper, D.K., 2003, Spleen transplantation in miniature swine: surgical technique and results in major histocompatibility complex-matched donor and recipient pairs, *Transplantation*, 75(11): 1799–1806.

Hom, D.B., Unger, G.M., Pernell, K.J., and Manivel, J.C., 2005, Improving surgical wound healing with basic fibroblast growth factor after radiation, *Laryngoscope*, 115(3): 412–422.

Hopewell, J.W., van den Aardweg, G.J.M.J., Morris, G.M., Rezvani, M., Robbins, M.E.C., Ross, G.A., Whitehouse, E.M., Scott, C.A., and Horrobin, D.F., 1994, Amerlioration of both early and late radiation induced damage to pig skin by essential fatty acids, *Int. J. Radiat. Oncol.*, 30(5): 1119–1125.

Kasper, M., Rudolf, T., Hahn, R., Peterson, I., and Müller, M., 1993, Immuno- and lectin histochemistry of epithelial subtypes and their changes in a radiation-induced lung fibrosis model of the mini pig, *Histochemistry*, 100: 367–377.

Kasper, M., Fuller, S.D., Schuh, D., and Müller, M., 1994, Immunohistological detection of the β subunit of prolyl 4-hydroxylase in rat and mini pig lungs with radiation induced pulmonary fibrosis, *Virchows Arch.*, 425: 513–519.

Lefaix, J.L. and Daburon, F., 1998, Diagnosis of acute localized irradiation lesions: review of the French experimental experience, *Health Phys.*, 75(4): 375–384.

Lefaix, J.L., Martin, M., Tricaud, Y., and Daburon, F., 1993, Muscular fibrosis induced after pig skin irradiation with single doses of ^{192}Ir -rays, *Br. J. Radiol.*, 66: 537–544.

Lefaix, J.L., Delanian, S., Lepat, J.J., Tricaud, Y., Martin, M., Nimrod, A., Baillet, F., and Daburon, F., 1996, Successful treatment of radiation induced fibrosis using Cu/Zn-SOD and Mn-SOD: an experimental study, *Int. J. Radiat. Oncol. Biol. Phys.*, 35(2): 305–312.

Li, J., Shan, Z., Ou, G., Liu, X., Zhang, C., Baum, B.J., and Wang, S., 2005, Structural and functional characteristics of irradiation damage to parotid glands in the miniature pig, *Int. J. Radiat. Oncol. Biol. Phys.*, 62(5): 1510–1516.

Martin, M., Lefaix, J.L., Pinton, P., Crechet, F., and Daburon, F., 1993, Temporal modulation of TGF-β1 and β-actin gene expression in pig skin and muscular fibrosis after ionizing radiation, *Radiat. Res.*, 134: 63–70.

Pennington, L.R., Popitz, F., Sakamoto, K., Pescovitz, M.D., and Sachs, D.H., 1986, Bone marrow transplantation in miniature swine: I. Autologous and SLA matched allografts, in Tumbleson, M.E., Ed., *Swine in Biomedical Research*, Vol. 1, New York: Plenum Publishers, pp. 377–380.

Radfar, L. and Sirois, D.A., 2003, Structural and functional injury in minipig salivary glands following fractionated exposure to 70 Gy of ionizing radiation: an animal model for human radiation induced salivary gland injury, *Oral Surg. Oral Med. Oral Path. Oral Radiol. Endodontics*, 96(3): 267–274.

Rezvani, M., Uzlenkova, N., Whitehouse, E., Frenkel, L., Wilkinson, J.H., Ross, G., Morris, G.M., Hopewell, J.W., and Pilipenko, N., 2000, Effects of lipochromin and levosinum in the modulation of radiation induced injury to pig skin, *Br. J. Radiol.*, 73(871): 771–775.

Robbins, M.E.C., Campling, D., Rezvani, M., Golding, S.J., and Hopewell, J.W., 1989, Nephropathy in the mature pig after irradiation of a single kidney: a comparison with the immature pig, *Int. J. Radiat. Oncol. Biol. Phys.*, 16: 15129–1528.

Robbins, M.E.C., Bywaters, T., Rezvani, M., Golding, S.J., and Hopewell, J.W., 1991a, Residual radiation induced damage to the kidney of the pig as assayed by retreatment, *Int. J. Radiat. Biol.*, 60(6): 917–928.

Robbins, M.E.C., Wooldridge, M.J.A., Jaenke, R.S., Whitehouse, E., Golding, S.J., Rezvani, M., and Hopewell, J.W., 1991b, A morphological study of radiation nephropathy in the pig, *Radiat. Res.*, 126: 317–327.

Robbins, M.E.C., Jaenke, R.S., Bywaters, T., Golding, S.J., Rezvani, M., Whitehouse, E., and Hopewell, J.W., 1993, Sequential evaluation of radiation induced glomerular ultrstructural changes in the pig kidney, *Radiat. Res.,* 135: 351–364.

Sabatier, L., Martin, M., Crechet, F., Pinton, P., and Dutrillaux, B., 1992, Chromosomal anomalies in radiation induced fibrosis in the pig, *Mutat. Res.*, 284: 257–263.

Scanff, P., Monti, P., Joubert, C., Grison, S., Gourmelon, P., and Griffiths, N.M., 1999, Modified bile acid profiles in mixed neutron and γ-irradiated pigs, *Int. J. Radiat. Biol.*, 75(2): 209–216.

Stepinac, T.K., Chamot, S.R., Rungger-Brandle, E., Ferrez, P., Munoz, J.L., van den Bergh, H., Riva, C.E., Pournaras, C.J., and Wagnieres, G.A., 2005, Light induced retinal vascular damage by Pd-porphyrin luminescent oxygen probes, *Invest. Opthal. Vis. Sci.*, 46(3): 956–966.

Takahashi, M., Balazs, G., Pipman, Y., Moskowitz, G.W., Palestro, C.J., Eacobacci, T., Khan, A., and Herman, P.G., 1995, Radiation induced lung injury using a pig model: evaluation by high resolution computed tomography, *Invest. Radiol.*, 30(2): 79–86.

Van den Aardweg, G.J.M.J., Arnold, M., and Hopewell, J.W., 1990, A comparison of the radiation response of the epidermis in two strains of pig, *Radiat. Res.*, 124: 283–287.

Van den Aardweg, G.J.M.J., Hopewell, J.W., Whitehouse, E.M., and Calvo, W., 1994, A new model of radiation induced myelopathy: a comparison of the response of mature and immature pigs, *Int. J. Radiat. Oncol. Biol. Phys.*, 29(4): 763–770.

Van den Aardweg, G.J.M.J., Hopewell, J.W., and Whitehouse, E.M., 1995, The radiation response of the cervical spinal cord of the pig: effects of changing the irradiated volume, *Int. J. Radiat. Oncol. Biol. Phys.*, 31(1): 51–55.

Zimmermann, A., Schubiger, P.A., Mettler, D., Geiger, L., Triller, J., and Rösler, H., 1995, Renal pathology after arterial Yttrium-90 microsphere administration in pigs: a model for superselective radioembolization therapy, *Invest. Radiol.*, 30(12): 716–723.

17 Imaging Techniques: CT, MRI, and PET Scanning

Aage Kristian Olsen, Dora Zeidler, Kasper Pedersen,
Michael Sørensen, Svend Borup Jensen, Ole Lajord Munk

SCANNERS

This chapter and the attached DVD deals with three different imaging techniques: computerized tomography (CT), magnetic resonance imaging (MRI), and positron emission tomography (PET).

CT is the use of x-ray equipment to obtain images from different angles of the body. A computer processes the data to develop a cross-sectional image of the body in a series of slices. CT can show different types of tissues and organs, such as bones and blood vessels, with good detail and contrast.

MRI involves the use of a magnetic field that forces the hydrogen cellular nuclei to align in different positions with the magnetic field. A radiofrequency pulse specific to hydrogen atoms is applied. When the magnetic field is removed and they move back into place, they transmit radio waves. The MRI scanner analyzes these signals and produces an image. The MRI signal derived from blood depends on the level of oxygenation and is therefore based on blood oxygen level dependent (BOLD) contrast. It is possible to get functional images of the cerebral blood flow and oxygen consumption.

PET utilizes radiation emitted from the pig after i.v. injection of a radioactive pharmaceutical that resembles a natural substance in the body and that produces positrons. When the positrons collide with electrons, gamma radiation from the tracer is emitted and detected by the scanner and a computer processes the data into a functional image. Thus, an image of the target organ's metabolism or such parameters as receptor density can be developed. It is also possible to image structures such as receptors for calculation of their density. Today, an increasing number of CT and PET scanners are combined in PET/CT scanners. This makes it possible to produce fusion images combining anatomy (CT) and function (PET).

All these scanners are expensive; consequently, human clinical scanners are often used for porcine studies. However, this requires that the scanners be cleaned and sanitized after use with animals. Urine, dander, and zoonotic organisms are the potential sources of contamination. Female pigs are often used because it is possible to catheterize their bladders, which helps prevent urinary contamination. Anesthetized pigs may be covered with blankets and plastic sheets to prevent contamination of the scanner and the scanner room. The protocol for sanitization and usage should be cleared by the hospital infection control department and the institutional veterinarian to prevent infections and allergies.

ANESTHESIA

Many kinds of anesthesia can be used for pigs during scanning procedures. A complete discussion of anesthetic techniques is provided in Chapter 2. Where short-term anesthesia can be used for CT and MR scans, long-term anesthesia is needed in most studies, including functional MR and PET scans. Stable physiological function is essential during these procedures. Good sedation and muscle relaxation are important to prevent movement artifacts in the images. This is especially important during PET scans, because a typical carbon-11 scan takes as long as 90 min. Bolus injections of neuromuscular-blocking agents are often needed to prevent spontaneous respiration; however, care must be taken to ensure the animal is under adequate anesthesia before these agents are used. The physiological function being studied should not be compromised by the anesthetic protocol. This is especially important in functional brain studies.

In many cases isoflurane anesthesia will fulfill most of the requirements. However, nonmagnetic equipment must be utilized for MRI studies or else the equipment must be shielded adequately from the magnetic field. Infusion protocols, as discussed in Chapter 2, may also be utilized to provide prolonged anesthesia. As an example, the center at our university (Aarhus University Hospitals, Denmark) is using the following anesthesia procedure for brain PET studies in 40-kg domestic pigs:

1. Premedication with 250 mg s-ketamine + 50 mg midazolam i.m.
2. Insertion of ear vein catheter (Venflon 20 or 22G)
3. Induction with 125 mg s-ketamine + 50 mg midazolam i.v.
4. Intubation with a size 7.0 endotracheal tube
5. Maintenance with either inhalation or infusion anesthesia; inhalation with 1 1/4–2% isoflurane in oxygen and N_2O (1:2) or oxygen and air (1:3) or infusion with 40 ml/h i.v. of a mixture containing 30-ml propofol (10 mg/ml), 10 ml s-ketamine (25 mg/ml) and 10 ml midazolam (5 mg/ml)
6. Bladder catheterization is performed and i.v. saline is administered

Many of the i.v. infusion protocols discussed in Chapter 2 may also be useful for long-term anesthesia. Spontaneous respiration may occur after many hours of anesthesia if the physiological parameters are not followed closely to ensure homeostasis. S-ketamine (ketamin) is the pure right-racemic isomer of ketamine and is used in order to decrease the dosage required by approximately 50% in the anesthetic protocol previously described.

SURGERY

In PET studies i.v. (rarely i.p.) tracer injections are always needed and often i.v. contrast injections are needed for MR and CT scans. Venous catheters are used for infusion of anesthetics, test drugs, and saline. It is possible to use the ear vein for tracer and contrast injection, but often a surgically placed central venous catheter is preferred. During dynamic PET studies arterial blood sampling is needed for the image calculations. Arterial catheters are also used for monitoring blood gases and blood pressure. Monitoring is especially important during functional brain scans because the cerebral blood flow is affected mainly by the partial CO_2 concentration, but also by the blood pressure. Catheters are often placed in the femoral artery and vein because both catheters can be placed at the same time. This site is ideal for brain studies, because of the long distance from the brain to the vessel access. During surgery and scanning procedures, the pigs are placed on an electric blanket to prevent hypothermia. The vascular access sites and the surgical procedures are detailed in Chapter 1 and Chapter 9.

MONITORING

During functional scans, stable physiological conditions are required. Also, the animal must be monitored to ensure that it is adequately anesthetized. In our laboratory, the following parameters are monitored during most PET and PET/CT scans: continuous blood pressure, electrocardiogram, heart rate, rectal temperature, oxygen saturation, blood gases every 30–60 min, blood glucose, and reflexes (intedigital, corneal, and palpebral).

Special equipment is needed during CT and MR scans because metal will interact with the scanners. Alternatively, the equipment can be placed outside the scanner room and connected to the pig by long tubes. For MR scans of the head or brain, the metal spring in the cuff of the tracheal tube must be removed prior to the scan. Even therapeutic iron injections or implants can be a problem. CT scanners are less sensitive to iron and other metals. In PET studies these substances are only a minor problem.

SCANNING PROCEDURES

CT scans are performed in only a few seconds to 1 min. MR scans require a few minutes, and functional MR scans often take up to 1 h. PET studies frequently take many hours. Prior to PET scans, a transmission scan (typically 15 min) is performed before the first emission scan. The transmission scan is used for photon attenuation correction of the emission recordings. Depending on the tracer used, the emission scans take from a few minutes to several hours. Tracers based on ^{15}O (H_2O^{15} for blood flow measurements and CO^{15} for blood volume measurements) take less than 10 min and ^{13}N (NH_3 for blood flow measurements) take 30 min. Tracers based on ^{11}C (^{11}C-raclopride for dopamine receptor measurements) and ^{18}F (^{18}F-FDG for glucose uptake) take from 90 min to several hours. We normally require 200–1000 MBq PET tracer for 40 kg Landrace pigs.

TECHNICAL INFORMATION FOR EACH OF THE IMAGES ON THE ATTACHED DVD

INSTRUCTIONS FOR THE DVD

Attached to the textbook is an IBM compatible DVD with a variety of images of pig anatomy which is explained in Chapters 17 and 18. Opening the textbook chapter to the corresponding area of the files on the DVD may be helpful.

Files on the DVD include Microsoft® Office PowerPoint® presentations, video clips and segmental MR images using a General Electric Centricity DICOM viewer from the internet. Additional instructions on viewing the programs are located within the folders on the DVD as well as in the introductory slides in the PowerPoint presentations.

Scan 1: Contrast Radiograph of the Cerebral Artery

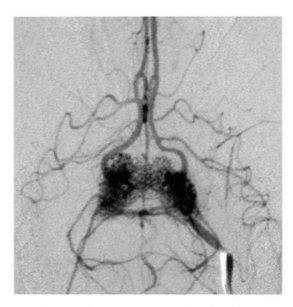

FIGURE 17.1 Sample image of CNS angiography on DVD (SCAN 1). (Aage Kristian Olsen, D.V.M., Ph.D., Aarhus PET Center, Denmark.)

Contrast angiography of the cerebral arteries performed by x-rays in a 40-kg female domestic Landrace pig under ketamine-midazolam anesthesia.

File: Scan 1
CT_contrast_brain_arteries

Scan 2: MRI (Magnetic Resonance Imaging)

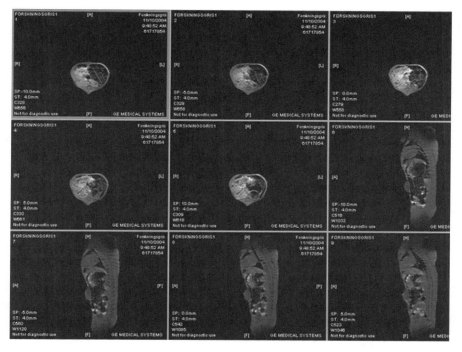

FIGURE 17.2 Sample image of MRI series on DVD (SCAN 2). (Aage Kristian Olsen, D.V.M., Ph.D., Aarhus PET Center, Denmark; and Dora Zeidler, C-FIN, Aarhus University, Denmark.)

Whole body	Head/brain	M,D
	Thorax	M
	Abdomen	M
	Legs	M
Head/brain	Nasal cavity	D

Note: M = Göttingen minipigs, D = domestic pigs (Landrace).

MR atlas of the male Göttingen minipig, 17 kg. The pig was killed with an overdose of pentobarbital 2 min prior to start of the MR scan. Imaging is performed using a 3-Tesla Excite HD, General Electric Medical Systems (Milwaukee, WI) MR scanner. The abdomen is scanned with a T2-weighted sequence with 4- and 2-mm slice thickness. This is followed by a 3D T1-weighted sequence with 1-mm slice thickness. The pelvic area is scanned with 3D T1 weighting in 1-mm slices and a T2-weighted sequence in 4-mm slice thickness. The thorax is scanned using a 3D T1 weighting with 1-mm slices and a T2-weighted sequence in 4-mm slice thickness. The heart is scanned in a 3D volume using 1-mm slices. The brain is scanned with a 3D T1 weighting and a T2-weighted sequence both with 1-mm slices. The caput is scanned with a 3D T1-weighted sequence with 1-mm slice thickness and a T2-weighted sequences using 3-mm slices.

The mucosa of the nasal cavity can be visualized by contrast MR, in this case a 40-kg female domestic pig under isoflurane-N_2O anesthesia. Imaging is performed using a 3-Tesla Excite HD, General Electric Medical Systems (Milwaukee, WI) MR scanner. Performing a 3D T1-weighted sequence with 1-mm consecutive slices followed by a comparable 3D T1-weighted sequence using Gd-DTPA visualizing the mucosa.

File: Scan 2
CDVIEWER
DICOM
AUTORUN
AUTORUN
DICOMDIR

Scan 3: PET (Positron Emission Tomography)

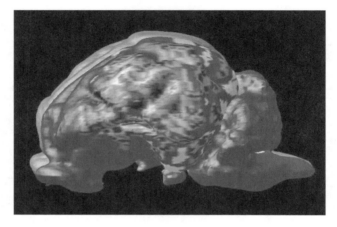

FIGURE 17.3 Sample image of PET image on DVD (SCAN 3).

Region	Tracer	Image	
	H$_2$O	Cerebral blood flow	D
	CO		

Water-PET: Cerebral blood flow (CBF) in a pig 6 h after acute stroke in left side of the brain. (Aage Kristian Olsen, D.V.M., Ph.D., Aarhus PET Center, Denkark.)

Cerebral blood flow can be measured with PET by use of the tracer [^{15}O] H$_2$O. This image was taken 6 h after permanently middle cerebral artery occlusion on the left side in a 40-kg female domestic pig. The tracer dose of [^{15}O] H$_2$O was 1000 MBq, and the pig was anesthetized with isoflurane and N$_2$O.

CO-PET: Parametric maps of cerebral blood volume (CBV) during hypercapnia in domestic pig. (Aage Kristian Olsen, D.V.M., Ph.D., Aarhus PET Center, Denmark.)

The PET tracer [^{15}O] CO binds to hemaglobin, and therefore it can be used to calculate the blood volume in different organs. In this case we were imaging the cerebral blood volume during the first 6 min after injection of 1000 MBq [^{15}O] CO in a 40-kg female domestic pig under isoflurane-N$_2$O anaesthesia.

File: Scan 3
PET_water_scan_strock
PET_CO-scan_hypercapnia

SCAN 4: DOPAMINE RECEPTORS

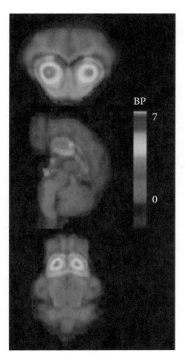

FIGURE 17.4 Sample image of PET images dopamine receptor on DVD (SCAN 4). (Kasper Pedersen, medical student, Aarhus PET Center, Denmark; and Aage Kristian Olsen, D.V.M., Ph.D., Aarhus PET Center, Denmark.)

RAC	Dopamine receptors	M
WAY	Serotonin system	M
MR-atlas	MR-atlas	M

Image of the voxelwise binding potential (BP) of the dopamine $D_{2/3}$ receptor radioligand [^{11}C] raclopride as a mean of four Göttingen minipigs (rainbow colors) superposed on the MRI-based common stereotaxic minipig brain atlas (gray colors). The BP values are proportional to the concentration of dopamine receptors. Anesthesia was performed with isoflurane and N_2O.

The common stereotaxic MRI atlas of minipig brain in three planes (left) on which is superposed a PET image showing the radioactivity concentration after injection of the serotonin 5-HT_{1A} radioligand [^{11}C]WAY-100635 in one Göttingen minipig (right). Isoflurane and N_2O anesthesia.

File: Scan 4
PET_RAC
PET_WAY
PET_RAC_WAY_legends

SCAN 5: PET SCAN OF A 40-KG FEMALE PIG AFTER INJECTION OF ^{18}F GALACTOSE

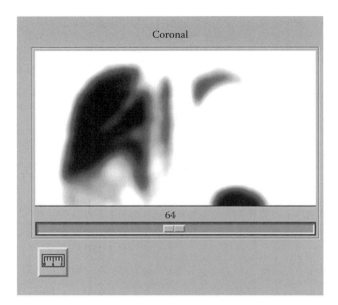

FIGURE 17.5 Sample image of PET images of the liver on DVD (SCAN 5). (Michael Sørensen, MD, Ph.D. student, Aarhus PET Center, Denmark; and Aage Kristian Olsen, D.V.M., Ph.D., Aarhus PET Center, Denmark.)

The tracer [^{18}F] F-galactose was used to test the liver galactose uptake; it is a marker for liver function. The image is from a 1-h PET scan with MBq [^{18}F] F-galactose in a 40-kg female domestic pig. Anesthesia was performed with propofol, ketamine, and midazolam IV.

File: Scan 5
PET_FDGal

Scan 6: CT and PET/CT of a Domestic Pig

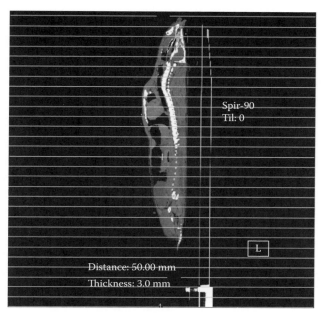

FIGURE 17.6 Sample image of PET/CT images on DVD (SCAN 6). (Ole L. Munk, M.Sc., Ph.D., Aarhus PET Center, Denmark; and Aage Kristian Olsen, D.V.M., Ph.D., Aarhus PET Center, Denmark.)

Images were acquired using a Siemens Biograph 16 HiRez PET/CT scanner. The scanner combines a 16-slice CT-scanner, and an LSO-based PET scanner with a spatial resolution approximately 4.6 mm.

Whole-body CT of a pig was acquired using 120 kV and 160 mAs as scan parameters. The images shown are 3-mm slices for each 5 cm.

PET/CT of the liver was acquired using 120 kV and 50 mAs as CT scan parameters (shown in grayscale). 50 min after injection of 200 MBq 18F-galactose, a PET image was acquired for 10 min (shown in red colorscale).

18 Ossabaw Island Miniature Swine: Cardiometabolic Syndrome Assessment

*Michael Sturek, Mouhamad Alloosh, James Wenzel,
James P. Byrd, Jason M. Edwards, Pamela G. Lloyd,
Johnathan D. Tune, Keith L. March, Michael A. Miller,
Eric A. Mokelke, and I. Lehr Brisbin, Jr.*

INTRODUCTION

Ossabaw swine were deposited on Ossabaw Island, GA, in the 1500s by Spanish explorers (Mayer and Brisbin, Jr., 1991) and, since then, the ocean has remained an impenetrable barrier to emigration of Ossabaw pigs to the mainland. Natural models of disease that arise from adaptation of animals to unique selection pressures can give insights into similar complex, multifactorial diseases in humans. Ossabaw miniature swine may recapitulate the natural pathogenesis of type 2 diabetes because of their "thrifty genotype" that enabled survival in the feast and famine ecology of Ossabaw Island. The thrifty genotype hypothesis is that in the hunter-gatherer stages of human development the ability to store excess fat enabled survival during periods of famine (Neel, 1962).

In the 1970s and early 1980s, Ossabaw miniature swine were studied by ecologists for their unique adaptations in their natural habitat on Ossabaw Island (Mayer and Brisbin, Jr., 1991; Stribling et al., 1984) and, after establishment of colonies on the mainland, Ossabaws were studied by animal scientists for their propensity to obesity (Buhlinger et al., 1978; Martin et al., 1973; Martin and Herbein, 1976; Weiss et al., 1974), insulin resistance (Wangsness et al., 1977), plasma lipoproteins (Etherton and Kris-Etherton, 1980), and renal physiology (Zervanos et al., 1983).

Renewed interest in Ossabaw miniature swine was sparked in 2001 with the realization of the obesity and diabetes epidemic (Bellenger et al., 2006; Mokdad et al., 2001) and Brisbin's timely appeal to the scientific community to save feral Ossabaw Island swine from eradication by the Georgia Department of Natural Resources for environmental reasons (Brisbin and Mayer, 2001; www.state.ga.us/dnr/wild/game_mgmt/theplan.pdf, 2000). Our laboratory obtained animals from the island in an expedition in 2002 and established a breeding colony at Indiana University. We have conducted studies involving diabetes and metabolic syndrome and have made comparisons to our Yucatan model (Boullion et al., 2003; Dixon et al., 1999, 2002; Edwards et al., 2006; Hainsworth et al., 2002; Kaser et al., 2004; Lloyd et al., 2006; Mokelke et al., 2003, 2005a, 2005b; Sheehy et al., 2006; Sturek et al., 2006; Witczak et al., 2004, 2005; Zafar et al., 2004).

The natural pathogenesis of type 2 diabetes involves a tendency to obesity with gradually increasing impairment of insulin action in a "prediabetes" condition, which has also been termed the *metabolic syndrome* or *cardiometabolic risk* (Eckel et al., 2005, 2006; Grundy et al., 2005; Kahn et al., 2005). In later stages, there is an increase in fasting blood glucose, which best defines diabetes. Intensive research is under way to meet the need for animal models to understand these comorbidities and develop therapies. The cardiometabolic risk or metabolic syndrome in the

Ossabaw pig could be an outstanding large animal model. Strategies involving transgenic manipulations in other species and other breeds of minipigs are under development.

The cardiometabolic syndrome in humans is actually a cluster of risk factors that includes (1) central (intra-abdominal) obesity, (2) insulin resistance, (3) impaired glucose tolerance, (4) dyslipidemia as measured by decreased plasma high-density lipoprotein (HDL) cholesterol compared to low-density lipoprotein (LDL), i.e., increased LDL/HDL ratio, (5) dyslipidemia as shown by increased plasma triglyceride, and (6) hypertension (Eckel et al., 2005; Ford et al., 2004; Grundy et al., 2004; McGill, Jr. et al., 2002). Although the definition and precise clinical utility have recently been controversial (Kahn et al., 2005), generally the presence of three of these characteristics renders a diagnosis of the cardiometabolic syndrome (Eckel et al., 2006; Grundy et al., 2004).

CHARACTERIZATION OF THE MODEL

The most critical question regarding the use of Ossabaw miniature swine is: Do recent removals from Ossabaw Island in 2002 have the thrifty genotype characteristics, i.e., "cardiometabolic risk," found in the early characterization during ~1970–1985? Data have been collected to study these characteristics, and it confirms the early data, thus providing a rationale for more cardiovascular characterization, which was not performed in the early studies. The attached DVD includes images of this data collection.

Genetic studies were performed on a repeating domain in the regulatory $\gamma 3$ subunit of the AMP-activated kinase (PRKAG3) gene. Hampshire pigs display a single amino acid difference at position 200 where arginine is mutated to glutamine (Arg200→Gln). The genotype is associated with high muscle glycogen, low intramuscular fat, and overall leanness (Andersson, 2003; Milan et al., 2000). In contrast, sequencing of the PRKAG3 gene in Ossabaw Island pigs revealed the majority to be homozygous for a different mutation, Val199→Ile, while the remainder of the pigs were heterozygous for the Val199→Ile mutation and the wild-type allele Val199–Arg200 (Lloyd et al., 2006). The Val199→Ile mutation is associated with low muscle glycogen and increased intramuscular fat, consistent with the obese Ossabaw pig phenotype (Andersson, 2003; Ciobanu et al., 2001).

Table A.32–Table A.34 in the appendix make systematic comparison of serum chemistry data from trapped pigs on Ossabaw Island and data derived from Yucatan and Ossabaw pigs housed long term (1 year) in a biomedical research facility on standard pig chow. Pigs were anesthetized with isoflurane to obtain blood samples for the latter group compared to the caval blood sampling that employed physical restraint for the clinical chemistry from trapped Ossabaw. For both breeds in captivity housed in the biomedical facility the anion gap, potassium, total bilirubin, creatine kinase, and CO_2 are normal compared to the trapped wild pigs, thus probably indicating a less stressful environment overall and less stressful blood sampling procedure. Notable differences are the increased triglycerides and glucose in Ossabaws compared to Yucatans, which reinforce the more extreme cardiometabolic risk factor profile of the Ossabaws. Another intriguing difference is the increased creatinine in Ossabaws, which suggests some mild renal impairment even under these controlled conditions. The decreased urea nitrogen is consistent with less muscle mass in the Ossabaw (Ezekwe and Martin, 1975; Hausman et al., 1983; Kasser et al., 1981) and argues against the increased creatinine being driven by possibly increased muscle mass in the Ossabaws. It is completely unknown whether the increased ability of the Ossabaw kidney to concentrate urine (Zervanos et al., 1983) for adaptation to high salt consumption renders it more susceptible to subsequent damage. Overall, there was no difference in hematology between Ossabaw and Yucatan pigs. The only striking value in both breeds is the low hematocrit of 27. This is explained entirely by the isoflurane anesthesia, as Ossabaws sampled in the conscious state had a hematocrit of 41.8 ± 2.6 (SD; N = 5), similar to conscious Yucatans in other studies.

Tables of normal values for Ossabaw minipigs are included in the appendix.

SUMMARY AND CONCLUSIONS

Ossabaw swine have been rediscovered as a valuable animal resource after the recent removal, in 2002, of feral swine from Ossabaw Island, following the first removal nearly 30 years ago. Ossabaw swine removed from the island must undergo a stringent quarantine to ensure health and absence of parasites and major infectious diseases. The pigs are thriving in captivity. It is hoped that "thrifty genotype" is maintained in captivity and the analogy to modern day humans suggests that the genotype will be maintained. Clearly, Ossabaw swine express the major components of the metabolic syndrome ("prediabetes," "cardiometabolic risk"), including extreme obesity, insulin resistance, impaired glucose tolerance, dyslipidemia, and hypertension. Selective breeding is under way to derive more general robust features of cardiometabolic risk and distinct lines of the AMP kinase mutation genotypes. This chapter has provided an overview of the evidence for metabolic properties and methods of assessment and has contrasted the Ossabaw with the characteristics of more genetically lean Yucatan swine and domestic swine. Vascular studies under way provide detailed methods and characterization of vascular anatomy and functional properties. Unique vascular calcification and excessive stenosis after coronary stenting suggest predisposition to vascular disease and utility of the Ossabaw swine model. Exercise training of obese pigs is described. These findings echo the consensus that pigs in general and Ossabaw swine specifically are anatomically and metabolically similar to humans. The cardiovascular system is almost indistinguishable from that of humans, and knowledge gained has much relevance to human medicine. Thus, the Ossabaw pig provides a unique animal resource to gain insight into multiple, complex factors involved in development of obesity and type 2 diabetes in humans and the resulting morbidity and mortality from cardiovascular disease. It is hoped that the future will see more widespread availability and use of Ossabaw swine in biomedical research.

Note: The attached DVD contains images and video clips of various aspects of the study of the cardiometabolic syndrome in Ossabaw Island minipigs (Figure 18.1–Figure 18.28). Complete figure legends are included with the images. The outlined titles as follows provide a guide to the illustrations on the DVD.

Figure 18.1 — Ossabaw Island pig and environment.

Figure 18.2 — Standard Ossabaw swine housing facility for biomedical research.

Figure 18.3 — Growth and adipose composition of lean and obese male Ossabaw pigs housed in biomedical research facility.

Figure 18.4 — Noninvasive imaging of adipose distribution in Ossabaw swine.

Figure 18.5 — Measurement of glucose regulation and cardiovascular parameters in conscious pig.

Figure 18.6 — Catheterization supplies and angiography equipment.

Figure 18.7 — Hind limb arteries, ventrodorsal view. Includes video clips 18.1–18.6.

Figure 18.8 — Hind limb, superficial femoral artery access for catheterization, and formation of collateral femoral arteries in ventrodorsal view. Includes video clips 18.7 and 18.8.

Figure 18.9 — Renal arteries in ventrodorsal view. Includes video clips 18.9 and 18.10.

Figure 18.10 — Major abdominal arteries in ventrodorsal view. Includes video clips 18.11 and 18.12.

Figure 18.11 — Forelimb and thoracic arteries in ventrodorsal view. Includes video clips 18.13 and 18.14.

Figure 18.12 — Left carotid and cerebral arteries in ventrodorsal view. Includes video clips 18.15 and 18.16.

Figure 18.13 — Schematic of heart and major epicardial coronary arteries and interventional devices.

ACKNOWLEDGMENTS

We acknowledge Rob Boullion, Kyle Henderson, Ph.D., Harold Laughlin, Ph.D., Dale Lenger, and Chris Downs of the University of Missouri, Bart Carter, D.V.M., M.S., formerly in the Office of Laboratory Animal Medicine at the University of Missouri and presently at Kansas State University, Clarence Bagshaw, D.V.M., Roger Parker, Allan Usher, the Ossabaw Island Foundation, Bob Monroe and the Georgia Department of Natural Resources, and Sandy West of Ossabaw Island for involvement in our initial removal of pigs from Ossabaw Island; Karan Singh, M.D., for earlier work on coronary flow; the Research Animal Angiography Laboratory of the Indiana Center for Vascular Biology & Medicine; and the Department of Radiology and Indiana Center of Excellence in Biomedical Imaging for positron emission tomography and magnetic resonance imaging. This work has been supported by National Institutes of Health grants RR013223 and HL062552, the American Diabetes Association, the Indiana Center of Excellence in Biomedical Imaging, Purdue-Indiana University Comparative Medicine Program, and the Fortune-Fry Ultrasound Research Fund of Indiana University. M. Sturek can be contacted regarding a tissue bank and availability of live Ossabaw swine.

REFERENCES

Andersson, L. 2003. Identification and characterization of AMPKg3 mutations in the pig. *Biochem. Soc. Trans.* 31:232–235.

Bellinger, D.A., E.P. Merricks, and T.C. Nichols. 2006. Swine models of type 2 diabetes mellitus: insulin resistance, glucose tolerance, and cardiovascular complications. *ILAR J.* 47:243–258.

Bergman, R.N., D.T. Finegood, and M. Ader. 1985. Assessment of insulin sensitivity *in vivo*. *Endocr. Rev.* 6:45–86.

Borkan, G., S. Gerzof, A. Robbins, D. Hults, C. Silbert, and J. Silha. 1982. Assessment of abdominal fat content by computed tomography. *Am. J. Clin. Nutr.* 36:172–177.

Boullion, R.D., E.A. Mokelke, B.R. Wamhoff, C.R. Otis, J. Wenzel, J.L. Dixon, and M. Sturek. 2003. Porcine model of diabetic dyslipidemia: insulin and feed algorithms for mimicking diabetes in humans. *Comp. Med.* 53:42–52.

Brisbin, Jr.I.L. and J.J. Mayer. 2001. Problem pigs in a poke: a good pool of data. *Science* 294:1280–1281.

Buhlinger, C.A., P.J. Wangsness, R.J. Martin, and J.H. Ziegler. 1978. Body composition, *in vitro* lipid metabolism and skeletal muscle characteristics in fast-growing, lean and in slow-growing, obese pigs at equal age and weight. *Growth* 42:225–236.

Ciobanu, D., J. Bastiaansen, M. Malek, J. Helm, J. Woollard, G. Plastow, and M. Rothschild. 2001. Evidence for new aAlleles in the protein kinase adenosine monophosphate-aActivated g3-subunit gene associated with low glycogen content in pig skeletal muscle and improved meat quality. *Genetics* 159:1151–1162.

Dixon, J.L., J.D. Stoops, J.L. Parker, M.H. Laughlin, G.A. Weisman, and M. Sturek. 1999. Dyslipidemia and vascular dysfunction in diabetic pigs fed an atherogenic diet. *Arterioscler. Thromb. Vasc. Biol.* 19:2981–2992.

Dixon, J.L., S. Shen, J.P. Vuchetich, E. Wysocka, G. Sun, and M. Sturek. 2002. Increased atherosclerosis in diabetic dyslipidemic swine: protection by atorvastatin involves decreased VLDL triglycerides but minimal effects on the lipoprotein profile. *J. Lipid Res.* 43:1618–1629.

Dyson, M.C., M. Alloosh, R.D. Boullion, E.A. Mokelke, and M. Sturek. 2004. Glucose intolerance and insulin resistance in Ossabaw compared to Yucatan swine (abstract). *FASEB J.* 18:A1224.

Dyson, M., M. Alloosh, J.P. Vuchetich, E.A. Mokelke, and M. Sturek. 2006. Components of metabolic syndrome and coronary artery disease in female Ossabaw swine fed excess atherogenic diet. *Comp. Med.* 56:35–45.

Eckel, R.H., S.M. Grundy, and P.Z. Zimmet. 2005. The metabolic syndrome. *Lancet* 365:1415–1428.

Eckel, R.H., R. Kahn, R.M. Robertson, and R.A. Rizza. 2006. Preventing cardiovascular disease and diabetes: a call to action from the American Diabetes Association and the American Heart Association. *Circulation* 113:2943–2946.

Edwards, J.M., J. Vuchetich, E.A. Mokelke, M. Alloosh, K.L. March, D. Hou, and M. Sturek. 2006. The Ossabaw swine model of the metabolic syndrome exhibits greater stenosis after coronary stenting than lean Yucatan swine (abstract). *FASEB J.* 20:A698.

Etherton, T.D. and P.M. Kris-Etherton. 1980. Characterization of plasma lipoproteins in swine with different propensities for obesity. *Lipids* 15:823–829.

Ezekwe, M.O. and R.J. Martin. 1975. Cellular characteristics of skeletal muscle in selected strains of pigs and mice and the unselected controls. *Growth* 39:95–106.

Ford, E.S., W.H. Giles, and A.H. Mokdad. 2004. Increasing prevalence of the metabolic syndrome among U.S. adults. *Diabetes Care* 27:2444–2449.

Georgia Department of Natural Resources, 2002. www.state.ga.us/dnr/wild/game_mgmt/theplan.pdf.

Grundy, S.M., H.B. Brewer, J.I. Cleeman, S.C. Smith, Jr., and C. Lenfant. 2004. Definition of the metabolic syndrome. *Circulation* 109:433–438.

Grundy, S.M., J.I. Cleeman, S.R. Daniels, K.A. Donato, R.H. Eckel, B.A. Franklin, D.J. Gordon, R.M. Krauss, P.J. Savage, S.C. Smith, Jr., J.A. Spertus, and F. Costa. 2005. Diagnosis and management of the metabolic syndrome: an American Heart Association/National Heart, Lung, and Blood Institute scientific statement. *Circulation* 112:2735–2752.

Hainsworth, D.P., M.L. Katz, D.A. Sanders, D.N. Sanders, E.J. Wright, and M. Sturek. 2002. Retinal capillary basement membrane thickening in a porcine model of diabetes mellitus. *Comp. Med.* 52:523–529.

Hausman, G.J., D.R. Campion, and G.B. Thomas. 1983. Semitendinosis muscle development in several strains of fetal and perinatal pigs. *J. Anim. Sci.* 57:1608–1617.

Kahn, R., J. Buse, E. Ferrannini, and M. Stern. 2005. The metabolic syndrome: time for a critical appraisal. Joint statement from the American Diabetes Association and the European Association for the Study of Diabetes. *Diabetologia* 48:1684–1699.

Kaser, S., E.A. Mokelke, M.N. Zafar, M.C. Dyson, and M. Sturek. 2004. Microvascular dysfunction after coronary stenting in a porcine model of the metabolic syndrome. *Diabetes* 53, Suppl. 2:A408–A409.

Kasser, T.R., R.J. Martin, J.H. Gahagan, and P.J. Wangsness. 1981. Fasting plasma hormones and metabolites in feral and domestic newborn pigs. *J. Anim. Sci.* 53:420–426.

Lloyd, P.G., M. Fang, I.L. Brisbin, Jr., L. Andersson, and M. Sturek. 2006. AMP kinase gene mutation is consistent with a thrifty phenotype (metabolic syndrome) in a population of feral swine (abstract). *FASEB J.* 20:A299.

Martin, R.J. and J.H. Herbein. 1976. A comparison of the enzyme levels and the in vitro utilization substrates for lipogenesis in pair-fed lean and obese pigs. *Proc. Soc. Exp. Biol. Med.* 151:231–235.

Martin, R.J., J.L. Gobble, T.H. Hartsock, H.B. Graves, and J.H. Ziegler. 1973. Characterization of an obese syndrome in the pig. *Proc. Soc. Exp. Biol. Med.* 143:198–203.

Mayer, J.J. and I.L. Brisbin, Jr. 1991. *Wild Pigs of the United States: Their History, Morphology, and Current Status,* Athens, GA: University of Georgia Press.

McGill, H.C., Jr., A. McMahan, E.E. Herderick, A.W. Zieske, G.T. Malcom, R.E. Tracy, J.P. Strong, and Pathobiological Determinants of Atherosclerosis in Youth (PDAY) Research Group. 2002. Obesity accelerates the progression of coronary atherosclerosis in young men. *Circulation* 105:2712–2718.

Milan, D., J.T. Jeon, C. Looft, V. Amarger, A. Robic, M. Thelander, C. Rogel-Gaillard, S. Paul, N. Iannuccelli, L. Rask, H. Ronne, K. Lundström, N. Reinsch, J. Gellin, E. Kalm, P.L. Roy, P. Chardon, and L. Andersson. 2000. A mutation in PRKAG3 associated with excess glycogen content in pig skeletal muscle. *Science* 288:1248–1251.

Mokdad, A., E. Ford, B. Bowman, D. Nelson, M. Engelgau, F. Vinicor, and J. Marks. 2001. The continuing increase of diabetes in the U.S. *Diabetes Care* 24:412–412.

Mokelke, E.A., Q. Hu, M. Song, L. Toro, H.K. Reddy, and M. Sturek. 2003. Altered functional coupling of coronary K$^+$ channels in diabetic dyslipidemic pigs is prevented by exercise. *J. Appl. Physiol.* 95:1179–1193.

Mokelke, E.A., N.J. Dietz, D.M. Eckman, M.T. Nelson, and M. Sturek. 2005a. Diabetic dyslipidemia and exercise affect coronary tone and differential regulation of conduit and microvessel K$^+$ current. *Am. J. Physiol. Heart Circ. Physiol.* 288:H1233–H1241.

Mokelke, E.A., R. Misra, and M. Sturek. 2005b. Caspase-3 levels are elevated in myocardium of hypercholesterolemic Ossabaw minipigs (abstract). *Diabetes* 54, Suppl. 1:A433.

Neel, J.V. 1962. Diabetes mellitus: a "thrifty" genotype rendered detrimental by "progress"? *Am. J. Hum. Genet.* 14:353–362.

Sheehy, A., E.A. Mokelke, P.G. Lloyd, J. Sturek, and M. Sturek. 2006. Reduced expression of leukemia inhibitory factor correlates with coronary atherosclerosis in the metabolic syndrome (abstract). *FASEB J.* 20:A698.

Stribling, H.L., Jr., I.L. Brisbin, J.R. Sweeney, and L.A. Stribling. 1984. Body fat reserves and their prediction in two populations of feral swine. *J. Wildl. Manage.* 48:635–639.

Wangsness, P.J., R.J. Martin, and J.H. Gahagan. 1977. Insulin and growth hormone in lean and obese pigs. *Am. J. Physiol.* 233:E104–E108.

Weiss, G.M., D.G. Topel, D.G. Siers, and R.C. Ewan. 1974. Influence of adrenergic blockage upon some endocrine and metabolic parameters in a stress-susceptible and a fat strain of swine. *J. Anim. Sci.* 38:591–597.

Witczak, C.A. and M. Sturek. 2004. Exercise prevents diabetes-induced impairment in superficial buffer barrier in porcine coronary smooth muscle. *J. Appl. Physiol.* 96:1069–1079.

Witczak, C.A., E.A. Mokelke, R.D. Boullion, J. Wenzel, D.H. Keisler, and M. Sturek. 2005. Noninvasive measures of body fat percentage in male Yucatan swine. *Comp. Med.* 55:445–451.

Zafar, M.N., E.A. Mokelke, S. Kaser, and M. Sturek. 2004. C-reactive protein is predictive of in-stent neointimal hyperplasia, but not atheroma at baseline, in swine with the metabolic syndrome (abstract). *Arterioscler. Thromb. Vasc. Biol.* 24:103.

Zervanos, S.M., W.D. McCort, and H.B. Graves. 1983. Salt and water balance of feral versus domestic Hampshire hogs. *Physiol. Zool.* 56:67–77.

Zygmont, S.M., V.F. Nettles, E.B. Shotts, W.A. Carmen, and B.O. Blackburn. 1982. Brucellosis in wild swine: a serologic and bacteriologic survey in the southeastern United States and Hawaii. *J. Am. Vet. Med. Assoc.* 181:1285-1287.

Appendix

TABLE OF CONTENTS

SECTION 1: GROWTH CHARTS, NUTRITION, AND PHYSIOLOGICAL PARAMETERS

TABLE A.1
Minipig Age–Weight Correlations

Hanford		Yucatan		Yucatan	
Age (in months)	Weight (kg)	Age (in months)	Weight (kg)	Age (in months)	Weight (kg)
1	4–7	1	3–6	1	3–5
2	8–11	2	7–9	2	6–8
3	12–19	3	10–15	3	9–12
4	20–27	4	15–20	4	12–14
5	25–33	5	20–25	5	14–16
6	34–42	6	25–30	6	16–20
8	40–50	8	35–45	8	25–35
10	45–55	10	45–55	10	30–40
12	55–70 (male)	12	55–65 (male)	12	55–65 (male)
	50–65 (female)		45–50 (female)		35–45 (female)

Source: Reprinted with permission from Sinclair Research, Auxvasse, MO.

TABLE A.2
Reproductive Physiological Parameters

	Microswine	Miniswine
Breed		
Growth	Yucatan	Hanford, Yucatan
Birth weight	600–700 g	600–1000 g
Weight as sexual maturity	15–20 kg	Hanford 28–42 kg; Yucatan 20–30 kg
Adult weight	40–60 kg (at 12–14 months)	68–80 kg (at 2 years)
Life span	10–15 years	10–15 years
Reproduction		
Gestation period	111–114 d	111–114 d
Average litter size	5–6	Hanford 6–8; Yucatan 5–6
Weaning age	28–35 d	28–35 d
Sexual maturity	5–6 months	5–6 months
Breeding age	6–8 months	6–8 months

Source: Reprinted with permission from Sinclair Research, Auxvasse, MO.

TABLE A.3
Recommended Diets

Age	Model	Recommended Diet[a]
Pigs 1–2 months old	Micro and mini	0.25–0.75 lb/d of a 50/50 mix of starter and maintenance and breeder diet
Pigs 2–3 months old	Micro and mini	0.75–1.25 lb/d, maintenance and breeder diet
Pigs over 3 months old	Micro	1.25–1.75 lb/d, maintenance and breeder
	Mini	1.75–2.2 lb/d, maintenance and breeder

[a] Individual animals and conditions vary, so new users of swine should be observant, especially at first, to get a feel for optimum feed levels. Weight loss and weight gain are the best indicators.

Source: Reprinted with permission from Sinclair Research, Auxvasse, MO.

TABLE A.4

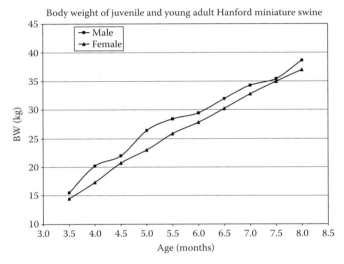

Source: Courtesy of Sinclair Research Center, Auxvasse, MO.

TABLE A.5

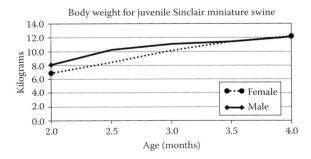

Source: Courtesy of Sinclair Research Center, Auxvasse, MO.

TABLE A.6
Weight Development (kg) of the Göttingen Minipig at the Full-Barrier Breeding Facility in Dalmose

Year	Body Weight (kg) 1995
Birth	0.45
1 month	2.7
2 months	5.3
3 months	7.2
6 months	13.7
9 months	17.7
12 months	23.9
18 months	32.4
24 months	34.9

Source: Courtesy of Peter Bollen, Ellegaard Göttingen Minipigs ApS, Dalmose, Denmark. Reprinted with permission from *Scand. J. Lab. Anim. Sci.*

TABLE A.7
Breeding Characteristics and Timing of Early Development in the Göttingen Minipig

Length of gestation	114 d
Placentation	Diffuse, epitheliochorial
Puberty	140–170 d
Cycle length	21–22 d
Oestrus length	3 d
Blastocyst formation	Day 5–6
Implantation	Day 11–13
Organogenesis period	Day 11–35

Source: Reprinted with permission from Jørgensen, K.D., 1998. *Scandinavian Journal of Laboratory Animal Science*, 25 (Suppl. 1), pp. 63–75.

TABLE A.8

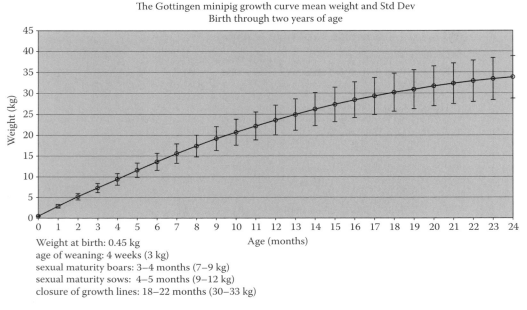

The Gottingen minipig growth curve mean weight and Std Dev
Birth through two years of age

Weight at birth: 0.45 kg
age of weaning: 4 weeks (3 kg)
sexual maturity boars: 3–4 months (7–9 kg)
sexual maturity sows: 4–5 months (9–12 kg)
closure of growth lines: 18–22 months (30–33 kg)

Source: Ellegaard Gottingen Minipigs ApS, Dalmose, Denmark

TABLE A.9
Feed Composition and Amount for Normal Growth of Ossabaw Miniature Swine

Age (months)	Feed Type	Feed (g)	kcal
Up to 1–1.5	Typical Creep Feed or LabDiet Mini-Pig Starter #5080	Ad Libitum	up to ~920
1.5	LabDiet Mini-Pig Grower #5L80 or Starter #5080	270	920
2	Lab Diet Mini-Pig Grower #5L80	300	990
3	Lab Diet Mini-Pig Grower #5L80	350	1155
4	Lab Diet Mini-Pig Grower #5L80	400	1320
5	Lab Diet Mini-Pig Grower #5L80	450	1485
6	Lab Diet Mini-Pig Grower #5L80	500	1650
7	Lab Diet Mini-Pig Grower #5L80	550	1815
8	LabDiet Mini-pig Breeder #5082 or Mini-Pig Grower #5L80	800	2400
>8	LabDiet Mini-pig Breeder #5082 or Mini-Pig Grower #5L80	~800	~2400–2700

Source: Courtesy of Michael Sturek, PhD, Indiana University.

SECTION 2: HEMATOLOGY AND SERUM CHEMISTRY

TABLE A.10
Biochemical and Hematologic Values (farm pigs, 3–4 months)

Parameter	Units	Baseline	Intraop	POD 1	POD 3	POD 7	POD 10
Na	mEq/l	142 ± 1	141 ± 1	142 ± 1	137 ± 4	143 ± 1	139 ± 1
K	mEq/l	4.8 ± 0.2	4.2 ± 0.1	4.7 ± 0.3	4.2 ± 0.3	4.1 ± 0.2	4.2 ± 0.2
Cl	mEq/l	101 ± 1	102 ± 1	98 ± 1	95 ± 6	103 ± 1	99 ± 2
Ca	mg/dl	10 ± 0.1	9.7 ± 0.1	8.8 ± 0.2	9.1 ± 0.3	9.4 ± 0.4	9.4 ± 0.0
P	mg/dl	9.5 ± 0.4	8.8 ± 0.4	8.6 ± 0.5	9.3 ± 1.6	7.5 ± 0.5	7.6 ± 0.7
Fe	μg/dl	137 ± 20	101 ± 21	40 ± 17	152 ± 105	78 ± 17	61 ± 6
Total protein	g/dl	5.6 ± 0.1	4.7 ± 0.1	5.3 ± 0.1	5.6 ± 0.8	5.3 ± 0.2	5.4 ± 0.1
Albumin	g/dl	3.1 ± 0.1	2.5 ± 0.1	2.8 ± 0.1	2.8 ± 0.2	2.7 ± 0.1	2.4 ± 0.1
Globulin	g/dl	2.5 ± 0.1	2.3 ± 0.1	2.4 ± 0.1	2.8 ± 0.5	2.5 ± 0.1	3.0 ± 0.0
Urea	mg/dl	10 ± 1	10 ± 1	12 ± 3	30 ± 19	11 ± 2	12 ± 1
Creatinine	mg/dl	1.2 ± 0..1	0.9 ± 0.1	1.1 ± 0.1	1.8 ± 0.9	1.0 ± 0.1	1.1 ± 0.2
Bicarbonate	mEq/l	26 ± 1	25 ± 1	30 ± 0.4	25 ± 1	28 ± 1	33
Hemoglobin	g/dl	11.2 ± 0.3	8.8 ± 0.2	12.2 ± 0.4	9.5 ± 0.8	9.0 ± 0.6	8.7 ± 0.7
Bilirubin	mg/dl	0.15 ± 0.04	0.09 ± 0.02	0.18 ± 0.02	.15 ± 0.02	0.13 ± 0.02	0.05 ± 0.05
Alkaline phosphatase	IU/l	164 ± 12	148 ± 14	164 ± 9	152 ± 23	126 ± 15	93 ± 4
ALT	IU/l	38 ± 3	32 ± 2	40 ± 7	36 ± 4	43 ± 8	28 ± 13
AST	IU/l	39 ± 3	35 ± 6	60 ± 17	137 ± 4	39 ± 13	24 ± 6
LD	IU/l	622 ± 51	446 ± 39	732 ± 155	654 ± 61	493 ± 18	365 ± 87
Prothrombin time	sec	11.2 ± 0.3	—	12.4 ± 0.7	10.8	—	—
Hematocrit	%	40 ± 1	30 ± 1	41 ± 1	37 ± 5	31 ± 2	30 ± 2
Leukocytes	×10³/μl	21 ± 1	15 ± 1	20 ± 3	19 ± 2	17 ± 1	18 ± 2
Neutrophils	%	57 ± 4	57 ± 3	60 ± 6	65 ± 7	51 ± 6	48 ± 19
Lymphocytes	%	39 ± 4	41 ± 3	37 ± 6	33 ± 8	41 ± 6	46 ± 16
Monocytes	%	3 ± 1	4 ± 1	1 ± 0	1 ± 1	5 ± 2	1 ± 0.3
Eosinophils	%	1 ± 0.4	2 ± 0.2	1 ± 1	2 ± 1	2 ± 0.3	2 ± 1
Band neutrophils	%	1 ± 0.4	1 ± 0.4	1 ± 1	0 ± 0	4 ± 2	—

Note: POD = postoperative day. Intraoperative values were from isoflurane-anesthetized pigs.

Source: Reprinted with permission from Drougas et al., *Lab. Anim. Sci.* 46(6): 648–655, 1996.

TABLE A.11

Blood Coagulation, Platelet, and Hematocrit Reference Values for Göttingen Minipigs

Parameter	Unit	Males	Females**	Fetal	Pregnant
Number of animals (n)		9	16	9	22
Age	Months	8 ± 2	11 ± 8	Gestation day 105 of 110	11 ± 3*
Hematocrit	%	32 ± 4	33+5	30 + 3	31.0+5
Platelets	10⁹/l	410 ± 90	420 ± 120	n.a.	440 ± 100
Fibrinogen	g/l	7.0 ± 2.0	7.5 ± 3.3	0.4 ± 0.1	4.0 ± 0.5
Fibrinmonomere	mg/l	60 ± 20	—	15 ± 10	40 ± 10
PTT	sec	30 ± 7	30 ± 4	45 ± 5	30 ± 8
PTI (Quick)	%human	160 ± 30	180 ± 30	110 ± 20	190 ± 30
AT III	%human	100 ± 10	110 ± 10	35 ± 10	110 ± 20
Factor II	%human	70 ± 10	±	40 ± 10	80 ± 15
Factor V	%human	370 ± 60	450 ± 150	360 ± 120	460 ± 160
Factor VII	%human	80 ± 20	140 ± 40	50 ± 10	100 ± 20
Factor VIII	%human	340± 60	340 ± 90	300 ± 160	380 ± 110
Factor IX	%human	200 ± 30	—	90 ± 10	190 ± 50
Factor X	%human	115 ± 15	—	55 ± 10	175 ± 50
Factor XI	%human	80 ± 20	—	20 ± 5	70 ± 20
Factor XII	%human	55 ± 20	—	20 ± 10	80 ± 40
Factor XIII	%human	40 ± 10	—	15 ± 5	40 ± 10
Protein C	%human	50 ± 10	76 ± 18	60 ± 5	80 ± 10
α2-APL	%human	80 ± 10	—	55 ± 5	70 ± 10

Note: Table entries are of the form: Mean ± SD.

* Samples were taken on gestation day 105 of 110.

** Petroianu, G.A., Maleck, W.H., 1997, Blood coagulation, platelets and haematocrit in male, female, and pregnant Göttingen minipigs, *Scandinavian Journal of Laboratory Animal Science,* 24, pp. 31–41.

Source: Petroianu, G.A., Maleck, W.H., Werth, W.A., Schummer, B., Rüfer, R., 1998, Blood coagulation, platelets and haemoatocrit in male, pregnant and fetal Göttingen minipigs, *Scandinavian Journal of Laboratory Animal Science,* Suppl. 1, pp. 211–219.

TABLE A.12
Hematology of the Göttingen Minipig

Parameter	Abbreviation	Unit		Male (3 months)	Female (3 months)	Male (6 months)	Female (6 months)
Eosinophils	EOS	%	Mean	0.87	0.93	1.33	2.13
			SD	1.25	1.53	1.18	2.26
Eosinophils	EOS	10^9/l	Mean	0.10	0.10	0.12	0.19
			SD	0.15	0.17	0.11	0.23
Basophils	BASO	%	Mean	0.67	0.53	0.73	0.33
			SD	0.90	0.74	0.88	0.62
Basophils	BASO	10^9/l	Mean	0.08	0.07	0.06	0.02
			SD	0.12	0.1	0.07	0.04
Monocytes	MONO	%	Mean	1.13	1.53	2.00	1.47
			SD	1.25	1.51	1.07	1.19
Monocytes	MONO	10^9/l	Mean	0.14	0.20	0.17	0.14
			SD	0.15	0.21	0.09	0.13
Platelet count	THROMB	10^9/l	Mean	513.1	490.3	348.3	364.5
			SD	88.34	115.2	79.47	51.72
Activated partial thromboplastin time	APTT	sec	Mean	45.86	44.08	42.65	43.22
			SD	5.77	9.99	8.17	9.83
Thrombin time	TT	sec	Mean	25.8	28.36	23.91	23.69
			SD	4.16	5.00	3.59	4.55
Prothrombin time	ptt	sec	Mean	11.71	11.54	11.94	11.65
			SD	0.34	0.46	0.62	0.41
Fibrinogen	FIBR	g/l	Mean	6.5	5.37	6.85	4.80
			SD	1.39	0.66	1.24	0.59

Source: Courtesy of Ellegaard Göttingen Minipigs ApS, Dalmose, Denmark. Reprinted with permission from Ellegaard, L. et al. 1995. Haematologic and clinical chemical values in 3- and 6-month-old Göttingen minipigs. *Scand. J. Lab. Anim. Sci.* 22(3): 239–248.

TABLE A.13
Red and White Blood Cell Parameters for Juvenile (7 weeks), Young (3 months)[a] and Adult (sexually mature — 6 months)[a] Male and Female Göttingen Minipigs and Pregnant Göttingen Minipigs in Gestation Weeks 8–9, 10–11, and 12–13

Parameter	Abbreviation	Unit	7 weeks		3 months		6 months		Pregnant		
			Male	Female	Male	Female	Male	Female	Week 8–9	Week 10–11	Week 12–13
Number of animals	n	—	20	20	15	15	15	15	5	5	5
Hemoglobin	Hb	mmol/l	7.7 ± 0.9	7.9 ± 0.8	7.5 ± 0.4	7.4 ± 0.5	7.9 ± 0.5	7.7 ± 0.6	7.9 ± 0.2	8.8 ± 0.4	7.0 ± 0.5
Red blood cell count	RBC	10^{12}/l	7.7 ± 0.8	7.7 ± 0.8	8.0 ± 0.4	8.1 ± 0.7	7.9 ± 0.6	8.0 ± 0.6	7.5 ± 0.4	7.8 ± 0.8	8.4 ± 0.5
Hematocrit	PCV	ml/100 ml	41 ± 4	42 ± 4	36.8 ± 1.5	36.7 ± 2.3	38.2 ± 1.8	37.6 ± 2.4	38 ± 1	42 ± 2	39 ± 2
Reticulocyte count	RETIC	%	—	—	1.3 ± 0.5	1.7 ± 0.8	1.7 ± 0.9	1.1 ± 0.5	1.1 ± 0.6	1.1 ± 0.4	1.0 ± 0.3
Reticulocyte count	RETIC	10^{12}/l	—	—	0.10 ± 0.04	0.13 ± 0.06	0.13 ± 0.07	0.09 ± 0.04	—	—	—
Mean cell volume	MCV	10^{15}/l	54 ± 4	55 ± 5	46.0+3	45.8 ± 4.3	48.4 ± 3.1	46.9 ± 2.3	51 ± 2	54 ± 5	57 ± 4
Mean cell hemoglobin	MCH	fmol	—	—	0.94 ± 0.06	0.93 ± 0.10	1.00 ± 0.09	0.97 ± 0.06	—	—	—
Mean cell hemoglobin concentration	MHCH	mmol/l	19 ± 1	19 ± 1	20 ± 1	20.2 ± 0.5	20.7 ± 0.7	20.4 ± 0.3	21 ± 0	21 ± 0	21 ± 0
White blood cell count	WBC	10^9/l	14.4 ± 3.6	13.8 ± 3.0	12.0 ± 2.5	11.4 ± 1.4	8.7 ± 1.5	8.6 ± 2.2	7.0 ± 1.0	8.2 ± 2.3	7.3 ± 2.7
Neutrophils	NEUTRO	%	35 ± 14	38 ± 11	29 ± 10	29 ± 14	34 ± 8	30 ± 10	36 ± 10	29 ± 9	34 ± 11
Lymphocytes	LYMPHO	%	61 ± 14	58 ± 11	68.8 ± 10.3	67.6 ± 13.9	61.8 ± 7.8	66.1 ± 8.8	59 ± 9	64 ± 9	59 ± 8
Lymphocytes	LYMPHO	10^9/l	—	—	8.19 ± 2.0	7.98 ± 1.4	5.34 ± 1.0	5.65 ± 1.4	—	—	—
Eosinophils	EOS	%	0.7 ± 1.2	0.5 ± 0.8	0.9 ± 1.3	0.9 ± 1.5	1.3 ± 1.2	2.2 ± 2.3	2.0 ± 2.1	2.4 ± 1.9	5.0 ± 3.3
Eosinophils	EOS	10^9/l	—	—	0.10 ± 0.15	0.10 ± 0.17	0.12 ± 0.11	0.19 ± 0.23	—	—	—
Basophils	BASO	%	0.4 ± 0.7	0.1 ± 0.2	0.7 ± 0.9	0.5 ± 0.7	0.7 ± 0.9	0.3 ± 0.6	1.2 ± 0.8	1.0 ± 1.0	0.6 ± 0.5
Basophils	BASO	10^9/l	—	—	0.08 ± 0.12	0.07 ± 0.10	0.06 ± 0.07	0.02 ± 0.04	—	—	—
Monocytes	MONO	%	2.9 ± 1.4	3.3 ± 1.6	1.1 ± 1.3	1.5 ± 1.5	2.0 ± 1.1	1.5 ± 1.2	1.4 ± 1.7	3.0 ± 1.9	0.6 ± 0.9
Monocytes	MONO	10^9/l	—	—	0.14 ± 0.2	0.20 ± 0.2	0.17 ± 0.1	0.14 ± 0.1	—	—	—
Platelet count	THROMB	10^9/l	532 ± 338	556 ± 173	513 ± 88	490 ± 115	349 ± 79	365 ± 52	320 ± 49	293 ± 53	313 ± 88
Activated partial thromboplastin time	APTT	sec	34+8	39 ± 11	45.9 ± 5.8	44.1 ± 10.5	42.7 ± 8.2	43.2 ± 9.8	33 ± 4	32 ± 13	26 ± 10
Thrombin time	TT	sec	23 ± 4	25 ± 4	25.8 ± 4.1	28.4 ± 5.0	23.9 ± 3.6	23.7 ± 4.6	21 ± 2	23 ± 3	19 ± 4
Prothrombin time	Prothr	sec	12 ± 1	11 ± 1	11.7 ± 0.3	11.5 ± 0.5	11.9 ± 0.6	11.7 ± 0.4	12 ± 0	12 ± 0	12 ± 1
Fibrinogen	Fibr	g/l	6.0 ± 1.3	5.2 ± 1.0	6.5 ± 1.3	5.4 ± 0.7	6.9 ± 1.3	4.8 ± 0.6	5.8 ± 0.8	5.6 ± 0.7	5.5 ± 0.9

Note: Table entries are of the form: Mean ± SD.

[a] Ellegaard, L., Damm Jørgensen, K., Klastrup, S., Kornerup Hansen, A., Svendsen, O., 1995. *Scand. J. Lab. Anim. Sci.*, 22 (3), pp. 239–248. Reprinted with permission.

Source: Jørgensen, K.D., Ellegaard, L., Klastrup, S., Svendsen, O., 1998. *Scand. J. Lab. Anim. Sci., Suppl.* 1, pp. 181–190. Reprinted with permission.

TABLE A.14
The Characteristics of Juvenile and Pregnant Göttingen Minipigs Compared with Young and Adult Individuals

	Hematology	Clinical Chemistry
Juvenile	High hemoglobin	Low serum carbamide
	Low red blood cell count	Low serum creatinine
	High hematocrit	High alkaline phosphatase
	High mean cell volume	High inorganic phosphorous
	Low mean cell hemoglobin	Low serum albumin
	Low percentage of eosinophils	High serum α_2-globulin
	High platelet count	Low albumin/globulin ratio
	Short activated partial thromboplastin time	
	Short thrombin time	
Pregnant	High hemoglobin	Low cholesterol
	Low red blood cell count	High triglyceride
	High mean cell volume	High creatine kinase
	Low white blood cell count	Low lactate dehydrogenase
	High percentage of eosinophils	High serum carbamide
	Low platelet count	High serum creatinine
	Short activated partial thromboplastin time	High serum total protein
	Short thrombin time	High serum β-globulin
	High plasma fibrinogen	High serum γ-globulin
		Low albumin/globulin ratio
		Low inorganic phosphorous

Source: Courtesy of Ellegaard Göttingen Minipigs ApS, Dalmose, Denmark.

TABLE A.15

Hematology Results for Juvenile and Young Adult Hanford Miniature Swine

Gender		Male[a]				Female[a]			
		Mean	SD	Minimum	Maximum	Mean	SD	Minimum	Maximum
Red Blood Cell									
Hematocrit	%	45.5	4.3	35.2	55.2	47.3	4.3	38.6	56.8
Hemoglobin	g/dl	14.5	1.3	11.2	17.5	15.0	1.3	12.3	17.9
Mean corpuscular hemoglobin	pg	18.4	1.1	16.4	21.1	18.8	1.0	15.8	20.3
Mean corpuscular hemoglobin concentration	g/dl	31.8	0.7	30.2	33.7	31.8	0.8	30.0	33.3
Mean corpuscular volume	fl	58.0	3.4	52.6	67.7	59.2	3.5	50.8	66.2
Red blood count	X10^6/µl	7.87	0.74	6.16	9.46	8.01	0.64	6.82	9.63
White Blood Cell									
Basophil	X10^3/µl	0.11	0.04	0.05	0.21	0.12	0.07	0.05	0.50
Eosinophil	X10^3/µl	0.32	0.30	0.01	1.49	0.28	0.22	0.01	1.19
Lymphocyte	X10^3/µl	11.98	2.41	7.19	17.98	11.36	2.75	5.59	17.33
Monocyte	X10^3/µl	0.68	0.22	0.24	1.32	0.66	0.24	0.14	1.47
Neutrophil	X10^3/µl	5.42	2.68	0.41	18.03	4.49	1.61	1.67	9.15
Large unstained cell	X10^3/µl	0.12	0.08	0.02	0.31	0.14	0.07	0.04	0.29
White blood count	X10^3/µl	18.6	3.6	13.0	30.4	17.1	3.1	11.1	25.8
Clotting Potential									
APTT	sec	18.3	2.6	13.9	26.0	18.3	2.8	13.3	26.0
Platelets	X10^3/µl	471.3	130.1	172.0	845.0	458.0	125.0	152.0	751.0
Prothrombin time	sec	14.2	1.0	11.8	17.1	14.1	1.1	12.1	17.6
Others									
Reticulocyte	X10^9/l	113.1	51.7	18.9	235.4	115.7	55.2	18.4	251.0

[a] N = 28 per gender group; age = ~4– 8 months.

Source: Courtesy of Sinclair Research Center, Auxvasse, MO.

TABLE A.16
Range[c] of Observed Hematologic Reference Values[d] for Sinclair Pigs

Analyte	Reference Value Range
WBC	4,700–15,300/µl
RBC	4.97–8.69 × 106/µl high
	9.8–17.3 g/dl
PCV (calculated)	27–49 vol%
PCV (centrifuged)	28–50 vol%
MCV	52–61 fl
MCH	18.6–21.4 pg
MCHC	34.0–35.7 g/dl
Neutrophil (S)	46.2–5,661/µl neutrophil (B)
	0–153/µl
Lymphocyte	3,102–8, 840/µl
Monocyte	0–1,572/µl
Eosinophil	0–544/µl
Basophil	0–162/µl platelets (n = 19)
	311–585 × 10³/µl
Plasma T. Protein	6.7–7.8 g/dl

Note: N = 20 for all analytes except platelets; 10 males and 10 females; all were 1.5 years old.

[a] Reference intervals were established by determining the nonparametric central 0.95 interfractile interval as recommended by the International Federation of Clinical Chemistry.

[b] Analtyes were measured using Kodak clinical chemistry systems except for serum osmolality, which was measured by a freezing point osmometer; some reference values were calculated from measured value.

[c] Too few reference values to establish reference interval by either parametric or nonparametric methods.

[d] WBC, RBC, Hgb, MCV, and platelets measured with Coulter 6-Plus 4; PCV (centrifuged) via microhematocrit method; 100 cell WBC differential counts; plasma total protein by refractometry; remaining values were calculated.

Source: Courtesy of Guy Bouchard, D.V.M., Sinclair Research Center, Auxvasse, MO. Values from the Clinical Pathology Laboratory, Department of Veterinary Pathology, University of Missouri.

TABLE A.17
Hematology Results for Juvenile Sinclair Miniature Swine

		Male				Female			
		Mean	SD	Minimum	Maximum	Mean	SD	Minimum	Maximum
Red Blood Cells									
Hematocrit	%	42.4	3.8	35.3	51.3	43.0	4.2	32.8	54.8
Hemoglobin	g/dl	13.4	1.3	11.2	16.4	13.6	1.3	10.7	17.2
Mean corpuscular hemoglobin	pg	17.9	1.1	15.0	19.4	18.7	1.0	16.4	20.7
Mean corpuscular hemoglobin concentration	g/dl	31.7	0.9	30.1	33.9	31.6	0.8	29.6	33.0
Mean corpuscular volume	fl	56.4	3.3	49.4	62.0	59.3	3.1	52.0	68.4
Red blood count	$X10^6/\mu l$	7.54	0.7	6.00	9.79	7.27	0.8	5.45	9.29
White Blood Cells									
Basophil	$X10^3/\mu l$	0.10	0.1	0.00	0.30	0.07	0.1	0.00	0.23
Eosinophils	$X10^3/\mu l$	1.44	1.3	0.00	6.00	1.38	1.1	0.00	5.00
Lymphocytes	$X10^3/\mu l$	11.62	3.8	4.95	20.46	9.96	2.8	5.41	17.65
Monocytes	$X10^3/\mu l$	0.98	0.5	0.31	2.69	0.82	0.4	0.13	1.77
Neutrophils	$X10^3/\mu l$	6.03	3.6	2.07	20.03	5.23	2.4	2.22	11.07
Large unstained cells	$X10^3/\mu l$	0.30	0.3	0.00	0.94	0.28	0.3	0.00	1.38
White blood count	$X10^3/\mu l$	19.31	5.2	9.21	30.59	16.62	4.1	9.44	26.73
Clotting Potential									
APTT	sec	16.3	2.0	12.1	21.8	16.9	2.8	12.1	29.3
Platelets	$X10^3/\mu l$	459	123.4	149	669	440	135.0	184	728
Prothrombin time	sec	14.4	1.6	10.9	18.4	14.4	2.0	10.5	19.1
Others									
Nucleated red cells	%	0	0.1	0	1	0	0.4	0	3
Reticulocyte	$X10^9/l$	130.4	61.8	37.3	276.3	136.7	57.6	52.2	326.8

Note: N = 47, age = ~3–4 months.

Source: Courtesy of Sinclair Research Center, Auxvasse, MO.

TABLE A.18
Hematologic Values of 30 Healthy, Mature Yucatan Miniature Swine

Value	Mean	Reference Range[a]	Range
RBC ($10^6/\mu l$)	7.0	5.4–8.6	5.6–8.8
Hemoglobulin (g/dl)	14.9	12.5–17.3	13.1–17.0
Hematocrit (%)	44.6	36.4–52.8	36.3–53.7
MCV[b] (fl)	64.4	57.0–71.8	58.2–72.5
MCH[c] (pg)	21.4	18.8–24.0	18.9–24.3
MCHC[d] (g/dl)	33.2	31.6–34.8	31.1–34.5
RDW	19.4	16.2–22.6	15.7–23.8
Platelets ($10^3/\mu l$)	440.6	201.4–679.8	217.0–770.0
WBC ($10^3/\mu l$)	12.6	6.6–18.6	6.9–21.2
100 cell manual differential			
% segmented neutrophils	41.9	17.5–66.3	18.0–64.0
% bands	0.2	0.0–1.2	0.0–2.0
% lymphocytes	45.6	19.2–72.0	21.0–71.0
% monocytes	7.5	1.1–13.9	2.0–15.0
% eosinophils	4.1	0.0–10.0	0.0–13.0
% basophils	0.5	0.0–2.5	0.0–5.0

[a] ×2 SD observed.

[b] Mean corpuscular volume.

[c] Mean corpuscular hemoglobin.

[d] Mean corpuscular hemoglobin concentration.

Source: Reprinted from Radin, M.J. et al., 1986. *Lab. Anim. Sci.*, 36(4): 425–427. With permission.

TABLE A.19
Clinical Chemistry of Göttingen Minipig

Parameter	Abbreviation	Unit		Male (3 months)	Female (3 months)	Male (6 months)	Female (6 months)
Alanine	ALAT	pkat/1	mean	1.12	1.00	0.92	0.96
			SD	0.16	0.17	0.07	0.27
Ornithine carbamyl	OCT	10/1	mean	4.49	4.13	4.43	4.79
transferase			SD	0.28	0.53	0.44	0.74
Sorbitol	SDH	pkat/1	mean	0.01	0.01	0.01	0.01
dehydrogenase			SD	0.01	0.01	0.01	0.01
Aspartate	ASAT	pkat/1	mean	0.38	0.34	0.36	0.34
aminotransferase			SD	0.13	0.09	0.10	0.07
Alkaline phosphatase	ALKPH	pkat/1	mean	4.29	3.88	3.49	2.71
			SD	0.92	1.11	0.75	0.98
Bilirubin	BILI	pmol/1	mean	2.69	2.27	2.32	1.87
			SD	0.49	0.74	0.48	0.56
Y-glutamyl transferase	GGT	pkat/1	mean	0.80	0.79	0.89	0.77
			SD	0.10	0.12	0.12	0.18
Cholesterol	CHOL	mmol/1	mean	1.72	2.40	1.33	0.96
			SD	0.33	0.49	0.20	0.43
Creatine kinase	CK	pkat/1	mean	5.99	1.17	7.89	9.38
			SD	2.25	2.20	4.85	3.88
Lactate dehydrogenase	LDH	pkat/1	mean	16.68	17.45	13.59	15.27
			SD	2.34	2.32	2.03	5.39
Amylase	AmYL	IU/1	mean	49.04	50.08	49.33	52.17
			SD	11.59	13.97	10.53	15.23
Protein (total)	PROT	g/l	mean	58.43	57.58	61.02	61.66
			SD	3.97	3.63	3.33	3.60
Triglicerides	TRIG	mmol/1	mean	0.40	0.59	0.36	0.47
			SD	0.07	0.12	0.07	0.12
Carbamid	UREA	mmol/1	mean	2.49	2.37	2.12	2.35
			SD	0.56	0.59	0.50	0.59

Source: Courtesy of Ellegaard Göttingen Minipigs. Reprinted from Ellegaard, L. et al. 1995. Haematologic and clinical chemical values in 3 and 6 months old Göttingen minipigs. *Scand. J. Lab. Anim. Sci.* 22(3): 239–248. With permission.

TABLE A.20
Serum Chemistry from Göttingen Breeding Facility (grouped by age)

| | | | | Values Grouped by Age of Animals | | | | | |
| | | | | 6 months | | 7 months | | 8 months[a] | |
Paramter	Abbreviation	Unit	Sex	Average	SD	Average	SD	Average	SD
Sodium	Na	mmol/l	Female	149.12	5.02	149.53	6.42	150.69	4.11
			Male	146.15	1.95	149.43	4.52	148.77	3.37
Potassium	K	mmol/l	Female	5.23	0.95	5.55	0.73	4.70	0.56
			Male	5.04	0.47	5.06	0.47	5.09	0.44
Chloride	Cl	mmol/l	Female	103.56	3.84	103.79	4.42	103.81	2.51
			Male	101.69	2.06	104.14	3.37	102.31	2.72
Alanine aminotransferase	ALAT	μkat/l	Female	0.83	0.14	0.78	0.25	0.78	0.14
			Male	0.87	0.15	0.89	0.15	0.85	0.12
Albumin	Albumin	g/l	Female	47.91	3.71	48.64	4.21	51.03	4.43
			Male	46.28	3.45	46.97	2.78	48.23	2.62
Alkaline phosphatase	AP	μkat/l	Female	2.95	1.03	3.23	0.90	3.21	0.72
			Male	3.34	0.85	3.64	0.66	3.91	0.78
Amylase	Amylase	μkat/l	Female	54.81	6.88	45.77	9.15	56.34	10.26
			Male	47.79	5.07	43.87	7.29	44.03	12.40
Aspartate aminotransferase	AST	μkat/l	Female	0.46	0.14	0.38	0.08	0.49	0.15
			Male	0.47	0.07	0.47	0.14	0.50	0.22
Calcium	Ca	mmol/l	Female	2.76	0.15	2.88	0.13	2.65	0.08
			Male	2.69	0.14	2.79	0.12	2.79	0.12
Cholesterol	Chol	mmol/l	Female	2.37	0.36	2.41	0.52	2.67	0.60
			Male	1.68	0.26	1.51	0.32	1.43	0.27
Inorganic phosphorus	Phosphor	mmol/l	Female	2.79	0.33	2.60	0.25	2.61	0.49
			Male	2.58	0.45	2.29	0.24	2.21	0.15
Total protein	T. Prot	g/l	Female	62.95	6.69	64.95	4.62	70.42	7.59
			Male	61.85	4.46	62.90	3.98	65.15	3.83
Triglycerides	Trigl.	mmol/l	Female	0.46	0.12	0.64	0.16	0.76	0.19
			Male	0.39	0.18	0.42	0.12	0.64	0.24
Carbamide	Urea	mmol/l	Female	2.59	0.53	3.68	0.51	3.96	0.90
			Male	2.56	0.75	3.22	0.48	4.12	0.93
Magnesium	Mg	mmol/l	Female	1.13	0.10	1.17	0.15	1.23	0.13
			Male	1.07	0.12	1.13	0.12	1.16	0.07

Note: Parameters measured on the following instrument: Advia 1200, Bayer Company. Blood samples obtained from the Ellegaard Göttingen Minipig ApS breeding facility, Dalmose, Denmark, 2006. The population of animals is the same in Table A.20, Table A.21, and Table A.22. It is the same data grouped differently.

[a] Also includes animals 8 months and 1 week of age.

Source: Data courtesy Altana Pharma AG, Barsbüttel, Germany.

TABLE A.21
Serum Chemistry from Göttingen Breeding Facility (grouped by gender)

Parameter	Abbreviation	Unit	Gender	Average	SD	N
Sodium	Na	mmol/l	Female	149.67	5.25	57
			Male	148.15	3.68	40
Potassium	K	mmol/l	Female	5.19	0.84	57
			Male	5.06	0.45	40
Chloride	Cl	mmol/l	Female	103.70	3.68	57
			Male	102.75	2.92	40
Alanine aminotransferase	ALAT	μkat/l	Female	0.80	0.18	58
			Male	0.87	0.14	38
Albumin	Albumin	g/l	Female	48.97	4.20	57
			Male	47.16	3.00	40
Alkaline phosphatase	AP	μkat/l	Female	3.10	0.91	57
			Male	3.64	0.78	40
Amylase	Amylase	μkat/l	Female	52.36	9.61	57
			Male	45.19	8.73	40
Aspartate aminotransferase	AST	μkat/l	Female	0.44	0.14	57
			Male	0.48	0.15	39
Calcium	Ca	mmol/l	Female	2.77	0.15	57
			Male	2.76	0.14	40
Cholesterol	Chol	mmol/l	Female	2.46	0.49	57
			Male	1.54	0.30	40
Inorganic phosphorus	Phosphor	mmol/l	Female	2.68	0.36	57
			Male	2.36	0.34	40
Total protein	T. Prot	g/l	Female	65.57	6.98	57
			Male	63.29	4.22	40
Triglycerides	Trigl.	mmol/l	Female	0.60	0.20	56
			Male	0.48	0.21	40
Carbamide	Urea	mmol/l	Female	3.31	0.89	56
			Male	3.32	0.96	39
Magnesium	Mg	mmol/l	Female	1.17	0.13	57
			Male	1.12	0.11	40

Note: Animals are from 6 months to 8 months + 1 week of age. Blood samples obtained from the Ellegaard Göttingen Minipig ApS breeding facility, Dalmose, Denmark, 2006; measured on the following instrument: Advia 1200, Bayer Company.

Source: Data courtesy Altana Pharma AG, Barsbüttel, Germany.

TABLE A.22
Serum Chemistry from Göttingen Breeding Facility
(grouped by parameter)

Parameter	Abbreviation	Unit	Average	SD	N
Sodium	Na	mmol/l	149.06	4.72	97
Potassium	K	mmol/l	5.14	0.71	97
Chloride	Cl	mmol/l	103.32	3.41	97
Alanine aminotransferase	ALT	μkat/l	0.83	0.17	97
Albumin	Albumin	g/l	48.25	3.86	97
Alkaline phosphatase	AP	μkat/l	3.32	0.90	98
Amylase	Amylase	μkat/l	49.49	9.88	96
Aspartate aminotransferase	AST	μkat/l	0.46	0.14	95
Calcium	Ca	mmol/l	2.77	0.15	97
Cholesterol	Chol	mmol/l	2.09	0.62	97
Inorganic phosphorus	Phosphor	mmol/l	2.55	0.39	97
Total protein	T. Prot	g/l	64.66	6.11	97
Triglycerides	Trigl.	mmol/l	0.55	0.21	97
Carbamide	Urea	mmol/l	3.31	0.91	97
Magnesium	Mg	mmol/l	1.15	0.12	96

Note: Animals are from 6 months to 8 months + 1 week of age. Average sex distribution: females 59%, males 41%. Serum chemistry measured on the following instrument: Advia 1200, Bayer Company. Blood samples obtained from the Ellegaard Göttingen Minipig ApS breeding facility, Dalmose, Denmark, 2006.

Source: Data courtesy Altana Pharma AG, Barsbüttel, Germany.

TABLE A.23

Clinical Chemistry Results for Juvenile and Young Adult Hanford Miniature Swine

		Male				Female			
		Mean	SD	Minimum	Maximum	Mean	SD	Minimum	Maximum
Electrolyte Balance									
Calcium	mg/dl	10.6	0.5	9.5	12.9	10.6	0.4	10.0	11.4
Chloride	mEq/l	102.6	3.3	96.0	120.0	102.1	1.9	97.0	107.0
Phosphorus	mg/dl	8.1	0.7	6.8	9.7	8.2	0.5	7.1	9.3
Potassium	mEq/l	6.0	0.8	4.3	7.8	6.0	0.8	4.7	8.6
Sodium	mEq/l	145	5	134	169	144	3	137	151
Carbohydrate Metabolism									
Glucose	mg/dl	89.2	11.0	72.0	123.0	89.5	11.9	68.0	131.0
Liver Function — Hepatocellular									
Alanine aminotransferase	U/l	41.4	8.9	26.0	74.0	44.2	10.6	26.0	75.0
Aspartate aminotransferase	U/l	50.2	31.6	20.0	164.0	58.4	50.7	20.0	286.0
Lactate dehydrogenase	U/l	564.7	239.9	338.0	1845.0	635.1	264.5	365.0	1768.0
Liver Function — Hepatobiliary									
Alkaline phosphatase	U/l	133.4	31.3	67.0	216.0	134.6	37.8	76.0	244.0
Total bilirubin	mg/dl	0.1	0.0	0.1	0.3	0.1	0.1	0.1	0.4
Kidney Function									
Creatinine	mg/dl	1.0	0.2	0.7	1.4	1.1	0.2	0.8	1.5
Urea nitrogen	mg/dl	8.2	2.2	4.0	14.0	9.5	2.4	5.0	14.0
Others									
Albumin	g/dl	3.7	0.4	2.8	4.5	3.7	0.3	3.1	4.5
Globulin	g/dl	2.7	0.5	2.0	3.8	2.9	0.4	2.1	4.0
A/G ratio		1.4	0.3	0.8	2.0	1.3	0.2	0.8	1.8
Total protein	g/dl	6.4	0.5	5.1	7.4	6.6	0.5	5.6	7.8
Cholesterol	mg/dl	73.3	12.0	45.0	108.0	90.6	16.2	56.0	142.0
Triglycerides	mg/dl	27.0	8.4	9.0	52.0	37.3	11.5	11.0	70.0
CO_2	mEq/l	26.5	3.3	21.0	35.0	24.3	2.5	17.0	28.0

Note: N = 28 per gender group; age = ~4–8 Months.

Source: Courtesy of Sinclair Research Center, Auxvasse, MO.

TABLE A.24
Reference Intervals for Clinical Chemistry Values of Sinclair Pigs

Analyte	Reference Interval	Analyte	Reference Interval
A/G ratio	0.9–1.7	CO_2 (total)	26–35 a mol/l
Albumin	3.3–4.8 g/dl	Creatinine	0.8–1.9 mg/dl
ALP	42–89 U/l	GGT	19–86 U/l
ALT	23–62 U/l	Glucose	48–290 mg/dl
AMS	365–1871 U/l	LDH	883–1450 U/l
Anion gap[a]	13.2–24.0 mmol/l	LPS	14–343 U/l
AST	16–43 U/l	Magnesium	1.7–2.3 mg/dl
Bilirubin (total)	0.1–0.3 mg/dl	Osmolality (meas)	285–324 mOsm/kg
Bilirubin (dir)	0.1–0.3 mg/dl	Osmolality (calc)[b]	276–307 mOsm/kg
Bilirubin (conj)	0.0–0.0 mg/dl	Osmolality gap[c]	3–20 mOsm/kg
Bilirubin (delta)	0.1–0.3 mg/dl	Phosphorus	5.8–7.8 g/dl
Calcium	10.0–11.3 mg/dl	Potassium	3.9–5.6 mmol/l
Chloride	98–106 mmol/l	Protein (total)	6.7–7.8 g/dl
Cholesterol	47–124 mg/dl	Urea nitrogen	7–13 mg/dl
CK	219–1411 U/l		

Note: N = 40 for all analytes; 20 males and 20 females; all were 1.5 years old.

[a] Anion gap = (Na + K) (Cl + CO_2).
[b] Calculated osmolality = 1.86 (Na + K) + UN/2.8 + Glucose/18.
[c] Osmolality gap = measured osmolality − calculated osmolality.

Source: Courtesy of Guy Bouchard, D.V.M., Sinclair Research Center, Auxvasse, MO.
Values from the Clinical Pathology Laboratory, Department of Veterinary Pathology.

TABLE A.25
Clinical Chemistry Results for Juvenile Sinclair Miniature Swine

		Male				Female			
		Mean	SD	Minimum	Maximum	Mean	SD	Minimum	Maximum
Electrolyte Balance									
Calcium	mg/dl	10.6	0.4	9.8	11.4	10.6	0.4	9.3	11.7
Chloride	mEq/l	103	3.2	96	110	104	3.3	97	110
Phosphorus	mg/dl	9.5	0.8	7.3	10.6	9.4	0.9	7.8	11.7
Potassium	mEq/l	5.8	0.9	4.1	8.0	5.8	0.8	4.3	8.3
Sodium	mEq/l	144	2.9	137	151	144	3.7	138	154
Carbohydrate Metabolism									
Glucose	mg/dl	86	12.1	58	112	80	17.6	42	118
Liver Function — Hepatocellular									
Alanine aminotransferase	U/l	32	8.3	20	55	31	8.0	19	55
Aspartate aminotransferase	U/l	37	17.0	18	91	37	16.9	13	89
Lactate dehydrogenase	U/l	538	172.0	338	1198	561	146.4	367	942
Liver Function — Hepatobiliary									
Alkaline phosphatase	U/l	102	26.4	51	168	96	18.5	51	140
Total bilirubin	mg/dl	0.2	0.1	0.1	0.6	0.2	0.1	0.1	0.8
Kidney Function									
Creatinine	mg/dl	0.9	0.2	0.6	1.4	0.9	0.2	0.5	1.3
Urea nitrogen	mEq/l	8	2.9	5	17	9	3.0	4	19
Others									
Albumin	g/dl	16.3	2.0	12.1	21.8	16.9	2.8	12.1	29.3
Globulin	g/dl	2.8	0.5	2.0	4.2	2.7	0.4	1.9	3.8
Bicarbonate	mEq/l	24	3.6	16	31	24	3.2	16	36
A/G ratio	mg/dl	1.28	0.3	0.59	1.90	1.31	0.3	0.71	2.05
Total protein	g/dl	6.2	0.5	5.1	7.2	6.1	0.5	4.6	8.0
Cholesterol	mg/dl	79	13.7	47	110	81	15.8	49	118
Triglycerides	mg/dl	50	26.8	18	139	56	31.2	22	150

Note: N = 51, age = ~3–4 Months.

Source: Courtesy of Sinclair Research Center, Auxvasse, MO.

TABLE A.26
Clinical Chemistry Reference Values for Fasted Yucatan Miniature Pigs

| Parameter | Unit | Mean | | SD | Pooled Values Observed | |
		Male	Female		Median	Range
Glucose	mmol/l	3.65	3.85	64	3.66	2.28–5.11
Urea	mmol/l	7.00	8.68	2.64	7.14	5.00–16.1
Creatinine	umol/l	106.1	123.8[a]	15.9	114.9	88.4–150.3
Uric acid	umol/1	3.6	7.1	7.1	5.9	0.0–29.7
Total protein	g/l	77.0	71.0	9.0	76.0	44.0–83.0
Albumin	g/l	53.0	46.0[a]	6.0	51.0	26.0–57.0
Globulin	g/l	24.0	25.0	4.0	24.0	18.0–36.0
Albumin/globulin		2.2	1.9[a]	0.3	2.1	1.3–2.7
Bilirubin total	umol/l	3.42	3.42	1.37	3.42	1.7–6.84
Triglyceride	mg/l	192	341[a]	134	235	100–530
Total cholesterol	mmol/l	1.81	1.89	0.38	1.85	1.03–2.67
Alkaline phosphatase	U/l	90.1	87.7	21.5	84.5	39.0–128.0
Gamma glutamyl transferase	U/l	61.1	62.1	11.2	61.5	41.0–86.0
Alanine aminotransferase	U/l	71.9	73.0	13.6	71.0	49.0–106.0
Lactate dehydrogenase	U/l	450.8	556.7[a]	88.0	492.0	389.0–727.0
Aspartate aminotransferase	U/l	38.7	41.8	5.9	39.0	32.0–55.0
Sodium	mmol/l	139.3	141.7	4.2	141.0	132.0–149.0
Potassium	mmol/l	4.0	4.2	.3	4.0	3.5–4.8
Chloride	mmol/l	101.2	105.0	4.3	102.0	96.0–111.0
Iron	umol/l	22.7	23.6	3.5	23.1	11.8–37.6
Calcium	mmol/l	2.72	2.52	.18	2.65	2.08–2.92
Phosphorus	mmol/l	2.42	2.39	.26	2.33	1.97–2.91

[a] Significant difference (P <.05) between sexes, N = 24.

Source: Reprinted from Parsons, A.H. and Wells, R.E. 1986. *Lab. Anim. Sci.,* 36(4):428–430. With permission.

TABLE A.27
Serum Biochemical Values of 30 Healthy Mature
Yucatan Miniature Swine

Value	Mean	Reference Range[a]	Range
Glucose (mg/dl)	79.8	36.4–123.2	56.0–153.0
SUN (mg/dl)[b]	19.2	9.2–29.2	10.0–29.0
Creatinine (mg/dl)	1.6	1.2–2.0	1.2–2.0
Total protein (gm/dl)	7.5	6.1–8.9	6.3–9.4
Albumin (gm/dl)	4.7	3.9–5.5	4.1–5.6
Globulin (gm/dl)	2.8	1.6–4.0	1.4–3.6
A-G[c]	1.8	0.8–2.8	1.11–3.49
Sodium (mEq/1)	147.0	144–152.6	142.0–153.0
Potassium (mEq/1)	4.6	4.0–5.2	3.9–5.2
Chloride (mEq/1)	104.2	94.4–114.0	95.0–114.0
Calcium (mg/dl)	10.6	9.6–11.6	9.3–11.6
Phosphorus (mg/dl)	6.9	5.1–8.1	5.0–8.3
Total bilirubin (mg/dl)	0.1	0.0–0.3	0.0–0.3
AST (IU/I)[d]	28.2	10.4–56.0	15.0–53.0
ALT(IU/I)[e]	33.6	20.4–46.8	20.0–48.0
CPK (IU/I)[f]	168.0	48.0–288.0	37.0–270.0
Cholesterol (mg/dl)	101.8	38.4–165.2	47.3–173.0

[a] X ± 2 SD observed.

[b] Serum urea nitrogen.

[c] Albumin globulin ratio.

[d] Aspartate aminotransferase.

[e] Alanine aminotransferase.

[f] Creatine phosphokinase.

Source: Reprinted from Radin, M.J. et al., 1986. *Lab. Anim. Sci.,* 36(4): 425–427. With permission.

TABLE A.28
Hematology for Male, Adult Yucatan and Ossabaw Miniature Swine

		Yucatan				Ossabaw			
		Mean	SD	Min	Max	Mean	SD	Min	Max
Erythrocytes	($\times 10^6$/ml)	4.4	0.2	4.0	4.7	4.8	0.5	4.2	5.4
Hematocrit[a]	%	26.6	1.6	24.0	29.0	26.6	2.7	23.0	29.0
Hemoglobin	g/dl	9.2	0.7	8.1	10.3	9.2	1.1	7.8	10.2
Mean corpuscular volume (MCV)	fl	60.7	2.2	58.0	64.0	55.7	1.3	54.0	57.0
Mean corpuscular hemoglobin (MCH)	Pg	21.1	1.1	19.9	22.6	19.1	0.6	18.6	20.0
Mean corpuscular hemoglobin concentration (MCHC)	g/dl	34.6	0.6	33.9	35.5	34.5	0.7	33.6	35.2
Leukocytes	($\times 10^3$/ml)	8.2	1.4	6.5	10.7	10.5	2.2	8.0	13.8
Semented neutrophils	($\times 10^3$/ml)	3.43	0.88	2.48	4.92	4.32	1.58	2.68	6.90
Banded neutrophils[b]	($\times 10^3$/ml)	0.09	0.02	0.08	0.11	0	0	0	0
Lymphocytes	($\times 10^3$/ml)	4.54	0.91	3.49	6.08	5.29	1.07	3.29	6.21
Monocytes	($\times 10^3$/ml)	0.29	0.17	0	0.50	0.79	0.44	0.37	1.40
Eosinophils	($\times 10^3$/ml)	0.04	0.05	0	0.11	0.07	0.10	0	0.27
Basophils	($\times 10^3$/ml)	0	0	0	0	0.11	0.20	0	0.40
Platelets[c]	($\times 10^3$/ml)	427.1	83.8	300	553	562.0	150.3	422.0	692.0

Note: N = 7 per breed group, except where noted; age = ~12–15 months.

[a] Hematocrit under anesthesia.

[b] Undetectable in all Ossabaws; detectable in 3 Yucatans.

[c] N = 4 Ossabaw.

Source: Courtesy of Michael Sturek, PhD, Indiana University.

TABLE A.29
Clinical Chemistry for Male, Adult Trapped Ossabaw Island Miniature Swine

		Mean	SD	Min	Max
Electrolytes					
Anion gap	mmol/l	28.5	5.5	21	40
Calcium	mg/dl	9.6	1.3	7.5	11.5
Chloride	mmol/l	95.2	9.1	80.0	107.0
Magnesium	mg/dl	2.8	0.6	2.1	4.5
Phosphorus	mg/dl	7.2	1.3	4.8	9.5
Potassium	mmol/l	7.3	1.2	4.8	9.6
Sodium	mmol/l	139.1	13.5	117	157
Carbohydrate Metabolism					
Glucose	mg/dl	136.5	75.4	82	436
Liver Function — Hepatocellular					
Alkaline phosphatase (ALP)	U/l	57.2	21.0	32.0	107.0
Aspartate aminotranferase (AST)	U/l	51.2	20.0	25	92
Gamma-glutamyl transferase (GGT)	U/l	59.0	9.6	42	77
Liver Function — Hepatobiliary					
Unconjugated bilirubin	mg/dl	0.005	0.02	0	0.1
Total bilirubin	mg/dl	0.27	0.16	0.1	0.6
Kidney Function					
Creatinine	mg/dl	1.8	0.4	1.1	2.7
Urea nitrogen	mg/dl	8.2	2.4	4.0	13.0
Others					
Albumin	g/dl	3.6	0.6	2.7	4.6
Globulin	g/dl	3.8	0.4	3.1	4.6
Albumin/globulin ratio		0.94	0.16	0.59	1.19
Total protein	g/dl	7.4	0.8	6.0	9.0
Creatine kinase	U/l	1031	638	179	2112
Total cholesterol	mg/dl	77.9	23.7	45	127
Triglycerides	mg/dl	33.2	13.2	18	74
Total CO_2	mmol/l	22.8	3.1	17	30
Body weight	kg	46.7	11.9	29.1	73.6

Note: N = 19; estimated age > 9 months. Mean, standard deviation (SD), and minimum (Min) and maximum (Max) values and units of measure are provided.

Source: Courtesy of Michael Sturek, PhD, Indiana University.

TABLE A.30
Clinical Chemistry for Male, Adult Yucatan and Ossabaw Miniature Swine

		Yucatan				Ossabaw			
		Mean	SD	Min	Max	Mean	SD	Min	Max
Electrolytes									
Anion gap	mmol/l	10.9	2.1	6.6	13.0	9.7	2.4	6.0	12.0
Calcium	mg/dl	10.0	0.44	9.5	10.6	10.0	0.18	9.8	10.2
Chloride	mmol/l	101.1	2.12	99.0	105.0	100.4	1.4	98.0	102.0
Magnesium	mg/dl	2.4	0.2	2.2	2.6	2.2	0.1	2.1	2.3
Phosphorus	mg/dl	6.63	0.5	6.4	7.2	7.1	0.4	6.5	7.5
Potassium	mmol/l	3.8	0.32	3.4	4.4	4.2	0.2	4.0	4.4
Sodium	mmol/l	142.7	2.1	139.0	145.0	142.0	1.5	140.0	143.0
Carbohydrate Metabolism									
Glucose	mg/dl	93.1	31.9	47	150	126.0	12.3	107	145
Liver Function — Hepatocellular									
Alkaline phosphatase (ALP)	U/l	58.1	13.5	42.0	83.0	67.0	7.6	62.0	75.0
Aspartate aminotranferase (AST)	U/l	29.1	5.1	19	34	24.0	4.2	19.0	26.0
Gamma-glutamyl transferase (GGT)	U/l	45.9	13.9	23	61	60.4	15.8	45.0	83.0
Liver Function — Hepatobiliary									
Unconjugated bilirubin	mg/dl	0.04	0.08	0.0	0.2	0	0	0	0
Total bilirubin	mg/dl	0.11	0.04	0.1	0.3	0.1	0.0	0.1	0.1
Kidney Function									
Creatinine	mg/dl	1.3	0.1	1.1	1.5	1.7	0.3	1.1	1.9
Urea nitrogen	mg/dl	15.1	2.4	11.0	18.0	10.7	2.6	7.0	14.0
Others									
Albumin	g/dl	3.3	0.2	2.9	3.5	3.4	0.3	3.1	3.7
Globulin	g/dl	3.0	0.2	2.9	3.2	2.8	0.2	2.6	3.0
Albumin/globulin ratio		1.11	0.15	0.94	1.4	1.20	0.08	1.13	1.35
Total protein	g/dl	6.3	0.3	6.0	6.6	6.2	0.4	5.8	6.7
Creatine kinase	U/l	303.1	114.4	203.0	469.0	450.3	94.6	397.0	570.0
Total cholesterol	mg/dl	73.3	12.0	45.0	108.0	90.6	16.2	56.0	142.0
Triglycerides	mg/dl	27.0	8.4	9.0	52.0	37.3	11.5	11.0	70.0
Total CO_2	mmol/l	33.3	1.11	32.0	35.0	35.4	3.2	32	40
Body weight	kg	60.7	6.2	53.2	68.9	74.1	4.8	68.6	81.4

Note: N = 7 per breed group; age = ~12-15 months. Mean, standard deviation (SD), and minimum (Min) and maximum (Max) values and units of measure are provided.

Source: Courtesy of Michael Sturek, PhD, Indiana University.

SECTION 3: ORGAN WEIGHTS AND MEASUREMENTS

TABLE A.31
**Percentage of Body Weight of Various Tissues
and Organs in the 12-Week-Old Pig**

Organ	Percentage of Body Weight
Body weight	100
Cerebrum	0.31 ± 0.06
Cerebellum	0.06 ± 0.02
Spinal cord	0.14 ± 0.08
Thyroid gland	0.02 ± 0.004
Larynx-trachea	0.21 ± 0.03
Lungs	1.09 ± 0.18
Heart	0.49 ± 0.06
Aorta	0.11 ± 0.05
Esophagus	0.13 ± 0.05
Stomach	1.22 ± 0.16
Small intestine	4.46 ± 0.38
Large intestine	2.74 ± 0.59
Liver	3.16 ± 0.41
Spleen	0.19 ± 0.05
Pancreas	0.29 ± 0.18
Kidneys	0.55 ± 0.01
Adrenal glands	0.0104 ± 0.0018
Skeletal muscle	35.97 ± 2.3
Fat	12.52 ± 1.04
Skeleton	16.73 ± 0.89
Rind	6.32 ± 0.54
Blood	5.53 ± 0.42
GI tract content	5.61 ± 2.22
Various connective tissues	3.33 ± 0.62

Note: Data are expressed as mean ± 1 SD; mean weight =
22.74 ± 3.45 kg. GI = stomach, small and large intestine.

Source: Reprinted from Elowsson et al., 1997, *Lab. Anim.
Sci.,* 47(2): 200–202. With permission.

TABLE A.32
**Percentage of Body Weight of Specified Muscles
(left and right sides) of the 12-Week Old Pig**

Muscle	Percentage of Body Weight
Longissimus dorsi	3.17 ± 0.27
Biceps femoris	2.14 ± 0.12
Quadriceps femoris	1.91 ± 0.17
Semitendinosus	0.66 ± 0.06
Semimembranosus	2.58 ± 0.21

Note: Mean weight = 22.74 ± 3.45 kg.

Source: Reprinted from Elowsson et al., 1997, *Lab. Anim. Sci.,*
47(2): 200–202. With permission.

TABLE A.33
Selected Organ Weights for Juvenile and Young Adult Hanford Miniature Swine

	Male				Female			
	Mean	SD	Minimum	Maximum	Mean	SD	Minimum	Maximum
Brain								
Absolute wt (g)	91.7	8.1	78.3	107.7	87.7	7.2	74.5	104.2
% BW	0.24	0.03	0.17	0.32	0.25	0.04	0.18	0.32
Adrenal (2)								
Absolute wt (g)	2.66	0.70	0.05	3.62	2.33	0.45	1.66	3.19
% BW	0.007	0.002	0.000	0.010	0.007	0.001	0.005	0.010
% Brain wt	2.93	0.89	0.06	4.60	2.68	0.57	1.80	4.10
Epididymis (2)								
Absolute wt (g)	86.3	10.8	65.7	105.0	NA	NA	NA	NA
% BW	0.22	0.03	0.16	0.27	NA	NA	NA	NA
% Brain wt	94.3	10.2	77.4	116.1	NA	NA	NA	NA
Heart								
Absolute wt (g)	159.1	20.8	128.0	215.4	144.4	19.9	110.7	178.5
% BW	0.41	0.05	0.34	0.51	0.40	0.03	0.36	0.47
% Brain wt	174	25	137	222	165	22	121	201
Kidney (2)								
Absolute wt (g)	153.9	22.3	115.9	198.6	123.0	13.9	96.9	146.1
% BW	0.39	0.05	0.31	0.49	0.35	0.04	0.27	0.41
% Brain wt	168	24	133	224	141	19	110	178
Liver								
Absolute wt (g)	672.9	61.1	533.2	798.7	677.5	67.8	561.1	866.7
% BW	1.7	0.2	1.4	2.2	1.9	0.2	1.7	2.4
% Brain wt	737	73	617	895	775	87	655	988
Lung								
Absolute wt (g)	263.0	38.3	222.5	354.9	230.5	43.5	184.1	348.3
% BW	0.67	0.09	0.52	0.88	0.65	0.12	0.52	1.03
% Brain wt	290	55	224	443	265	56	183	428
Pituitary Gland								
Absolute wt (g)	0.21	0.05	0.11	0.37	0.16	0.04	0.07	0.22
% BW	0.00050	0.00001	0.00030	0.00100	0.00050	0.00010	0.00020	0.00070
% Brain wt	0.23	0.07	0.14	0.47	0.19	0.05	0.08	0.24
Prostate								
Absolute wt (g)	4.0	1.4	2.1	6.6	NA	NA	NA	NA
% BW	0.010	0.004	0.01	0.02	NA	NA	NA	NA
% Brain wt	4.4	1.5	1.9	7.7	NA	NA	NA	NA
Seminal Vesicle (2)								
Absolute wt (g)	148.2	49.0	72.3	252.7	NA	NA	NA	NA
% BW	0.38	0.12	0.20	0.59	NA	NA	NA	NA
% Brain wt	163	56	70	301	NA	NA	NA	NA

Continued.

TABLE A.33 *(Continued)*
Selected Organ Weights for Juvenile and Young Adult Hanford Miniature Swine

	Male				Female			
	Mean	SD	Minimum	Maximum	Mean	SD	Minimum	Maximum
Spleen								
Absolute wt (g)	202.6	105.2	53.3	414.5	148.0	94.9	38.3	379.5
% BW	0.51	0.25	0.15	0.99	0.43	0.29	0.12	1.12
% Brain wt	222	118	62	480	171	114	50	466
Testis (2)								
Absolute wt (g)	211.8	35.1	133.6	273.3	NA	NA	NA	NA
% BW	0.54	0.09	0.37	0.68	NA	NA	NA	NA
% BW	0.14	0.05	0.08	0.30	0.11	0.04	0.05	0.18
% Brain wt	57.9	19.7	31.5	121.4	46.0	20.0	20.0	85.8
Thyroid (2)								
Absolute wt (g)	3.3	1.0	2.0	6.1	2.5	0.7	1.5	4.7
% BW	0.0083	0.0027	0.0000	0.0200	0.0071	0.0016	0.0000	0.0100
% Brain wt	3.6	1.3	2.1	7.4	2.9	0.9	1.7	5.3
Uterus								
Absolute wt (g)	NA	NA	NA	NA	262.5	97.9	117.5	551.0
% BW	NA	NA	NA	NA	0.72	0.23	0.35	1.24
% Brain wt	NA	NA	NA	NA	302	115	121	608
Ovaries								
Absolute wt (g)	NA	NA	NA	NA	6.4	2.4	1.8	10.2
% BW	NA	NA	NA	NA	0.018	0.006	0.006	0.030
% Brain wt	NA	NA	NA	NA	7.4	2.8	2.0	11.5

Note: N = 28, age = ~6-8 months, NA = not applicable.

Source: Courtesy of Sinclair Research Center, Auxvasse, MO.

TABLE A.34
Age-Related Whole Body Composition and Body Weight
of the Female Sinclair Miniature Swine[1]

Age (in years)	Bone Mineral Content (kg)[2]	Lean Mass (kg)[2]	Total Fat (kg)[2]	Body Weight (kg)[2,3]
1.0	0.806[a]	25.000[a]	9.014[a]	34.819[a]
1.5	1.216[b]	33.812[b]	16.702[a,b]	51.730[b]
2.0	1.556[c]	43.853[c]	24.396[b,c]	69.806[c]
2.5	1.745[c,d]	44.710[c]	30.384[c,d]	76.839[c,d]
3.0	1.849[d,e]	49.552[d]	37.071[d,e]	88.472[d,e]
3.5	1.804[d,e]	49.319[d]	28.140[b,c,d]	79.262[c,d,e]
4.0	1.991[e]	52.427[d]	37.665[d,e]	92.083[e,f]
>6.0	2.021[e]	52.115[d]	47.892[e]	102.029[f]

Note: [1] Whole-body composition measured using a Dual Energy X-ray Absorptiometer (QDR 2000-Plus, Hologic, Waltham, MA).

[2] [a,b,c,d,e,f] Means with different superscripts within the same column are different at $p < 0.05$.

[3] Body weights of miniature swine older than 2.5 years of age are exaggerated due to obesity.

Source: Reprinted with permission from Bouchard et al., 1995, Retrospective evaluation of production characteristics in Sinclair miniature swine — 44 years later, *Lab. Anim. Sci.,* 45(4): 408–414.

TABLE A.35
Selected Organ Weights for Juvenile Sinclair Miniature Swine

	Male				Female			
	Mean	SD	Minimum	Maximum	Mean	SD	Minimum	Maximum
Brain								
Absolute wt (g)	76.7	4.78	67.7	85.2	72.2	3.16	64.9	77.9
% BW	0.61	0.086	0.51	0.77	0.59	0.068	0.47	0.71
Adrenal (2)								
Absolute wt (g)	1.39	0.197	1.04	1.71	1.23	0.150	1.04	1.48
% BW	0.011	0.002	0.009	0.015	0.010	0.002	0.008	0.015
% Brain wt	1.81	0.26	1.32	2.30	1.71	0.22	1.42	2.06
Epididymis (2)								
Absolute wt (g)	11.4	3.69	5.16	15.6				
% BW	0.087	0.019	0.058	0.113				
% Brain wt	14.8	4.70	7.61	21.1				
Heart								
Absolute wt (g)	59.4	8.75	43.4	73.1	53.3	7.31	39.2	64.8
% BW	0.47	0.033	0.39	0.52	0.43	0.029	0.39	0.50
% Brain wt	77.3	9.67	62.0	89.2	73.8	9.64	60.4	88.4
Kidney (2)								
Absolute wt (g)	58.9	6.92	48.3	72.6	53.2	4.10	46.2	59.3
% BW	0.47	0.10	0.34	0.71	0.43	0.05	0.36	0.52
% Brain wt	77.1	9.98	66.1	93.8	73.8	5.56	63.0	80.7
Liver								
Absolute wt (g)	324	44.5	246	394	312	29.1	268	363
% BW	2.59	0.52	1.76	3.67	2.53	0.31	2.09	3.13
% Brain wt	423	56.1	332	516	433	42.6	365	513
Lung								
Absolute wt (g)	165	64.8	115	354	202	98	103	448
% BW	1.29	0.44	0.92	2.57	1.65	0.83	0.80	3.44
% Brain wt	215	85.7	161	469	280	135	140	611
Pituitary Gland								
Absolute wt (g)	0.103	0.034	0.072	0.191	0.081	0.019	0.057	0.118
% BW	0.001	0.0002	0.001	0.001	0.001	0.0002	0.000	0.001
% Brain wt	0.13	0.047	0.090	0.26	0.11	0.028	0.082	0.17
Prostate								
Absolute wt (g)	1.00	0.412	0.595	1.74				
% BW	0.008	0.003	0.004	0.015				
% Brain wt	1.32	0.56	0.71	2.35				
Seminal Vesicle (2)								
Absolute wt (g)	8.93	3.81	2.03	12.6				
% BW	0.069	0.028	0.023	0.11				
% Brain wt	11.6	5.01	3.00	17.3				

Continued.

TABLE A.35 *(Continued)*
Selected Organ Weights for Juvenile Sinclair Miniature Swine

	Male				Female			
	Mean	SD	Minimum	Maximum	Mean	SD	Minimum	Maximum
Spleen								
Absolute wt (g)	44.6	19.7	12.5	86.1	48.6	17.2	22.2	72.5
% BW	0.34	0.13	0.14	0.58	0.40	0.15	0.17	0.62
% Brain wt	57.4	23.6	18.4	105	67.6	24.4	30.2	104
Testis (2)								
Absolute wt (g)	49.9	19.6	21.2	78.5				
% BW	0.38	0.11	0.21	0.52				
% Brain wt	64.6	24.3	31.4	95.8				
Thymus								
Absolute wt (g)	26.4	12.0	9.85	48.6	22.5	8.58	13.1	44.1
% BW	0.20	0.089	0.11%	0.41%	0.18	0.061	0.10	0.30
% Brain wt	34.4	16.2	14.5	65.2	31.3	12.3	18.3	62.2
Thyroid (2)								
Absolute wt (g)	1.22	0.274	0.744	1.73	1.04	0.282	0.653	1.51
% BW	0.010	0.002	0.007	0.014	0.008	0.002	0.006	0.012
% Brain wt	1.58	0.31	1.10	2.15	1.44	0.38	1.00	2.06

Note: N = 12, age = ~4 months.

Source: Courtesy of Sinclair Research Center, Auxvasse, MO.

TABLE A.36
Visceral Composition of Male Yucatan and Ossabaw Miniature Swine

	Diet		
Breed	**Control Chow**	**46% kcal Fat**	**75% kcal Fat**
Ossabaw	N = 7	N = 8	N = 3
% Protein	12.2 ± 0.4	11.7 ± 0.3	9.9 ± 0.5
% Fat	19.9 ± 1.9	23.4 ± 0.8	28.9 ± 0.6
Yucatan	N = 6	N = 5	N = 3
% Protein	13.2 ± 0.5	13.4 ± 0.5	11.9 ± 0.2
% Fat	12.5 ± 2.1	16.2 ± 2.8	20.3 ± 2.0

Note: Values are mean ± standard error.

Source: Courtesy of Michael Sturek, PhD, Indiana University.

SECTION 4: REPRODUCTIVE PARAMETERS

TABLE A.37
Effect of Parity on Reproductive Parameters of Sinclair Miniature Swine

Parity	N	Litter Size	Stillborn H	Weaned Piglets	N	Litter Weight (kg)
1	150	6.5 ± 2^a	$0.64 \pm 09^{a,b}$	5.0 ± 0.2^a	124	3.5 ± 0.1^a
2	100	$7.6 \pm 0.2^{b,c}$	$0.47 \pm 0.11^{a,b}$	$6.4 \pm 0.2^{b,c}$	85	$4.4 \pm 0.2^{b,c}$
3	60	$7.9 \pm 0.3^{b,c}$	$0.52 \pm 0.14^{a,b}$	6.7 ± 0.3^c	55	4.5 ± 0.2^c
4	35	$7.2 \pm 0.4^{a,b}$	0.91 ± 0.18^b	5.4 ± 0.4^a	34	$3.9 \pm 0.2^{a,b}$
5	16	$7.5 \pm 0.5^{a,b,c}$	$0.63 \pm 0.27^{a,b}$	$5.5 \pm 0.6^{a,b}$	13	$4.0 \pm 0.4^{a,b,c}$
>6	10	8.9 ± 0.7^c	1.90 ± 0.34^c	$5.8 \pm 0.7^{a,b,c}$	9	$4.3 \pm 0.5^{a,b,c}$

Note: Data collected between 1985 and 1993, expressed as mean ± SEM; N, number of litters applies to the columns on the right; under certain circumstances some litters were not weighted.

[a,b,c]Means with different superscripts within column are different at $p < 0.05$.

Source: Reprinted from Bouchard G. et al., 1995, *Lab. Anim. Sci.,* 45(4): 408–414. With permission.

TABLE A.38
Effect of the Sow Age on Reproductive Parameters of Sinclair Miniature Swine

Sow	N	Litter Size	Stillborn H	Weaned Piglets	N	Litter Weight (Kg)
1	72	6.4 ± 3^a	0.39 ± 0.13^a	5.2 ± 0.3^a	69	3.4 ± 2^a
2	164	$7.4 \pm 0.2^{b,c}$	$0.54 \pm 0.8^{a,b}$	6.2 ± 0.2^b	142	4.2 ± 0.1^b
3	88	$7.2 \pm 0.2^{b,c}$	$0.72 \pm 0.12^{b,c}$	$5.7 \pm 0.2^{a,b}$	68	4.1 ± 0.2^b
4	34	$7.7 \pm- 0.4^{b,c}$	1.09 ± 0.19^c	$5.6 \pm 0.4^{a,b}$	30	4.1 ± 0.3^b
5	6	$6.0 \pm 0.9^{a,b}$	$0.67 \pm 0.44^{a,b,c}$	$4.5 \pm 0.9^{a,b}$	5	$3.8 \pm 0.6^{a,b}$
>6	7	8.6 ± 0.8^c	2.00 ± 0.41^d	4.4 ± 0.9^a	6	$3.3 \pm 0.6^{a,b}$

Note: Data collected between 1985 and 1993, expressed as mean ± SEM; N, number of litters applies to the columns on the right; under certain circumstances some litters were not weighted.

[a,b,c]Means with different superscripts within column are different at $p < 0.05$.

Source: Reprinted from Bouchard G. et al.. 1995. *Lab. Anim. Sci.,* 45(4): 408–414. With permission.

TABLE A.39
Correlation between Morphology and Motility of Göttingen Minipig Sperm

	Motility		
Morphology	Vigorous Progressive (%)	Weak Progressive (%)	No Progressive (%)
Normal (n = 520)	95	4	1
Distal drop (n = 200)	10	83	7
Coiled flagellum and distal drop (n = 200)	0	20	80

Source: Reprinted from Jørgensen, K.D. et al., 1998, *Scand. J. Lab. Anim. Sci.,* Suppl. 1, 161–169. With permission.

TABLE A.40
Minipig Sperm Morphology of Göttingen Minipig
Breeding Boars

	From Ejaculates (n = 37)	From Cauda Epididymis (n = 9)
Normal sperm	50 ± 23%	17 ± 7%
Proximal drop	2 ± 2%	15 ± 22%
Distal drop	6 ± 9%	24 ± 17%
Coiled flagellum and distal drop	10 ± 11%	34 ± 15%
Coiled flagellum	23 ± 10%	6 ± 5%
Extremely coiled flagellum	6 ± 7%	1.4 ± 1.0%
Bent flagellum	4 ± 4%	0.9 ± 0.9%
Detached flagellum	0.5 ± 1.0%	0.5 ± 0.4%
Detached normal head	1.8 ± 4.3%	1.8 ± 1.7%
Detached abnormal head	0.01 ± 0.08%	0 ± 0%
Small head	0.2 ± 0.4%	0.1 ± 0.2%
Abnormal shape of head	0.1 ± 0.3%	0.1 ± 0.2%
Acrosom changes	0.01 ± 0.08%	0 ± 0%

Source: From Jørgensen, K.D. et al., 1998, *Scand. J. Lab. Anim. Sci.*, Suppl. 1, 161–169. With permission.

TABLE A.41
Reproductive Data for Göttingen Minipig Breeding Boars (n = 6)

	Ejaculate (ml)	Sperm Count in Ejaculate × 10⁶/ml	Gilts Mated	Gilts Pregnant	Number of Mating Days (mean)	Testes Weight (g) Left	Testes Weight (g) Right
	91	52.4	17	11 (65%)	2.6	38.81	38.91
	120	68.9	12	8 (67%)	2.5	50.15	48.71
	81	38.8	16	9 (56%)	2.6	42.88	43.36
	89	108.5	13	10 (77%)	1.8	43.03	46.44
	63	43.7	7	6 (86%)	2.3	—	—
	116	73.1	7	5 (71%)	1.9	—	—
Mean	93	64.2	12	8 (70%)	2.3	43.72	44.36
SD	22	25.6	4	2 (10%)	0.4	4.71	4.24
Range	81–120	38.8–108.5	7–17	5–11 (56–86%)	1.8–2.6	38.81–50.15	38.91–48.71

Source: Jørgensen, K.D. et al., 1998, *Scand. J. Lab. Anim. Sci.*, Suppl. 1, 161–169. With permission.

TABLE A.42
Reproductive Data for Cryptorchid Göttingen Minipigs

	Ejaculate (ml)	Sperm Count in Ejaculate (× 10⁶/ml)	Weight of Testis in Scrotum (g)	Weight of Epididymis in Scrotum (g)	Weight of Testis in Abdominal Cavity (g)	Weight of Epididymis in Abdominal Cavity (g)
	72	18.7	25.80 (l)	12.50	6.03 (r)	4.76
	49	0.3	17.68 (l)	14.90	6.59 (r)	8.09
	88	39.9	19.09 (r)	7.64	5.01 (l)	3.37
	43	31.7	31.56 (r)	17.33	10.12 (l)	12.23
	83	13.7	24.70 (l)	9.56	7.75 (r)	4.76
	—	—	42.13 (r)	12.39	1.04 (l)	3.48
	—	—	37.95 (l)	12.43	7.72 (r)	5.45
	69	16.3	31.73 (r)	10.83	5.06 (l)	7.13
	—	—	24.54 (l)	10.61	— (r)	—
	86	31.9	29.68 (r)	13.26	3.34 (l)	5.28
Mean	70	21.8	28.49	12.15	5.85	6.06
SD	18	13.5	7.74	2.73	2.66	2.77
Range	43–88	0.3–39.9	17.68–42.13	7.64–17.33	1.04–10.12	3.37–8.09

Note: N = 11, l = left, r = right.

Source: Reprinted from Jørgensen, K.D. et al., 1998, *Scand. J. Lab. Anim. Sci.*, Suppl. 1, 161–169. With permission.

SECTION 5: FETAL PARAMETERS

TABLE A.43
Fetal Skeletal Diagnoses in Göttingen Minipigs

M	Palatoschisis	1%
M	Gnathoschisis	1%
m	Short nasal bone	1%
m	Incomplete ossification of frontal and parietal bones	1%
m	Four sternebrae	3%
m	One or more sternebrae small	5%
m	Irregular shape of one or more sternebrae	4%
m	Misaligned sternebrae	1%
m	Incomplete ossification of vertebrae	1%
m	Extra ossification centre between vertebrae	2%
m	Fused vertebrae	2%
m	Irregular shape of one or more vertebrae	2%
m	Kinky tail	3%
m	Wavy ribs	1%
m	Misaligned ribs	2%
m	Three metacarpals	1%
m	Five or less carpals	4%
m	Seven carpals	1%
M	Hexadactyly, forelegs	1%
M	Tridactyly, forelegs	1%
m	Incomplete ossification and irregular shape of sacral bones	1%

Note: Day 110–112; n = 220. M = Major malformations/abnormalities (obviously detrimental). m = Minor malformations/abnormalities (of little consequence).

Source: Reprinted from Jorgensen, K.D., 1998, *Scand. J. Lab. Anim. Sci.,* 25 (Suppl 1): 63–75. With permission.

TABLE A.44
Fetal Skeletal Diagnoses in Göttingen Minipigs

	Day 68–70 n = 78 (%)	Day 110–112 n = 220 (%)
Sternebrae		
6 Sternebrae	13	30
5 Sternebrae		67
4 Sternebrae	60	3
3 Sternebrae	23	
< 3 Sternebrae	4	
One or more sternebrae small	63	5
Irregular shape of one or more sternebrae	23	4
Misaligned sternebrae	1	1
Ribs		
15 Ribs or rudimentary 15th rib	18	15
14 Ribs	51	68
13 Ribs	6	6
Cervical rib	25	11
14th Rib rudimentary	15	20
One cleft rib	16	10
Fused ribs	6	8

Source: Reprinted from Jorgensen, K.D., 1998, *Scand. J. Lab. Anim. Sci.*, 25 (Suppl 1): 63–75. With permission.

TABLE A.45
Fetal Skeletal Diagnoses in Gottingen Minipigs

Common Skeletal Variants

Day 68–70; n = 78

One or more sternebrae small	63%
Irregular shape of one or more sternebrae	23%
Three sternebrae	23%
Five or six sternebrae	13%
Cervical rib or rudimentary rib close to C7	25%
Fifteen ribs or rudimentary fifteenth rib	18%
One cleft rib	16%
Fourteenth rib rudimentary	15%
Thirteen ribs	6%
Fused ribs	6%
Small ossification centers in the muscles between scapulae (spinous processes of thoracic vertebrae)	22%
Pentadactyly, forelegs	6%
Two ossification points in 1st and/or 4th toe	27%

Day 110–112; n = 220

Six sternebrae	30%
Fused sternebrae	12%
Fourteenth rib rudimentary	20%
Fourteen ribs or rudimentary fifteenth rib	15%
Cervical rib or rudimentary rib closed close to C7	11%
One cleft rib	10%
Fused ribs	8%
Thirteen ribs	6%
Fused coccygeal vertebrae	8%
Five metacarpals	6%
Pentadactyly, foreleg(s)	9%
One or more carpals small	12%
One or more tarsals small	27%
Six tarsals	10%
Four or less tarsals	16%

Source: Reprinted from Jorgensen, K.D., 1998, *Scand. J. Lab. Anim. Sci.*, 25 (Suppl 1): 63–75. With permission.

TABLE A.46
Population Data for Fetal Values That Follow in Yucatan Minipigs

	Pigs (n = 54)			
	Early Gestation (n = 11)	Late Gestation (n = 43)	Sows (n = 12)	
No. of females	8	25	No. of early gestation	3
No. of males	3	18	No. of late gestation	9
Body weight (g)	366 ± 26	653 ± 200	Body weight (kg)	61 ± 15
Gestation			Age (months)	17 ± 9
Days	82 ± 6	104 ± 6		
Range	(76–88)	(98–110)		

Source: Reprinted from Schantz, L.J. et al., 1995, *Lab. Anim. Sci.*, 45(3): 285–289. With permission.

TABLE A.47
Erythrocytic Data for Fetal Pigs

	Pigs (n = 54)		
	Early Gestation (n = 11)	Late Gestation (n = 43)	Sows (n = 12)
Erythrocytes ($\times 10^6$/μl)	4.30 ± 0.49	4.74 ± 0.55	4.22 ± 0.39
Hemoglobin (g/dl)	9.3 ± 0.7	10.3 ± 1.1	9.0 ± 1.3
Hematocrit (%)	32.7 ± 2.4	34.6 ± 3.9	27.3 ± 3.4
MCV[a] (fl) 77 ± 7	73 ± 4	65 ± 2	
MCH[b] (pg)	22.0 ± 2.8	21.8 ± 0.9	21.2 ± 1.0
MCHC[c] (%)	28.6 ± 1.2	29.8 ± 1.5	32.9 ± 0.5
Nucleated erythrocytes (/100 leukocytes)[d]	148 ± 26	11 ± 18	0

[a] Mean corpuscular volume (femtoliters).
[b] Mean corpuscular hemoglobin (picograms).
[c] Mean corpuscular hemoglobin concentration.
[d] Age differences were significant ($P < .05$).

Source: Reprinted from Schantz, L.J. et al., 1995, *Lab. Anim. Sci.*, 45(3): 285–289. With permission.

TABLE A.48
Leukocytic Data for Fetal Pigs

| | Pigs (n = 54) | | |
	Early Gestation (n = 11)	Late Gestation (n = 43)	Sows (n = 12)
Leukocytes[a] ($\times 10^3/\mu l$)	21 ± 0.3	4.1 ± 2.1	9.7 ± 0.6
Neutrophils[a] (%)	28 ± 1.0	35 ± 17	66 ± 4
Bands (%)	0 ± 1.0	0	1 ± 1
Lymphocytes[a] (%)	70 ± 2	63 ± 18	31 ± 4
Monocytes (%)	1 ± 1	1 ± 1	2 ± 0
Eosinophils (%)	0	0	0
Basophils (%)	0	0	0
Metamyelocytes (%)	0	0	0

[a] Age differences were significant between sow and fetal values ($P < .05$).

Source: Reprinted from Schantz, L.J. et al., 1995, *Lab. Anim. Sci.*, 45(3): 285–289. With permission.

TABLE A.49
Serum Electrolyte Data for Fetal Pigs

| | Pigs (n = 54) | | |
	Early Gestation (n = 11)	Late Gestation (n = 43)	Sows (n = 12)
Ca[a] (mg/dl)	10.8 ± 0.7	11.4 ± 0.9	9.7 ± 0.1
P (mg/dl)	8 ± 0.8	8.7 ± 0.9	7.4 ± 0.2
Na[b] (mEq/l)	130 ± 1.0	141 ± 5.0	139 ± 1.0
K[a] (mEq/l)	8.1 ± 2.3	6.5 ± 1.0	4.7 ± 0
Cl (mEq/l)	95 ± 3.0	100 ± 4.0	103 ± 2.0

[a] Age differences were significant ($P < .05$).
[b] Age differences were significant between sow and fetal values ($P < .05$).

Source: Reprinted from Schantz, L.J. et al., 1995, *Lab. Anim. Sci.*, 45(3): 285–289. With permission.

TABLE A.50
Serum Enzyme Data for Fetal Pigs

	Pigs (n = 54)		
	Early Gestation (n = 11)	Late Gestation (n = 43)	Sows (n = 12)
ALP[a] (IU/l)	333 ± 145	531 ± 230	66 ± 31
LD[b] (IU/l)	1,207 ± 545	491 ± 174	497 ± 26
AST[c] (IU/l)	178 ± 129	47 ± 40	46 ± 10
ALT[d] (IU/l)	15 ± 11	6 ± 3	29 ± 9
GGT[e] (IU/l)	94 ± 23	65 ± 15	42 ± 1
Amylase[f] (U/l)	641 ± 171	1,044 ± 281	1,711 ± 39

[a] Alkaline phosphatase; age difference was significant between sow and fetal values ($P < .01$).
[b] Lactate dehydrogenase.
[c] Aspartate transaminase.
[d] Alanine transaminase; age difference was significant between sow and fetal values ($P < .05$).
[e] γ-Glutamyltransferase.
[f] Age differences were significant ($P < .05$).

Source: Reprinted from Schantz, L.J. et al., 1995, *Lab. Anim. Sci.* 45(3): 285–289. With pemission.

TABLE A.51
Serum Metabolite Data for Fetal Pigs

	Pigs (n = 54)		
	Early Gestation (n = 11)	Late Gestation (n = 43)	Sows (n = 12)
Glucose[a] (mg/dl)	32 ± 5.0	65 ± 42	79 ± 1.0
BUN[b] (mg/dl)	20 ± 2.0	15 ± 5.0	19 ± 4.0
Uric acid (mg/dl)	0	0.3 ± 0.3	0
Cholesterol[a] (mg/dl)	44 ± 7.0	59 ± 11	60 ± 3.0
Bili[c,e] (mg/dl)	0.4 ± 0.1	0.2 ± 0.1	0.3 ± 0.1
Creatinine[a,d] (mg/dl)	0.7 ± 0.0	1.4 ± 0.4	1.3 ± 0.3
Triglyceride[a,e] (mg/dl)	18 ± 3.0	20 ± 4.0	42 ± 1.0
BUN/creatinine[f] ratio	28 ± 1.0	13 ± 8.0	12 ± 4.0

[a] Age difference was significant between early fetal group and sow ($P < .05$).
[b] Blood urea nitrogen.
[c] Total bilirubin.
[d] Age difference was significant between early and late fetal groups ($P < .05$).
[e] Age difference was significant between late fetal group and sow ($P < .05$).
[f] Age differences were significant ($P < 0.05$).

Source: Reprinted from Schantz, L.J. et al., 1995, *Lab. Anim. Sci.*, 45(3): 285–289. With permission.

TABLE A.52
Population Data for Protein Electrophoresis for Fetal Pigs

| | Pigs (n = 44) | | | |
	Early Gestation	Late Gestation	Sows	
n	9	35	n	8
No. of females	7	19	No. of early gestation	2
No. of males	2	16	No. of late gestation	6
Body weight (g)	380 ± 15	641 ± 220	Body weight (kg)	59 ± 14
Gestation			Age (months)	15 ± 6
Days	86 ± 1	0.3 ± 7		
Range	(85–87)	(96–110)		

Source: Reprinted with permission from Schantz, L.J. et al., 1995, *Lab. Anim. Sci.*, 45(3): 285–289. With permission.

TABLE A.53
Serum Protein Electrophoresis Data for Fetal Pigs

| | Pigs (n = 44) | | Sows (n = 8) | |
	Early Gestation	Late Gestation	Early Gestation	Late Gestation
Tp[a] (g/dl)	1.75 ± 0.04	2.22 ± 0.39	5.44 ± 0.08	6.32 ± 0.67
ALP[b] (g/dl)	0.24 ± 0	0.50 ± 0.25	2.64 ± 0.09	2.93 ± 0.37
GLOB[c] (g/dl)	1.52 ± 0.05	1.73 ± 0.30	2.81 ± 0.01	3.39 ± 0.53
α_1[d,e] (g/dl)	0.42 ± 0.02	0.24 ± 0.11	0.14 ± 0.06	0.04 ± 0.03
α_2[d,e] (g/dl)	0.66 ± 0.13	0.94 ± 0.25	1.01 ± 0.13	1.27 ± 0.24
β[d,f] (g/dl)	0.30 ± 0.02	0.41 ± 0.14	0.85 ± 0.07	1.04 ± 0.35
γ[d,f] (g/dl)	0.15 ± 0.17	0.14 ± 0.13	0.81 ± 0.01	1.15 ± 0.54
ALB/GLOB[f]	0.16 ± 0.01	0.31 ± 0.18	0.94 ± 0.04	0.89 ± 0.20

[a] Total protein concentration; difference between sow groups was significant ($P <.05$). Age difference was significant between early and late fetal groups ($P < 0.05$).

[b] Albumin; age difference was significant between sow and fetal values ($P <.05$).

[c] Total globulin concentration; difference between sow groups was significant ($P <.05$). Age difference was significant between sow.and fetal values ($P < 0.05$).

[d] Globulin fraction.

[e] Age difference was significant between early fetal group and sows ($P <.05$).

[f] Age difference was significant between sow and fetal values ($P <.05$).

Source: Reprinted with permission from Schantz, L.J. et al., 1995, *Lab. Anim. Sci.*, 45(3): 285–289. With permission.

SECTION 6: ANIMAL HEALTH AND GENERAL REFERENCES

TABLE A.54
Health Monitoring Report (HMR) for Ellegaard
Göttingen Minipigs

	Method
Viral Infections	
Aujeszky's disease	ELISA
Classical swine fever	ELISA
Encephalomyocarditis virus	IPT
Hemagglutinating encephalomyelitis	IPT
Porcine epidemic diarrhea	ELISA
Porcine influenza	
H1N1	HI
H3N2	HI
Porcine parvovirus	ELISA
Porcine reproductive and respiratory disease (EU type +U.S. type)	ELISA
Porcine reproductive and respiratory disease (EU type + U.S. type)	IPT
Porcine respiratory coronavirus	ELISA
Porcine rotavirus	Latex aggl.
Porcine rotavirus	ELISA
Transmissible gastroenteritis	ELISA
Porcine circovirys type 2 (PCV2)	IPT
Bacterial Infections	
Actinobacillus pleuropneumoniae	
Serotype 1, 2, 5, 6, 7, 8, 10, 12	ELISA/CF
Bordetella bronchiseptica	Culture
Brachyspira (Serpulina) *hyodysenteriae*	Culture
Campylobacter spp.	Culture
Clostridium perfringens	
Type A	Culture
Type C	Culture
Erysipelothrix rhusiopathiae	Culture
Eubacterium suis	Culture
Haemophilus parasuis	Culture
Lawsonia intracellularis	PCR
Leptospira spp.	
L. pomona	MAT
L. bratislava	MAT
Listeria monocytogenes	Culture
Mycoplasma hyopneumoniae	ELISA
P. multocida (toxin producing)	Culture
P. haemolytica (M. haemolytica)	Culture
P. pneumotropica	Culture
Other pasteurellae	Culture
Salmonella spp.	Culture
Staphylococcus hyicus	Culture
β-haemolytic Streptococci [*]	Culture

TABLE A.54 *(Continued)*
Health Monitoring Report (HMR) for Ellegaard Göttingen Minipigs

	Method
Streptococcus pneumoniae	Culture
Streptococcus suis	Culture
Yersinia enterocolitica	Culture
spp. Associated with lesions:	

Fungal Infections

Candida albicans	Culture
Microsporum spp.	Culture
Trichophyton spp.	Culture

Parasitological Infections

Arthropods	Micr. insp.
Helminths	Flotation
Coccidiea (Eimeria, Isospora)	Flotation
Toxoplasma gondii	IFA

Note: Abbreviations for methods: CF = complement binding; latex aggl. = latex agglutination; ELISA = enzyme linked immuno-sorbent assay; micr. insp. = microscopical inspection; HI = hemagglutination inhibition; NE = not examined in current screen; IFA = immunofluorescence assay; MAT = micro agglutination test; IPT = immunoperoxidase test; PCR = polymerase chain reaction. HMR is performed twice per year in each breeding colony and done under FELASA recommendations.

Source: From Rehbinder et al., 1998, *Laboratory Animals*, 32(1): 1–17. Courtesy of Ellegaard Göttingen Minipigs, Dalmose, Denmark.

TABLE A.55
Drug Formulary

Antibiotics[a]

Amoxicillin	10 mg/kg bid p.o.
Ampicillin	2–5 mg/kg bid i.m.
Ceftiofur	3–5 mg/kg sid i.m.
Ceftriaxone	50–75 mg/kg tid i.m. or i.v.
Cephaloridine	10 mg/kg bid i.m. or s.c.
Cephradine	25–50 mg/kg bid p.o.
Enrofloxacin	5 mg/kg bid i.m. or p.o.
Erythromycin	2–5 mg/kg bid i.m. or i.v.
Gentamicin	2 mg/kg sid p.o.
Griseofulvin	20 mg/kg sid p.o.
Kanamycin	6 mg/kg bid i.m.
Lincomycin	5–10 mg/kg bid p.o.
	2–5 mg/kg i.m.
Penicillin, procaine/benzathine	10,000–40,000 units i.m. every 3 d
Tetracycline/oxytetracycline	10–25 mg/kg p.o. bid; 2-5 mg/kg sid i.m.
Trimethoprim/sulfadiazine	5 mg/kg sid i.m.
	25–50 mg/kg sid p.o.
Metronidazole	66 mg/kg sid p.o.
Tylosin	8.8 mg/kg p.o. bid
	2–4 mg/kg bid i.m.

Anthelmintics

Amprolium	10 mg/kg p.o.
Fenbendazole	5 mg/kg p.o.
Ivermectin	200 µg/kg i.m.
Levamazole	8 mg/kg p.o.
Thiabendazole	75–100 mg/kg p.o.

[a] Life-saving antibiotics are banned for use in animals that may enter the human food chain or for treatments that may result in microbial resistance to antibiotics.

Source: Code of Federal Regulations, Title 21, Vol. 6, pg. 339–340 (21 CFR556.1), 2005. http://www.avma.org.

GENERAL REFERENCE TEXTBOOKS FOR SWINE

1. Bollen, P.J.A., Hansen, A.K., Rasmussen, H.J., and Suckow, M.A., 2000, *The Laboratory Swine*, Boca Raton, FL: CRC Press.
2. Cramer, D.V., Podesta, L.G., and Makawka, L., 1994, *Handbook of Animal Models in Transplantation Research*, Boca Raton, FL: CRC Press.
3. Flecknell, P.A., 1996, *Laboratory Animal Anaesthesia*, 2nd ed., New York: Academic Press.
4. Getty, R., Ed., 1975, *Sisson and Grossman's The Anatomy of the Domestic Animals — Porcine*, Vol. 2, Philadelphia, PA: W.B. Saunders, pp. 1215–1422.
5. Gilbert, S.G., 1966, *Pictoral Anatomy of the Fetal Pig*, 2nd ed., Seattle, WA: University of Washington Press.
6. Hawk, C.T., Leary, S.L., and Morris, T.H., 2005, *Formulary for Laboratory Animals*, 3rd ed., Ames, IA: Blackwell Publishing.
7. Jensen, S.L., Gregersen, H., Shokouh-Amiri, M.H., and Moody, F.G., 1996, *Essentials of Experimental Surgery: Gastroenterology*, U.K.: Harwood Academic Publishers.
8. Kohn, D.H., Wixson, S.K., White, W.J., and Benson, G.J., Eds., 1997, *Anesthesia and Analgesia in Laboratory Animals*, New York: Academic Press.
9. Lindberg, J.E. and Ogle, B., 2001, *Digestive Physiology of Pigs: Proceedings of the 8th Symposium*, New York: CABI Publishing.
10. Pond, W.G. and Mersmann, H.J., 2001, *Biology of the Domestic Pig*, Ithaca, NY: Comstock Publishing Associates.
11. Popesko, P., 1977, *Atlas of Topographical Anatomy of the Domestic Animals*, Vol. 1, 2nd ed., Philadelphia, PA: WB Saunders.
12. Sack, W.O., 1982, *Essentials of Pig Anatomy and Harowitz/Kramer Atlas of Musculoskeletal Anatomy of the Pig*, Ithaca, NY: Veterinary Textbooks.
13. Stanton, H.C. and Mersman, H.J., Eds., 1986, *Swine in Cardiovascular Research*, Vol. 1 and 2, Boca Raton, FL: CRC Press.
14. Svendsen, O., 1998, The minipig in toxicology: proceedings of the satellite symposium to Eurotox 97, *Scand. J. Lab. Anim. Sci.*, 25(Suppl. 1).
15. Swindle, M.M., 1983, *Basic Surgical Exercises Using Swine*, Philadelphia, PA: Praeger Press.
16. Swindle, M.M., Ed., 1992, *Swine as Models in Biomedical Research*, Ames, IA: Iowa State University Press.
17. Swindle, M.M., 1998, *Surgery, Anesthesia and Experimental Techniques in Swine*, Ames, IA: Iowa State University Press.
18. Swindle, M.M. and Adams, R.J., Eds., 1988, *Experimental Surgery and Physiology: Induced Animal Models of Human Diseases*, Baltimore, MD: Williams and Wilkins.
19. Tumbleson, M.E., Ed., 1986, *Swine in Biomedical Research*, Vol. 1–3, New York: Plenum Press.
20. Tumbleson, M.E. and Schook, L.B., Eds., 1996, *Advances in Swine in Biomedical Research*, Vol. 1 and 2, New York: Plenum Press.

REVIEW ARTICLES

1. Swindle, M.M., Wiest, D.B., Smith, A.C., Garner, S.S., Case, C.C., Thompson, R.P., Fyfe, D.A., and Gillette, P.C., Fetal surgical protocols in Yucatan miniature swine, *Lab. Anim. Sci.*, 46(1): 90–95, 1996.
2. Swindle, M.M. and Smith, A.C., Comparative anatomy and physiology of the pig, *Scand. J. Lab. Anim. Sci.*, 25(Suppl. 1): 1–10, 1998.
3. Swindle, M.M., Smith, A.C., and Goodrich, J.G., Chronic cannulation and fistulation procedures in swine: a review and recommendations, *J. Invest. Surg.*, 11(1): 7–20, 1998.
4. Swindle, M.M., Nolan, T., Jacobson, A., Wolf, P., Dalton, M.J., and Smith, A.C., Vascular access port (VAP) usage in large animal species, *Contemp. Top. Lab. Anim. Sci.*, 44(3): 7–17, 2005.

WEB SITES

1. Contains swine literature database from Animal Welfare Information Center
   http://www.nal.usda.gov/awic/pubs/swine/swine.htm
2. Contains reviews of models and Sinclair, Hanford and Yucatan information
   http://www.sinclairresearch.com/
3. Tutorial on swine procedures in research: Laboratory Animal Training Association
   http://www.latanet.com/online/onlinetr.htm
4. Biology and diseases of swine
   http://www.ivis.org/advances/Reuter/swindle/chapter_frm.asp?LA=1
5. Basic information on swine
   http://www.aphis.usda.gov/vs/ceah/cahm/Swine/swine.htm
   http://www.nal.usda.gov/awic/pubs/swinehousing/swinehousing2.htm
6. Göttingen minipig background information
   http://minipigs.dk
7. CD-rom training series on husbandry, handling, injection techniques, anesthesia, analgesia and perioperative care
   http://www.latanet.com/desktop/drs.html
   http://www.latanet.com
8. National Swine Research Resource Center
   http://www.nsrrc.missouri.edu/

Index

F

Face mask, use for anesthetic induction, 60
Facial artery, 330
Fallopian tubes, 175, 176, 178. *See also* Tubal ligation
  histology, 176
  laparoscopic procedures, 357
Farrowing, defined, 6
Fasciocutaneous flaps, 94
  location of, 92
Fasting
  and clinical chemistry values for Yucatan minipigs, 425
  for endoscopic and laparoscopic procedures, 345
  in liver transplantation, 134
  preoperative, 42, 101
Fat tissue, inability to hold sutures, 87
Feeding chart
  for farm pigs, 8
  for minipigs, 7
Female urogenital tract, 28, 29
  dorsal view, 29
  surgical anatomy, 175
  surgical approaches, 177–179
Femoral arterial ligation, 233
Femoral arteriovenous fistula, 234
Femoral artery/vein
  access site, 24
  catheterization, 228
  in Ossabaw minipigs, 499
  Seldinger technique, 300–303
  surgical approaches, 228
  surgical cutdown, 227
Femoral head, surgical approach, 294
Femoral vessels, peripheral vascular access to, 299
Femur, surgical approaches, 293, 294
Fentanyl, 57
  for postoperative analgesia, 66
Fentanyl patches, 66
Fetal catheterization, 184–187
Fetal parameters, 439–445
Fetal pigs
  enzyme data, 444
  erythrocytic data, 442
  leukocytic data, 443
  protein electrophoresis, 445
  serum electrolyte data, 443
  serum metabolite data, 444
Fetal position, 182
Fetal sepsis, 186
Fetal sizes, by breed, 181
Fetal skeletal diagnoses, in Göttingen minipigs, 439–440, 442
Fetal surgery, 180–187
  complications of, 186
  heart and lung blocks, 190
  pacemaker implantation, 189
  silastic band on pulmonary artery, 189
Fiber, in minipig diets, 7
Fistulation, 234
Flank approach
  to expose kidney, 162

  to nephrectomy, 161–162
  suturing urethra into psoas from, 168
Flexible endoscopic research. *See also* Endoscopy
  anatomic considerations, 345–346
  training in, 351–353
Flooring standards, 9, 12
  recommendations for agricultural research, 11
Flumazenil, 69
Fluoroscopic imaging, 299, 310
  artificially created aneurysm, 313
  coil after VSD placement, 311
  stent in circumflex coronary artery, 312
Fogarty embolectomy catheters, 315
Foley catheter, 167
Food bowls, securing, 13
Foreleg
  lymphatics of, 151
  surgical approaches to bones/joints, 294
Fractional shortening (FS), 335
Frontal sinus, surgical approaches, 275
Full-thickness wounds, 95
Fungal infections, in Göttingen minipigs, 447
Furosemide, 240, 248
  after intracranial procedures, 272
Fusiform aneurysms, 244
  surgically created, 243

G

Gallbladder, 128
  cholecystectomy, 126–127
  laparoscopic view, 355
  size and volume, 123
  surgical anatomy, 123–125
  surgical approach, 126–127
  surgical view, 142
Gallstones, endoscopic implantation, 350
Gastric antrum, endoscopic view, 348
Gastric ulceration, with NSAIDs, 68
Gastric varices, 350
Gastroesophageal reflux, porcine model of, 107–108
Gastrointestinal bleeding, and endoscopic hemostasis, 350
Gastrointestinal effects, of opioid analgesics, 67
Gastrointestinal endoscopy, 352. *See also* Endoscopy
Gastrointestinal procedures
  abdominal surgery principles, 101–104
  colonic anastomosis and fistulation, 115–116
  enterotomy, 108–110
  Gastrotomy and gastrostomy techniques, 106–108
  GI surgical anatomy, 97
  hemorrhagic shock, 120
  intestinal anastomosis, 112–113
  intestinal and multivisceral transplantation, 117–119
  intestinal diversion/bypass, 113–115
  intestinal fistulation, 108–110
  intestinal infusion catheter implantation, 110–112
  intraperitoneal sepsis, 120
  postoperative care, 104–106
  pyloroplasty, 108
  rectal prolapse, 116–117

Q

R